pharmaceutical chemistry

pharmaceutical chemistry

SECOND EDITION

edited by

Chris Rostron • Jill Barber

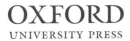

OXFORD

UNIVERSITY PRESS

OXFORD

UNIVERSITY PRESS

Great Clarendon Street, Oxford, OX2 6DP,
United Kingdom

Oxford University Press is a department of the University of Oxford.
It furthers the University's objective of excellence in research, scholarship,
and education by publishing worldwide. Oxford is a registered trade mark of
Oxford University Press in the UK and in certain other countries

1st Edition 2013

Impression: 1

Published in the United States of America by Oxford University Press
198 Madison Avenue, New York, NY 10016, United States of America

British Library Cataloguing in Publication Data
Data available

Library of Congress Control Number: 2020945107

ISBN 978–0–19–877978–0

Printed in Great Britain by
Bell & Bain Ltd., Glasgow

Oxford University Press makes no representation, express or implied, that the
drug dosages in this book are correct. Readers must therefore always check
the product information and clinical procedures with the most up-to-date
published product information and data sheets provided by the manufacturers
and the most recent codes of conduct and safety regulations. The authors and
the publishers do not accept responsibility or legal liability for any errors in the
text or for the misuse or misapplication of material in this work. Except where
otherwise stated, drug dosages and recommendations are for the non-pregnant
adult who is not breast-feeding

Links to third party websites are provided by Oxford in good faith and
for information only. Oxford disclaims any responsibility for the materials
contained in any third party website referenced in this work.

PREFACE

Pharmaceutical Chemistry

In this textbook we hope to persuade you that *Pharmaceutical Chemistry* is fundamental to the discipline of pharmacy. The chemistry we present here is illustrated using real drug molecules and the reactions that they undergo in the body, in the laboratory, and on storage in the pharmacy and in the home. The text aims to explain how a drug molecule is made; the process that turns it into a medicine; the role the pharmacist has when dispensing that medicine; and what happens in the body when it is taken. Most importantly, the text shows how each of these aspects are integrated, reflecting the most up-to-date teaching practices.

Do please *read* this book. It can be used as a reference book, especially in the run-up to examinations, but the authors would like to think that you will curl up on a winter's evening and just read it, and it has been written with that use in mind.

ACKNOWLEDGEMENTS

The editors wish to acknowledge the support of the contributing authors, all experts in the field of pharmacy or medicinal chemistry education, who have spent a considerable amount of time writing and reviewing their chapters. We would also like to extend our thanks to the staff at Oxford University Press, especially Jonathan Crowe, who has supported this project from the outset and displayed great patience during its progress.

We would also like to thank the reviewers of the first and second edition who devoted their time and shared their expertise in order to influence the final form of the book and ensure it remains accurate and relevant.

CONTENTS

CHAPTER 1

THE IMPORTANCE OF PHARMACEUTICAL CHEMISTRY

Jill Barber And Chris Rostron

CHAPTER 2

ORGANIC STRUCTURE AND BONDING

Alastair Mann

CHAPTER 3

STEREOCHEMISTRY AND DRUG ACTION

Rosaleen J. Anderson, Adam Todd, Mark Ashton And Lauren Molyneux

MASTERING THE MATERIAL

> **Box 9.1   Bacteria versus archaea**
>
> Archaea are often found living in some of th
> ditions where humans would not be able to
> above 100 °C, such as those seen in deep-se
> out by archaea are similar to those of bacte
> to those of eukaryotes. More recently, a nu

BOXES

Additional material that adds interest or depth to concepts covered in the main text is provided in the Boxes.

> All our cells contain identical genetic inf
> up the various types of tissues, organs ar

KEY POINTS

The important 'take-home messages' that you must have a good grasp of are high-lighted in the Key points. You may find these form a helpful basis for your revision.

> **Self-check 2.1**
>
> In tetrachloromethane, the Cl–C–Cl bond an
> gles are in the range 107.5° to 108.5°, while
> explain these differences?

SELF-CHECK QUESTIONS

Questions are provided throughout the chapters in order for you to test your un-derstanding of the material. Take the time to complete these, as they will allow you to evaluate how you are getting on, and they will undoubtedly aid your learning. Answers are provided on the Online Resource Centre.

> **FURTHER READING**
>
> Clayden, J., Greeves, N. and Warren, S. (
> A student friendly undergraduate textb
> key concepts of organic chemistry.
> McMurry, J. *Fundamentals of Organi*
> 9781439049730. Another student friendly
> Sykes, P., *A Primer to Mechanisms in O*
> simpler treatment of organic reaction

FURTHER READING

In this section we direct you to additional resources that we encourage you to seek out in your library or online. They will help you to gain a deeper understanding of the mat-erial presented in the text.

> **Absorption** (*verb*, **to absorb**) The taking up ⌐
> electromagnetic radiation by matter.
>
> **ACE inhibitor** Angiotensin-converting enzym
> inhibitors inhibit the conversion of angiotensin
> to angiotensin II; they may be used to treat hea
> failure and hypertension.
>
> **Acetylcholinesterease** An enzyme that catalyse

GLOSSARY

You will need to master a huge amount of new terminology as you study pharmacy. The glossaries in each volume should help you with this. Glossary terms are shown in pink.

ONLINE RESOURCES

Visit the Online Resource Centre for related materials, including ten multiple-choice questions for each chapter, with answers and feedback.

Go to: www.oup.com/he/rostron-barber2e

SEEING THE CONNECTIONS

> **Case study 9.1**
>
> Angela has told Ravi she is pregnant and ⌐
> parents. However, Angela had an older bro
> 25, and she does not want this for her chil
> cannot remember if there is a history of CF i
> a chance their baby inherits CF.

CASE STUDIES

Case studies show how the science you learn at university will impact on how you might advise a patient. Reflection questions and sample answers encourage you to think critically about the points raised in the case study.

LECTURER SUPPORT MATERIALS

For registered adopters of the volumes in this series, the online resources also feature figures in electronic format, available to download, for use in lecture presentations and other educational resources.

To register as an adopter, visit www.oup .com/he/rostron-barber2e, select the volume you are interested in, and follow the on-screen instructions.

> **ANY COMMENTS?**
>
> We welcome comments and feedback about any aspect of the series. Just visit www.oxfordtextbooks.co.uk/orc/feedback and share your views.

ABOUT THE EDITORS

Editor, Dr Chris Rostron, graduated in Pharmacy from Manchester University and completed a PhD in Medicinal Chemistry at Aston University. He gained Chartered Chemist status in 1975. After a period of post-doctoral research he was appointed as a lecturer in Medicinal Chemistry at Liverpool Polytechnic. He is now an Honorary Research Fellow in the School of Pharmacy and Biomolecular Sciences at Liverpool John Moores University. Prior to this he was an Academic Manager, and then a Reader in Medicinal Chemistry at the school. He was a member of the Academic Pharmacy Group Committee of the Royal Pharmaceutical Society of Great Britain and chairman for five years. He was chairman of the Academic Pharmacy Forum and deputy chair of the Education Expert Advisory Panel of the Royal Pharmaceutical Society. He has been an external examiner in Medicinal Chemistry at a number of Schools of Pharmacy both in the UK and abroad. In 2008 he was awarded honorary membership of the Royal Pharmaceutical Society of Great Britain for services to Pharmacy education.

Editor, Dr Jill Barber, studied Natural Sciences at the University of Cambridge and completed a PhD in Bio-organic Chemistry at the same university. She then spent five years in some of the oldest universities in Europe, learning Biochemistry, German, and Renaissance Music. She settled in Manchester, with a permanent position in the School of Pharmacy and Pharmaceutical Sciences, where she teaches chemotherapy and its underlying chemistry and biochemistry. Her current research involves using mass spectrometry to quantify the proteins involved in the response to drugs, both in bacteria and in humans. She has also published several teaching-related research papers about the factors influencing student success. She is a Lady Grandmaster of the International Correspondence Chess Federation and enjoys singing and playing the trombone.

Contributors

Professor Rosaleen J. Anderson, Faculty of Applied Science, University of Sunderland, UK

Dr Mark Ashton, School of Pharmacy, Newcastle University, UK

Dr Jill Barber, School of Pharmacy and Pharmaceutical Sciences, University of Manchester, UK

Dr Helen Burrell, School of Pharmacy and Biomolecular Sciences, Liverpool John Moores University, UK

Dr Andrew Evans, School of Pharmacy and Biomolecular Sciences, Liverpool John Moores University, UK

Dr Andrew J. Hall, Medway School of Pharmacy, UK

Dr Geoff Hall, Leicester School of Pharmacy, De Montfort University, UK

Dr Matthew Ingram, School of Pharmacy and Biomolecular Sciences, University of Brighton, UK

Dr Alastair Mann, Faculty of Science, Engineering and Computing, Kingston University, UK

Dr Lauren Molyneux, School of Pharmacy, Newcastle University, UK

Dr Chris Rostron, School of Pharmacy and Biomolecular Sciences, Liverpool John Moores University, UK

Dr Tim Snape, School of Pharmacy and Biomedical Sciences, University of Central Lancashire, UK

Dr Mike Southern, School of Chemistry, Trinity Bioscience Institute, Trinity College, Dublin, Ireland

Dr Adam Todd, School of Medicine, Pharmacy and Health, Durham University, UK

Dr Alex White, Cardiff School of Pharmacy and Pharmaceutical Sciences, Cardiff University, UK

ABBREVIATIONS

ABO	ABO blood groups
ACE	angiotensin-converting enzyme
ADME	absorption, distribution, metabolism and excretion
ADP	adenosine diphosphate
ADR	adverse drug reactions
AMP	adenosine monophosphate
API	active pharmaceutical ingredient
ATP	adenosine triphosphate
AZT	azidothymidine
BNF	British Nation Formulary
BP	British Pharmacopoeia, or blood pressure
CFC	chlorofluorocarbon
CNS	central nervous system
CoA	coenzyme A
COMT	catechol-O-methyltransferase
CYP	cytochrome P450
DMSA	dimercaptosuccinic acid
DNA	deoxyribonucleic acid
EAS	electrophilic aromatic substitution
EDTA	ethylenediamine tetraacetic acid
EHC	emergency hormonal contraception
EI	electron ionization
EMA	European Medicines Agency
Et	ethyl
FDA	Food and Drug Administration
GABA	gamma-aminobutyric acid
GC	gas chromatography
GLC	gas–liquid chromatography
GORD	gastro-oesophageal reflux disease
HPLC	high-performance liquid chromatography
HTS	high-throughput screening
ICI	Imperial Chemical Industries
INR	international normalized ratio
IPA	isopropyl alcohol
IR	infrared
IUD	intrauterine contraceptive devices
IUPAC	International Union of Pure and Applied Chemistry
MDMA	3,4-methylenedioxy-N-methylamphetamine (ecstasy)
Me	methyl
MHRA	Medicines and Healthcare products Regulatory Agency
mRNA	messenger RNA
MRSA	meticillin-resistant strains of *Staphylococcus aureus*
MS	mass spectrometry
NAS	nucleophilic aromatic substitution
NMR	nuclear magnetic resonance
NSAID	non-steroidal anti-inflammatory drug
ODS	octadecylsilane
OTC	over the counter
RMM	relative molecular mass
RNA	ribonucleic acid
ROS	reactive oxygen species
rRNA	ribosomal RNA
SAM	S-adenosylmethionine
SAR	structure–activity relationship
SHU	Scoville heat units
SLS	sodium lauryl sulfate
SSRI	selective serotonin reuptake inhibitors
THC	Δ^9-tetrahydrocanabinol
TLC	thin-layer chromatography
tRNA	transfer RNA
USP	United States Pharmacopoeia
UV	ultraviolet
WHO	World Health Organization

THE IMPORTANCE OF PHARMACEUTICAL CHEMISTRY

Jill Barber And Chris Rostron

Pharmacy is all about drugs: how drugs are made, how to get them into the body, how they work, their **metabolism**, their side-effects, their interactions with other drugs, and how we communicate with patients and other healthcare professionals about drugs. At the heart of the discipline of pharmacy is chemistry, because drugs are, of course, chemicals.

This chapter is an overview of the importance of pharmaceutical chemistry. Every living organism is like a test tube, carrying out huge numbers of chemical reactions; in this chapter we will explore some of these reactions. Every drug is made using chemical reactions, some of these are in a laboratory, but some are in nature; we will study both. Every drug needs to be made up into a **formulation**: perhaps a tablet, or a cream or an injectable solution, and sometimes the formulation process needs chemistry as well. Many drugs are metabolized, and drug metabolism is chemistry. We will briefly overview these processes.

Learning objectives

Having read this chapter you are expected to be able to:

- draw chemical structures the way organic chemists draw them
- give examples of chemical reactions that take place in the human body
- give examples of the importance of chemistry in the manufacture and formulation of drugs.

1.1 CHEMICAL STRUCTURES AND NOMENCLATURE

Before we consider the importance of pharmaceutical chemistry in detail, it is important that you understand the chemical structures and some of the nomenclature used in this book. Most students who study organic chemistry at university (whether in a chemistry course or as part of a biological sciences or health sciences course) get confused by two things.

- University chemists use 'old-fashioned' names for simple chemicals like ethanoic acid (they call it acetic acid).
- University chemists hardly ever label carbon atoms or count hydrogen atoms.

It is tempting to conclude either that school teachers are just wrong, or that organic chemists know very little about their own subject. Neither is true. When you started primary school you learnt to print your letters very carefully, using wide-lined paper. Some years later you learnt how to do joined-up writing on unlined paper and eventually you learnt to use a word-processing package on a computer. For most students, writing is quite different at the age of 18 from the age of 5. It is similar with chemistry.

Trivial and IUPAC systematic nomenclature

The International Union of Pure and Applied Chemistry (IUPAC) has defined systematic names for organic compounds, and you may be familiar with many of these. Nevertheless, very common substances retain their trivial (non-systematic) names because lots of people, including cooks, gardeners and biologists, use these names. Some trivial names (such as valeric acid for 3-methylbutanoic acid) have already gone out of fashion but other very common trivial names (such as acetic acid) remain, at least for the time being. A few systematic names are so similar to other systematic names that they are inconvenient or even dangerous. Chemical laboratories are noisy places, so trichloromethane can sound like dichloromethane, and ethanal can sound like ethanol. To prevent accidents we continue to use the trivial names for these chemicals: chloroform for trichloromethane and acetaldehyde for ethanal. Even IUPAC does not recommend systematic names when they might be dangerous! In this book we will use systematic names, except where trivial names are required either for safety or for communication with members of the public. This means that you will use more trivial names than when you were at school.

> In Chapter 4, 'Properties of aliphatic hydrocarbons', the nomenclature of organic compounds is introduced.

Chemical structures

Consider a simple drug molecule, aspirin, as shown in Figure 1.1. All the structures (A–E) are correct, but most chemists would normally use A or B.

Structures A and E (the professional structure and the college structure) are both right, but have three important differences.

- Structure A has no carbons represented by C. Carbons-7, -8 and -9 are represented by the ends or conjunctions of bonds.

- Structure A has only one hydrogen atom drawn in. The remaining hydrogens are implied— you know that carbon must have four bonds or charges; the hydrogen atoms on the benzene ring and at carbon-9 are not drawn in.

Figure 1.1 The chemical structure of aspirin, drawn in several different ways

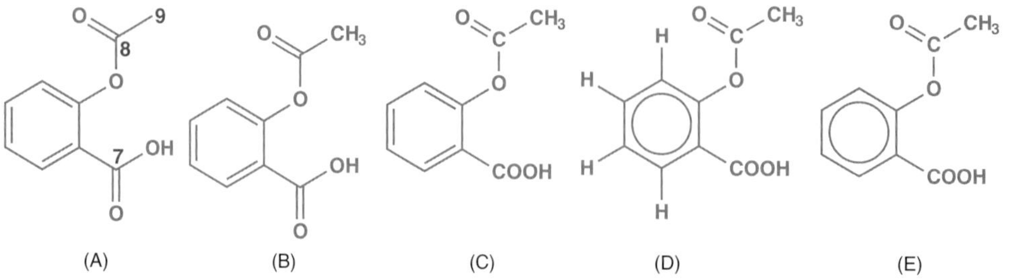

(A)   (B)   (C)   (D)   (E)

> **Self-check 1.1**
>
> Check that you understand how chemical structures can be pictured, by redrawing the following structures with all the hydrogens and carbons labelled: (a) the painkiller, paracetamol (Figure 1.2A), (b) metronidazole, an antibacterial agent used to treat some important infections of the stomach and intestines (Figure 1.2B), and (c) naproxen, another painkiller, available over the counter in the USA but only on prescription in Europe (Figure 1.2C).

- Finally, in structure A, a Kekulé ring structure is drawn. You may have learnt that the two Kekulé structures are in very rapid equilibrium, so that all the bond lengths in a benzene ring are equal. This is absolutely correct, but it is much easier to draw mechanisms using a Kekulé structure, so most chemists use these most of the time.

So professional chemists abbreviate structures for speed and convenience, whereas school teachers draw in carbons and hydrogens to help less experienced students understand exactly which atoms are present in a given molecule. You will not usually be forced to abbreviate your structures, but you will need to recognize and understand structures drawn like Figure. 1.1A.

> Aspirin is used as a painkiller, as an anti-inflammatory and to reduce the risk of blood clots. Like many drugs, it is an aromatic molecule, containing a benzene ring. Chapter 7, 'Introduction to aromatic chemistry', introduces compounds with benzene rings, and explains how their structures influence their physical and chemical properties.

Now have a look at Figure 1.3(A–C) and compare it with Figure 1.2(A–C). Do you see what has happened? A chemical structure can be drawn correctly from any angle and different people have their preferred angles. If you are drawing out a chemical reaction, it is usually easiest to

> **Self-check 1.2**
>
> The OCH_3 group on the naproxen molecule is sometimes written OMe instead. How could you represent $O-CH_2CH_3$ using the same convention?

Figure 1.2   A, paracetamol; B, metronidazole; C, naproxen

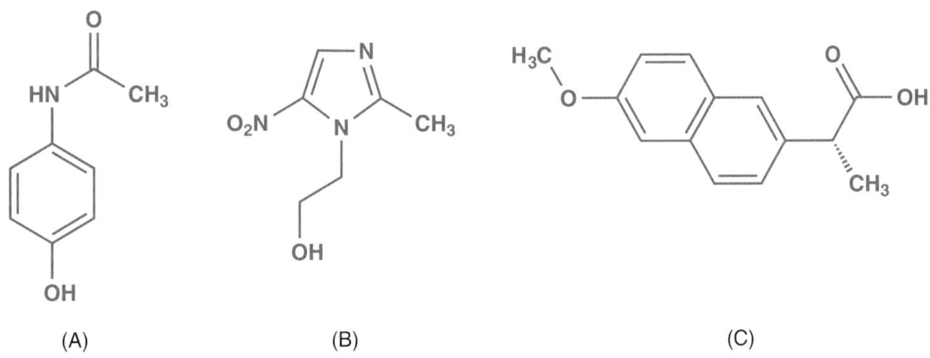

(A)   (B)   (C)

Figure 1.3   A, paracetamol; B, metronidazole; C, naproxen

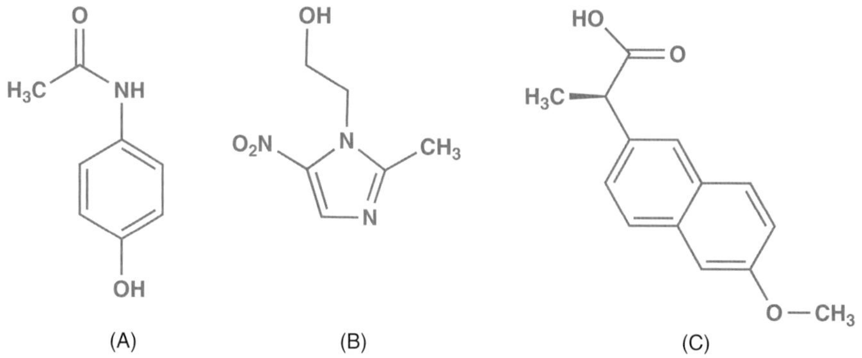

(A)   (B)   (C)

put the reactive groups on the right if you are writing in English or another language that goes from left to right, but you do not have to.

> Chapter 3, 'Stereochemistry and drug action', introduces the three-dimensional structures of molecules. Studying this chapter will help you to visualize molecules from different angles. It will also explain the importance of three-dimensional structure in drug action.

1.2 THE HUMAN TEST TUBE

This section introduces some of the chemical reactions that take place in the body. The human body carries out simple chemistry on complex structures. The same chemical reactions can also take place outside the body, and they are discussed in greater detail in later chapters.

Vision

'I am fearfully and wonderfully made' wrote King David of Israel nearly 3,000 years ago, despite the fact that he knew little or no chemistry! King David was in awe of the way the human body works, and one of the most exciting things a body can do is see. He would have been amazed to learn that vision is based on a simple chemical reaction, in which 11-*cis*-retinal is **isomerized** to *trans*-retinal (see Figure 1.4), catalysed by the action of light.

This reaction and the reverse reaction are fast. The human brain can detect changes in colour and light within a few milliseconds and distinguish movement at nearly 1,000 frames per second. Films in the cinema and on television run at about 50–60 frames per second. Our brains are clever at filling gaps; were they not, our favourite movies would judder like old news footage.

Opsin is a protein involved in vision; retinal binds to it. Opsin comes in three forms, absorbing light in the red, green and yellow regions of the electromagnetic spectrum, and enabling us to see colours. The red and green opsins are very similar indeed, and it is easy for one to mutate so that it absorbs light in the wrong region. This leads to red–green colour blindness.

> The terms *cis*- and *trans*-retinal are used here. A *cis* double bond is a special case of a Z double bond, and a *trans* double bond is a special case of an E double bond. Chapter 3, 'Stereochemistry and drug action', introduces stereochemistry, and these terms are discussed in more detail there.

Figure 1.4 The chemistry of vision. Light catalyses the conversion of 11-*cis*-retinal (bound to the protein opsin) to *trans*-retinal, starting a signalling cascade that leads to an image being perceived in the brain. The mechanism of this geometrical isomerization is still being investigated; however, we know that free rotation can only occur about single bonds, so the mechanism shown is possible

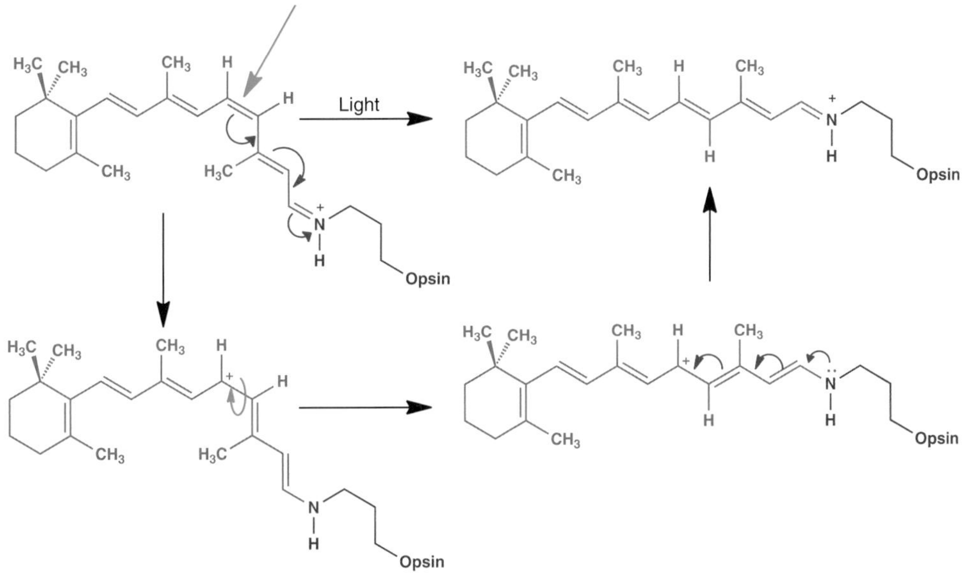

Energy

Vision is remarkable, but energy metabolism is perhaps even more astonishing. Why do we get tired when we do not eat? Why is it possible to starve to death?

The answer, of course, is chemistry. Most of our food gets broken down to a small molecule called acetate, CH_3COO^-. In its protonated form, CH_3COOH, acetate is found in vinegar (acetic or ethanoic acid), but in the body it is normally deprotonated. Acetate takes part in numerous chemical reactions, which enable us to derive energy from food, as well as to make vital components of our bodies. Central to acetate metabolism is the citric acid cycle (Figure 1.5). You may have come across this cycle when learning biology.

Acetate is activated in the body to give the **thioester** acetyl coenzyme A, which reacts with oxaloacetate (a 4-carbon molecule derived from two molecules of acetate). This reaction is a standard carbon–carbon bond forming reaction, yielding citryl coenzyme A, another thioester. Citryl coenzyme A is hydrolysed to give citrate. The concentration of citric acid (protonated citrate) can be as high as 0.3 M in lemons and limes, but is a lot lower in our bodies. Citrate then undergoes many more chemical reactions, eventually yielding proteins, nucleic acids, fats, and all the other molecules we need to live.

> Citric acid is a tricarboxylic acid. It contains three carbonyl groups. The chemistry of the carbonyl group and its importance in drugs and in biological systems is introduced in Chapter 6, 'The carbonyl group and its chemistry'. In Chapter 8, 'Inorganic chemistry in pharmacy', the

Figure 1.5 The formation of citrate from acetate in the citric acid cycle. The carbon–carbon bond-forming reaction in which citrate is formed is discussed in Chapter 6, 'The carbonyl group and its chemistry'. This reaction is catalysed by citrate synthase, an enzyme that speeds up the reaction. (If you find the structures a bit daunting at this stage, do not worry—all will become clear in the next few chapters.)
Lemon: © André Karwath / Wikimedia Commons / CC BY-SA 2.5
Vinegar: source Stockbyte

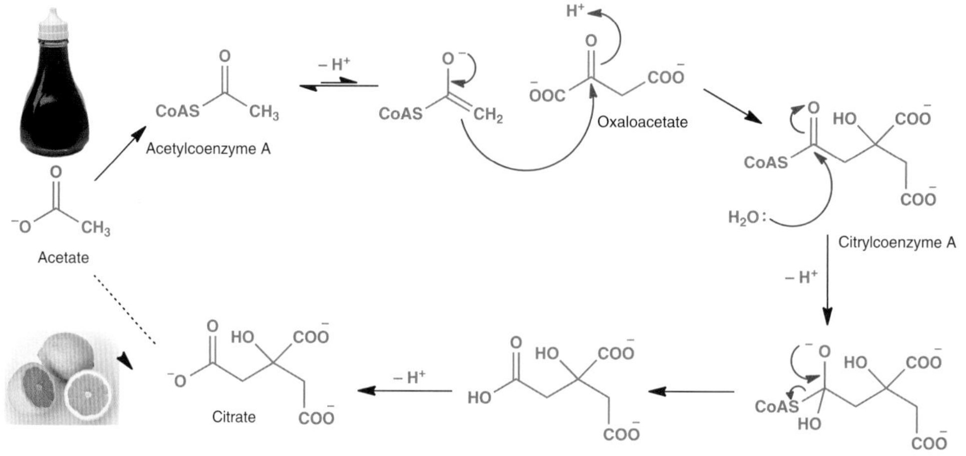

chemistry of sulfur, phosphorus, and metals important in biology is introduced. Thioesters are very important in biological systems, but are seldom found in the chemical laboratory.

The citric acid cycle and coenzymes are covered in Chapter 11, 'Carbohydrates and carbohydrate metabolism'.

You will have noticed the curly arrows on the structures in Figure 1.5. These represent the movement of a pair of electrons. If you are not familiar with curly arrows, do not worry; by the end of Chapter 2, you will be.

The citric acid cycle does not only make molecules though. It also converts food into energy using, of course, chemistry. The chemical reactions of the citric acid cycle indirectly generate ATP (adenosine triphosphate), the universal currency of energy. The body drives chemical reactions by hydrolysing ATP. This reaction is shown in Figure 1.6.

So if we do not eat, we get tired, because we cannot do the chemical reactions to make ATP, and if we do not eat for a long time, we starve, because we cannot replace the bits of us that are continuously made and replaced.

> Chapter 8, 'Inorganic chemistry in pharmacy', introduces phosphorus chemistry, including the chemistry of phosphoesters, such as ATP.

Self-check 1.3

In the citric acid cycle, citrate is isomerized to isocitrate (see Figure 1.7). Redraw isocitrate with all its carbon and hydrogen atoms labelled.

Figure 1.6 The hydrolysis of ATP. This reaction has a large negative ΔG, and is able to drive less favourable reactions

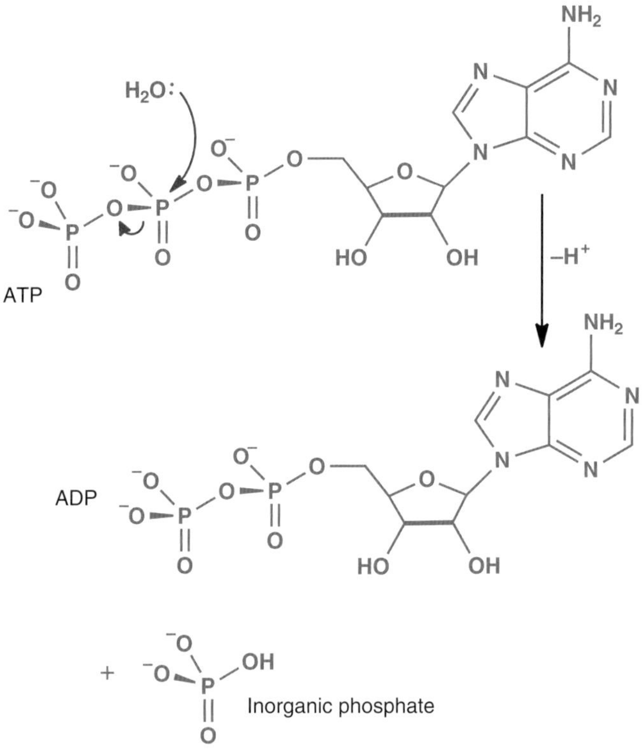

Figure 1.7 The conversion of citrate to isocitrate

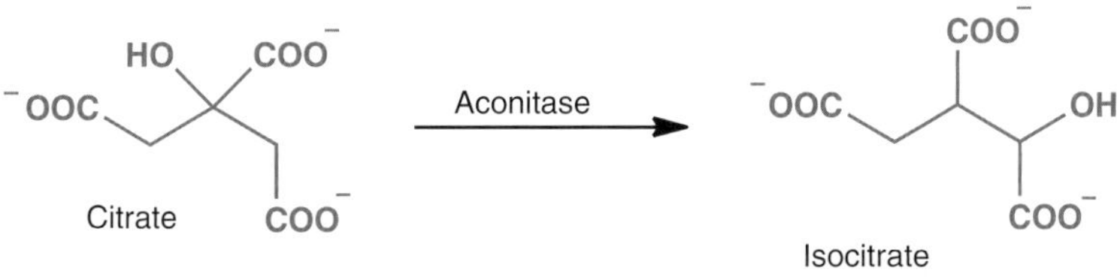

Self-check 1.4

The conversion of citrate to isocitrate is a two-stage process, catalysed by the enzyme aconitase (Figure 1.7). Draw a mechanism (use curly arrows) for the conversion of citrate to isocitrate. The intermediate is known as *cis*-aconitate. This is a much harder question. If you find it too difficult, try again after working through Chapter 5, 'Alcohols, phenols, ethers, organic halogen compounds, and amines'.

❯ Isocitrate is another intermediate in the citric acid cycle, which you will learn about in Chapter 11, 'Carbohydrates and carbohydrate metabolism'.

The liver

Even in ancient times, people thought that the liver had a role in well-being. We now know that this is because the liver carries out quite complex chemistry. The liver recognizes **xenobiotics** (substances that are not normally in the blood stream, see Box 1.1) and processes them. Oxidation is a common reaction in the liver, since oxidized products are often more easily excreted than the parent xenobiotics. For example, ethanol is oxidized in the liver (Figure 1.8).

> Chapter 5, 'Alcohols, phenols, ethers, organic halogen compounds, and amines', introduces the chemistry of important functional groups such as hydroxyl groups, amines, and halogen compounds. Oxidation and dehydration of alcohols such as ethanol are among the reactions described.

In the liver, ethanol is oxidized to acetate via acetaldehyde (ethanal), and acetate is used to produce energy. When it is metabolized properly, alcohol is just food, and is very high in calories; however, the real problems come when it is not metabolized properly. Oxidation of ethanol is slow, so most people can only process about one unit (about 8g) per hour. The ethanol that is not metabolized acts on the central nervous system, causing all the familiar effects of alcohol consumption (slow reactions, lack of inhibition, difficulty in controlling speech or movement). You can slow down the absorption of alcohol by eating, helping your liver to keep up, but that is pharmaceutics, not chemistry.

The effects of alcohol are, however, less harmful than the effects of acetaldehyde. Acetaldehyde, like other aldehydes, causes the symptoms of hangover: nausea, vomiting, shortness of breath, and accelerated heart-rate. The oxidation of alcohol is a two-stage process, as shown in Figure 1.8, and if you drink too much alcohol, acetaldehyde can accumulate, causing a hangover. The drug disulfuram, used in the treatment of chronic alcoholism, works by inhibiting the enzyme aldehyde dehydrogenase which converts acetaldehyde to acetate. Patients taking disulfuram (usually alcoholics) experience severe hangover symptoms within 30 minutes of consuming alcohol, which usually dissuades them from further alcohol consumption.

> More information on the metabolism of alcohols can be found in Chapter 5, 'Alcohols, phenols, ethers, organic halogen compounds, and amines'.

Box 1.1   Terms containing 'xeno' and 'philius'

Xenophilius Lovegood, a character in *Harry Potter and the Deathly Hallows*, has a name meaning 'love of the strange' or stranger, from the Greek 'xeno' meaning 'strange' and 'philius' meaning 'love'. He should help you remember xenobiotic and words such as hydrophilic (water-loving).

Figure 1.8   The oxidation of ethanol to acetate in the liver

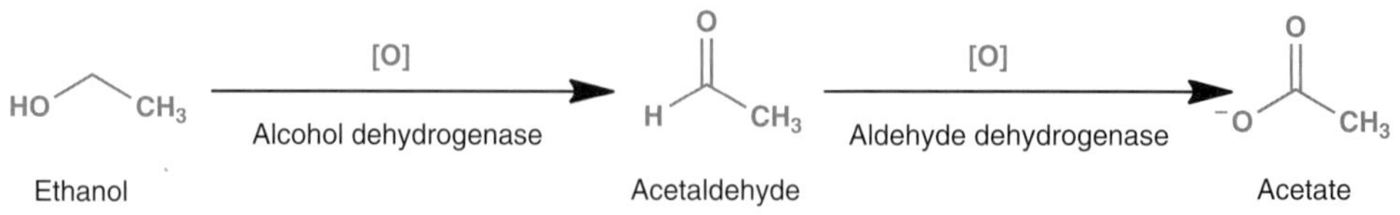

Self-check 1.5

Methanol is very toxic, because it is oxidized by the liver to become an aldehyde, which cannot be further oxidized. Draw the structure of this aldehyde. (It is known as formaldehyde, but its IUPAC name is methanal.)

Self-check 1.6

How would you treat methanol poisoning? (This is a harder question.)

Protein synthesis

King David worried about his hair going grey but he did not know how hair is made. Hair, nails, muscles, tendons and ligaments are all made largely from proteins. Enzymes are also usually proteins, and proteins are made by chemical reactions. Proteins are polymers of amino acids, and amino acids are just carboxylic acids with amino groups (see Figure 1.9). To make proteins, these amino acids are joined together (polymerized) using amide bonds. In proteins these bonds are known as peptide bonds. The carboxylic acid group of one amino acid and the amino group of another amino acid react together, and straightforward carbonyl chemistry leads to the formation of an amide bond.

The amide bond is very strong, so it is absolutely perfect for hair and nails. Your hair does not fall out in the rain, because this bond is so strong. To break it requires boiling in acid, or catalysis by enzymes.

> The chemistry of amides is covered in more detail in Chapter 6, 'The carbonyl group and its chemistry'.

Figure 1.9 (A) General structure of an amino acid. (B) Formation of a peptide bond, shown in green. R can be any of twenty different groups. At its simplest, R is H, which gives the amino acid glycine; when R is CH_3, the amino acid is alanine

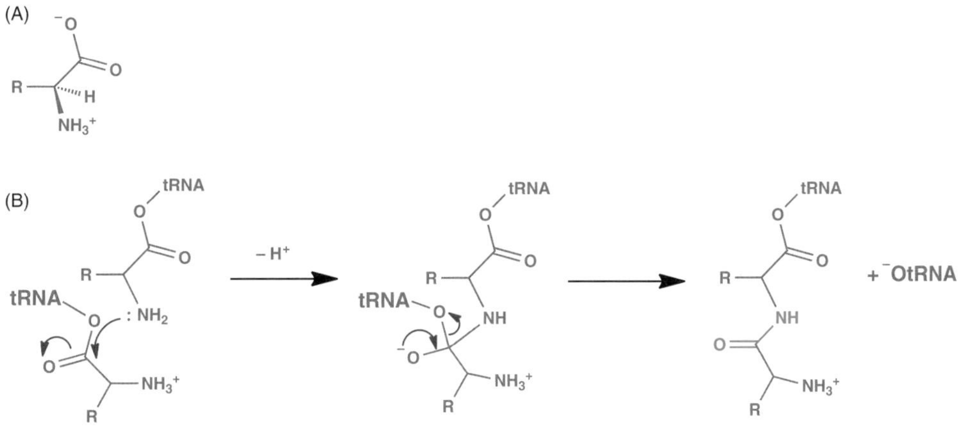

9

> **Self-check 1.7**
>
> Draw the structure of the tripeptide glycine-alanine-glycine (usually abbreviated gly-ala-gly or GAG).

🔑 Human cells carry out a vast array of chemical reactions that are vital to the body's normal processes, such as energy production, protein synthesis, and protection against toxic xenobiotics.

The formation of peptide bonds is very simple chemistry, yet the cell uses up to 40% of its energy making proteins, and the machinery that makes proteins can constitute up to 30% of the cell's dry weight (the weight of everything except the water). Look at Figure 1.9 and see if you can see why.

The point is that R can be any of twenty different groups, and to make a particular protein of perhaps 300 amino acids, the correct amino acid needs to be selected each time. The vast machinery of the ribosome, and other associated enzymes, is required to ensure that proteins are produced accurately.

❯ More information on the mechanism of operation of ribosomes is given in Chapter 9, 'Nucleic acids'.

❯ You may have noticed that alanine is a **chiral** molecule. The four groups surrounding the carbon-2 are all different, and this means that the mirror image of the structure shown cannot be superimposed on that structure. Chirality is discussed in detail in Chapter 3, 'Stereochemistry and drug action'.

1.3 MORE TEST TUBES: PLANTS AND MICROORGANISMS

Like humans and other animals, plants and microorganisms depend on chemistry for their normal function. Sometimes this chemistry is adapted in surprising ways to produce compounds that we can use as drugs.

Antimalarial drugs

Every 45 seconds a child dies of malaria—a protozoal illness common in Africa, the Indian subcontinent, and parts of South America. Like many tropical illnesses, research into its treatment has been badly underfunded, and there are few effective drugs for treating the disease. The first effective drug against malaria was quinine (see Figure 1.10), isolated from the bark of the *Cinchona* tree, where it can accumulate at up to 13% dry weight. Quinine is a remarkable structure, but you will not be surprised to learn that it is made using (enzyme–catalysed) chemistry. The biosynthesis of quinine is far from straightforward, but you should pay some attention to the structure. To study chemistry effectively, you need to be able to draw structures, even complex

Figure 1.10 Quinine, artemisinin, and the Anopheles mosquito. When an infected mosquito bites a human, it passes the malaria parasite into the human blood stream, causing fever and sometimes death. This is why insect nets and insect repellent are very important in the prevention of malaria. Drugs such as quinine and artemisinin can be used to treat malarial infections
Image by skeeze from Pixabay

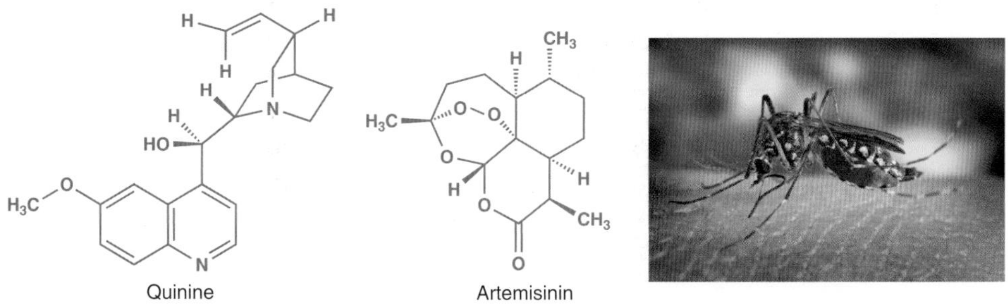

Quinine   Artemisinin

structures, quickly and neatly. Quinine is a good structure to practise drawing (you can copy it—there is no need to memorize it).

Quinine changed the course of history, allowing Europeans to colonize much of Africa in Victorian times. Thousands of troops died during the Second World War because they were cut off from the supply of quinine, most of which came from Indonesia. The best organic chemists in the world tried to synthesize the drug, to develop an alternative supply, but this is the sort of molecule that plants make much more efficiently than chemists, and synthetic quinine is not commercially successful.

The malaria parasite readily develops resistance to drugs, and quinine is not widely used today. The most important antimalarial drug now is artemisinin, which, traditionally, is extracted from the Chinese herb *Artemisia annua*. Modern production methods, however, use genetically modified yeast. The enzymes that catalyse the synthesis of artemisinic acid have been copied into ordinary baker's yeast; artemisinic acid is then chemically converted into artemisinin (see Figure 1.11). This is very modern chemistry, at the interface with biology.

> In Chapter 13, 'Origins of drug molecules', we ask how drugs are made. Some drugs are made by nature (plants, fungi or bacteria typically), some are made in the chemical laboratory, and an increasing number, like artemisinin, are made by a combination of chemistry, biology, and genetic engineering.

Nystatin

Fungal infections can be very dangerous, but more usually they are just uncomfortable. Thrush and Athlete's Foot are among the most common. Soil bacteria are a rich source of drugs to treat such infections—a fact recognized by Elizabeth Lee Hazen, a microbiologist working in New York in the middle of the twentieth century. Hazen was clearly a generous person; when she discovered a promising strain of soil bacterium in a friend's garden, she did not name it after herself, but after her friend. The bacterium is called *Streptomyces noursei*, after the Nourse family. Hazen and her colleague Rachel Fuller Brown, a biochemist, isolated the first clinically

Figure 1.11 Farnesyl pyrophosphate is converted into a cyclic structure (amorpha-4,11-diene) then oxidized to artemisinic acid in genetically engineered yeast. The remainder of the artemisinin synthesis is carried out in the laboratory. This work was funded by the Bill and Melinda Gates Foundation

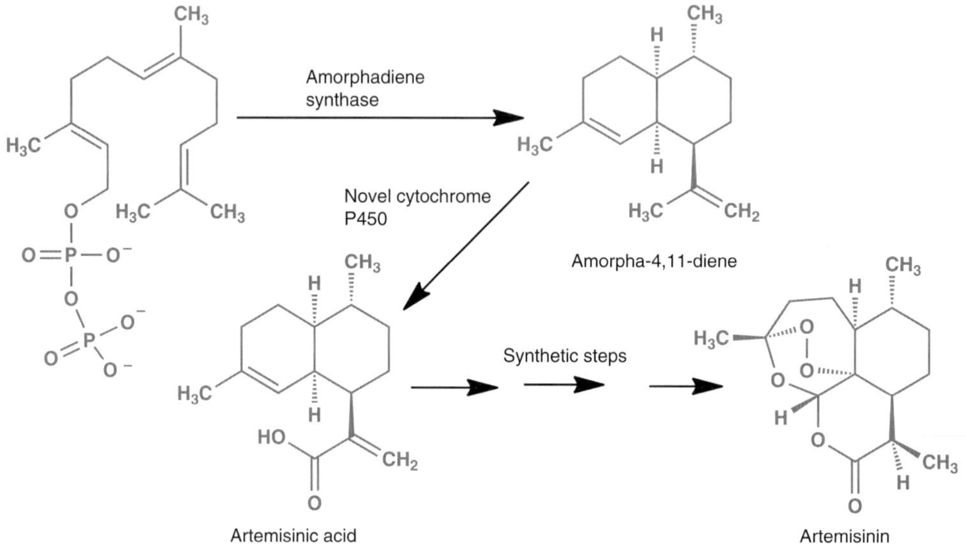

Amorphadiene synthase

Amorpha-4,11-diene

Novel cytochrome P450

Synthetic steps

Artemisinic acid

Artemisinin

useful antifungal agent from *S. noursei* cultures. They named this drug nystatin, in honour of their employer, the New York State Department of Public Health. After its launch in 1954 the drug was a huge success, and Hazen and Brown collected $13 million in royalties, which they donated to a trust fund for advancing women in science.

The large ring of nystatin (see Figure 1.12) is derived from acetate and propionate units, linked head-to-tail. These are modified so that one side of the molecule is covered in hydroxyl residues and attracts water (is hydrophilic) and the other side of the molecule contains hydrophobic alkene groups. This structure enables the molecule to interact with hydrophobic molecules in the centre of the fungal cell membrane and with hydrophilic groups on the outside, thus disrupting the membrane. The disrupted membrane leaks and the fungal cell dies.

Linking together acetate and propionate molecules is a recurring theme in microbial chemistry. Figure 1.13 shows the reaction in which two acetate molecules are joined. It is very similar to the formation of citrate as shown in Figure 1.5. This reaction can be repeated many times and is used to form fatty acids, drugs, and other molecules. The microbial cell expends a lot of energy in these processes, which require many different enzymes; nevertheless, each enzyme catalyses a quite ordinary chemical reaction.

> In Chapter 4, 'Properties of aliphatic hydrocarbons', we consider the properties of hydrocarbons, including alkenes, like nystatin. The structure of the cell membrane can be seen in Chapter 9, 'Nucleic acids'.

In 1966 the River Arno flooded, and the city of Florence was devastated. Numerous collections of artworks in churches, libraries and private collections were affected, and the science of

Figure 1.12 (A) Nystatin. Acetate units are represented in blue and propionate units in purple. (B) Diagram of a cell membrane. The nystatin molecule is able to interact with the hydrophobic inside of the membrane and the hydrophilic outside. Adapted from *Human Physiology: The Basis of Medicine*, 2nd edn, by Gillian Pocock and Christopher D. Richards (2006), by permission of Oxford University Press

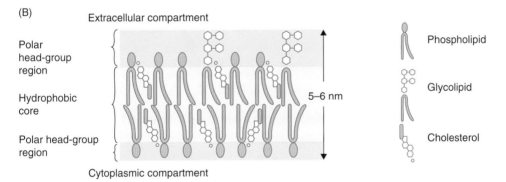

Self-check 1.8

Can you draw the mechanism of addition of another acetate unit to the four-carbon unit shown in Figure 1.13?

---

restoration advanced under the threat of the loss of priceless art treasures. There was a fear that fungi would colonize the priceless painted wooden panels, so they were sprayed with nystatin!

Penicillin

Penicillin is a hugely successful antibiotic made by fungi from three amino acids, as shown in blue, green, and pink in Figure 1.14.

The discovery of penicillin is perhaps the most famous drug discovery story ever told. The Scottish microbiologist, Alexander Fleming, went on holiday leaving some bacteria growing on nutrient plates. When he returned, zones of bacteria had been killed, close to where a fungus had fallen on the plates. There is no doubt that the discovery of penicillin was a lucky accident, but Fleming was prepared to work very hard to isolate penicillin from the fungal culture he had discovered.

Figure 1.13 Head-to-tail polymerization of acetate units. Acetyl coenzyme A is activated, by conversion to malonyl coenzyme A. Both acetyl coenzyme A and malonyl coenzyme A become enzyme-bound and are able to react together, giving a four-carbon unit that can interact with another molecule of malonyl coenzyme A, and so on

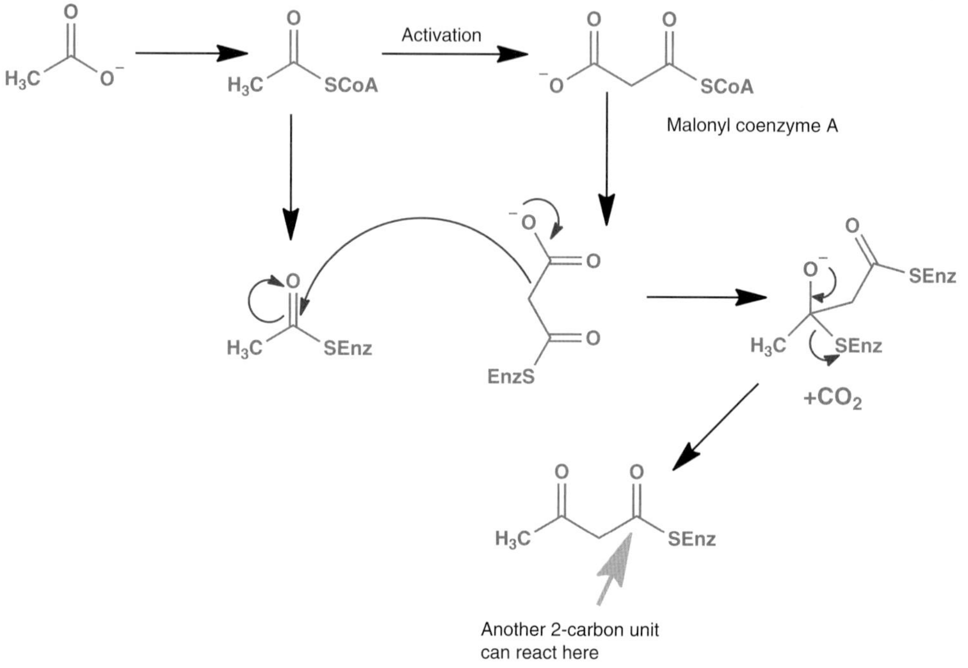

Figure 1.14 Biosynthesis of benzylpenicillin and 6-aminopenicillanic acid and semi-synthesis of amoxicillin

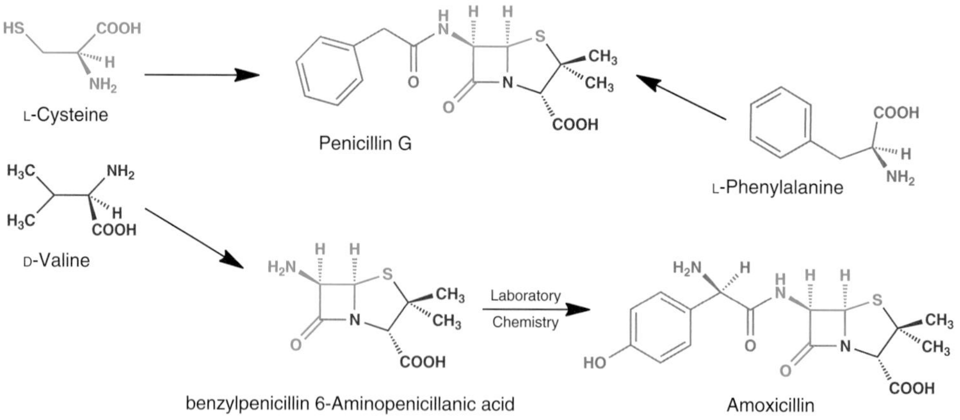

Penicillin itself (now called benzylpenicillin to distinguish it from other penicillins) has saved countless lives, but the fungi that produce penicillin can do something even cleverer than that. They can produce 6-aminopenicillanic acid—a molecule that can be modified by chemists to give numerous different penicillins, including amoxicillin, the yellow medicine usually given to children with respiratory tract infections.

Box 1.2 Nature is good at chirality

When nature makes a chiral molecule, it makes just one isomer, in the case of alanine, the one drawn in blue. Chemists will nearly always make a 50:50 mixture of the two possible isomers, the blue one and the purple one.

When you have four chiral centres, as in penicillin, instead of two possible isomers, there are 2^4, that is 16, only one of which works as a drug, but the fungus makes the right one every time. This is the main reason why so many drugs are still isolated from fungi, bacteria, and plants.

Self-check 1.9

Since penicillin is made from amino acids it contains amide bonds. Can you find them?

In 1957 the American chemist John Sheehan synthesized phenoxymethylpenicillin (penicillin v) in the laboratory, but no laboratory synthesis has ever been as efficient as the fungal synthesis, so they are not used to produce penicillin. We can see why by looking at the molecule, as explained in Box 1.2.

> Chirality is discussed in Chapter 3, 'Stereochemistry and drug action', and penicillin is discussed in more detail in Chapter 13, 'Origins of drug molecules'.

Insulin

Insulin is a small protein that most human beings and other mammals produce quite successfully in the pancreas. It enables us to take up glucose from blood into tissues. If we do not do this, the high levels of glucose become toxic. People with Type 1 diabetes (which normally begins in childhood) are unable to synthesize adequate amounts of insulin and need to take it as a medicine (usually as a subcutaneous injection). Initially, individuals were treated with pig insulin, which differs by only one amino acid from human insulin. Some people, however, developed an allergic reaction to pig insulin, because it is not identical with human insulin, and so recognized by their immune systems as 'foreign'.

Insulin is now produced in microbes (see Figure 1.15). The human gene has been inserted into bacterial cells using genetic engineering, and these bacteria are able to produce insulin cheaply and in a pure, safe form. It is much easier to purify a single protein from bacteria than from mammalian sources.

> Chapters 9, 10, 11 and 12 discuss biological macromolecules and their importance in pharmacy. Very often these compounds (proteins, nucleic acids, lipids, carbohydrates) are targets for drugs. Insulin, however, is not a target, but a drug itself.

15

Figure 1.15 How a microbe produces a human protein. (A) A gene is synthesized and inserted into a small circular DNA called a plasmid. (B) Many copies of the plasmid are then inserted into bacterial cells, and these cells produce the required human protein

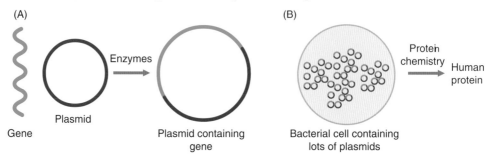

(A)

Enzymes

Gene

Plasmid

Plasmid containing gene

(B)

Protein chemistry

Human protein

Bacterial cell containing lots of plasmids

Box 1.3 Fred Sanger

Fred Sanger is the only living person to have won two Nobel Prizes, and the only person to win the Chemistry Prize twice. His 1958 Nobel Prize was for the development of the chemistry of protein sequencing. He chose insulin as his first sequencing project.

Plants and microorganisms use chemical reactions to produce a wide range of interesting molecules. Many of these substances can be used as drugs or can be modified to make drugs.

1.4 GLASS AND PLASTIC TEST TUBES

Quinine, artemisinin, nystatin and penicillin are all found in nature and are called natural prod-ucts. Morphine, tetracycline, and chloramphenicol are also natural products (see Figure 1.16). This is not to say that you buy them in a health food shop in the form of dried leaves. They are drugs that have been tested properly and are administered in carefully regulated forms. Many plants, bacteria and fungi carry out complex chemistry and so produce many (perhaps a third) of the drugs we use today.

Figure 1.16 Morphine, chloramphenicol, tetracycline

Morphine

Chloramphenicol

Tetracycline

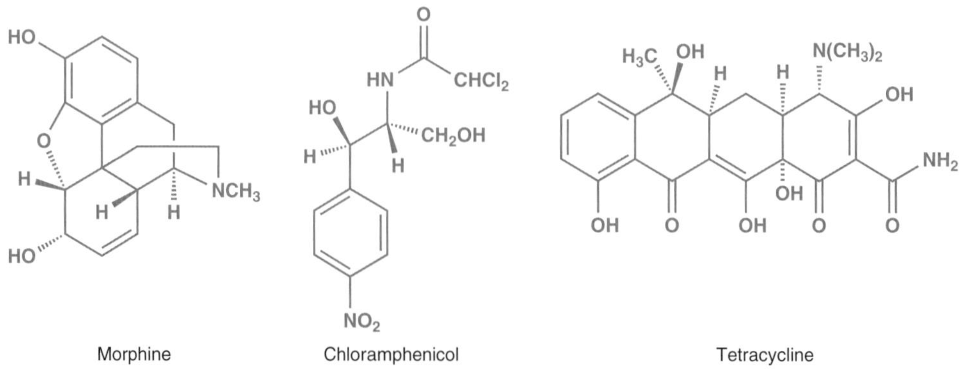

Figure 1.17 Do you know this molecule?

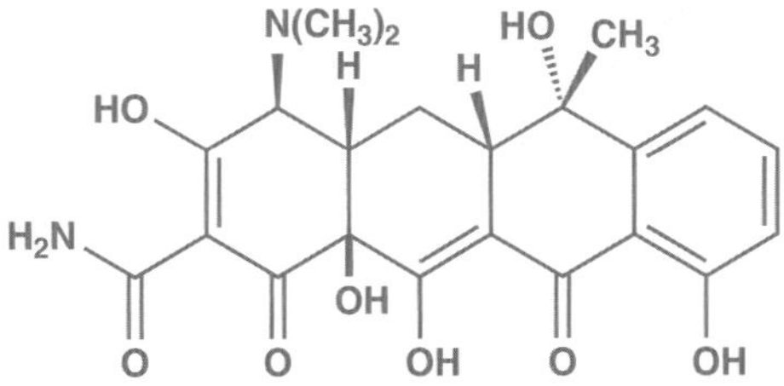

Self-check 1.10

Look at Figure 1.17. What molecule is this?

Self-check 1.10

Look at Figure 1.17. What molecule is this?

17

There is an increasing demand for genetically engineered protein drugs, produced in microbes or in cell culture. These include insulin, clotting Factor VIII (used to treat haemophilia) and several anti-cancer drugs. Other drugs are synthetic—they are made entirely in the laboratory by chemists. Others still, such as amoxicillin, are semi-synthetic—nature provides a complex starting material and laboratory chemists modify it.

Semi-synthetic drugs

Semi-synthetic drugs are very common. Microbes or plants put together a complex structure with medicinal activity. Chemists in laboratories then modify the drug to make new molecules that are more active drugs, or drugs that are better tolerated by patients.

Figure 1.18 shows the structure of erythromycin, a very important antibiotic isolated from a soil bacterium. This molecule is made in the same way as nystatin, except that propionate units, rather than acetate units, are bolted together. Erythromycin is very effective, but has a few problems. For example, it is very acid-sensitive and rather hydrophilic. Together, these two factors mean that erythromycin typically needs to be taken four times per day for seven days because the drug is quickly degraded and eliminated in the body. The acid-sensitivity also means that erythromycin cannot be used to treat infections of the stomach, such as *Helicobacter pylori*, the bacterium that causes stomach ulcers.

A Croatian research group, led by Dr. Slobodan Djokic, developed azithromycin in 1980. Erythromycin is used as the starting material, so all the chiral centres (eighteen of them) and the sugars are already present. Erythromycin is very cheap, because the soil bacteria can make tonnes of it. Figure 1.18 shows the simple chemistry by which erythromycin can be modified to make azithromycin (it is simplified slightly but all the concepts are present).

Azithromycin was a blockbuster drug with sales of more than $1 billion per year. It can be given once daily for just three days, and is not acid-sensitive.

Synthetic drugs

We have considered some examples of natural products that have been made in the laboratory. Penicillin, quinine, and even erythromycin have been synthesized, but these syntheses are not economical sources of the drugs. There are, however, a few drugs that are now made purely in

Figure 1.18 The main steps of the elaboration of erythromycin to produce the blockbuster drug azithromycin

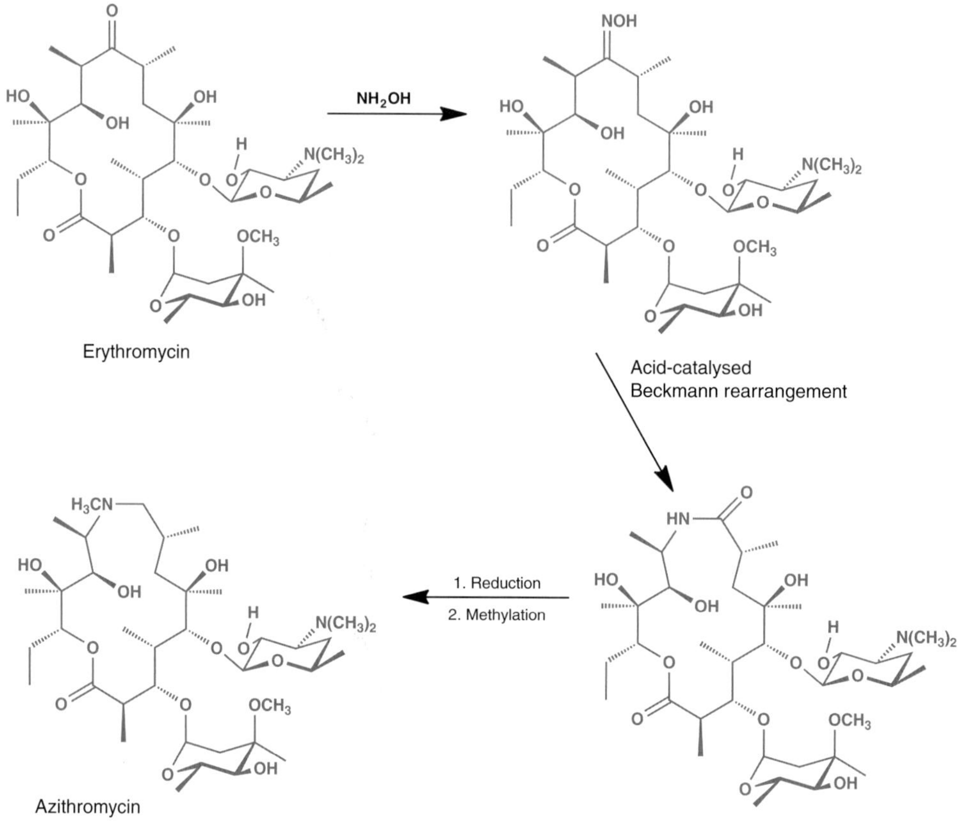

Erythromycin

NH$_2$OH

Acid-catalysed
Beckmann rearrangement

1. Reduction
2. Methylation

Azithromycin

the laboratory, even though they were originally isolated from nature. These include the antibiotic chloramphenicol (see Figure 1.19), which was originally isolated from the soil bacterium *Streptomyces venezuelae*, but is now synthesized in the laboratory. Chloramphenicol is a good choice for laboratory synthesis because it has very few chiral centres, and it is therefore not too difficult to make the correct isomer (see Figure 1.19).

Figure 1.19 Chloramphenicol

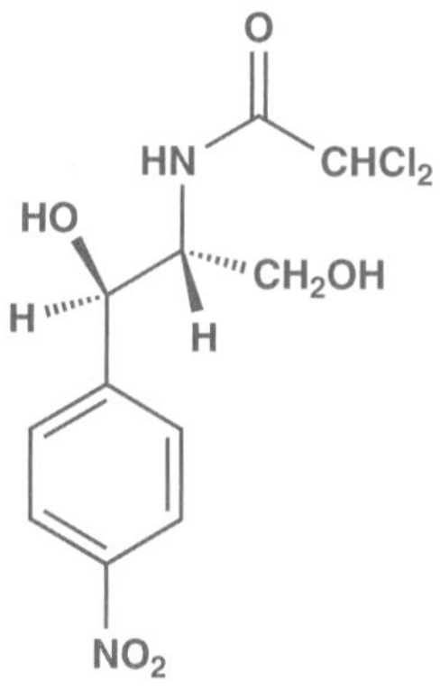

Self-check 1.11

How many chiral centres does chloramphenicol have?

Figure 1.20 The synthesis of aspirin from salicylic acid

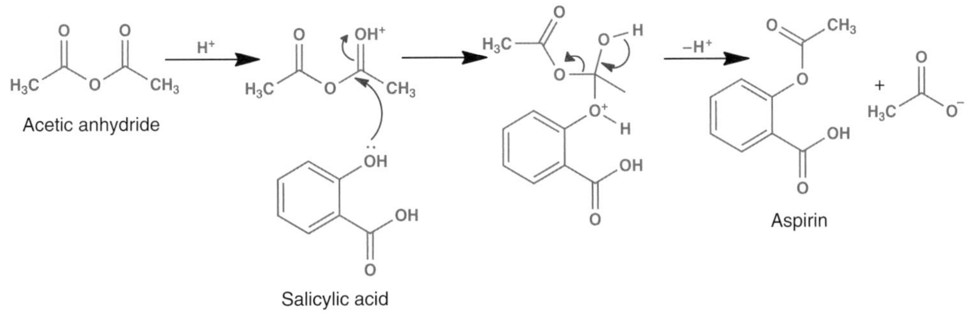

Acetic anhydride

Salicylic acid

Aspirin

About half of the drugs in use today are not found in nature, but are made in laboratories. If you have not already made aspirin yourself, you probably will, by treating salicylic acid with acetic anhydride, as shown in Figure 1.20.

Ibuprofen is a painkiller first developed by the Boots company in 1960, and strongly recommended by dentists (among others); it is extremely effective and has fewer side-effects than other common painkillers (see Box 1.4). The original synthesis was eight steps and generated quite a lot of waste. In the mid-1980s a new company (BHC) developed a new 'green' synthesis of ibuprofen, as shown in Figure 1.21.

Self-check 1.12

If you store aspirin in your bathroom cabinet for some months, it may smell of vinegar. Why is that?

Box 1.4   Common pain-killers

If you work in a pharmacy you will almost certainly have to advise about painkillers. Aspirin is not recommended for children because it is associated with Reyes Syndrome, a disease that causes multiple organ failure and which can be fatal. In some adults, aspirin can cause gastric bleeding. Paracetamol is therefore often preferred, but the tablets are huge (500 mg), and for many people they are difficult to swallow. In addition, it is relatively easy to overdose on paracetamol, and an overdose can lead to a slow, painful death from liver failure. Ibuprofen has a similar mechanism of action to aspirin, but the side-effects are comparatively rare. An effective dose is normally a single 200 mg tablet. For severe, but non-dangerous, pain (dental or post-operative pain), ibuprofen and paracetamol can both be taken safely because their modes of action are different. Do not take aspirin and ibuprofen at the same time though!

Figure 1.21 Green synthesis of ibuprofen. The three catalysts can be recovered, so there is very little waste of material

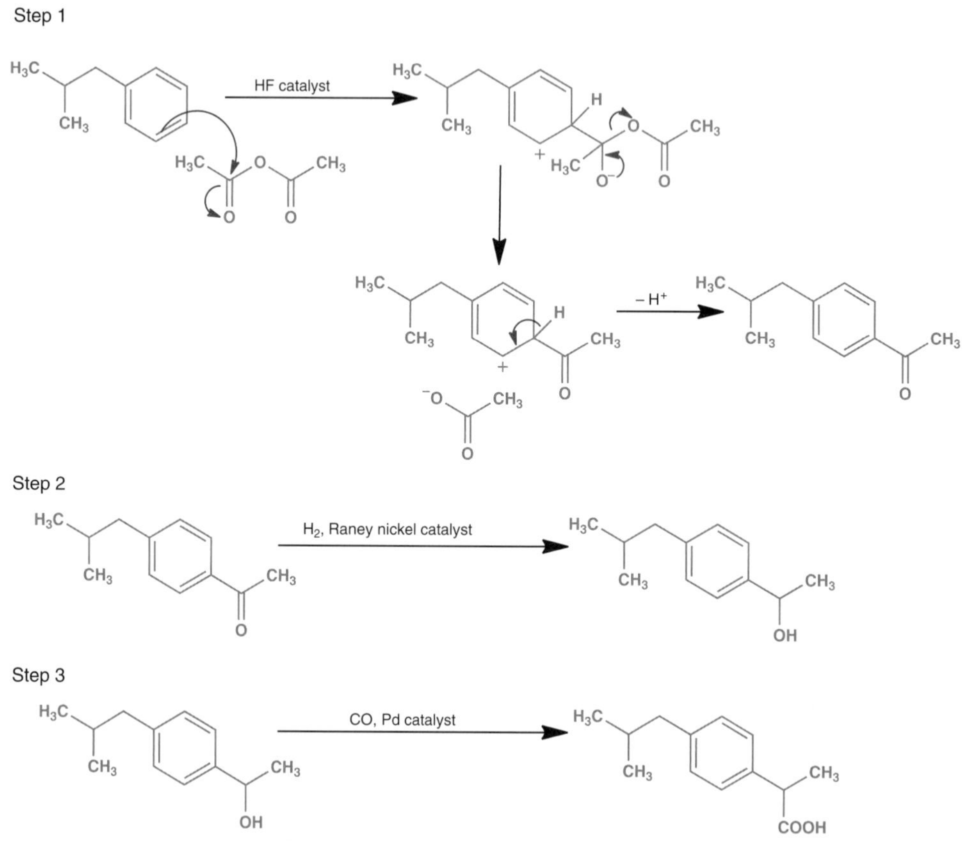

Step 1

Step 2

Step 3

Self-check 1.13

There is one small waste molecule in the synthesis of ibuprofen. What is it?

A 'green' synthesis aims to minimize its impact on the environment, for example, through reducing the use of hazardous materials such as organic solvents, and reducing by-products, thereby achieving a lower wastage of carbon or other materials. Green synthesis is increasingly important in the twenty-first century, with global temperatures rising and the population increasing. Green chemistry is chemistry that has a minimal impact on the environment.

Atorvastatin

In 2017, atorvastatin generated sales of $1.9 billion. It is a statin used for lowering blood cholesterol levels. Some medical professionals recommend statins for everyone over about 55 years old (sometimes 50 for men, 65 for women) to reduce the risk of heart attack and stroke.

Figure 1.22 Atorvastatin. The active part of the drug molecule is shown in red

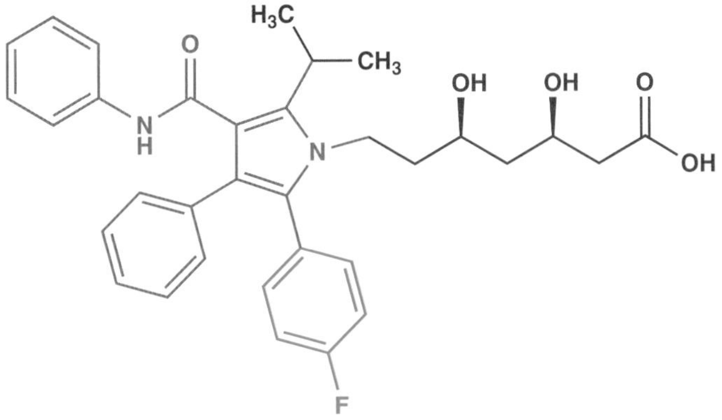

Others feel that statins are already over-used. These drugs make a lot of money for drug companies because they are taken by people who are not sick, every day for years or decades. Contrast this with antibiotics which are taken for a few days until the patient gets well or dies.

Statins work by inhibiting 3-hydroxy-3-methylglutaryl-coenzyme A reductase (HMGR), a key enzyme in the production of cholesterol. The synthesis of atorvastatin illustrates a major advantage of the glass test tube over the microbial test tube. You can see, in Figure 1.22, how lots of different compounds could be made from the same route. The red part of the molecule is essential and very few variations can be made, but each of the other four substituents can be changed independently. For example, the fluoro-substituted aromatic ring (shown in green) needs to be a hydrophobic group (otherwise the drug does not bind to the target), but there are lots of possibilities. Twenty different **analogues** were tested before the fluoro-substituted aromatic ring was chosen. The isopropyl group (shown in purple) was chosen similarly, followed by the two remaining substituents. The analogues that can be made starting from a natural product are usually much more limited. (Note that chemists cannot always predict whether an analogue is likely to improve a drug molecule; very often they make lots of analogues and choose the best after testing.)

Self-check 1.14

How many chiral centres does atorvastatin have?

Self-check 1.15

Draw atorvastatin with all its carbon and hydrogen atoms labelled, and then work out the molecular formula of the drug.

Many drug molecules are made by chemists in laboratories. Simple molecules are made wholly in the laboratory, whereas more complex drugs are often made by chemical modification of natural products.

1.5 FROM TEST TUBE TO PHARMACEUTICAL

Drugs are chemicals and are made using chemistry. Usually, however, a drug has to be converted into a medicine. The pharmacist does not hand out white powders; instead, the drugs are converted into tablets, solutions, suspensions, or creams—and sometimes this conversion process relies on chemistry.

Chloramphenicol palmitate

We have already met chloramphenicol as an example of a drug which is a natural product but is now made principally in the laboratory. However, chloramphenicol has an unpalatable bitter taste and so some chemistry has to be carried out in order to produce a palatable medicine. To mask the intense bitter taste, the primary alcohol of chloramphenicol is esterified with palmitic acid (see Figure 1.23) to produce chloramphenicol palmitate. This chemical reaction (esterification) reduces the water solubility of chloramphenicol such that it can be formulated as a suspension that does not interact with the taste receptors on the tongue. Once the suspension reaches the intestinal tract the ester linkage is hydrolysed (more chemistry) by enzymes (esterases) to the active chloramphenicol and the dietary fatty acid, palmitic acid. Chloramphenicol palmitate is therefore a pro-drug.

Metabolic reactions

We have already seen that the major site of drug metabolism is the liver. The role of liver metabolism is to recognize and remove xenobiotics from the body. Most drugs are xenobiotics and so will be subject to these metabolic reactions. Although largely enzyme-controlled, these reactions are simply chemical reactions which make the xenobiotics more water soluble and, therefore, easier to eliminate from the body. Knowledge of these chemical reactions can be used

Figure 1.23   Chloramphenicol palmitate

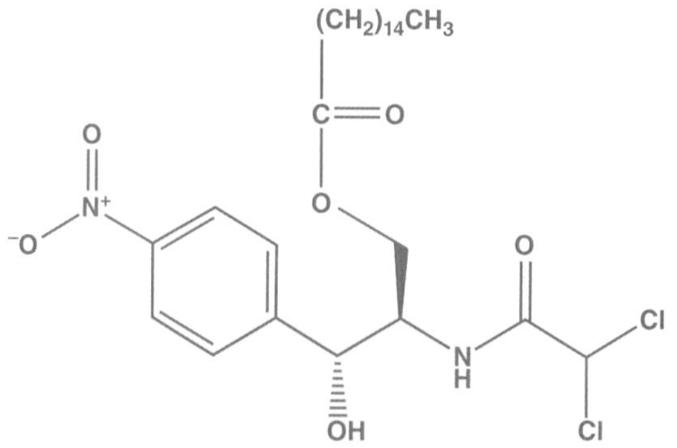

chloramphenicol palmitate

> ### Case study 1.1
>
> A parent comes into the pharmacy where you are working and comments that their child does not like taking erythromycin because of the taste. Children's erythromycin is an ester that hydrolyses when it gets warm. When this happens, the medicine still works but it leads to the bad taste.
>
> #### Reflection questions
> 1. What would you suggest to this parent?
>
> 2. The hydrolysis of erythromycin esters is base-catalysed, so why cannot you make them up in acidic solution to prevent the hydrolysis?
>
> *For answers, visit the online resources which accompany this textbook.*

to improve the activity profile of therapeutic agents. For example, the duration of action can be increased or decreased by introducing chemical functionalities which are more resistant or susceptible to metabolic inactivation. We can also use metabolic chemistry to convert an inactive molecule into an active one—so-called 'pro-drugs'.

> Examples of all these situations can be found in Chapter 14, 'Absorption, distribution, metabolism, and excretion'.

Sunscreen

When the sun shines on pale skin and turns it brown (or red), chemical reactions are taking place. Cells in the skin produce melanin, a pigment that absorbs ultraviolet as well as visible light. By absorbing energetic ultraviolet rays, it protects the skin from DNA damage. Because melanin is coloured, it turns the skin brown or tanned. Sunscreen is designed to reduce the exposure of the skin to damaging ultraviolet rays and may use organic or inorganic chemicals, or both. You may have seen cricketers wearing inorganic sunscreen on their faces. The zinc oxide or titanium dioxide reflects both ultraviolet and visible light so that the skin appears bright white. It is now possible to make inorganic sunscreen clear by using smaller particles, which are not nearly so bright.

Organic sunscreens work by absorbing ultraviolet light and converting it to harmless infrared radiation. To do this, an organic molecule requires a **chromophore** that absorbs over the right range of wavelengths. Organic molecules that absorb light in the ultraviolet or visible range have several adjacent double bonds and/or lone pairs of electrons; the larger the number of double bonds present, the higher the wavelength of most efficient absorption.

Para-aminobenzoic acid is one compound able to absorb harmful UV-B rays, and it is used in organic sunscreens. Figure 1.24 shows the structure of *para*-aminobenzoic acid and its alternate double bonds. However, Figure 1.24 also shows that *para*-aminobenzoic acid does not absorb over the whole ultraviolet range. If this were the only compound in sunscreen, people would still get burned. So a sunscreen contains lots of different compounds, all absorbing at different wavelengths and between them covering the whole UV-B range (280–320 nm), and often the UV-A range (320–400 nm) as well.

Figure 1.24 The ultraviolet spectrum of *para*-aminobenzoic acid, a constituent of organic sunscreens

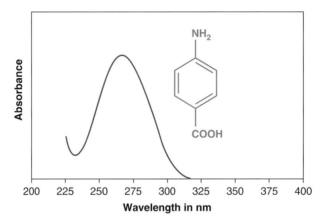

Drug substances themselves are of little use if they cannot be delivered appropriately to the patient in an appropriate form. This means that drugs are converted into appropriate dosage forms, thus becoming a medicine.

CHAPTER SUMMARY

This chapter is an overview, and most of the material will be covered in more detail elsewhere in the book. You should now understand that:

• Pharmacy is the science of drugs and all drugs are chemicals.

• Chemicals, whether in a body, in a plant or microbe, or in a test tube, do chemistry, not magic.

• Chemical structures can be drawn without labelling carbons and without drawing in hydrogens.

• Drugs are made by plants and microbes, by chemists, or by a mixture of the two.

• Chemistry can contribute to converting a drug into a medicine.

FURTHER READING

At this stage of your career, you should be finding out a little bit about every drug you encounter. Find out what medicines your grandparents are taking, and ask:

• What is it for?

• How does it work?

• What is its chemical structure?

If you watch medical dramas on the television, ask yourself the same questions about the drugs that are mentioned. You will find most of the answers in the British National Formulary at http://bnf.org/bnf or in Wikipedia at http://en.wikipedia.org/wiki. Wikipedia is written by members of the public and is not systematically peer-reviewed like a scientific journal, but it is *much* more reliable and impartial than most web pages. Use it to find out the basics about non-controversial subjects, including diseases and drugs. (Do not, however, use it as a major source for your final year project!) If you want to know more about the chemistry described here, try a good organic chemistry textbook, such as *Organic Chemistry* by Clayden, Greeves, and Warren.

You should also just read. Pharmacy is where science meets communication, and reading really helps effective communication. Dorothy L. Sayers' novel *The Documents in the Case* will help you understand the difference between a synthetic drug and a natural product. If you do not like fiction, try reading Ben Goldacre's *Bad Science* or Atul Gawande's *Complications*.

Clayden, J., Greeves, N. and Warren, S. *Organic Chemistry*, 2nd edn. Oxford University Press, 2012.

Djokic, S., Kobrehel, G., Lopotar, N., Kamenar, B., Nagl, A. and Mrvos, D. 'Erythromycin series. Part 13. Synthesis and structure elucidation of 10-dihydro-10-deoxo-11-methyl-11-azaerythromycin A', *J. Chem. Res. (S)* 1988:152–3.

Ibuprofen, a case study in green chemistry. Royal Society of Chemistry. http://intechemistry. files.wordpress.com/2010/09/ibuprofen-rsc-booklet.pdf

This is a resource produced by the Royal Society of Chemistry which you may like to work through, perhaps when you are revising for examinations.

Penniston, K. L., Nakada, S. Y., Holmes, R. P. and Assimos, D. G. 'Quantitative assessment of citric acid in lemon juice, lime juice, and commercially-available fruit juice products,' *J. Endourology* 2008, 22(3):567–70.

Psalm 139 vs 13 and Psalm 71 vs 18.

Both attributed to King David, although many Biblical scholars think that they were written by someone else.

Ro, D. K., Paradise, E. M., Ouellet, M., Fisher, K. J., Newman, K. L., Ndungu, J. M., Ho, K. A., Eachus, R. A., Ham, T. S., Kirby, J., Chang, M. C., Withers, S. T., Shiba, Y., Sarpong, R. and Keasling, J. D. 'Production of the antimalarial drug precursor artemisinic acid in engineered yeast', *Nature* 2006, 440:940–3.

Self-check

For the answers to the Self-Check questions in Chapter 1, visit the online resources which accompany this textbook.

CHAPTER 2

ORGANIC STRUCTURE AND BONDING

Alastair Mann

The modern periodic table now shows the existence of over one hundred elements, and while each of them is unique in its own way it is fair to say that carbon is the most unique of them all. Indeed, one of the traditional branches of chemistry—organic chemistry—is essentially the chemistry of compounds based on this one element.

In this chapter we will explore how carbon is able to become a part of such a diverse range of organic compounds. We will consider how we can rationalize the bonding, structure and, with particular relevance to pharmacy, the shapes of organic molecules. We will also examine the types of forces and interactions that occur *between* molecules, as opposed to the covalent bonds which hold them together. Finally, we will look at the idea of reaction mechanisms, which allow us to explain and even predict how such compounds will react in the presence of others.

Learning objectives

Having read this chapter you are expected to be able to:

- explain the structure and bonding of organic molecules
- recognize the hybridization state of carbon atoms in molecules of pharmaceutical interest and describe how this hybridization influences molecular shape
- describe the types of intermolecular forces that operate between organic molecules
- show how curly arrows may be used to describe mechanisms in organic chemistry.

2.1 WHAT IS ORGANIC CHEMISTRY?

Today, most scientists have little doubt about what they mean by the term 'organic chemistry'. The term 'organic' is used to refer to carbon-based compounds such as alcohols, amines, esters and so on, in which carbon is covalently combined with other elements, particularly hydrogen, oxygen, nitrogen and sulfur. Two hundred years ago, however, the picture was different.

The idea of there being organic compounds and inorganic compounds has its roots in the theories of the early nineteenth-century Swedish chemist, Berzelius. Berzelius was in turn reflecting the division of the kingdoms, by the ancient Greek philosopher Aristotle, into mineral

Jons Jacob Berzelius, Friedrich Wohler and Aristotle. All public domain images. Wikimedia Commons/Public Domain

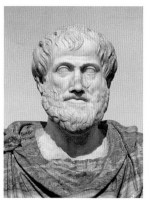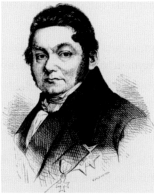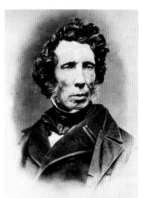

| Aristotle: 384–322 BC | Jöns Jacob Berzelius 1779–1848 | Friedrich Wöhler 1800–1882 |

(inorganic) and into animal and vegetable (organic). Berzelius felt that there was some kind of 'vital force' which must exist in organic compounds, making them distinct from inorganic compounds. This concept of vitalism was strong and can be found in both Asian and Western cultures. Indeed it was so strong that it was believed that organic compounds could not be synthesized from inorganic compounds—an idea which, if true, would have profound implications in the manufacturing sector of the modern pharmaceutical industry!

The idea started to be eroded in 1828 by the German chemist Friedrich Wöhler, who succeeded in synthesizing the organic compound, urea, from the inorganic substance, ammonium cyanate, shown in Figure 2.1.

As is so often the case in science, **serendipity** played a part. Wöhler did not set out to undermine the theory of vitalism, even though that was the eventual effect of his work. In fact, this was not the first time Wöhler had converted an inorganic compound to an organic compound. Four years earlier, in 1824, he had converted the inorganic substance cyanogen $(CN)_2$ to the organic compound, oxalic acid. This toxic compound with the formula HO_2CCO_2H is found in wood sorrel (belonging to the genus *Oxalis*, hence the name of the compound), rhubarb and black tea. Although the production of urea from ammonium cyanate is more famous, the synthesis of oxalic acid from cyanogen is generally regarded as the first synthesis of an organic compound from an inorganic compound.

Many other examples followed, notably the synthesis of ethanoic (acetic) acid from carbon disulfide (CS_2) by Kolbe in 1845, and the idea of a vital force in organic chemistry faded away. We are left with the modern idea that organic chemistry is the chemistry of the compounds of carbon, and typically involves covalent bonding of carbon to H, O, N, S, P and the halogens, with important contributions from many other elements in the periodic table too.

Figure 2.1   Wöhler's synthesis of urea via ammonium cyanate

$$Pb(NCO)_2 + 2NH_3 + 2H_2O \longrightarrow Pb(OH)_2 + 2NH_4(NCO)$$

Lead cyanate   Ammonium cyanate

$$NH_4(NCO) \longrightarrow [NH_3 + HNCO] \longrightarrow (NH_2)_2CO$$

Ammonia and isocyanic acid   Urea

What is so special about carbon?

There are a number of features that make carbon such an important and unique element, which can be summarized as follows:

- It forms a huge variety of compounds. Alkanes and alkenes (see Chapter 4), alcohols and amines (see Chapter 5), carboxylic acids (see Chapter 6) are just some examples.

- It is able to bond with many other elements in the periodic table, including s block elements such as lithium and magnesium, p block elements such as nitrogen, oxygen and the halogens, d block elements such as iron, copper and zinc, and even f block elements such as cerium and uranium.

- It can 'catenate'. In other words, it can form long chains of carbon atoms in a way that very few other elements can. (Sulfur also forms chains of atoms, as do selenium, tellurium and silicon to some extent.)

- It can take part in different types of homonuclear bond; carbon can form single, double or triple bonds with a neighbouring carbon atom. This leads to different shapes of molecules, which becomes of considerable importance when designing medicines and thinking about how they interact with other molecules present in the body. Carbon nearly always takes part in covalent, rather than ionic, bonding.

Allotropes of carbon

Although this chapter is much more concerned about the *compounds* that carbon forms, we should briefly note that even as an element, carbon is not as straightforward as it might first appear. Like many other elements, it can exist as a number of different *allotropes*, or different forms of the element where the atoms are bonded together in different arrangements. For a long time, the only known forms, or allotropes, of carbon were diamond and graphite.

In 1985, a third allotrope was discovered in which sixty carbon atoms were found to be arranged in the shape of a football. For the discovery of these so-called buckminsterfullerenes (often nicknamed 'buckyballs'), Harry Kroto and his co-workers were awarded the Nobel Prize for chemistry in 1996. Variations on these structures, where carbon atoms are arranged in long tubes (nicknamed 'buckytubes') have since been reported. More recent developments in material science have led to the reporting of another allotrope of carbon. This consists of single sheets of carbon atoms and is known as graphene. These can even be produced by physically separating the layers of atoms that make up graphite with adhesive tape, leaving the bonding *within* the sheet itself, which is now one atom thick, intact. In 2010, the Nobel Prize for Physics was awarded to Andre Geim and Kostya Novoselov for this ground-breaking work.

2.2 THE SHAPE OF MOLECULES

The shape of a molecule is very important. In pharmacy, it may govern the way in which a substrate binds to an enzyme, and in turn, the way in which a molecule may act as a drug. That a molecule can act as a drug when given to a patient is of huge importance. It relies on a correct fit between the drug and the receptor binding sites in the patient. Most receptor sites involve proteins, and drugs interact with specific amino acids in these proteins. These interactions trigger a series of reactions in the body which lead to the beneficial effect of the drug (see Box 2.1).

The hormone adrenaline will trigger **bronchodilation** during an asthma attack, so you might think it would be a good treatment for this condition. However, when used as a drug, it has unwanted side-effects such as increasing the heart rate. The synthetic compound, salbutamol, was first introduced by Allen and Hanburys (part of GlaxoSmithKline) in 1968, as an alternative treatment for the symptoms of asthma and is still used today. Because the shapes of the two molecules—adrenaline and salbutamol—have similarities (see Figure 2.2), salbutamol will fit into the adrenaline receptors in the muscles in the bronchiole walls, alleviating the well-known feelings of shortness of breath in the asthma sufferer, yet without producing many of the unwanted side-effects.

Figure 2.2   The structures of adrenaline and salbutamol

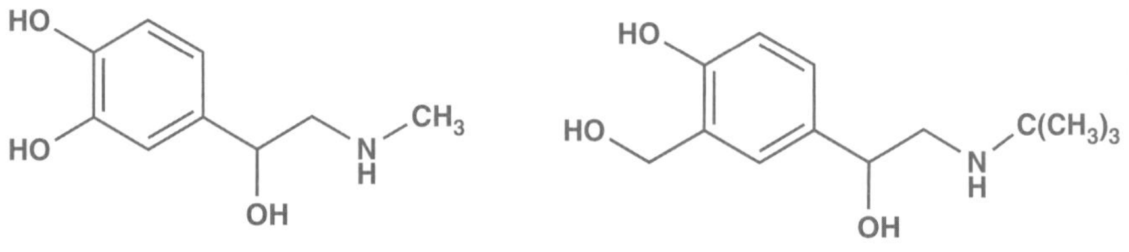

Adrenaline

Salbutamol

Changes in the three-dimensional arrangement of atoms in a molecule can cause significant differences in its properties in the human body. Arranged correctly, ibuprofen is a nonsteroidal anti-inflammatory drug; the mirror-image form, however, has no useful effect at all. Similarly, the mirror-image form of S-penicillamine, a drug used to treat rheumatoid arthritis, would not improve the patient's condition. Much worse, in fact, it would have a toxic effect on the body. The structures of ibuprofen and penicillamine are shown in Figure 2.3.

2.3 THE ELECTRONIC CONFIGURATION OF CARBON

Carbon is the sixth element in the periodic table (atomic number Z = 6) and therefore an isolated carbon atom contains six electrons. We can use a combination of the *aufbau principle* and *Hund's rule* to predict how these electrons will be accommodated in the available atomic orbitals. The *aufbau principle* tells us that we start with the lowest energy **orbital** (the 1s orbital) and fill it with electrons first, before moving onto the next lowest energy orbital (the 2s orbital) and repeating the process. Once the three 2p orbitals (identified as $2p_x$, $2p_y$ and $2p_z$) are reached, we need to apply *Hund's rule* and place electrons into each of these orbitals separately, rather than pairing up two electrons in any single 2p orbital. As a result, we can write the ground state electronic configuration of carbon as $1s^2\,2s^2\,2p^2$ just based on the aufbau principle, or more fully as $1s^2\,2s^2\,2p_x^1\,2p_y^1$, applying Hund's rule as well. The third 2p orbital, $2p_z$ is empty, and by convention we do not write $2p_z^0$; we leave out any empty orbitals.

Alternatively, it may be illustrated as a series of boxes, shown either horizontally or, as in Figure 2.4, vertically in order of increasing energy. Arrows are then used, pointing either up or down to represent the opposite spins of two electrons occupying the same orbital (in the case of

Figure 2.3 The structures and properties of ibuprofen and penicillamine

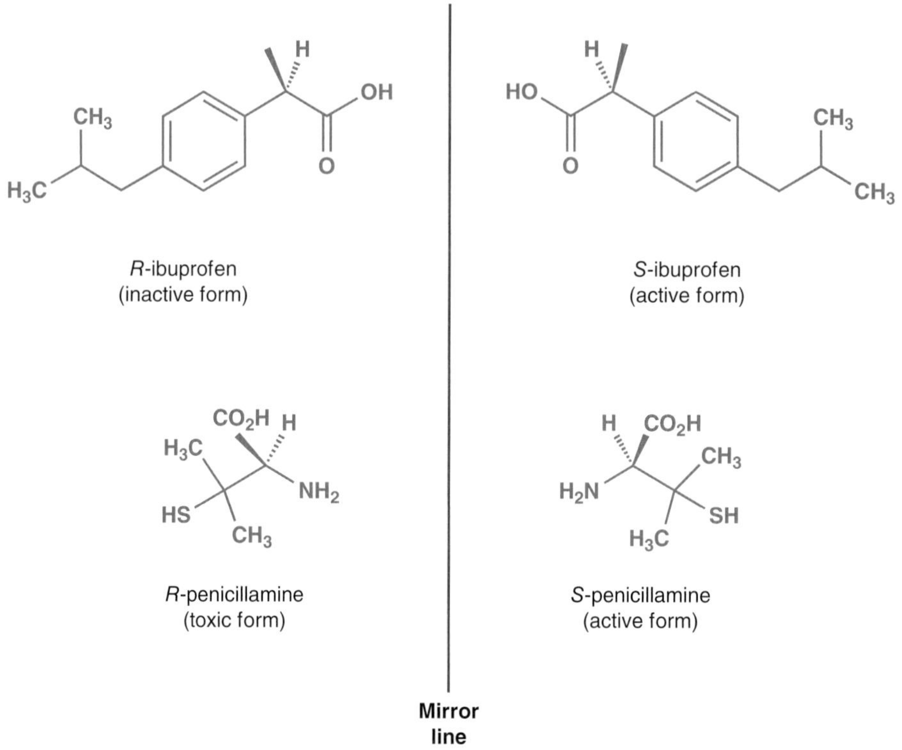

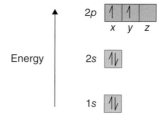

R-ibuprofen
(inactive form)

S-ibuprofen
(active form)

R-penicillamine
(toxic form)

S-penicillamine
(active form)

**Mirror
line**

Figure 2.4 The ground state electronic configuration of carbon. Note that the $2p_x$ and $2p_y$ orbitals each contain one electron, but the $2p_z$ orbital is empty

Energy

2p ⬆ ⬆
   x y z

2s ⬆⬇

1s ⬆⬇

the 1s and 2s orbitals). In the singly occupied 2p orbitals, the fifth and sixth electrons have parallel spins and so are shown pointing in the same direction in the lowest energy, or so-called *ground state*.

At this point, we should describe the shapes of the atomic orbitals that have already been referred to in this section. The 1s and 2s orbitals are spheres (they are spherically symmetric about the nucleus). The 2s orbital is bigger than the 1s orbital and the bulk of the electron density is therefore further from the nucleus. The shape of the 2p orbitals is sometimes described as a *dumbbell*, or perhaps more simply, a solid figure of eight. All three 2p orbitals are identical and are the same distance from the nucleus. They all have the same energy and therefore are said to be **degenerate**. As a result of mutual repulsion between them, the three 2p orbitals are arranged mutually perpendicular to each other (all at right angles), lying along the *x*, *y* and *z* axes that originate at the nucleus. The shapes of these are shown in Figure 2.5.

Figure 2.5 The shapes of s and p orbitals. Note that the shapes of 1s and 2s orbitals are the same but the 2s orbitals are bigger

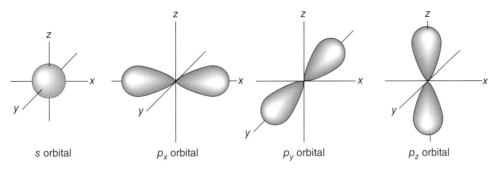

s orbital　　　　p_x orbital　　　　p_y orbital　　　　p_z orbital

2.4 THE SHAPE OF ORGANIC MOLECULES

The ideas outlined in Section 2.3 are not immediately consistent with experimental observations of organic molecules. For example, the various representations of the ground state electronic configuration of atomic carbon all indicate that there are only *two* unpaired electrons, suggesting that carbon might only be **divalent**, yet we know that it is normally **tetravalent**. (In fact, there are some species known as carbenes in which carbon does behave as if it is divalent, though these are very unusual).

Furthermore, if we look at the relative orientation of the 2p orbitals, it is clear that these are arranged at right angles to each other, so we might expect to find 90° bond angles in carbon compounds. With the possible very rare exception of the so-called cubanes, where eight carbon atoms are arranged at the corners of a cube, these are never observed. Angles of around 109°, 120° or 180° are much more common.

A third difficulty arising from the $1s^2\ 2s^2\ 2p_x^1\ 2p_y^1$ orbital model concerns the observed bond lengths. How can we explain why all four C–H bonds in methane are identical in terms of bond length and bond strength? We would also find it difficult to explain why the C–H and C–C bonds in alkanes, alkenes and alkynes vary in terms of their length and strength. Variability in the length and strength of bonds between carbon and other elements, such as oxygen, nitrogen and sulfur, is also seen.

This variability in bond angle and bond length can be illustrated by looking at three simple hydrocarbons: ethane, ethylene (systematic name, ethene) and acetylene (systematic name, ethyne), shown in Figure 2.6.

Figure 2.6 Bond angles and bond lengths in ethane, ethene and ethyne

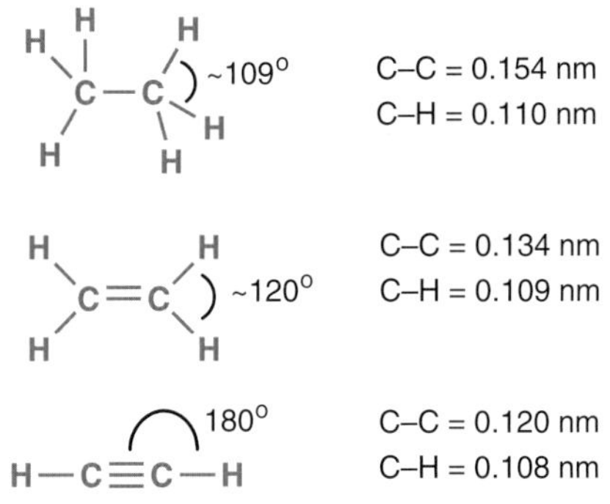

C–C = 0.154 nm
C–H = 0.110 nm
~109°

C–C = 0.134 nm
C–H = 0.109 nm
~120°

180°
C–C = 0.120 nm
C–H = 0.108 nm
H—C≡C—H

Excited states and hybridization

Our understanding of how electrons are accommodated in an isolated carbon atom and the known shapes of molecules, such as the hydrocarbons shown in Figure 2.6, do not match. To overcome these differences between theory and observation, we need to introduce two further ideas.

The first idea is the *excited state* of atomic carbon. In the excited state, energy has been supplied and, as a result of this, one of the 2s electrons has been promoted (raised to a higher orbital) and now sits in the previously unoccupied $2p_z$ orbital. This is shown in Figure 2.7.

This excited state now contains four unpaired electrons, which are available for bonding to other elements. So carbon now has the potential to be tetravalent, which is consistent with observation. However, if these electrons were used to form bonds while occupying the three 2p orbitals we could still not account for the known shapes of organic molecules. In such a scenario, three of the hydrogen atoms in a compound such as methane (CH_4) would be attached to the carbon atom via a 2p orbital and so would be arranged at right angles to each other, while the fourth, attached to a spherical 2s orbital, would have no preferred orientation. To make matters worse, because of the different energies of the 2s and 2p orbitals and their different distances from the nucleus, the four C−H bonds in methane would not all be of equal length, in contrast to what is well established by physical measurements.

So although the production of an excited state is a useful start, something further is needed. This is the concept of hybridization of the atomic orbitals to produce new hybrid orbitals.

Hybridization is effectively a mixing process, in which combinations of atomic orbitals are taken and blended together to produce the same number of new, hybrid orbitals. These display properties that are somewhere between those of the original atomic orbitals used to produce them. Hybridization is used to rationalize the observed shapes and structures of real molecules, allowing us to overcome the difficulties that we encountered when we tried to explain these observed properties in terms of the atomic orbitals available.

At a more advanced level, hybridization can be described using some sophisticated mathematics. However, a less intimidating, qualitative description of hybridization was first put forward by the American chemist Linus Pauling in the 1930s, and works perfectly adequately here.

There are three possible ways that the 2s and 2p atomic orbitals in carbon can be combined, or hybridized, differing only in how many 2p orbitals are involved. These are described as:

- **sp³ hybridization**: here all four orbitals (2s and three 2p) are mixed to produce four new hybrid orbitals, which are labelled sp³. These hybrid orbitals are used to rationalize the observed shapes of saturated organic molecules such as CH_4, C_2H_6 and many others.

- **sp² hybridization**: here only three orbitals (2s and two of the 2p orbitals) are mixed to produce three new hybrid orbitals, which are labelled sp². The third 2p orbital remains unhybridized, although it still plays a part in bonding. These hybrid orbitals are used to rationalize the observed shapes of unsaturated organic molecules such as the alkene, ethene (ethylene).

Figure 2.7 Formation of an excited state of carbon

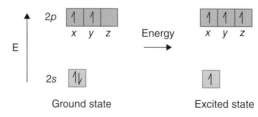

- **sp hybridization**: here only two orbitals (2s and just one of the 2p orbitals) are mixed to produce two new hybrid orbitals, which are labelled sp (there is no need to put a superscript 1 on this; the correct notation is sp, not sp^1). The other two 2p orbitals remain unhybridized, although they still play a part in bonding. These hybrid orbitals are used to rationalize the observed shapes of unsaturated organic molecules such as the alkyne, ethyne (acetylene).

Let us now consider the three types of hybridization in more detail, in all cases starting from the excited state of carbon illustrated in Figure 2.7. In each case, the following properties of the hybrid orbitals have to be considered:

- the *energy* of the hybrid orbitals with respect to the starting atomic orbitals
- the *shape* of the hybrid orbitals
- the *relative orientation* of the hybrid orbitals with respect to each other and also with respect to any unhybridized orbitals that may be present
- their *use in bonding* in organic compounds.

sp^3 hybridization

The way in which the 2s and three 2p orbitals in the excited state of atomic carbon are combined to give four sp^3 hybrid orbitals is shown in Figure 2.8. (The 1s orbital is not shown in this diagram as it is much lower in energy and so is not directly involved in bonding.) The result is the production of four new, degenerate orbitals, each one of which accommodates a single electron from carbon. This makes carbon tetravalent and allows it to form four bonds to itself or other elements. Because these new orbitals are three parts p and one part s, they lie somewhere between the original 2s and 2p orbitals in terms of energy, though rather closer to the original 2p level. Looking ahead, we can imagine that the sp^2 and sp hybrids will progressively drop in energy, as the percentage of s character increases each time. (It is 25% in sp^3, 33% in sp^2 and 50% in sp hybridization.)

The shape of these hybrids is rather harder to explain in detail without adopting a fuller, more mathematical approach. However, we can adopt a simpler, more pictorial approach, seeing what would happen in just one dimension when an s orbital is combined with a p orbital. This is illustrated schematically in Figure 2.9, where the effect of adding a 2s orbital to a 2p

Figure 2.8   sp^3 hybridization of carbon

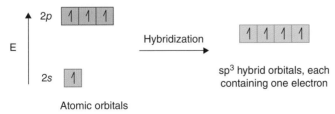

Figure 2.9   Shape of a hybrid orbital: same coloured regions add together and different coloured regions cancel

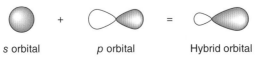

orbital is shown. As a result, the size of the hybrid orbital is reduced on the left of the nucleus, as shown in the diagram, and is increased on the right. The resulting shape is sometimes de-scribed as looking a bit like a tadpole.

Again looking ahead, we can predict that as the relative contribution of the s orbital increases as we go to sp^2 and finally to sp hybridization, the resulting hybrid orbital will be a broadly similar shape, though it will become slightly shorter and slightly rounder each time. We will see later that this shortening of the orbital is the reason that C−H bonds become progressively shorter as we go from alkanes to alkenes and finally to the alkynes (see Figure 2.6 for details).

The relative orientation of the four sp^3 hybrid orbitals is determined by mutual repulsion, which maximizes the separation between four identical and similarly charged objects in space. The optimum way of doing this is to have them pointing towards the corner of a tetrahedron, which results in an angle between them of 109.5°.

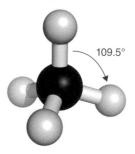

This is the angle observed between the C−H bonds in methane illustrated here, or between the C−Cl bonds in tetrachloromethane. However, if the four groups or atoms attached to the central carbon atom are not identical, there are small deviations from the perfect tetrahedral angle to allow for the difference in sizes and electronegativities of the substituent groups sur-rounding the carbon atom. These deviations are typically only about one or two degrees.

We learn more about bond angles in organohalogen compounds such as tetracholorometh-ane in Box 2.2.

Box 2.2 Halothane, an anaesthetic

Halothane (2-bromo-2-chloro-1,1,1-trifluoroethane) is an organohalogen compound, first syn-thesized by Charles Suckling in 1951 while he was working for ICI (Imperial Chemical Indus-tries). It is trademarked under the name *Fluothane*® and was used as a general anaesthetic from the mid-1950s onwards, administered by inhalation. Although it is still used in veteri-nary medicine and in some parts of the developing world, in many developed countries it has now been superseded by other compounds. These often also contain CF_3 groups, though they tend also to contain ether functions. Halothane and tetrachloromethane are illustrated in Fig-ure 2.10, though without representing the full, three-dimensional aspects of their structures.

Self-check 2.1

In tetrachloromethane, the Cl−C−Cl bond angle is 109.5°. In halothane, the F−C−F bond an-gles are in the range 107.5° to 108.5°, while the Br−C−Cl bond angle is nearly 112°. Can you explain these differences?

Figure 2.10 Halothane and tetrachloromethane

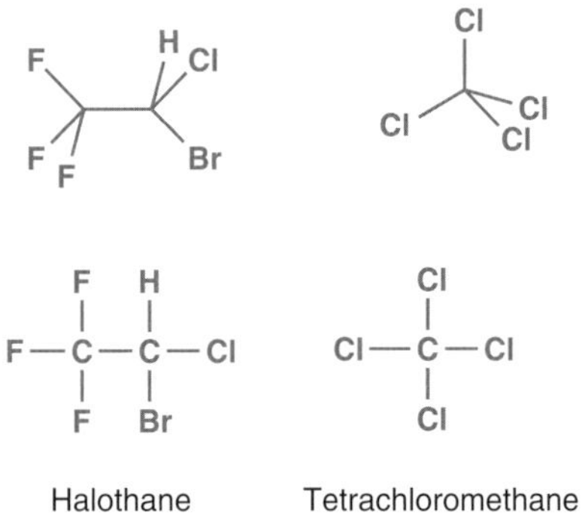

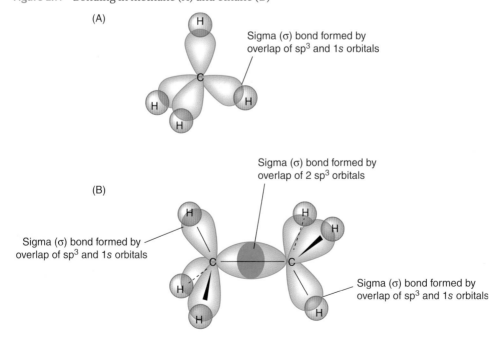

Halothane   Tetrachloromethane

The four sp³ hybrid orbitals are used to form σ- (sigma) bonds (often synonymous with the term 'single bond') by an 'end-on' or 'head-on' overlap of one of these orbitals with another suitable orbital in a second atom. The term 'end-on' implies that these orbitals are pointing straight at each other, along the internuclear axis. Sigma (σ) bonds are the strongest type of covalent chemical bonds and are radially symmetric about the internuclear bond axis—in other words, if you sliced through a σ bond at right angles to the internuclear axis, you would 'see' a circle.

In methane, each sp³ hybridized orbital on carbon overlaps with a 1s orbital on a hydrogen atom, which also contains a single electron. This leads to the formation of four conventional covalent σ-bonds, sometimes more rigorously described as sp³–s σ-bonds to reflect the contributing orbitals. This is illustrated in Figure 2.11. In ethane, three of the sp³ hybrid orbitals on carbon overlap with 1s orbitals on hydrogen, while the fourth overlaps (again end-on) with the

Figure 2.11 Bonding in methane (A) and ethane (B)

(A)

Sigma (σ) bond formed by
overlap of sp³ and 1s orbitals

Sigma (σ) bond formed by
overlap of 2 sp³ orbitals

(B)

Sigma (σ) bond formed by
overlap of sp³ and 1s orbitals

Sigma (σ) bond formed by
overlap of sp³ and 1s orbitals

sp^3 hybrid on a second carbon atom. This gives a sp^3–sp^3 C–C σ-bond, or more simply, a carbon–carbon single bond.

Alkanes (and many other molecules), employ exclusively single, σ-bonds. Simple alcohols and amines, such as ethanol and ethylamine, also employ only single, σ-bonds. C–O and C–N bonds are formed by end-on overlap of a sp^3 hybrid orbital on carbon with an appropriate orbital on either oxygen or nitrogen. However, carboxylic acids, ketones, alkenes, nitriles and alkynes require the other two types of hybridization – sp^2 and sp—to account fully for their bonding and structures.

There is generally completely free rotation about σ-bonds, even when there are different (sometimes quite bulky) groups attached to the atoms making the bond. (An exception to this is in most cyclic compounds, as is discussed in Chapter 3.) We will see in the following section, 'sp^2 hybridization', that free rotation is prevented when other types of bonds, termed pi (π) bonds, are formed.

sp^2 hybridization

The way in which the 2s and *two* of the three 2p orbitals in the excited state of atomic carbon are combined, to give three sp^2 hybrid orbitals, is shown in Figure 2.12 (again, the 1s orbital is not shown in this diagram as it is much lower in energy and so is not involved in bonding). The result is the formation of three new, degenerate orbitals, in addition to the unhybridized 2p orbital. Each one of these orbitals accommodates one of the four valence electrons, so again carbon is tetravalent and able to form four bonds to other elements.

Given that these new hybrid orbitals are two thirds p and one third s, they again lie somewhere between the 2s and 2p orbitals in terms of energy. They are still closer to the original 2p level, though this time slightly lower in energy than the sp^3 hybrids we saw previously (because the orbitals now have 33% s character).

The shape of these hybrids is broadly similar to the sp^3 hybrids described earlier. However, they are slightly shorter and rounder than the sp^3 hybrids, reflecting the increased contribution from the 2s atomic orbital. As was suggested previously and shown in Figure 2.6, the C–H bond in an alkene is slightly shorter than in an alkane because the sp^2 hybrid orbital is shorter than an sp^3 hybrid orbital.

The relative orientation of the three sp^2 hybrid orbitals and the unhybridized 2s orbital is again governed by mutual repulsion, with their orientations maximizing their separation in space. However, this time the argument is not quite as simple, because the four objects we need to separate are not all identical. This time, the three sp^2 hybrids point towards the corners of an equilateral triangle (in a so-called *trigonal planar* arrangement), with the unhybridized 2p orbital placed perpendicular to these. This results in an angle of 120° between the three sp^2 hybrids, which of course is approximately the angle observed between C–H bonds in an alkene

Figure 2.12 sp^2 hybridization of carbon

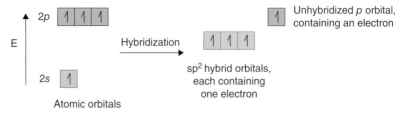

such as ethylene. In fact, this H−C−H angle is closer to 118° because of the greater bulk of the rest of the molecule compared with the two hydrogen atoms, so the angles have to adjust slightly to accommodate this (see Figure 2.6).

The three sp² hybrid orbitals are able to form σ-bonds to other elements in exactly the same way as sp³ hybrid orbitals can. A σ-bond is formed by end-on overlap of the appropriate orbitals, and the C−H bonds may be described this time as sp²−s, while the C−C bonds are described as sp²−sp².

The unhybridized 2p orbital on a carbon atom can also become involved in bonding between two adjacent carbon atoms. However, end-on overlap is not possible because the orbitals are pointing the wrong way. Instead, a weaker, 'side-on' overlap between the two parallel orbitals is all that is possible. This leads to the formation of a π-bond between the two carbon atoms, where the electron density is now located above and below the internuclear axis rather than along it. This time a slice through the internuclear axis would reveal two areas of electron density, one above and one below the axis, rather than the radial distribution seen in the case of a σ-bond. This overall bonding scheme is shown in Figure 2.13.

Side-on overlap is not as effective as end-on overlap, so the π-bond in a so-called double bond—which comprises one σ-bond and one π-bond—is weaker than a σ-bond. This is often reflected in the chemistry of an alkene. Chapter 4 introduces several reactions in which the π bond is lost, perhaps by addition across it, while the σ-bond remains intact. Critically, however, the π-bond is strong enough to prevent free rotation about the C−C axis, whereas this rotation readily occurs when there is only a σ-bond holding the two atoms together. This is what permits the formation of geometric, or *cis* and *trans* isomers in alkenes, and is discussed more in Chapters 3 and 4.

Figure 2.13   Bonding in ethene

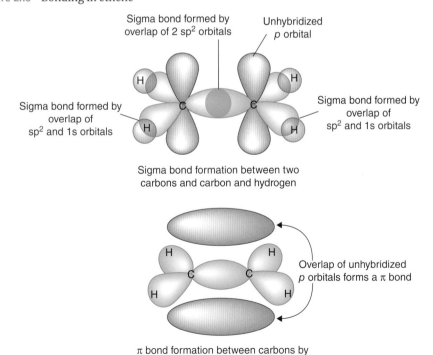

Sigma bond formed by overlap of 2 sp² orbitals

Unhybridized p orbital

Sigma bond formed by overlap of sp² and 1s orbitals

Sigma bond formed by overlap of sp² and 1s orbitals

Sigma bond formation between two carbons and carbon and hydrogen

Overlap of unhybridized p orbitals forms a π bond

π bond formation between carbons by overlap of unhybridized p orbitals

So far, we have only considered the formation of double bonds between two carbon atoms, though in fact a similar description can be used for the double bonds observed between carbon and oxygen in a carbonyl group, C=O (for example, in a ketone), or in the C=N bond, for example, in an imine. In these cases, the carbon atom is sp² hybridized (as is the heteroatom, O or N), with angles of about 120° between any other atoms attached to it.

sp hybridization

The way in which the 2s and just *one* of the three 2p orbitals in the excited state of atomic carbon are combined to give two sp hybrid orbital, is shown in Figure 2.14. (Once again, the 1s orbital is not involved in this process and so is not shown in the diagram.) The result is the formation of two new, degenerate orbitals, in addition to the two unhybridized 2p orbitals. Each orbital accommodates one of the four valence electrons in carbon, so carbon is again tetravalent and is able to form four bonds to other elements. Given that these new hybrid orbitals are now made up of equal parts s and p, they lie half way between the 2s and 2p orbitals in terms of energy, below both the sp³ and sp² hybrids seen in the previous two sections.

The shape of these sp hybrids is broadly similar to the sp³ and sp² hybrids already described (and the same reasons are used to account for their shapes). However, they are slightly shorter and rounder than the sp³ and sp² hybrids, reflecting the increased contribution from the 2s atomic orbital. As was discussed earlier and shown in Figure 2.6, the C–H bond in an alkyne is slightly shorter than the C–H bonds in either an alkane or an alkene, because it is an sp hybrid orbital that is involved in the formation of the C–H bond.

Once again, the relative orientation of the two sp hybrid orbitals and the two unhybridized 2p orbitals is governed by their mutual repulsion, to maximize their separation in space, and, once again, the four objects being separated are not identical. The optimum arrangement is to have the two sp hybrids pointing away from each other with a bond angle of 180° between them. The two unhybridized 2p orbitals are then placed mutually perpendicular to these (see Figure 2.15). Having the two sp hybrids 180° apart is consistent with the shape of a simple alkyne like acetylene (ethyne), where the four H–C–C–H atoms are found in a linear arrangement (see Figure 2.6).

The two sp hybrid orbitals are able to form σ-bonds to other elements in exactly the same way as sp³ and sp² hybrid orbitals, with a σ-bond being formed by end-on overlap of the appropriate orbitals. The C–H bonds are described this time as sp–s, while the C–C bonds are described as sp–sp.

The two unhybridized 2p orbitals on a carbon atom also become involved in bonding between two adjacent carbon atoms and, again, weaker side-on overlap occurs because end-on overlap is not possible. This leads to formation of two π-bonds between the two carbon atoms, which

Figure 2.14   sp hybridization of carbon

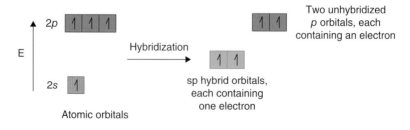

Figure 2.15   Bonding in ethyne (acetylene)

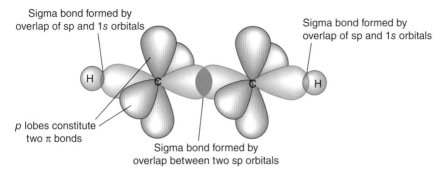

Sigma bond formed by overlap of sp and 1s orbitals

Sigma bond formed by overlap of sp and 1s orbitals

p lobes constitute two π bonds

Sigma bond formed by overlap between two sp orbitals

Formation of two π bonds between the carbons by overlap of two pairs of unhybridized p orbitals

Self-check 2.2

What kind of chemical reaction would occur between acetylene (ethyne) and bromine? Draw the structure of the compound that would be produced when ethyne reacts with two moles of Br_2. The names acetylene and ethyne are both acceptable; see Box 2.3.

lie in planes arranged at right angles to each other. The electron density associated with these is now located in front and behind the internuclear axis, as well as above and below it. This time, a slice through the internuclear axis would reveal four areas of electron density associated with the π-bonds, in addition to the radial distribution around the axis arising from the C–C σ-bond. This overall bonding scheme is shown in Figure 2.15.

As we saw with bonding in the alkenes in the section discussing 'sp² hybridization', side-on overlap is not as effective as end-on overlap, because the orbitals cannot get close enough to maximize it. As a result, the second and third bonds (the π-bonds) in a so-called triple bond are both weaker than the σ-bond, which influences the chemistry of the alkynes.

So far we have only considered the formation of triple bonds between two carbon atoms, though in fact a similar description can be used for the triple bonds observed between carbon and nitrogen in a nitrile (C ≡ N) group. In this case, the carbon atom is still regarded as being sp hybridized (as is the nitrogen atom), with angles of 180° forming between any other atoms or groups attached to it.

Box 2.3   Systematic nomenclature and trivial names

By the time you have studied this book you will be familiar with both systematic nomenclature and the trivial names of many common organic molecules. In the early chapters, we will normally give both. Later, we will use whichever is more appropriate in the context.

Self-check 2.3

Why does carbon, generally, not form triple bonds to oxygen?

Recognizing hybridization states and the shapes of molecules

The previous sections have described how we can rationalize the experimentally observed bonding and structure of organic molecules by invoking different patterns of hybridization of the valence shell orbitals, 2s and 2p. However, it is also important to think about this the other way round: to be able to look at the structure of a molecule, recognize the hybridization states of its carbon atoms, and hence begin to visualize the three-dimensional shape of the compound.

While such visualization may seem difficult initially, there are some simple guidelines that will help you to do this reliably. You should look at an individual carbon atom and count the number of atoms it is bonded to. This is a reflection of the number of σ-bonds that have been formed to it and hence the number of hybrid orbitals that were required to make this bonding possible. For example, in methane or ethane we can see that carbon is bonded to four separate atoms and so it needs to be sp^3 hybridized. The bond angles between these various attached atoms, or groups, will be about 109°. Likewise, we saw that there are three separate atoms attached to the central carbon in an alkene and that sp^2 hybridization was required to rationalize this. The corresponding bond angles around the carbon atom are seen to be about 120°. Finally, there are only two separate atoms attached to each carbon atom in an alkyne and so sp hybridization is required to account for this. The associated bond angles are 180°.

We also extended these ideas, which were discussed in most detail for the hydrocarbons, to include other atoms, for example O and N, but equally S, P and the halogens too. In other words, it does not matter what other element carbon is attached to when we come to assess its hybridization state in this way.

These guidelines are summarized in Table 2.1.

Some compounds of interest and relevance in pharmacy are shown in Figure 2.16. The three drug structures shown here all contain carbon atoms in all three possible hybridization states!

Self-check 2.4

Now draw all the structures in Figure 2.16 as 'stick' structures (See Chapter 1 if you are not sure how to do this).

Table 2.1 Hybridization state and bond angles around carbon atoms

Number of separate atoms attached to a carbon atom	Hybridization state of the carbon atom	Approximate bond angles around the carbon atom
4	sp^3	109°
3	sp^2	120°
2	sp	180°

Figure 2.16 Structures of drugs and hybridization states of carbon in them

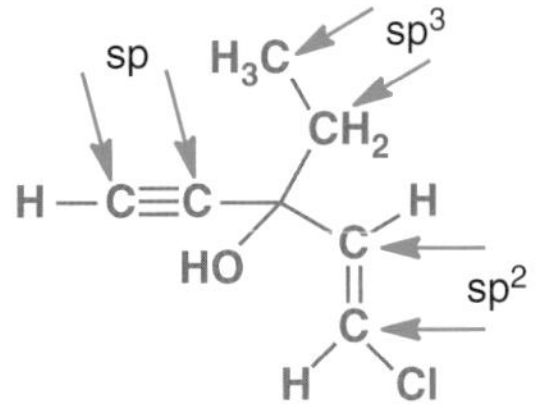

Ethchlorvynol – a sedative

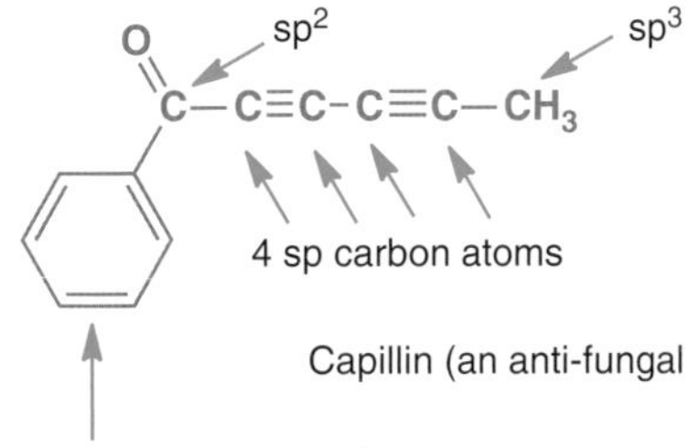

All 6 ring carbons are sp^2

4 sp carbon atoms

Capillin (an anti-fungal agent)

All 6 ring carbons are sp^2

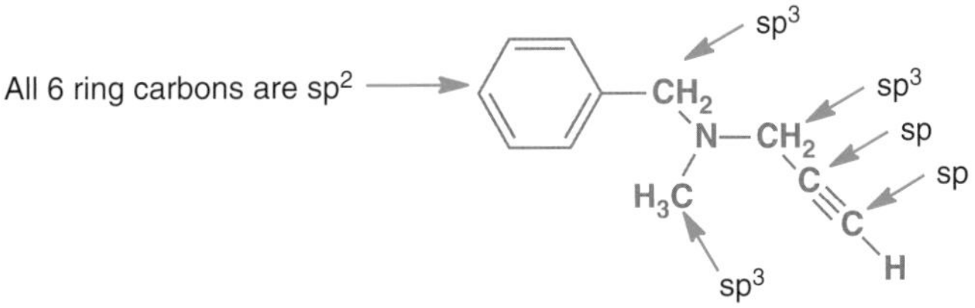

Pargyline (an anti-hypertensive)

Figure 2.17 Structures of paracetamol, ethinylestradiol Methylpentynol

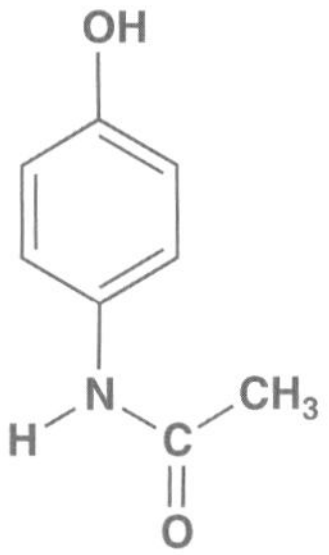

Paracetamol
(an analgesic)

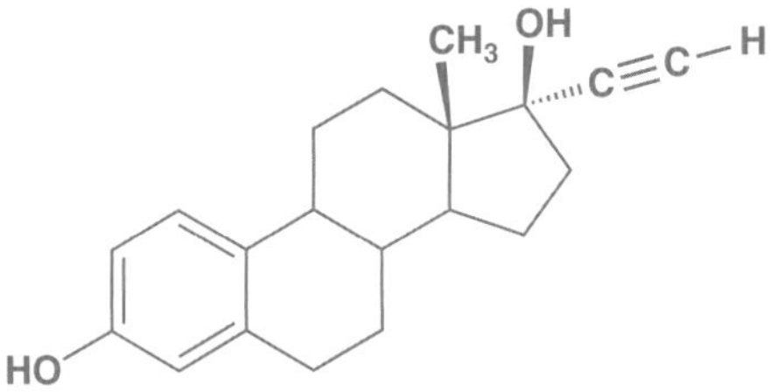

Ethinylestradiol
(oral contraceptive)

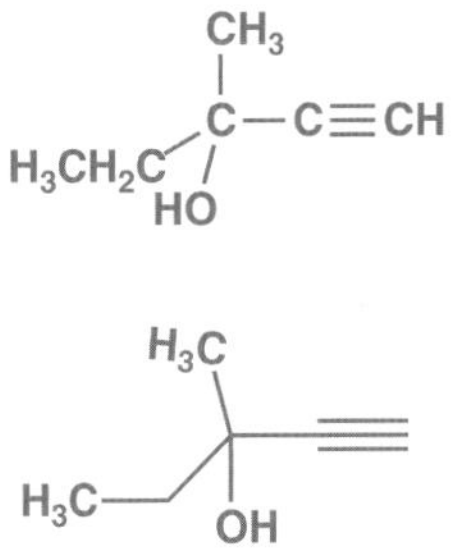

methylpentynol (a sedative)
alternative representations

Self-check 2.5

Figure 2.17 shows the structures of three more drugs. What are the hybridization states of each of the carbon atoms in them? What are the bond angles around each of the carbon atoms? Note that in two of the structures, paracetamol and oblivon, only two of the three possible hybridization states are observed. However, the other example, ethynylestradiol, is more complicated and all three hybridization states of the carbon atom are present.

Carbon utilizes hybrid electronic orbitals to bond covalently to other atoms. These orbitals determine the overall molecular shape. The shape of a molecule is very important with respect to its chemical and biological activities.

2.5 INTERMOLECULAR FORCES

So far we have only considered the covalent bonds *within* a molecule that hold it together—in other words, the *intra*molecular forces. Before going on to look at how we can describe the reactions of these molecules, we need to be aware of the forces that occur *between* molecules, holding one molecule to the next—in other words, the *inter*molecular forces.

The importance of these forces is shown by thinking about the physical properties of one of the substances most familiar to us: water. For such a small molecule, water has an unexpectedly high boiling point. It is approximately 200° higher than might be predicted by comparison to the boiling points of the other hydrides in the same group of the periodic table: H_2Te (-2.2 °C), H_2Se (-41.5 °C) and H_2S (-60.7 °C). Simple extrapolation of this trend might suggest that the boiling point of water would be around -100 °C, not +100 °C, which we know it to be. Its melting point is also considerably higher than would be expected from comparison to other, related substances.

Relatively strong intermolecular forces exist between water molecules in all of its physical states (solid, liquid and gas), causing its apparently anomalous properties, and without these unusual properties life could never have evolved in the way that is familiar to us. Although we have used water as an extreme example, in fact intermolecular forces of varying types and strength must exist between the atoms and molecules of *all* substances—otherwise we would never be able to observe them in the liquid or solid states.

There are a number of different types of intermolecular force that can act between covalently bonded molecules, holding them in contact with one another. All are very much weaker than the covalent forces that operate in a σ-bond or π-bond, or the ionic forces that operate in a substance such as sodium chloride. Those that we will examine, and an indication of their strength, are given in Table 2.2. (Values for covalent bonds and ionic lattice energies are also given as a comparison, but you can see that these are at least an order of magnitude stronger.)

London (van der Waals) forces

These are the weakest forces that occur between molecules. They are referred to both as London dispersion forces (after Fritz London, a German-American physicist), or as van der Waals forces, although, strictly speaking, van der Waals forces also include other types of intermolecular interaction. London forces occur in substances where there is no permanent dipole. Because the electrons in a molecule are moving continuously, even the electrons in a non-polar molecule can become unevenly distributed within the molecule, causing it to have a temporary dipole. This temporary polarization in a molecule causes neighbouring molecules to become

Table 2.2 Strengths of intermolecular and intramolecular forces

Type of intermolecular force	Approximate strength (kJ mol⁻¹)
London (van der Waals) forces	<2
Dipole–dipole interactions	1–3
Hydrogen bonding	10–30
Intramolecular forces for comparison	
Covalent bonds	300
Ionic bonds (lattice energy)	~760 for NaCl

temporarily polarized as well, and so the molecules can be weakly attracted to each other. These temporary dipoles are induced, and, therefore, the interactions are also known as induced dipole-induced dipole interactions.

Dipole–dipole interactions

The second type of intermolecular interaction we need to consider are dipole–dipole interactions, which are described as electrostatic interactions. These affect molecules in which there is a *permanent* dipole, as opposed to the temporary ones described in the previous section. The polarization in a bond, and hence in a molecule, is the result of differences in the electronegativity between the two atoms in a covalent bond, leaving partial positive ($\delta+$) and negative ($\delta-$) charges on the two atoms concerned. Molecules with permanent dipoles are attracted to each other because the molecules can align themselves in such a way that the positive end of one dipole is close to the negative end of another dipole, resulting in an overall attractive force between two adjacent molecules, as shown in Figure 2.18.

Hydrogen bonding

A hydrogen bond is a particularly strong type of electrostatic interaction, or dipole–dipole interaction, which occurs specifically between an H–X bond (where X is an electronegative atom, normally F, O or N) and another electronegative atom, X'. X' is not only highly electronegative but possesses one or more lone pairs of electrons. In practice, this means that X' is also nitrogen, oxygen or fluorine. The interaction is typically about one tenth the strength of a covalent bond, and is strong enough to make the interatomic distance less than the sum of the van der Waals radii. (In other words, the two atoms are closer together than they should be, based on their diameters, which implies there is some degree of covalent character in these bonds.)

Figure 2.19 illustrates the hydrogen bonding present between two adjacent water molecules and between two adjacent ethanol molecules. In the liquid phase, a molecule of water, or ethanol, may take part in more than one hydrogen bond by involving both lone pairs of electrons on the oxygen atoms or both hydrogen atoms on the water molecule (though only the single H atom on the OH group of the ethanol). Extensive hydrogen bonding is the reason water has such a high boiling point (100 °C) compared with other hydrides in the same group of the periodic table. Sulfur, for example, is much less electronegative than oxygen and cannot form strong hydrogen bonds. Consequently, H_2S, a pungent-smelling gas with an aroma of rotten eggs, has a boiling point of -60.7 °C. Several other important properties of water, including its unusual expansion on freezing, may also be attributed to hydrogen bonding.

Figure 2.18 Dipole–dipole interactions

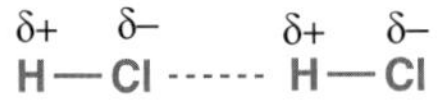

$$\overset{\delta+ \quad \delta-}{H-Cl} \cdots\cdots \overset{\delta+ \quad \delta-}{H-Cl}$$

Dipole-dipole interaction
between two HCl molecules

$$\overset{\delta+ \quad \delta-}{H_3C-OH} \qquad \overset{\delta+ \quad \delta-}{H_3C-NH_2}$$

Polarisation in ethanol and ethylamine

Figure 2.19   Hydrogen bonding between water molecules and ethanol molecules

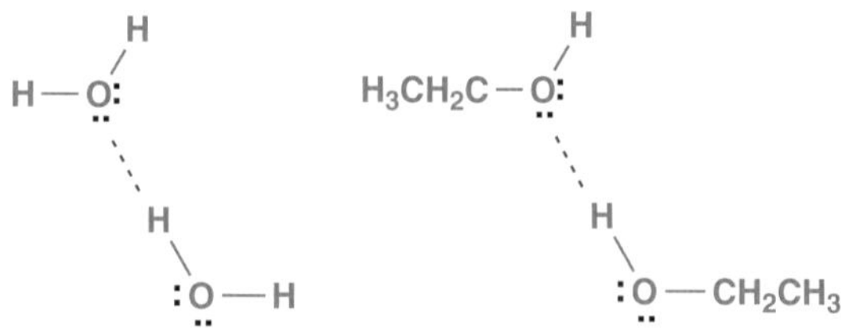

Hydrogen bonding turns out to be extremely important in organic molecules, many of which contain N−H and O−H bonds (amines, alcohols and carboxylic acids, for example). Even molecules without N−H or O−H bonds may become involved in hydrogen bonding, as the C=O group in a ketone, for example, contains an oxygen atom with two lone pairs of electrons that may become hydrogen bonded to the O−H or N−H group in a second molecule. The importance of these types of electrostatic bonds in describing how drugs may become attached to receptor sites in the body (or in the holding together of the two strands in a nucleic acid) is immense.

We can also use Figure 2.19 to illustrate two important ideas—those of a *hydrogen bond donor* and a *hydrogen bond acceptor*. In the case of water, the O−H bond is regarded as the hydrogen bond *donor* (it donates the hydrogen), while the oxygen atom with the lone pair is the hydrogen bond *acceptor* (it accepts the hydrogen). In the case of amines, the N−H bond is the *donor* and the N atom with the lone pair is the *acceptor*.

> For more information about the significance of hydrogen bonding in alcohols, see Chapter 5.

Self-check 2.6

Consider the two structural isomers with the formula C_2H_6O. One of these has a boiling point of 78 °C and the other a boiling point of –24 °C. Give the names and structural formulae of both isomers and explain the difference in their boiling points.

Self-check 2.7

The structure of the anaesthetic, halothane, was shown in Figure 2.10. Can you identify any part of this structure that might act as a hydrogen bond acceptor?

Self-check 2.8

The structures of water and ethanol are both shown in Figure 2.19. Can you show how hydrogen bonding can occur between a molecule of ethanol and a molecule of water; how might this account for the high solubility of ethanol in water, and vice versa? This ability of an organic molecule to dissolve in water is very important in the distribution of a drug around the body.

Self-check 2.9

The structures of diethyl ether and triethylamine are shown here. How might these two compounds hydrogen bond to water? Why can they not hydrogen bond to each other?

$$CH_2CH_3$$

$$H_3CH_2C-\overset{..}{\underset{..}{O}}:$$

Diethyl ether

$$\overset{CH_2CH_3}{\underset{CH_2CH_3}{\overset{|}{\underset{}{N}}}}$$

$$H_3CH_2C$$

Triethylamine

Whereas atoms in organic molecules are held together by covalent bonds, the intermolecular forces between molecules can take a variety of forms, depending on the nature of the molecules. Intermolecular forces comprise van der Waals forces, dipole–dipole attraction and hydrogen bonds.

2.6 REACTION TYPES AND THE MAKING AND BREAKING OF BONDS

Chemical reactions involving organic compounds can be classified into four types. These are listed below and illustrated in Figure 2.20.

1. *substitution*—where one group is replaced by another; an example of this is the formation of propanenitrile in the reaction of bromoethane with potassium cyanide

2. *elimination*—where two groups are lost, to create a double (or perhaps triple) bond; an example of this is the formation of propene in the reaction of 1-bromopropane with a base

3. *addition*—the reverse of elimination, where two groups are added across a double (or perhaps triple) bond; an example of this is the formation of 2-bromocyclohexanol when cyclohexene is shaken with bromine water

4. *rearrangement*—where reordering of the structure occurs and the atoms are now bonded to each other in a different arrangement; an example of this is the Fries rearrangement in which an aromatic ester rearranges in the presence of an aluminium trichloride catalyst to give a mixture of hydroxy aromatic ketones.

These classifications are useful, but they only describe what has happened, rather than *how* it has happened. The latter consideration of 'how' is the stuff of organic reaction mechanisms and is introduced in Section 2.7.

All reactions involve some sort of bond cleavage (breakage) and bond formation. If bond cleavage results in the formation of anions and cations, it is described as heterolytic cleavage. In heterolytic cleavage, the two electrons in the σ-bond between the two atoms move as a *pair* and end up on either one or other of the two atoms involved. Of course, with an example represented just as X−Y, this could be illustrated as occurring in two possible ways—both electrons going to X or both to Y. However, with 'real' molecules the two electrons will always go to the more electronegative of the two atoms, which is where the negative charge will reside at the

Figure 2.20 Examples of the four classes of organic reactions

Substitution:

$$CH_3CH_2Br + KCN \longrightarrow CH_3CH_2CN + KBr$$

Elimination:

$$CH_3CH_2CH_2Br + KOH \longrightarrow CH_3CH=CH_2 + H_2O + KBr$$

Addition:

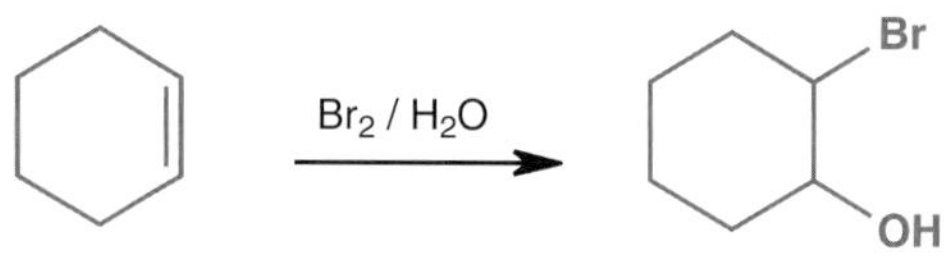

Rearrangement:

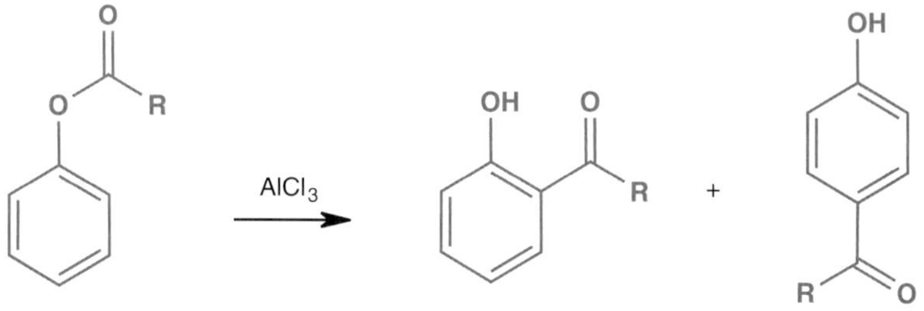

end of the process. Thus, for example, HCl will undergo heterolytic cleavage to give H$^+$ and Cl$^+$, rather than H$^-$ and Cl$^+$. (You can think of this as arising from the partial polarization, represented as δ+ and δ− in Figure 2.18, being taken to an extreme, resulting in a complete separation of the charges into +and −).

On the other hand, in homolytic cleavage, the two electrons in the σ-bond separate and one goes onto each of the two atoms that were originally involved in the bond. The result is the formation of two neutral species called free radicals (or just radicals), each with an unpaired electron.

Simple illustrations of what is meant by the terms *heterolytic cleavage* and *homolytic cleavage* are shown in Figure 2.21.

There are also some more complex but very important processes—particularly in some of the rearrangement reactions—where bonds do not appear to break in either of these ways, but nevertheless migration of atoms and bonds has occurred. These are grouped together as the so-called pericyclic reactions, though they are not discussed further here.

Figure 2.21 Homolytic and heterolytic cleavage

$$X-Y \longrightarrow X^{\bullet} + Y^{\bullet} \quad \text{(Homolytic cleavage)}$$

$$X-Y \longrightarrow X^{+} + Y^{-} \quad \text{(Heterolytic cleavage)}$$

$$X-Y \longrightarrow X^{-} + Y^{+} \quad \text{(Heterolytic cleavage)}$$

$$H-Cl \longrightarrow H^{+} + Cl^{-} \quad \text{(Heterolytic cleavage, controlled by electronegativities)}$$

Chemical reactions involve the making and breaking of covalent bonds. Reactions between organic molecules are classified into four types—substitution, elimination, addition and rearrangement.

2.7 **THE PRINCIPLES OF ORGANIC REACTION MECHANISMS**

In the introduction to this chapter, the reasons why carbon might be regarded as a unique element were outlined. Perhaps we can now add a further reason. Our understanding of the way in which carbon-based (organic) compounds react, using the ideas of mechanisms to explain them, is particularly well developed—certainly more so than for the chemistry of any other single element. By understanding and using mechanisms, organic chemistry ceases to be an endless list of unrelated reactions—which of course it is definitely not, though it can sometimes be perceived in that way! Instead, it becomes something that can be rationalized and which very often has quite predictable outcomes.

The vast majority of reactions encountered in the early stages of any organic chemist's, or indeed pharmacist's, career involve the motion of electron pairs. However, radical processes involving the motion of single electrons are extremely important in biological systems (see, for example Box 2.4). They are often oxidation and reduction (redox) processes involving some of the transition metals that have variable oxidation states.

Twice in the preceding paragraph, the word *motion* has been used in the context of electrons in reaction mechanisms. When describing, or illustrating, reaction mechanisms, this motion has to be represented somehow. Conventionally this is done using so-called 'curly arrows', and their use in this way gives rise to the often-used expressions 'curly arrow theory' or 'curly arrow description' of mechanism.

The correct use of these curly arrows is explained below, but before that it is useful to review *all* the types of arrow that are commonly encountered in chemistry. These are shown together in Figure 2.22.

The most important point to come out of the last two arrows shown in Figure 2.22 is quite simply that they illustrate the motion of electrons, either singly or in pairs. Therefore, they start at the place where the electrons *are* and they point towards where the electrons *end up* (in that way showing the direction of motion of the electrons). It is a simple idea, but one that is all

Figure 2.22   The different types of arrow used in chemistry

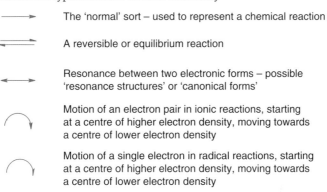

The 'normal' sort – used to represent a chemical reaction

A reversible or equilibrium reaction

Resonance between two electronic forms – possible 'resonance structures' or 'canonical forms'

Motion of an electron pair in ionic reactions, starting at a centre of higher electron density, moving towards a centre of lower electron density

Motion of a single electron in radical reactions, starting at a centre of higher electron density, moving towards a centre of lower electron density

Box 2.4 The hydroxyl radical

One of the most significant radical species in the body is the hydroxyl radical (HO·). It is one of a group of species referred to as *reactive oxygen species* (ROS), which includes hydrogen peroxide (H_2O_2) and the superoxide ion (O_2^-). Of these, the hydroxyl radical is the shortest lived and most reactive species and is the one that is capable of causing the most damage to organisms. It can be formed by the breakdown of peroxides in the body (sometimes mediated by the presence of iron or other transition metals), but also, importantly, by the action of ionizing radiation on water. It is this reaction that leads to much of the tissue damage that is observed as a result of exposure to ionizing radiation, particularly X-rays or gamma rays.

The hydroxyl radical cannot be eliminated from the body by any enzymatic reaction and it will react quickly and destructively with all types of macromolecules found in living organisms—for example, carbohydrates, lipids and nucleic acids.

It may lead to breaking of nucleic acid strands, or to the alteration of the bases within them so that the nucleic acids will no longer correctly replicate. At a chemical level, this may either involve the hydroxyl radical removing a hydrogen atom from the structure, or alternatively the substitution of an aromatic ring with an OH group.

Lipids and carbohydrates are also attacked, generally by removal of a hydrogen atom from the macromolecule, followed by subsequent attack by O_2 to give a hydroperoxyl (ROO·) radical. It is the reactions that occur with this peroxyl radical that lead to the breakdown of the macromolecule.

There is, therefore, a lot of interest in the role of antioxidants in the body, which can quench the effect of free radicals and interrupt the destructive chemical processes that would otherwise take place. These antioxidants include compounds such as vitamin C, vitamin E and, more generally, the polyphenols found in a wide variety of foodstuffs (including red wine).

too often confused. However, once they are understood, mechanisms become a very powerful tool in explaining and even predicting organic chemical reactions.

Examples of 'curly arrows' in ionic and radical processes

The purpose of these examples is *not* to describe in detail the major classes of organic reactions—for example, the S_N1 and S_N2 substitution processes observed in the haloalkanes, the electrophilic addition across a double bond in an alkene, or the electrophilic aromatic substitution of an aromatic compound such as benzene. Rather, it is to show *how arrows work* and what they can do; the specific reactions cited perviously will all be explained in later chapters of this book. Our purpose here is only to establish the ground rules for using these arrows to describe reactions. We need to begin by restating that where ionic reactions and electron pairs are involved we use *double headed* arrows to describe them, and where radical reactions and single electrons are involved we use *single headed* arrows to describe them.

More information can be found in Chapter 5, 'Alcohols, phenols, ethers, organic halogen compounds and amines'.

The role of radical reactions in the ageing process is another fascinating area, but mostly lies outside the scope of this chapter.

While waiting for her prescription in Tu's pharmacy, a customer is browsing the cosmetics counter. Upon collecting her prescription she remarks that most of the 'anti-ageing' creams contain vitamin E and asks Tu why this is.

Reflection questions
1. What possible role might vitamin E possess in anti-ageing preparations?
2. Are there any side-effects related to an overdose of vitamin E?

For answers, visit the online resources which accompany this textbook.

Neutralization of an acid and a base

One of the simplest (and also one of the fastest) of all chemical reactions is the neutralization of an acid by a base, and this provides an excellent starting point for showing how curly arrows work. Figure 2.23 illustrates this reaction, showing the arrow starting at the region of high electron density (the negatively charged hydroxide ion) and moving towards the region of low electron density (the positively charged proton), exactly as the electrons would do in this reaction. In this figure, the lone pairs of electrons around the oxygen atom have been omitted and the arrow is just shown starting from the negatively charged oxygen atom. It is not wrong to draw in the lone pairs, but they do not participate in this reaction, so they are not normally drawn.

Conversion of bromomethane to methanol by hydroxide

This is a simple example of a substitution reaction that serves to illustrate how a reaction can be described using more than one curly arrow. In this case, shown in Figure 2.24, the C–Br bond breaks at the same time as the C–O bond forms, and *both* processes need to be shown. The

Figure 2.23   Mechanism of neutralization

$$HO^- \quad \curvearrowright \quad H^+ \quad \longrightarrow \quad H_2O$$

Figure 2.24   Mechanism of nucleophilic substitution

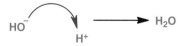

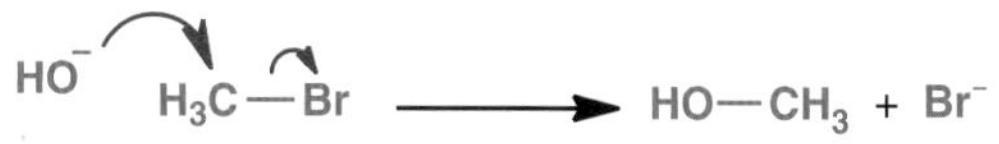

$$HO^- \quad H_3C-Br \quad \longrightarrow \quad HO-CH_3 + Br^-$$

Since the mid-nineteenth century, diethyl ether ($CH_3CH_2OCH_2CH_3$) has been used as an inhalation anaesthetic. It can be prepared by the Williamson synthesis, which involves the reaction of the ethoxide ion ($CH_3CH_2O^-$), used as the sodium salt, sodium ethoxide, and bromoethane (CH_3CH_2Br). Draw the curly arrow mechanism of the substitution reaction involved in the formation of this ether.

Self-check 2.11

Methoxypropane ($CH_3OCH_2CH_2CH_3$) is an isomer of diethyl ether and has also been used as an anaesthetic. It too could be synthesized from a suitable combination of an alkoxide ion and a haloalkane. Can you suggest what the starting materials might be here, and, again, propose a mechanism for the reaction?

arrow coming from the hydroxide ion is acting in exactly the same way we saw in Figure 2.23 — electrons flow towards an area of low electron density. Note how the second arrow, showing the heterolytic cleavage of the C–Br bond, starts in the middle of the bond and moves towards the Br. The two bonding electrons leave the C–Br bond and move to (become *localized onto*) the bromine atom, converting it to a bromide ion.

Electrophilic addition to an alkene

The electrophilic addition reactions that occur with the alkenes are described in more detail in Chapter 4. However, Figure 2.25 shows the first step in such a reaction — in this case, the addition of a proton to the double bond, which is typically what happens when an alkene is hydrated under acid conditions to give an alcohol. The point here is to clarify an apparent contradiction between the idea of 'electrophilic attack *on* an alkene', yet the arrow is going *away* from it. These ideas are surprisingly often confused, yet there is no contradiction here. The attack is electrophilic; in other words, the proton is attracted to a region of high electron density associated with the π-bond between the two carbon atoms, while the curly arrow is doing precisely what it is meant to do, showing the flow of electrons *away* from the alkene, towards the positively charged proton. Both parts of the description of this reaction are therefore perfectly correct.

Figure 2.25   First step in the mechanism of electrophilic addition of water to an alkene

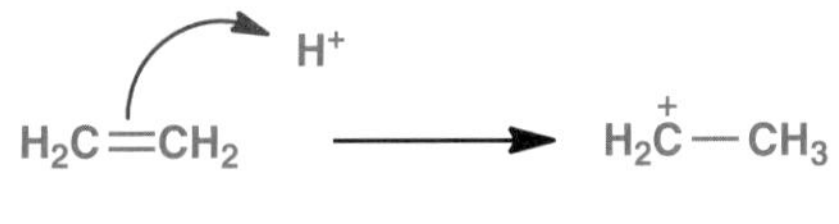

Self-check 2.12

Figure 2.25 shows how addition of a proton to an alkene gives an ethyl carbocation. If this was then attacked by water, the product would be $CH_3CH_2OH_2^+$, which is a protonated form of the final product, ethanol. Show how this might be produced, using a curly arrow to indicate the motion of electrons involved.

Self-check 2.13

If the ethyl carbocation in Figure 2.25 was attacked by a bromide ion rather than water, what would the final product be? Again, use a curly arrow to show the motion of the electrons involved.

Delocalization of electrons in a carboxylate ion

The three previous examples have shown curly arrows representing the reaction between two separate species. However, they may also be used to represent the motion, or delocalization, of electrons within a single species. The carboxylate anion is a good example of this.

The conventional drawing of this carboxylate ion might imply that the two carbon–oxygen bonds are different—with one shorter, stronger double bond and one longer, weaker single bond. However, we know from spectroscopic and crystallographic studies that these two bonds are in fact identical.

Acetate (ethanoate) is usually written as shown in Figure 2.26A with a complete octet of eight electrons around each oxygen. We could also place the negative charge on the other oxygen to give the structure shown in Figure 2.26B. However, neither of these structures represents the compound completely accurately. These are referred to as **resonance structures** or **canonical forms**. The actual structure of the compound, or intermediate, is an average of these and is referred to as a **resonance hybrid**. In the resonance hybrid, electrons are delocalized within the CO_2^- part of the structure, producing bonds that are intermediate in character between single and double bonds, and with lengths that are intermediate too.

Once again, the curly arrows show the flow of the electrons and, where appropriate, they start in the middle of the bond that is being broken, in this case a π-bond. In this example, you can also see the use of the double-ended arrow to indicate the resonance between the two forms.

Figure 2.26 Mechanism of delocalization in a carboxylate anion

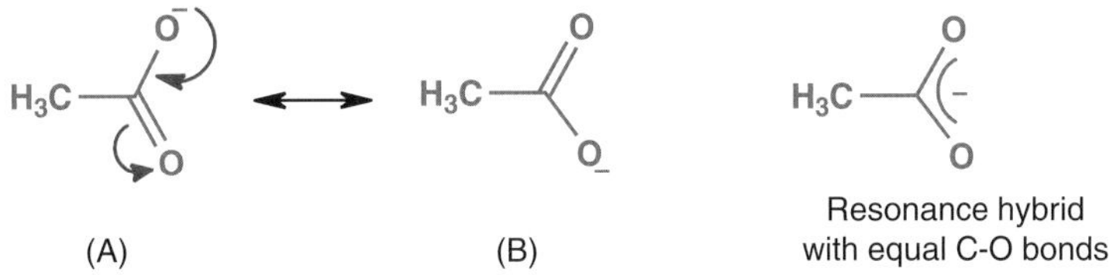

(A)   (B)   Resonance hybrid with equal C-O bonds

Addition of a bromine atom to an alkene

It is possible to add HBr to an asymmetric alkene such as propene ($CH_3CH=CH_2$) in two different ways. Under ionic conditions, Markovnikov's Rule (see Box 2.5) is obeyed, and in the major product the H goes onto the CH_2 group, while the Br goes onto the middle carbon atom. The product is 2-bromopropane. However, under free radical conditions, the H and the Br add the opposite way round and the product is 1-bromopropane and is described as the anti-Markovnikov product.

While we will not enter into a full explanation of this difference, the first step of the anti-Markovnikov reaction—the addition of a bromine atom to propene—is shown in Figure 2.27. This shows how curly arrows may be used to show the flow of electrons in a *freer-adical* process. Three electrons are involved—one from the bromine atom and the two in the carbon–carbon π-bond—so this time we need three, single-headed curly arrows to show the process in full. However, their sense is exactly the same as we have seen previously, and, again, all they are doing is showing the direction of motion of the electrons.

Figure 2.27   Mechanism of radical addition to an alkene

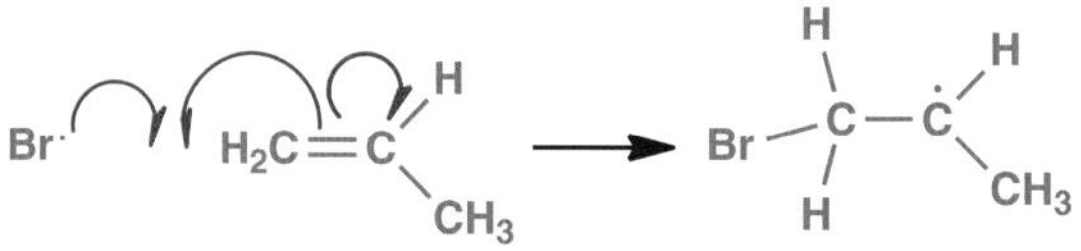

Box 2.5   Markovnikov's rule—a reminder

The expression 'Markovnikov's rule' refers to the conclusions derived from a series of empirical observations made by the Russian chemist, Vladimir Markovnikov, which were published around 1870. They allow us to predict the outcome of a chemical reaction when a compound of general formula HX (for example HCl, HBr or even H_2O, which we might regard as H-OH) is added to an asymmetric alkene such as propene.

When we look at the double bond in propene, we can see that it has one H attached to one end and two H atoms attached to the other end of it. There are various ways in which Markovnikov's rule can be expressed, but one form is: in the addition of HX to an asymmetric alkene, the H from the HX goes onto the carbon atom in the double bond which already has the greater number of H atoms.

In fact a *mixture* of products is generally produced, but Markovnikov's rule allows us to identify the *major* product. In this case, it is 2-bromopropane, with 1-bromopropane present as the minor product. It is now perfectly possible to rationalize these original empirical observations in terms of the stabilities of the carbocation intermediates in the reaction, and this is done in Chapter 4.

While Markovnikov's rule works well under ionic conditions, it is possible to vary the reaction conditions so that the major and minor products are reversed—a process often referred to as anti-Markovnikov addition. Typically this will occur if the reaction is carried out under free radical conditions, though, again, the outcome may be rationalized by considering the stability of the radical intermediates that are formed.

The two processes are summarized in Figure 2.28.

Figure 2.28   Markovnikov and anti-Markovnikov addition of HX to an alkene

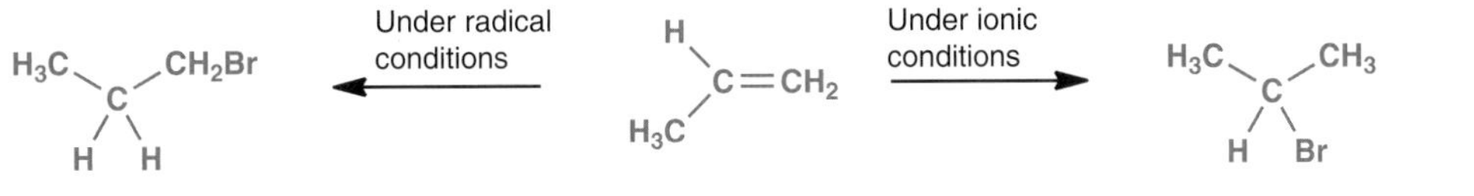

1-bromopropane
anti-Markovnikov product

2-bromopropane
Markovnikov product

The way in which organic molecules react has been extensively studied and detailed reaction mechanisms are widely used and accepted. The movement of electrons during these reaction mechanisms are represented by curly arrows.

CHAPTER SUMMARY

- Organic chemistry can be regarded as, essentially, the chemistry of carbon compounds.
- The chemical properties of carbon allow it to form an enormous variety of compounds. It can bond with many other elements and with itself, utilizing different types of bonds, to form chains and rings.
- Carbon utilizes hybrid orbitals to form covalent bonds with itself and other atoms.
- These hybrid orbitals are sp^3, sp^2 and sp and form single, double and triple bonds respectively. These orbitals determine the overall shape of a molecule.
- There are a variety of intermolecular forces such as hydrogen bonds, dipole–dipole attractions and van der Waals forces.
- Most chemical reactions can be classified as one of four types—substitution, elimination, addition and rearrangement.
- The way in which these reactions take place can be represented by reaction mechanisms which demonstrate the movement of electrons by means of curly arrows.
- An understanding of reaction mechanisms and the nature of intermolecular forces is essential to drug synthesis, drug-receptor interactions and drug metabolism.

FURTHER READING

Clayden, J., Greeves, N. and Warren, S. *Organic Chemistry*, 2nd edn. Oxford University Press, 2012. A student friendly undergraduate textbook with an emphasis on clarity and understanding of the key concepts of organic chemistry.

McMurry, J. *Fundamentals of Organic Chemistry*, 7th edn. Cengage Learning, 2011. ISBN 9781439049730. Another student friendly organic chemistry textbook.

Sykes, P., *A Primer to Mechanisms in Organic Chemistry*. Longman, 1995. ISBN 9780582266445. A simpler treatment of organic reaction mechanisms providing a basic understanding of organic reactions. Although out of print it is still widely available.

Self-check

For the answers to the Self-Check questions in Chapter 2, visit the online resources which accompany this textbook.

CHAPTER 3

STEREOCHEMISTRY AND DRUG ACTION

Rosaleen J. Anderson, Adam Todd, Mark Ashton And Lauren Molyneux

The common analgesic ibuprofen, which you met in Chapter 1, actually consists of two forms. One of these forms is used to treat headaches, the other is completely inactive. The two forms have mostly identical physical properties, but their three-dimensional shapes are different—they are mirror images of one another. The three-dimensional shape of biological molecules and drugs is profoundly important for their action, as we will explore in this chapter.

This chapter introduces the concepts of isomerism, structure and shape, particularly with reference to the activity of drugs, and relates strongly to the hybridization and bonding you studied in Chapter 2.

Learning objectives

Having read this chapter you are expected to be able to:

- recognize, differentiate and discuss the key features of constitutional isomers, conformational isomers and stereoisomers (geometric and optical isomers)

- assign the stereochemistry of asymmetric alkenes and chiral molecules using the IUPAC nomenclature

- explain how molecular shape, size and stereochemistry affect the biological activity and pharmaceutical action of drugs.

3.1 INTRODUCTION

The term 'isomerism' is used to describe the ways in which molecules can have identical compositions in terms of carbon, hydrogen, nitrogen etc., but differences in their patterns of bonding or **conformation** that may lead to dramatically different three–dimensional shapes. There are many drugs used in medicine that exhibit isomerism. For example, it is essential to have a good understanding of isomerism to explain why:

- the selective serotonin reuptake inhibitors (SSRIs) escitalopram and citalopram are used at different doses to treat depression, or

- the antibiotic metronidazole interferes with the anticoagulant agent warfarin (and thus increases the risk of a patient having a haemorrhage), or

- thalidomide—an anti-angiogenesis drug used in the treatment of multiple myeloma—is contraindicated in pregnancy.

> You will find explanations of these first two points in the online resources which accompany this book (www.oup.com/he/rostron-barber2e) and you will learn about the third point, relating to thalidomide, during this chapter.

The structures of citalopram, warfarin and thalidomide are shown in Figure 3.1. It is their stereoisomerism that imparts their particular pharmacological properties; we will consider this property in more detail in this chapter.

By the time you have read through this chapter, you should realize the impact these concepts have on the everyday practice of a pharmacist and how important it is to have an understanding of isomerism. We will also explore how different isomers can display dramatically different physical, chemical and biological properties, discussing these as examples throughout this chapter.

Figure 3.1   The chemical structures of citalopram, warfarin and thalidomide; all of these molecules have one thing in common—a chiral (or stereogenic) carbon

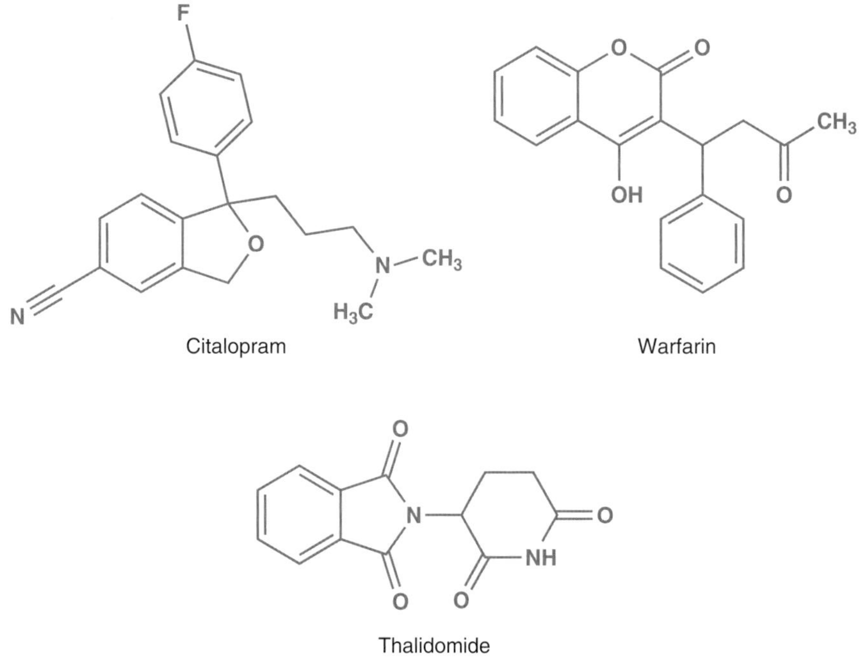

Citalopram

Warfarin

Thalidomide

As we look at the effects of isomerism on pharmaceutical science, we will consider how iso-mers can act differently on **receptors**, which are physiological species such as proteins and nucleic acids, and can be activated by natural molecules and drugs to cause specific effects. Molecules that activate a receptor to produce a specific response are called **agonists**; molecules that bind to a receptor, but do not trigger the response (and block the binding of an agonist at the same receptor in doing so) are called **antagonists**. You will meet these concepts in greater detail when you study pharmacology.

3.2 CONSTITUTIONAL ISOMERISM

Isomers are molecules that contain the same atoms but which are bonded together differently. If the atoms in the isomers are connected in different ways (i.e. their *connectivity* is different), then they are called **constitutional isomers** (sometimes called structural isomers). Consider the structure of paracetamol, $C_8H_9NO_2$ (structure A), shown in Figure 3.2. Paracetamol is an **analgesic**, which also has **antipyretic** properties and is therefore often given to children after immunizations to reduce fever.

If we swap the position of the acetyl (ethanoyl) group from the nitrogen atom to the phenol oxygen of paracetamol (that is the oxygen bonded to the benzene ring), we obtain another com-pound, as shown in Figure 3.2 (structure B). This compound has the same molecular formula as paracetamol ($C_8H_9NO_2$), but is not paracetamol; it is an example of a **constitutional isomer**. In fact, there are many constitutional isomers for paracetamol, some of which are shown in Figure 3.3. You will meet the different functional groups in the other chapters in this book; here, our focus is that these constitutional isomers may have different physical and chemical prop-erties from paracetamol and probably will not treat your headache.

Constitutional isomers are sometimes formed as by-products of organic synthesis and may even be toxic to the patient. The British Pharmacopoeia (BP) is responsible for setting assays and standards for the purity of pharmaceuticals and has limit tests for such by-products.

Self-check 3.1

Figure 3.3 shows ten different constitutional isomers of paracetamol. There are many more; can you draw some more examples?

Figure 3.2   Paracetamol (*para*-acetylaminophenol) (A) and a constitutional isomer (B)

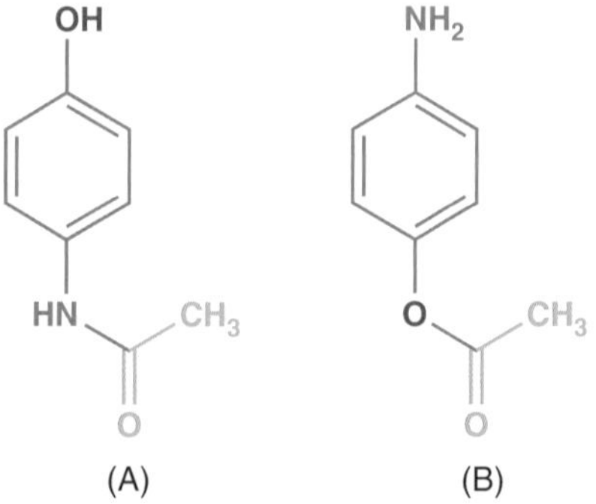

(A)   (B)

Figure 3.3 Some examples of constitutional isomers of paracetamol, $C_8H_9NO_2$

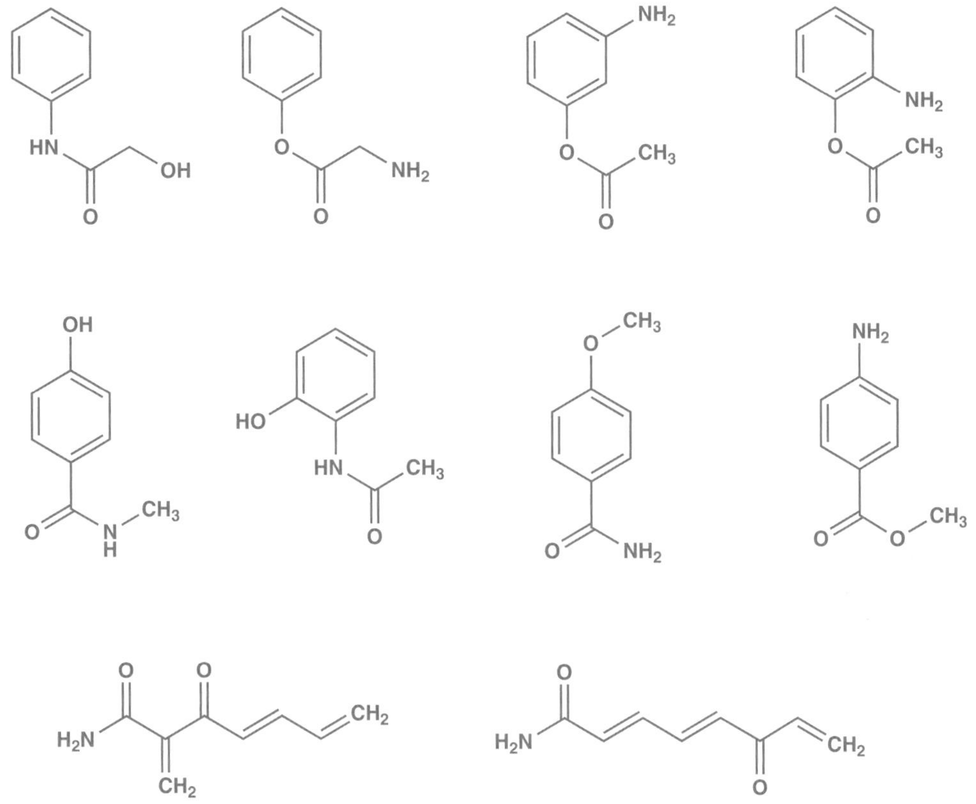

3.3 CONFORMATIONAL ISOMERISM

Conformational isomerism arises because rotation is possible about σ-bonds, allowing molecules to adopt a variety of shapes. Conformational isomers are just different shapes adopted by the same molecule. Rotation about σ-bonds allows a molecule to find its most stable conformation or to adopt a shape that can bind to an enzyme or receptor. Conformational isomerism is therefore very important for pharmaceuticals and their medicinal action. Restricting conformation is an important strategy in drug design and discovery—by using structures and groups that have a limited range of conformations available to them, a desired shape for binding to a particular medicinal target can be promoted, with the resulting prize of strong interactions with the receptor and greater potency of the drug.

Conformations of linear molecules

Let us look, firstly, at a relatively simple molecule; we can apply the principles we consider here to larger molecules. Nabumetone is a pro-drug that is activated by liver enzymes to a non-steroidal anti-inflammatory drug (NSAID), which acts to reduce pain and inflammation in osteoarthritis and rheumatoid arthritis.

Conformational isomers can interconvert by the rotation of bonds and movement of atoms, without the need to break any bonds. This makes conformational isomerism distinct from other forms of isomerism.

There are two methylene (CH_2) carbon atoms (C2 and C3) in nabumetone, C2 with a ketone substituent, $COCH_3$, and C3 with a substituted aromatic naphthyl group. We can draw the structure as shown, with an extended (spread out) CH_2-CH_2 central unit; but does this represent the actual conformation? How are the ketone and aromatic groups arranged around this central unit?

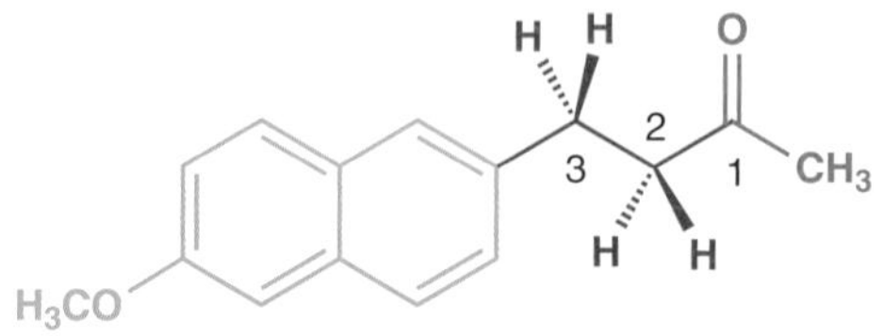

Nabumetone

We can represent and view this structure in a number of ways; the two most popular, when considering conformation, are the 'sawhorse' and Newman projections, Table 3.1. The sawhorse form views the molecule from one end of the C2–C3 bond, slightly from the side, whereas the Newman projection looks directly along the C3–C2 bond, with C2 behind C3. The circle in the Newman projection represents C2 and the point at which the bonds from 'naph' and the two H atoms meet is C3.

When the atoms or groups on the front carbon atom are lined up with the atoms or groups on the back carbon atom (i.e. on the same 'side' of the carbon–carbon bond), they are said to be **eclipsed**. When the atoms or groups on the two carbon atoms lie on opposite sides of the carbon–carbon bond, they are said to be **staggered**; this type of conformation is generally lower in energy than the eclipsed forms, as there is less repulsion of spatially close atoms and bonding electrons (which cause *steric* and *torsional* strain, respectively) in the molecule. Other

Table 3.1 Sawhorse and Newman projections for two conformations of nabumetone (naph represents the substituted naphthyl unit)

Linear structure	Sawhorse projection	Newman projection
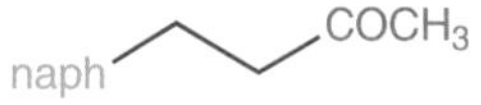 Staggered	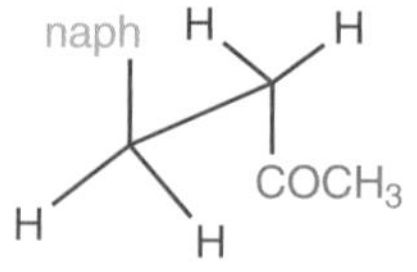	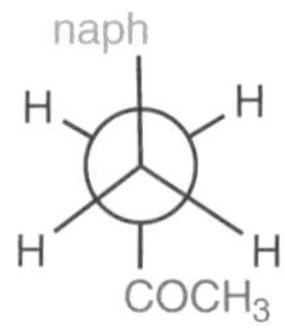
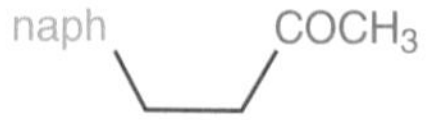 Eclipsed	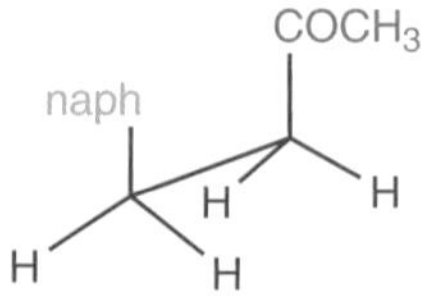	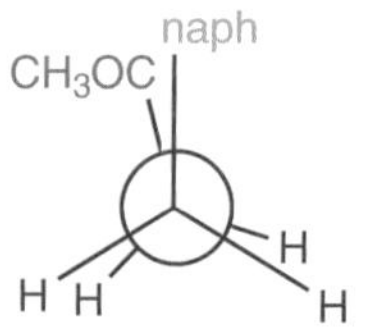

nomenclature is sometimes used to describe conformations of linear molecules; you can read about them on the online resource website which accompanies this book (www.oup.com/he/rostron-barber2e)

We can use the Newman projection to look along the C3–C2 bond and consider the possible conformations nabumetone can adopt (see Figure 3.4). If we start with the two substituents arranged one behind the other, we have our starting point, conformation **A**; then, keeping the front carbon and its attached atoms/groups stationary and rotating the rear carbon atom clockwise around the C–C bond, we can trace the energy changes in this molecule as it passes through several high and low energy conformations (see Figures 3.4A and 3.4B).

The most stable conformations for simple linear molecules are generally those that involve a staggered arrangement of substituents on the central C–C bond, most often in the antiperiplanar form; however, other features in some molecules, such as hydrogen bonding, can result in alternative conformations becoming more stable.

> Another example, that of cysteamine, $NH_2CH_2CH_2SH$, is discussed in the online resources which accompany this book.

Conformations of cyclic molecules

Of course, cyclic molecules do not have total freedom of rotation around their bonds—they are fixed by the cyclic structure. However, if at all possible, these molecules minimize their potential energy by adopting the lowest energy conformation available to them. Aromatic molecules are cyclic and planar, so they cannot readily change conformation. Aliphatic cyclic compounds,

Self-check 3.2

Study Figures 3.4A and B and explain why each of conformations A to F gives rise to an energy maximum or minimum. Why is A the highest energy conformation, while D is the minimum energy conformation?

Figure 3.4A Key conformations around a substituted two carbon unit; in this case, nabumetone

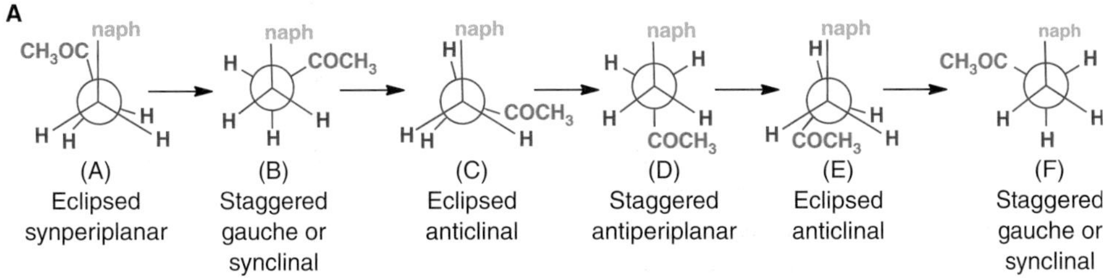

(A)	(B)	(C)	(D)	(E)	(F)
Eclipsed synperiplanar	Staggered gauche or synclinal	Eclipsed anticlinal	Staggered antiperiplanar	Eclipsed anticlinal	Staggered gauche or synclinal

Figure 3.4B Plot of energy changes as a function of dihedral angle calculated at every whole degree between 0 and 360° for nabumetone. [Calculations performed by Dr. Peter Dawson using Gaussian software.] The dihedral angle between two substituents, X and Y, is the angle between the two planes in which the substituents lie and is described by θ (theta)

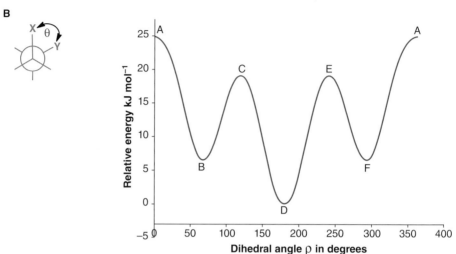

by comparison, can adopt different conformations, within the restrictions imposed by their cyclic nature. As far as possible, the energy in these molecules is minimized by adopting conformations in which the substituents are staggered, rather than eclipsed, and the bond angles are as normal as possible for the hybridization of the atoms. In this chapter we are concentrating on six-membered rings, particularly cyclohexane and its related structures; however, there are many examples of pharmaceuticals containing aliphatic cyclic systems with seven, five, four and three atoms in the ring. You will find some of these examples in the online resources accompanying this book.

Let us consider a cyclohexane ring. We often draw it in the same way as a benzene ring, as a hexagon, but without the π-system. However, a regular hexagon has internal angles of 120°, whereas an sp³ hybridized carbon atom has a preferred bond angle of 109.5°. In addition, the two H atoms on each cyclohexane carbon would be eclipsed with those on the adjacent carbon atoms, so this is obviously not the best conformation. If you make a model of cyclohexane with a molecular model kit, you find that it naturally adopts a non-planar structure to achieve carbon bond angles of about 109.5°. There are two main conformations adopted by a cyclohexane ring: a *chair* form and a *boat* form, as shown in Figure 3.5.

> More information on hybridization can be found in Chapter 2, 'Organic structure and bonding'.

In the chair form of cyclohexane, each carbon bears one hydrogen vertically either up or vertically down from the ring. These are termed the axial bonds, because of their position parallel to the symmetry axis of the ring, as seen in Figure 3.6, structure **A**. The second hydrogen atom on each carbon is sited around the plane of the ring, and these are termed equatorial bonds, structure **B**. To draw the equatorial bonds, note that they are parallel to the ring bond on the adjacent carbon atom: in **C** they are shown in pink, in **D** as green, and in **E** as turquoise.

In general, substituents in an **equatorial** position are favoured over the **axial** position, as there is less steric strain. In Figure 3.7: **A** views cyclohexane from the same plane as the ring; **B** shows how two axial substituents can be co-planar and close in space, even though they are on non-adjacent ring atoms; **C** shows how equatorial substituents on adjacent ring atoms do not lie in the same plane, which reduces steric strain. Because of the possibility of *ring flip*, which interconverts the two chair forms, the axial and equatorial positions are often interchangeable, allowing the most stable conformation to be adopted. This is very important in pharmaceuticals, as it makes a significant difference to the shape of the molecule.

> This is a broad generalization, as there are several factors to consider when studying the conformations of cyclic molecules. You will find a more detailed discussion of the factors affecting the preferred conformation of cyclic molecules in this book's online resources, along with an explanation of ring flip.

An interesting example is provided by pethidine, an opioid and potent analgesic (see Figure 3.8). In this molecule, the six-membered ring is a piperidine, with two substituents on the same carbon atom. Does the molecule prefer the phenyl ring to be equatorial, or the ester group? It was argued that the larger phenyl ring would cause greater steric strain than the ester group if it was axial, which agreed with the crystal structure of pethidine showing the phenyl ring in

Figure 3.5 Representations of cyclohexane (the hydrogen atoms are omitted for clarity in the last three structures; see Figure 3.6 for structures with H atoms included)

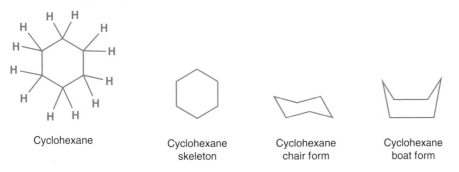

Cyclohexane

Cyclohexane skeleton

Cyclohexane chair form

Cyclohexane boat form

Figure 3.6 The position of the bonds on a six-membered ring in the chair conformation

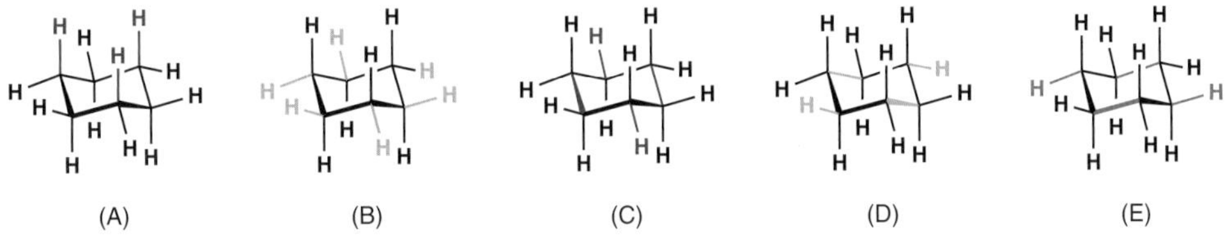

(A)   (B)   (C)   (D)   (E)

Figure 3.7   Arrangement of bonds around the chair conformation of a six-membered ring

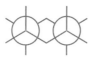
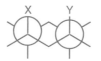
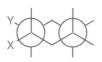

(A) Chair conformation: all bonds on adjacent carbon atoms are staggered

(B) X and Y both axial sited in the same plane, they are close together

(C) X and Y both equatorial in different planes, they are further away in space

the preferred equatorial position (see Figure 3.8), which also puts the N-methyl group into the preferred equatorial position.

Six-membered rings with a chair conformation are common in biological systems and in pharmaceuticals. Examples include the anticancer agents, doxorubicin and daunomycin; many steroids, such as cholesterol; and the aminoglycosides, an important class of antibiotics. Figure 3.9 shows two aminoglycosides, gentamicin (a natural product) and amikacin (a semi-synthetic drug consisting of a three-ring microbial product to which a side chain is added synthetically). In both of these antibiotic examples, the central cyclohexane ring adopts a chair conformation that puts all of the substituents into equatorial positions. The pyranose rings also adopt chair conformations that put as many as possible of their substituents into equatorial positions.

Figure 3.8   The two chair conformations of pethidine: the crystal structure shows that the second conformation, with the phenyl ring in the equatorial position, is preferred

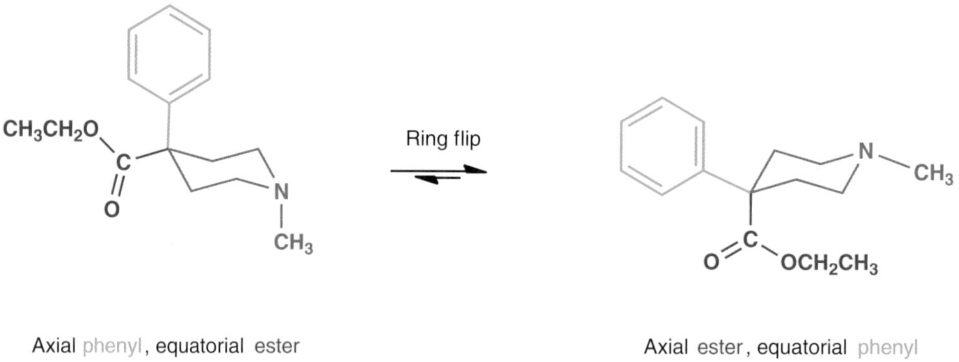

Axial phenyl, equatorial ester

Ring flip

Axial ester, equatorial phenyl

Figure 3.9   Chair conformations of cyclohexane and pyranose rings in two examples of aminoglycoside antibiotics, gentamicin and amikacin

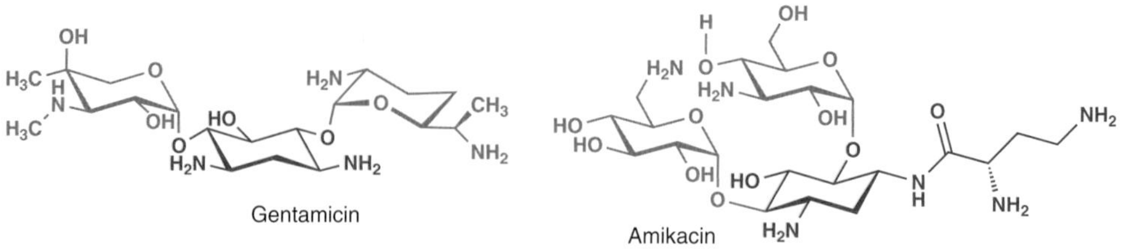

Gentamicin

Amikacin

The boat conformation for six-membered rings is much less common due to adverse strain and interactions (see Figure 3.10). The *geminal* H atoms on one end of the structure are coloured to show their spatial relationship. (Geminal H atoms are bonded to the same central atom; a CH_2 group has two geminal H atoms attached to the same carbon atom. The term comes from the Latin word *Gemini*, meaning twins). As you can see in the 'end view' conformation, this results in several bonds lying in the same plane, giving rise to torsional strain, and the 'flagpole' atoms are very close in space, causing steric strain, particularly if one or both of these atoms is not H. In fact, the boat conformation is usually only seen when there are few or no conformational options.

The importance of conformation on shape can be seen in the case of donepezil, one of the leading treatments for Alzheimer's disease. This drug inhibits the enzyme acetylcholinesterase by binding snugly into a defined cavity or 'pocket' in the enzyme—the active site. (The active site of an enzyme is the region of the enzyme that carries out the catalytic activity; it usually has a defined three-dimensional size and shape to which the substrate binds with strong affinity.) Fortunately, this involves the most stable chair conformation for the central piperidine ring with the large substituents in the equatorial positions (see Figure 3.11). If the diaxial conformation had been a better fit in the active site, donepezil is unlikely to have been a good inhibitor, as it would have to adopt a less favourable, higher energy, conformation to bind.

Figure 3.12 shows how donepezil binds to the acetylcholinesterase enzyme. Look at this figure, and notice how donepezil fits snugly into the active site, whose shape is emphasized by the surface plot of the enzyme depicted here. The favoured conformation with the substituents in the equatorial positions is relatively horizontal and has good complementarity to the size and shape of the active site of this enzyme. The diaxial substituted conformation would not be able to fit into this site.

> Other cyclic systems, based on five-membered and four-membered rings, are important in medicine. They also have defined preferred conformations, which you can study on the online resources website.

Figure 3.10   The boat conformation of a six-membered ring suffers from steric and torsional strain

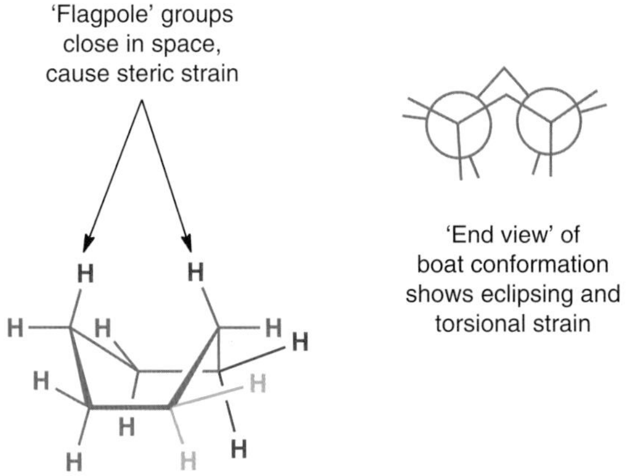

'Flagpole' groups
close in space,
cause steric strain

'End view' of
boat conformation
shows eclipsing and
torsional strain

Figure 3.11 The two chair conformations of donepezil: the most stable chair conformation of the piperidine ring puts the two substituents into equatorial positions (shown on the left)

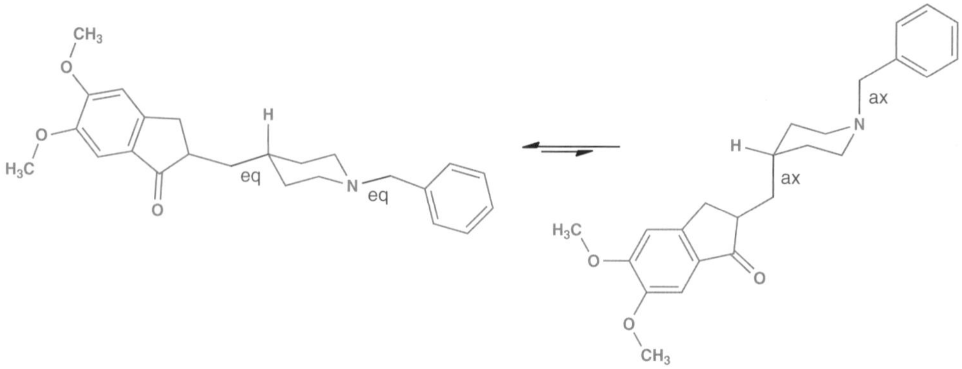

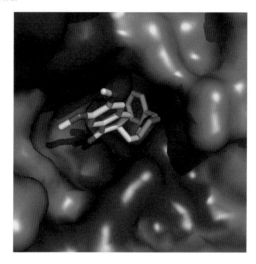

Figure 3.12 Complementarity of the stable chair conformation of donepezil to the active site of acetylcholinesterase

Copyright Jonathan Crowe.

3.4 STEREOISOMERISM

Many drugs used in medicine exhibit stereoisomerism, so it is important that, as pharmacists/pharmaceutical scientists, we are familiar with this subject. In this part of the chapter we will meet some more concepts that relate to the three-dimensional (3D) shape of molecules and the way this affects their properties, including their pharmacological actions.

Stereoisomers of a molecule have the same connectivity of atoms to each other, but these can be arranged differently in three dimensions. Unlike conformational isomers, stereoisomers cannot usually interconvert easily. In this section we will consider geometric isomers and optical isomers; for both cases we will consider the effects of this type of isomerism on shape and pharmaceutical action.

Geometric isomerism

Geometric isomers occur when groups of atoms are arranged asymmetrically across a double bond. We will use the drug, tamoxifen, an oestrogen receptor antagonist used in the treatment of breast cancer, as an example; the structures of two isomers of this molecule—we call them the Z and E isomers—are shown in Figure 3.13. (This situation is actually an oversimplification, as tamoxifen exerts the majority of the antioestrogen effect via its metabolite, (Z)-4-hydroxytamoxifen.)

As you can see, tamoxifen contains an alkene group. In Chapter 2 you learnt that the alkene group has two kinds of bond—a **strong** σ-bond and a **weaker** π-bond. The weaker π-bond has an area of electron density both above and below the σ-bond and, as a result, rotation is not usually possible about a double bond (in other words, the double bond is 'locked' in place). Look at (Z)-tamoxifen again, and notice how the two unsubstituted phenyl rings are on either side of the double bond, diagonal to each other. If we want the two phenyl rings to be on the same side of the double bond, as in (E)-tamoxifen, we have to break and reform the π-bond, which requires a lot of energy. (Z)-Tamoxifen and (E)-tamoxifen cannot easily interconvert and are therefore classed as configurational isomers, specifically geometric isomers.

But what do the letters Z and E actually tell us? They relate to the Cahn–Ingold–Prelog system, which is used to name or classify geometric isomers; it was published in 1966 and adopted later by IUPAC. This system enables scientists to communicate about stereochemical isomers without ambiguity. The Cahn–Ingold–Prelog system is explained in more detail later in this chapter when we discuss enantiomers and chirality. These assignments come from German: Z stands for zusammen, which (roughly translated) means together, while E stands for entgegen, which means opposite.

To use the Cahn–Ingold–Prelog system, we must first assign a priority to the groups at either end of the alkene based upon the atomic number of each of the atoms. The atom with

Figure 3.13 (Z)-Tamoxifen (left), the active drug used clinically (Z isomer), and the inactive (E)-isomer (right)

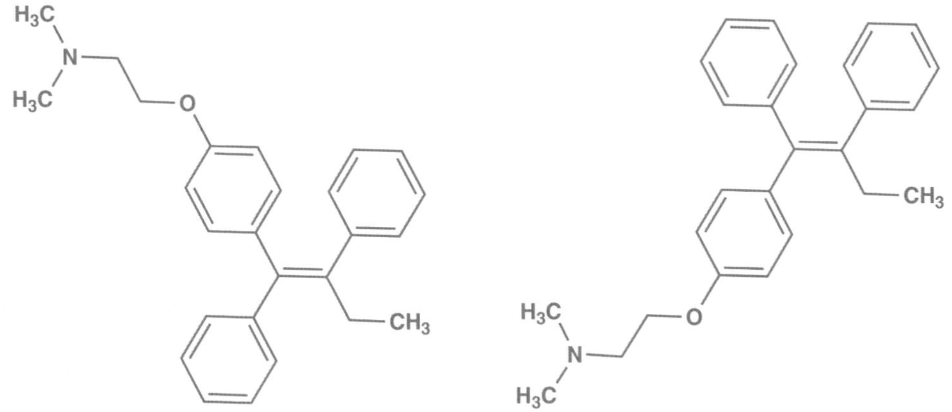

highest atomic number is given top priority. If the two highest priority groups are on the *same* side of the alkene, the alkene is assigned as Z (= together = on the same side); if the groups given top priority are on *different* sides, the alkene is assigned as E (= opposite = on different sides).

Let us take the structure of tamoxifen as an example.

1. Firstly, draw an imaginary line through the centre of the double bond (we now have two parts to the molecule—shown in red and blue). Now we need to assign priority to each atom at either side of the double bond, based on the atomic number.

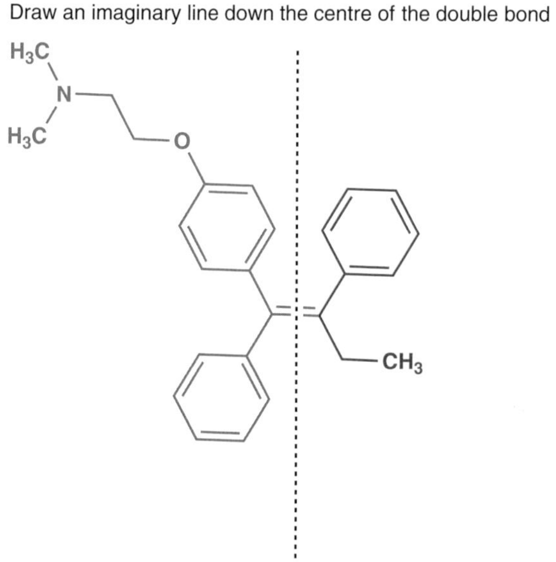

Draw an imaginary line down the centre of the double bond

2. Let us concentrate on the red half of the molecule first. We have two carbon atoms bonded directly to the alkene; one atom is part of the ethyl group and the other is part of the benzene ring. Fortunately, there is a way of differentiating between them.

   The carbon atom which forms part of the benzene ring is bonded to another two carbon atoms, while the carbon atom which forms part of the ethyl group is bonded to two hydrogen atoms and only one carbon atom. The carbon atom with more atoms of higher atomic number attached to it takes higher priority; the carbon atom in the benzene ring therefore takes priority 1, and the carbon atom in the ethyl group takes priority 2.

3. We now follow the same principles with the blue half of the molecule: both carbon atoms attached to the alkene are part of aromatic rings, and the 2 and 3 positions of the aromatic rings are identical. The oxygen atom on carbon-4 (attached to the top benzene ring) eventually makes the difference. Oxygen on the substituted aromatic ring has a higher atomic number than hydrogen in the unsubstituted ring, so the top ring (as drawn) is given priority 1.

4. We can now decide whether this molecule is E or Z. In the case of tamoxifen, the two groups given priority 1 are on the same side of the alkene, so it is assigned as the Z isomer.

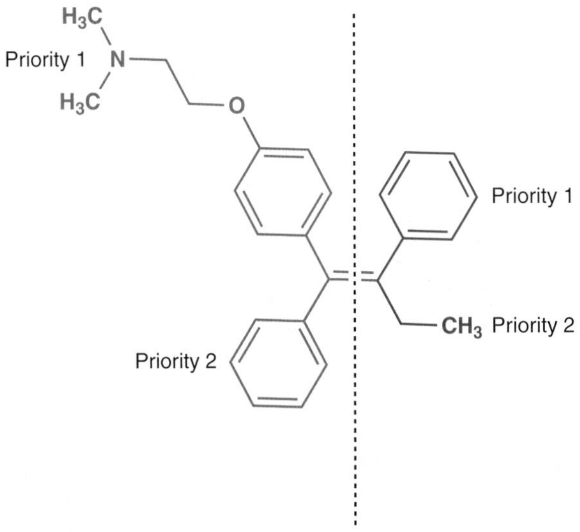

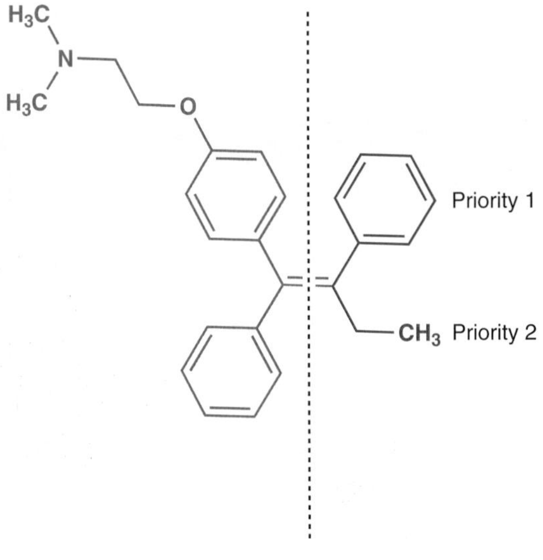

If you have previously met *cis* and *trans* nomenclature, you might name (Z)-tamoxifen as *trans*-tamoxifen because the two identical phenyl rings are on opposite faces at either end of the double bond (these terms come from the Latin translation; *cis* means 'on the same side' and *trans* means 'on the other side'). You would be correct! The *cis* and *trans* system predates the (Z) and (E) system, and is limited to alkenes in which one of the substituents on each alkene C is the same. (This is a rare example in the pharmaceutical world, when *cis* does not correlate with (Z) or *trans* with (E).) Although you will occasionally meet *cis* and *trans* nomenclature, alkene groups in pharmaceuticals are assigned explicitly using the (Z) and (E) system adopted by IUPAC. It is essential that there is no doubt that the correct form of a drug is being used.

Let us return to the world of medicine and see how geometric isomerism can have an impact on the patient. The 3D shape of a drug molecule is crucial to the desired therapeutic response in the body. To recap, tamoxifen is an oestogen receptor antagonist and is given as the Z isomer. In Figure 3.14, you can see tamoxifen drawn in three dimensions, as a 'stick' diagram and with an added surface. The E isomer is shown in the same way. The two isomers differ dramatically

Figure 3.14 (A) Stick structures of (Z)-tamoxifen (left) and (E)-tamoxifen (right); (B) surface representations of (Z)-tamoxifen (left) and (E)-tamoxifen (right) showing the dramatic difference to shape imparted by geometric isomerism. The colour represents partial charge on individual atoms: at one extreme, blue atoms have a partial negative charge, while at the opposite extreme, pink represents atoms with a partial positive charge. The shades of purple represent atoms that are close to being neutral

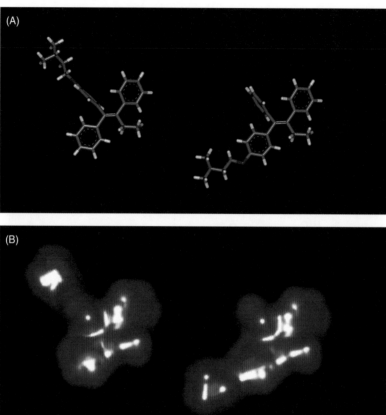

in 3D shape. In fact, they differ so much that the *E* isomer cannot bind to the oestrogen receptor. It is quite useless in the treatment of breast cancer.

> When considering aliphatic cyclic systems, the *cis* and *trans* nomenclature is still used to describe the relationship of ring substituents; as the bonds in the ring are tethered and unable to rotate, the relative orientation of the substituents is fixed. This is discussed more, along with several examples of such molecules, in the online resources.

Optical isomers

Optical isomers are so-called because of the different way the isomers interact with plane-polarized light. We will look at this property later in this section; first, we will consider how these isomers arise structurally.

Let us consider the structure of a natural amino acid, 2-aminopropanoic acid (alanine), whose structure is shown in Figure 3.15, to illustrate how the property of chirality can arise.

In Chapter 2 we saw that an sp³ hybridized carbon atom has a tetrahedral shape. To represent the tetrahedral 3D shape in the 2D medium of paper, we use hashed line bonds (these represent the bonds going away from you) and bold wedge bonds (these represent the bonds coming towards you), in addition to the bonds in the plane of the paper.

These compounds both have the molecular formula $C_3H_7NO_2$ and the atoms are connected together in the same order; however, you cannot arrange these molecules side by side so that they look identical. If you do not believe us, make models of the two compounds and try to superimpose them! The two structures are actually non-superimposable mirror images of each other (similar to the way in which your hands are mirror images of one another—providing you are not wearing any jewellery!) and are called **enantiomers** (see Figure 3.16). Again, if we use our hands as an example, each hand would be an enantiomer. One simple test for chirality considers whether two mirror images are superimposable or not; if the mirror images are superimposable (the pair can be overlaid exactly onto each other, like most socks), then those articles or compounds are **achiral** (meaning, not chiral)—while non-superimposable mirror images (like most shoes) are enantiomers of a chiral species.

Note: In this book, we mostly use the terms 'chiral' and 'achiral', these being currently more common. A chiral molecule exhibits 'handedness'—it exists as optical isomers that, like our hands, are non-superimposable mirror images. An achiral molecule does not exhibit handedness. The terms **stereogenic** and **non-stereogenic**, respectively, may be used instead.

Enantiomers are non-superimposable and are called chiral because they have no internal plane of symmetry. An equimolar mixture of enantiomers is called a **racemate**, or a **racemic** mixture. **Racemization** occurs when a sample of 100% of one enantiomer is converted into the racemate. Any carbon atom bonded to four different groups has no plane of symmetry and is therefore chiral—we say the molecule has a chiral or stereogenic carbon. A molecule containing one or more chiral atoms is usually chiral, except for examples with an internal plane of

Figure 3.15   2-Aminopropanoic acid (alanine)—a simple molecule that displays chirality

$$CO_2^-$$

H₃C ⁺NH₃ H

$$CO_2^-$$

H H₃N⁺ CH₃

Figure 3.16   The chirality of hands and asymmetric molecules

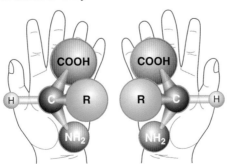

symmetry (for example, see the section on 'Molecules with more than one chiral centre'). A molecule with a plane of symmetry is achiral and therefore **cannot** exist as enantiomers.

Molecules with chiral carbon atoms are the most common form of chirality observed in medicine, but other forms of chiral centre do exist. For example, on the online resources website you will meet omeprazole, a 'proton pump' inhibitor that is used to prevent and treat stomach and duodenal ulcers, which has a chiral sulfur atom; and cyclophosphamide, an anticancer agent with a chiral phosphorus atom.

As we have seen previously, many drugs work by interacting with receptors that are formed from building blocks that are chiral (such as a protein or nucleic acid), or by binding to and inhibiting enzymes; the 3D shape of a molecule is therefore crucial if the molecule is going to 'fit' into the enzyme active site or receptor and elicit a therapeutic response. To illustrate this, let us consider morphine—an opioid analgesic extracted from the poppy, *Papaver somniferum*, which you will meet again in Chapter 13. *Papaver somniferum* (sometimes called the opium poppy) is a source of opium from which many clinically useful alkaloids are obtained, including morphine, codeine, papaverine and noscapine. Codeine and morphine are analgesics; papaverine is used for the treatment of erectile dysfunction; and, noscapine acts as a cough suppressant. Morphine has a very complex structure, including several chiral centres (see Figure 3.17); it binds to opioid receptors in the brain where it elicits an analgesic (pain-killing) effect.

For morphine to bind to the opioid receptor in the brain it has to have a specific shape, illustrated in Figure 3.18A (left). If we invert all of the chiral centres in morphine, we change its shape (see Figure 3.18A (right)); the two 'stick' structures of morphine look quite similar, but, if we put a surface on the molecules (see Figure 3.18B), you can see how the charge (shown in different colours) and 3D shape varies between the two structures.

We learn more about the importance of understanding the impact of enantiomers on the pharmaceutical industry in Box 3.1.

Stereochemical nomenclature of chiral compounds

Now you can identify molecules with a chiral carbon atom and can see that one chiral carbon in a molecule leads to two, non-superimposable, mirror image isomers called enantiomers, we need a method to communicate which enantiomer is under consideration at any particular time—we need some standard nomenclature.

IUPAC nomenclature is used internationally by the majority of scientists, most of the time (one specific exception will be discussed later); for stereochemistry, we use the same Cahn–Ingold–Prelog system of nomenclature introduced in the earlier section on geometrical isomers. So how do we go about using this system in the context of chiral molecules? First, we must represent a three-dimensional chiral sp³ carbon in two dimensions on paper. In Figure 3.15 we met alanine

Figure 3.17   The chemical structure of morphine

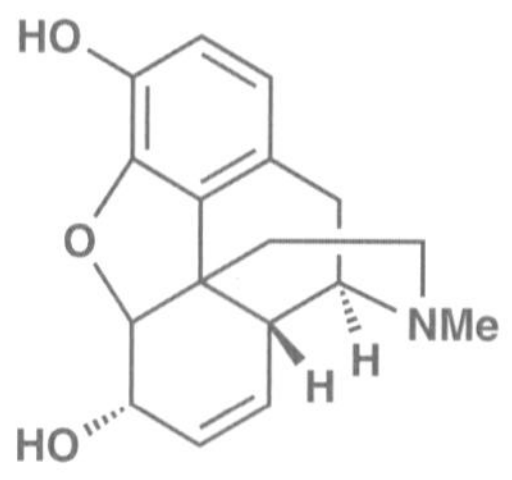

Figure 3.18 The structure of morphine ((A) left) and with a surface to show molecular shape ((B) left); the structures on the right in (A) and (B) belong to the mirror image form of morphine in which the chiral centres have been inverted. Again, the atoms are coloured according to their partial charge: blue/cyan represents partial negative charge, and red/pink atoms have a partial positive charge

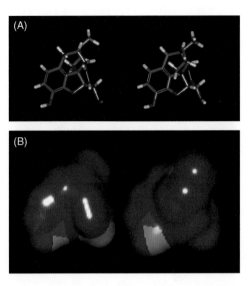

Self-check 3.3

How many chiral carbon atoms can you find in the structure of morphine?

drawn in 3D, with two adjacent bonds in the plane of the paper, a hashed bond behind the plane and a wedge bond in front of the plane.

With four atoms or groups attached to the chiral carbon drawn in a correct tetrahedral format, we can follow a procedure to identify the stereochemistry:

1. Assign a priority to each atom attached directly to the chiral carbon, based upon the atomic number Z of each of the atoms. The atom with highest atomic number has top priority (number 1), the atom with the second highest atomic number gets number 2 priority, the third highest atomic number gets number 3 priority, and the atom with the lowest atomic number is given the lowest priority (number 4).

2. Once identified, the number 4 priority atom or group is put to the back of the tetrahedral structure. This is the hashed wedge bond on our stick diagram, leaving the other three atoms or groups in the foreground (like the steering wheel of a car)—the assignment of stereochemistry is based upon these three atoms or groups.

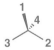

Self-check 3.4

We have been looking at molecules with a chiral centre that are drawn in 3D, where it is easier to identify which is the chiral carbon. Of course, molecules are not always drawn in 3D, so it is important to be able to identify which are the chiral carbons in stick diagrams. Look at the examples below and identify the chiral carbon atoms in each structure; some may have more than one.

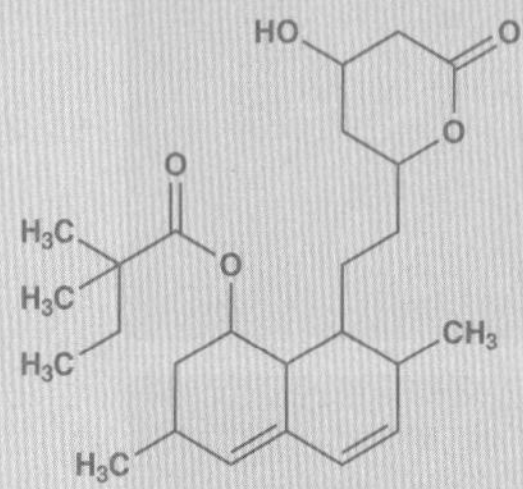

Simvastatin

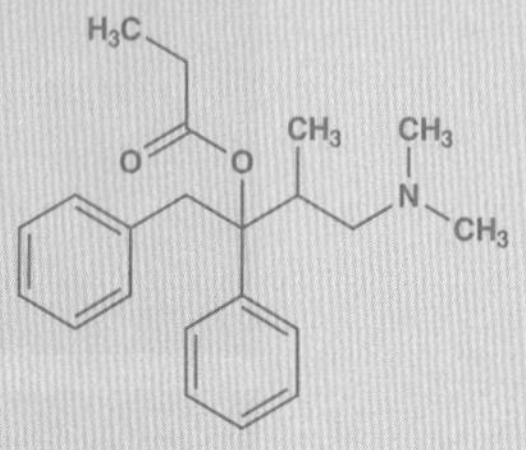

Dextropropoxyphene

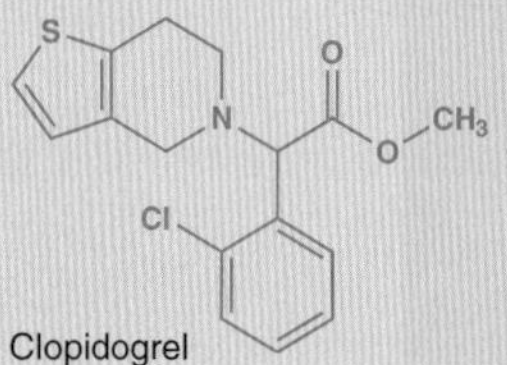

Clopidogrel

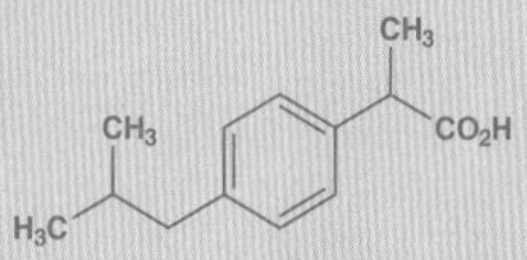

Ibuprofen

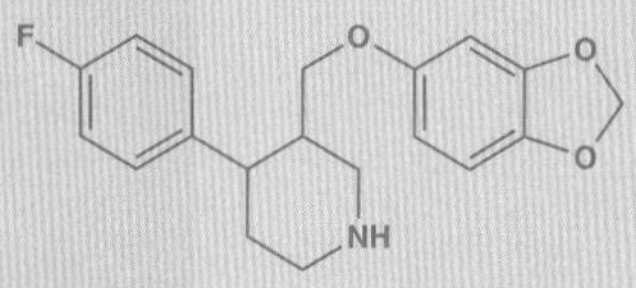

Paroxetine

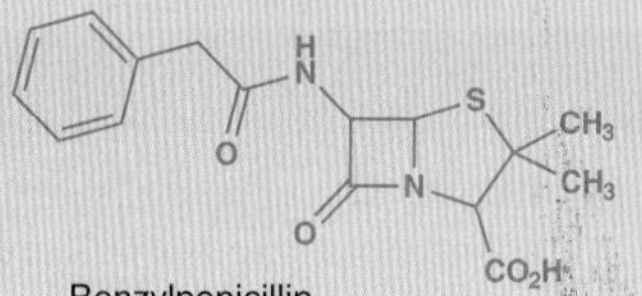

Benzylpenicillin

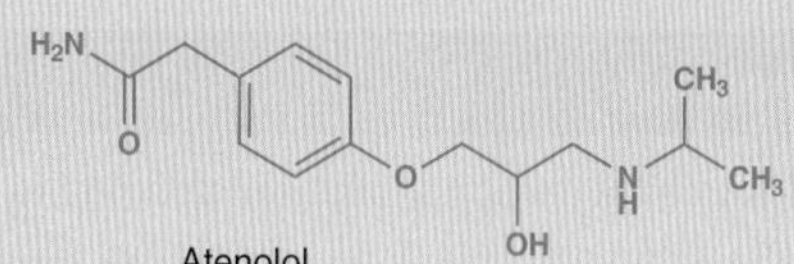

Atenolol

Self-check 3.5

There are many ways to draw a tetrahedral shape correctly; two are shown (see Figure 3.19), next to an incorrect structure. Why is the third drawing incorrect? [Hint: examine a tetrahedral model!]

Figure 3.19   Two different ways of correctly representing a chiral atom in three dimensions

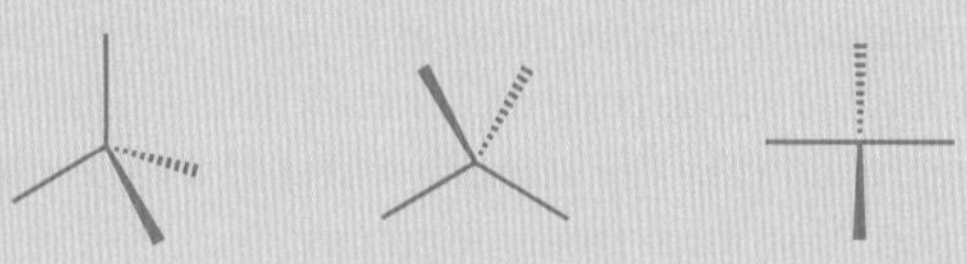

3. If the order of the atoms proceeds 1,2,3 in a clockwise direction, the nomenclature *R* (from the Latin *rectus*, meaning 'right-handed') is used, as in the example here; if the atoms prioritized as 1,2,3 follow an anticlockwise direction, then the nomenclature *S* (from the Latin *sinister*, meaning 'left-handed') is used. It is convention to use italicized capital *R* and *S* for this nomenclature.

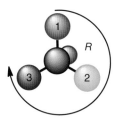

Worked example

In our example, alanine, there are four atoms or groups arranged around the chiral carbon (indicated with a *): the methyl (CH_3) group and the carboxylate (CO_2^-) group are both in the plane of the paper, while the ionized amine (NH_3^+) group is at the front and the H atom is at the back. We can see that the chiral C has four different atoms/groups attached to it: CH_3, CO_2^-, NH_3^+ and H.

$$CO_2^-$$
$$H_3C \overset{*}{\diagup}\!\!\!\overset{\cdots\cdots H}{\underset{+NH_3}{\Big|}}$$

1. To prioritize them, we need the atomic numbers Z, which you can obtain from a periodic table: **N**, Z=7; **C**, Z=6; **H**, Z=1. (It is tempting to assign stereochemistry using the relative atomic masses of each element to prioritize the atoms; however, be aware that doing this can result in the wrong priorities being assigned. The only way to be correct with certainty is to use the atomic number, Z.)

$$CO_2^-$$
$$H_3C \overset{*}{\diagup}\!\!\!\overset{\cdots\cdots H \, 4}{\underset{\underset{1}{+NH_3}}{\Big|}}$$

2. We can immediately see that **N** takes priority 1 and **H** priority 4. Adding the priority numbers to the structure, we find that the number 4 priority atom is already at the back, on the hashed wedge bond.

3. To assign priorities 2 and 3, we need to distinguish between the two carbon atoms, by taking account of the atoms that are attached to each one. Once again, we consider the atomic numbers of the next attached atoms to identify which has highest priority. In our example, one C atom has three hydrogen atoms attached (**H** Z=1), while the other has oxygen atoms (**O** Z=8); we therefore assign the carboxylate group (CO_2^-) as priority 2 and the CH_3 as priority 3. **An atom with multiple bonds, such as a carbonyl group (C=O), is given the same priority as multiple single bonds to the same atom or group**; in the case of a carbonyl, the carbon is equivalent to a carbon having two bonds to oxygen (O–C–O).

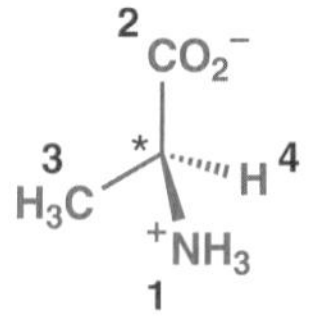

$$\overset{2}{CO_2^-}$$

$$\overset{3}{H_3C} \overset{*}{\underset{\overset{|}{\underset{1}{^+NH_3}}}{\diagup}} \cdots H \ 4$$

4. We can now ignore the H at the back, and look at the direction of the 1,2,3 priority groups. In this molecule they go anticlockwise from NH_3^+ to CO_2^- to CH_3, so the nomenclature S is assigned. We can distinguish this enantiomer from its mirror image by naming it (2S)-2-aminopropanoic acid. This conveys the exact formula and connectivity, along with the correct stereochemistry around the chiral carbon.

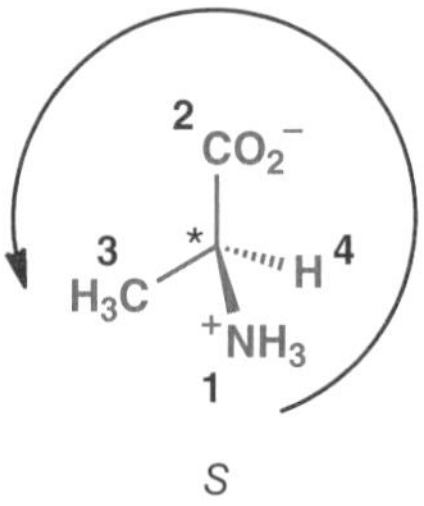

$$\overset{2}{CO_2^-}$$

$$\overset{3}{H_3C} \overset{*}{\underset{\overset{|}{\underset{1}{^+NH_3}}}{\diagup}} \cdots H \ 4$$

S

A more complex example is provided by vigabatrin, an anti-convulsant drug. Only one of the two enantiomers is credited with its anti-convulsant activity.

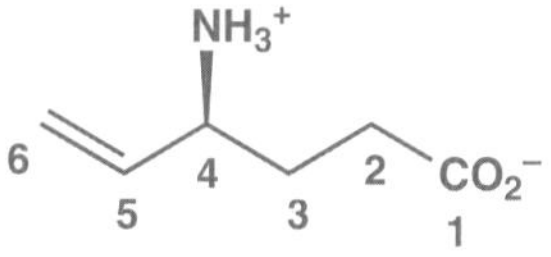

$$NH_3^+$$

$$\overset{6}{\diagup}\overset{}{\underset{5}{=}}\overset{}{\underset{4}{\diagup}}\overset{}{\underset{3}{\diagdown}}\overset{}{\underset{2}{\diagup}}\overset{}{\underset{1}{CO_2^-}}$$

Active enantiomer
of vigabatrin

First, we need to identify the chiral carbon atom (C4); it is often highlighted by the stereo-chemistry shown around it. In this case, we need to add a H on a hashed wedge bond that is not currently shown on the structure. Then we can prioritize the atoms attached to C4, the chiral carbon.

There is a N atom, two C atoms and a H atom, with atomic numbers Z of 7, 6 and 1, respectively. We can immediately assign the N as priority 1 and the H as priority 4, but we need to differentiate between the two carbons atoms (C3 and C5) to decide which has higher priority.

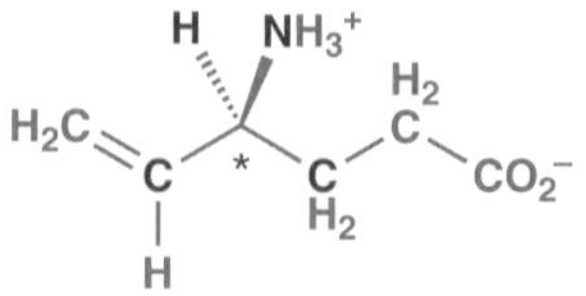

$$H \quad NH_3^+$$

$$H_2C \overset{}{\underset{\overset{|}{H}}{=}} C \overset{*}{\diagup} \underset{H_2}{C} \overset{H_2}{\diagup} C \diagdown CO_2^-$$

The methine alkene carbon (C5) has a double bond to the terminal CH_2 group, equivalent to two single bonds to carbon, plus one bond to an H atom. The other carbon atom C3, shown to the right of the chiral carbon, has one single bond to another carbon atom (C2) and two bonds to H atoms. We can summarize the bonding to each of C3 and C5 to help us assign the priority:

- C3 has 1C and 2H bonded to it,
- C5 has the equivalent of two single bonds to C and 1H bonded to it (remember we consider a multiple bond, such as the alkene to C5, as multiple single bonds to the same atom or group, so that we consider C5 as having two bonds to C);
- therefore,
- C5 has higher priority than C3, as it has more carbon atoms (higher atomic number) attached to it, so
- C5 gets priority 2, with C3 getting priority 3.

The priority 4 group (H) is at the back, so we can now ignore it and look at the order of the 1,2,3 priority groups: the sequence goes anticlockwise, so this has the nomenclature S.

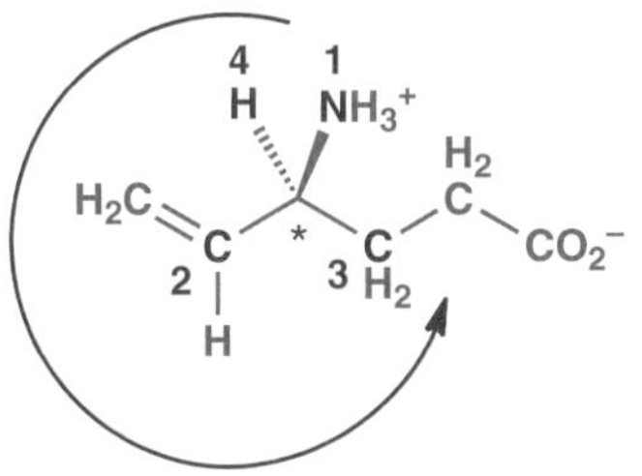

The S enantiomer of vigabatrin irreversibly inhibits gamma-aminobutyric acid (GABA) transaminase and is the active drug with the desired pharmacological properties.

Sometimes, a chiral molecule is drawn with the number 4 priority group at the front, instead of at the back. In this case you are seeing the structure reversed, so you can reverse the stereochemistry to get the correct assignment. For example, if you were given the structure of fluoxetine shown on the left in Figure 3.20, with the H at the front, it only needs the whole molecule to be turned around through 180° to move the H to the back as in the structure on the right. The stereochemistry looks like it will be R on the structure shown on the left, but this is viewing it

Figure 3.20 (S)-Fluoxetine viewed from front and back faces

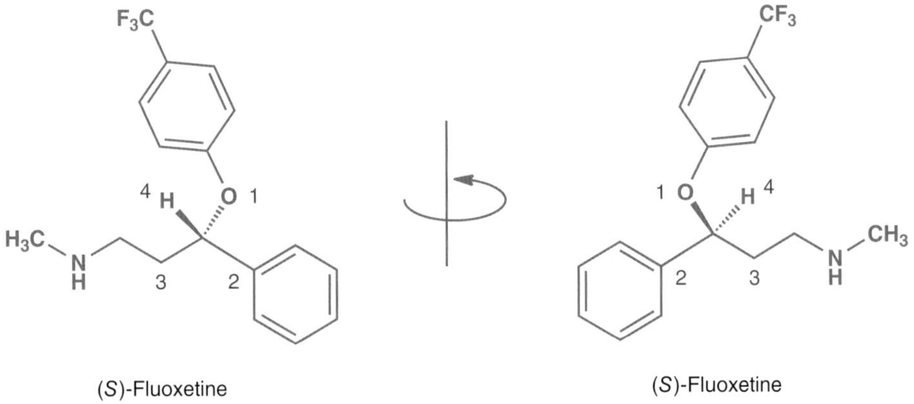

(S)-Fluoxetine

(S)-Fluoxetine

from the wrong side. When the whole molecule has been rotated, the correct stereochemistry, as shown on the structure on the right, is *S*.

When a chiral molecule is drawn so that the number 4 priority group is in the plane of the paper, you can imagine looking along the bond from the chiral carbon to the number 4 priority group (the C–H bond in this example). If you find this challenging, you could try redrawing the molecule, but this requires great care so that you do not invert it while redrawing.

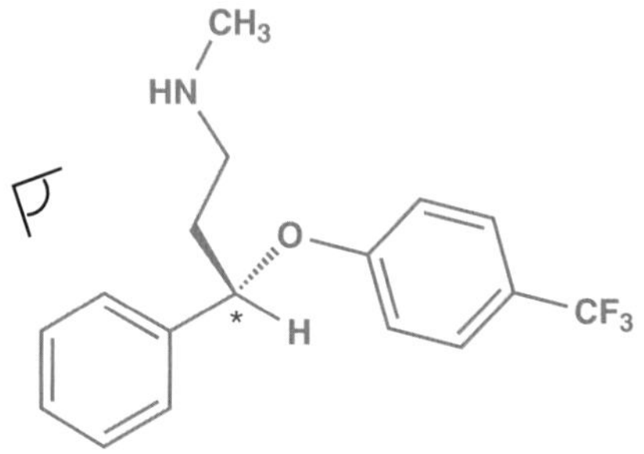

Fluoxetine

> If you want to try this approach, you will find fluoxetine as a worked example in the online resources. Other practice examples, including the rules for assigning the stereochemistry of cyclic compounds can also be found in the online resources.

Stereoisomerism in helices

Helical structures are commonly found in biological systems and are a source of chirality on the macromolecular scale; notable examples include the double helix of DNA and the α-helix structural motif that is commonly found in proteins.

Box 3.1 The pharmaceutical impact of stereochemistry—Thalidomide

You may be asking yourself why it should matter whether or not a drug has any chiral centres. That is a good question, and one that arose as a consequence of a drug approved for human use and then later withdrawn because it caused horrendous adverse effects. You may have heard of thalidomide and that it caused severe deformities in children born to mothers who had taken this drug early in their pregnancy, but you may not be aware that it was a turning point in drug development and regulation worldwide.

Thalidomide was first synthesized and patented in 1953 by the pharmaceutical company Chemie Grünenthal, then licensed as a hypnotic sedative in 1957. It was thought to be so safe that it was released in Germany as an 'over the counter' agent in 1960 and promoted as an entirely safe remedy for morning sickness and restless sleep in pregnancy. More than forty other countries worldwide introduced this new wonder-drug with many indications, including asthma, hypertension and migraine, as well as morning sickness. In the USA, regulation was stricter, following a tragedy involving a toxic taste-masking agent, and the Food and Drug Administration (FDA) refused to license thalidomide.

Over the next two years there were numerous reports of deformities in children born to mothers who had taken thalidomide. It is estimated that between 10,000 and 20,000 foetuses were affected. Thalidomide was taken off the market worldwide in 1961–62.

At that time, the concept that the enantiomers of a drug could have different activities in the body, or that their effects could be different in a foetus to the responses in an adult, was not recognized. After thalidomide was withdrawn from the UK market in 1962, an enquiry was initiated to investigate how such a huge mistake could have been made. It was eventually found that the (R)-enantiomer of thalidomide possessed the anti-emetic, anxiolytic properties that promoted sleep and benefited morning sickness, while the (S)-enantiomer had teratogenic properties, which meant it resulted in severe adverse effects to a foetus.

Although it is easy to think of rescuing the situation by marketing only the (R)-thalidomide, it was shown that each enantiomer of thalidomide is racemized *in vivo*, so that administration of the pure (R)-enantiomer leads to production of some of the teratogenic (S)-thalidomide.

As a result of this tragedy, the yellow card reporting system of adverse drug reactions (ADR) was introduced in the UK in 1964, and the Medicines Act of 1968 established a Medicines Commission and strict standards on the efficacy and safety of drugs. Many years later, in the 1990s, the regulatory bodies[1] with control of the registration of new drugs introduced new regulations that require the absolute stereochemistry of the active form(s) of a chiral agent to be identified early in drug development and justification for the use of a racemic mixture over a pure enantiomer. Such requirements usually entail stereoselective synthesis of each single enantiomer, or sometimes a pair of diastereoisomers, and the pharmacological properties of each individual chiral species to be established independently.

Thalidomide has now been reintroduced for the treatment of multiple myeloma and certain skin diseases, such as leprosy. Care is taken to ensure no patients on thalidomide are, or may become, pregnant.

[1] The regulatory body for the UK is the MHRA—the Medicines and Healthcare products Regulatory Agency, while the corresponding body in Europe is the EMA—the European Medicines Agency—and in the USA is the FDA—the Food and Drug Administration.

77

There are many examples of helical stereoisomerism beyond biology: a spiral staircase is a helix, as is a corkscrew. If you are familiar with the use of a corkscrew, you will know that they are designed for use by the right hand; in fact, if you are left-handed, you may have already searched for a 'left-handed corkscrew' (yes, they do exist!). Right-handed and left-handed corkscrews are mirror images of each other and are non-superimposable: they meet the criteria we used earlier to identify chiral molecules and are, in fact, stereoisomers. The double helix usually found in DNA is right-handed, although a left-handed form is known; the α–helix found in proteins is also right-handed (see Figure 3.21).

Figure 3.21   Left- and right-handed helices

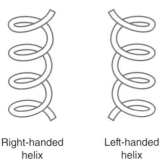

Right-handed   Left-handed
helix   helix

Self-check 3.6

Asthma is a condition that causes the airways to become inflamed, and in the UK alone there are over 5 million people receiving treatment for asthma—this equates to a staggering 1 in 12 adults and 1 in 11 children. Thankfully, there are many drug treatments available for managing asthma, some of which are shown below. You will notice that each drug contains a chiral centre—can you assign them as either *R* or *S*? In practice, some of these drugs are given as an equimolar mixture of both enantiomers (the racemate).

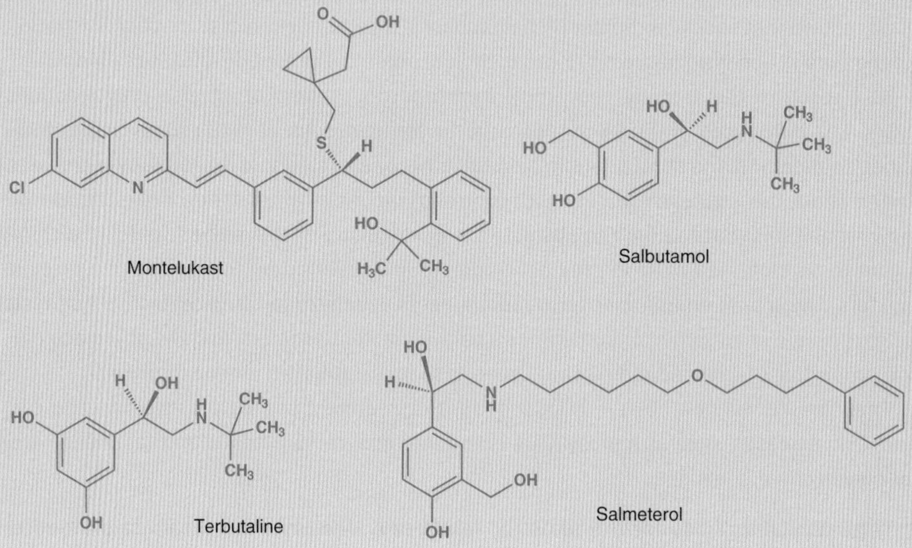

Montelukast

Salbutamol

Terbutaline

Salmeterol

Fischer's nomenclature: D and L

When you study macromolecules, such as sugars, peptides and proteins (see Chapters 10 and 11), you will learn that they are based on chiral building blocks; the way in which substrates, inhibitors or receptors bind to them is crucial to the biochemical processes that go on in our bodies. Biologists often talk about L–amino acids or D–sugars, not mentioning *R* or *S*; you may wonder why these molecules use a different system and why you have to learn about two sets of nomenclature for chiral molecules.

It is true that using the single IUPAC system streamlines the learning process, but the 'old' (or 'trivial') nomenclature system is retained because it simplifies the names of biological molecules; see Figure 3.22 for some examples.

The system of D and L nomenclature is based upon the work of Emil Fischer, who studied sugars, such as glucose, mannose and fructose, between 1884 and 1894. His careful work showed that they are isomers of each other and he established their stereochemistry. To achieve this aim, he synthesized each sugar from a known molecule with established stereochemistry, D–glyceraldehyde, using a reaction that partly bears his name—the Kiliani–Fischer reaction; C2 of D–glyceraldehyde becomes C5 in each sugar.

Comparison of the stereochemistry of natural glucose, mannose and fructose showed they had the same stereochemistry at C5 as observed at C2 of D–glyceraldehyde; by carrying out many reactions with each sugar and characterizing the products, he used the results to solve the absolute stereochemistry at each chiral centre. This was a seriously impressive achievement, particularly when you remember that he did it without the use of modern characterization techniques, like IR and NMR spectroscopy, mass spectrometry and X-ray crystallography! (Fischer also studied the chemistry of purines and the nature and structure of peptides and proteins, discovering that the amino acid building blocks were held together by amide (peptide) bonds. He was awarded the Nobel Prize in 1902 for his contributions to chemistry.)

Note that the convention is to use small capitals for the Fischer nomenclature: D and L rather than D and L. However, we use 'full size' capitals for IUPAC Z/E and R/S nomenclature.

In Figure 3.22, the upper chemical name under each structure is the IUPAC name, while the lower name is the old name. You can see that there are sometimes advantages to using the trivial name—sugars are very well known molecules and D-glucose is much easier to use, and type, than (2R, 3S, 4R, 5R)-2,3,4,5,6-pentahydroxyhexanal!

What do D and L stand for and how do we decide which to use? Fischer devised a way of representing sugars to make their stereochemistry clear and unambiguous. He placed the most oxidized carbon atom, numbered C1, at the top of a page and the chain of carbon atoms vertically down. As a result, the two other groups on every carbon atom stuck up away from the paper and towards the viewer. With a light held above the structure, the 2D shadow of the 3D molecule was cast on the paper below, illustrated for D-glyceraldehyde in Figure 3.23, and is called a **Fischer projection**. When drawn according to Fischer's rules, the shadow (and so the drawing) of a particular chiral molecule will always be the same.

This system is most usually applied to sugars and amino acids, which have either aldehyde and hydroxyl (OH), or carboxylic acid and amino groups (NH_2) in common. **If the OH or NH_2 on the** *highest numbered chiral carbon* (the one nearest the bottom of the page) **is on the right of the**

Figure 3.22 Carbohydrate examples of IUPAC and Fischer nomenclature. Although glucose, fructose and mannose are represented as acyclic molecules here, in aqueous solution the cyclic form of each predominates: the hemiacetal forms of glucose and mannose and the hemiketal form of fructose. You will meet these structures in more detail in Chapter 11

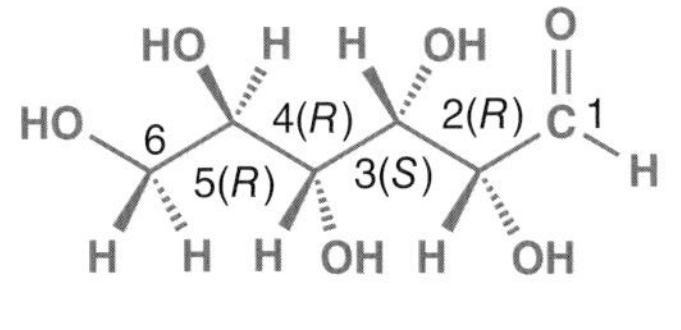

(2R, 3S, 4R, 5R)-2,3,4,5,6-pentahydroxyhexanal
[D-glucose]

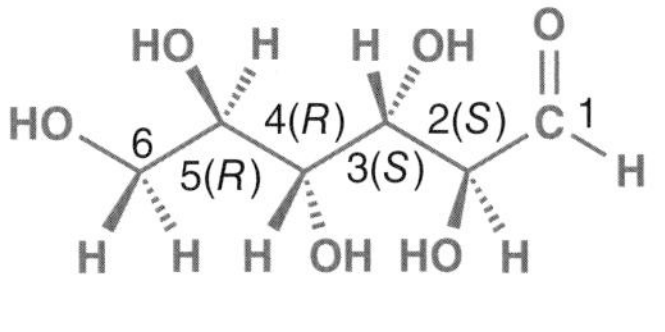

(2S, 3S, 4R, 5R)-2,3,4,5,6-pentahydroxyhexanal
[D-mannose]

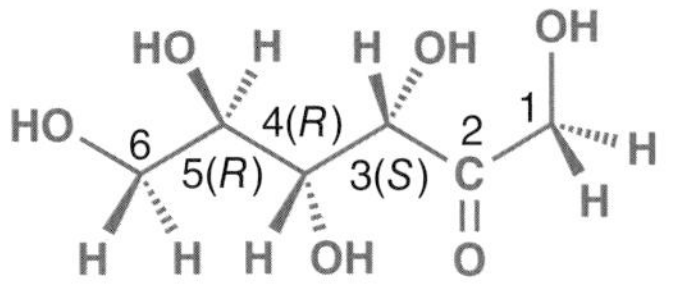

(3S, 4R, 5R)-1,3,4,5,6-pentahydroxy
hexan-2-one [D-fructose]

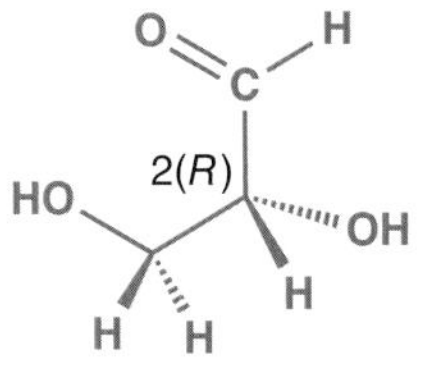

(2R)-2,3-dihydroxypropanal
[D-glyceraldehyde]

vertical carbon chain, then the molecule is designated D, if it is on the left of the vertical carbon chain, then it is designated as L. The D and L forms of a compound are **enantiomers**, that is, they are mirror images. The notation comes from the Latin; D for dextro, meaning 'right', and L meaning laevo (or levo) for 'left'.

You can try this for yourself using a molecular model kit and a torch (or the torch application on your phone), using Figure 3.23 as a guide.

Figure 3.23 The origin of the Fischer system of nomenclature for chiral biological building blocks, such as sugars and amino acids, demonstrated for D-glyceraldehyde

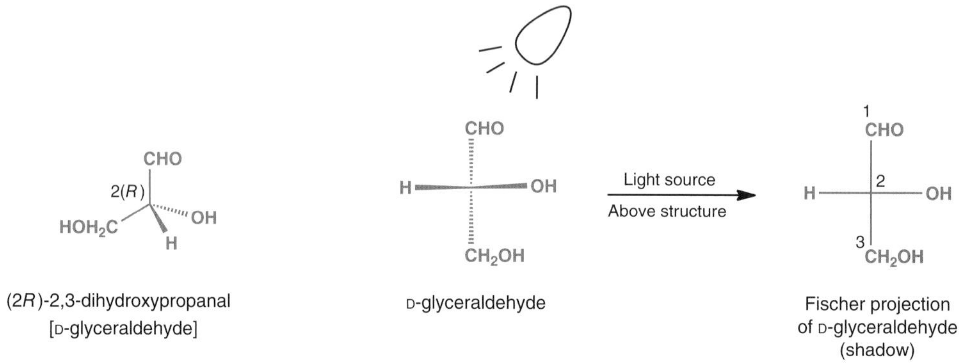

(2R)-2,3-dihydroxypropanal
[D-glyceraldehyde]

D-glyceraldehyde

Fischer projection
of D-glyceraldehyde
(shadow)

Self-check 3.7

The same rules as those described above are applied to glucose, any other sugar, and a range of other molecules, such as amino acids. The two enantiomers of glucose are shown in Figure 3.24; can you use Fischer's rules to decide which is the natural D-glucose and which is the L-form? Two natural amino acids, alanine and serine, are also shown in Figure 3.24; use Fischer's rules to decide if the D- or L-form is the naturally occurring form of each.

Figure 3.24 The enantiomers of glucose and two natural amino acids as Fischer projections

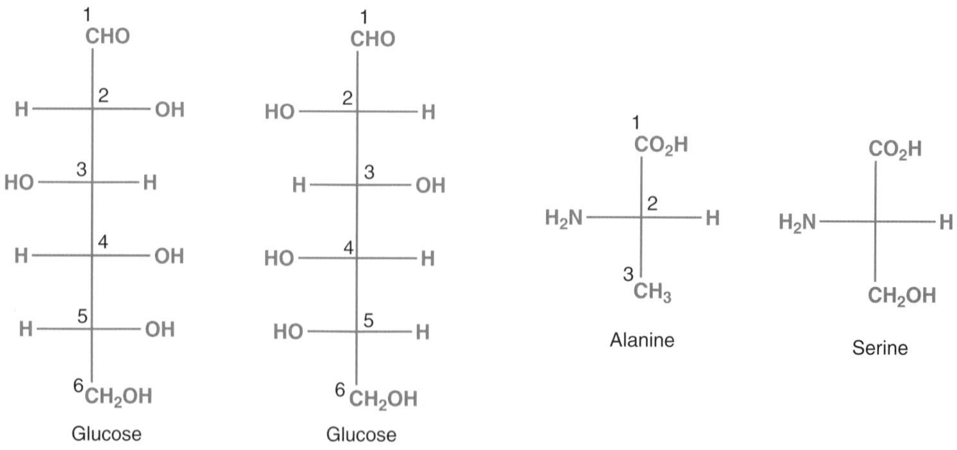

Glucose

Glucose

Alanine

Serine

Manipulating Fischer projections

There are some rules to using Fischer projections that must be adhered to for accuracy: if you turn an entire Fischer projection through 90° on paper, then the stereochemistry inverts. You can check this by making models of each structure below (remembering the horizontal bonds always stick up out of the paper towards you) and putting each into the Fischer projection with the most oxidized carbon at the top and the carbon chain vertically down, then check where the OH group is—left (L) or right (D) (see Figure 3.25).

The stereochemistry also inverts if you swap the positions of any two groups; in the examples shown in Figure 3.26 the two groups that have been swapped are highlighted. Again, you can convince yourself by making the models.

Properties of enantiomers

Constitutional isomers and geometric isomers have different physical and chemical properties: their melting points, boiling points etc., are different. In contrast, a pair of enantiomers has identical physical and chemical properties: they have the same melting points, boiling points, solubilities, and even have the same NMR spectra. There are only two key differences in their dynamic properties; we will look at these distinguishing features in some detail in this section.

In Table 3.2, some physical properties of the enantiomers of ibuprofen, whose structures are shown in Figure 3.27, are listed.

Notice how the melting points of the enantiomers are the same, whereas the melting point of the racemate is different. It is common for the melting point of the racemate to be higher than either of the enantiomers from which it is formed; the enantiomers combine in a 1:1 ratio with high affinity to form an ordered crystalline solid, requiring greater energy (a higher temperature) to separate the enantiomers. The tight crystal packing can also contribute to lower solubility of the racemate. You may wonder why the racemate of ibuprofen is used, when the activity resides largely in the (S)-enantiomer. There are three main reasons:

1. Economics: the racemic mixture is cheaper to synthesize.

2. Toxicology: the (R)-enantiomer does not have any significant adverse effects.

Figure 3.25 Illustration of inversion of Fischer projection nomenclature by rotation of the structure

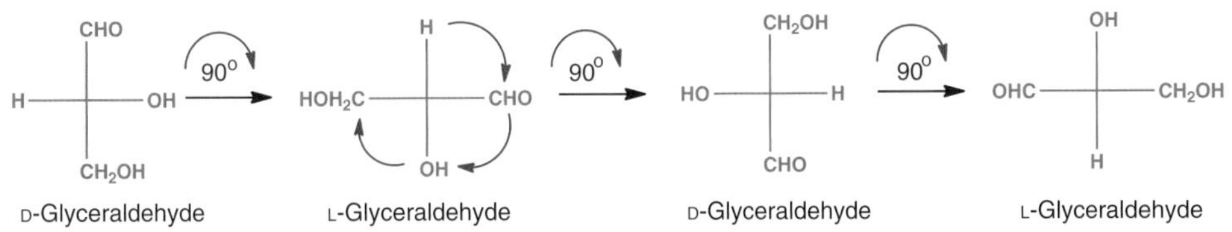

Figure 3.26 Each reversal of two adjacent groups inverts Fischer stereochemical assignment

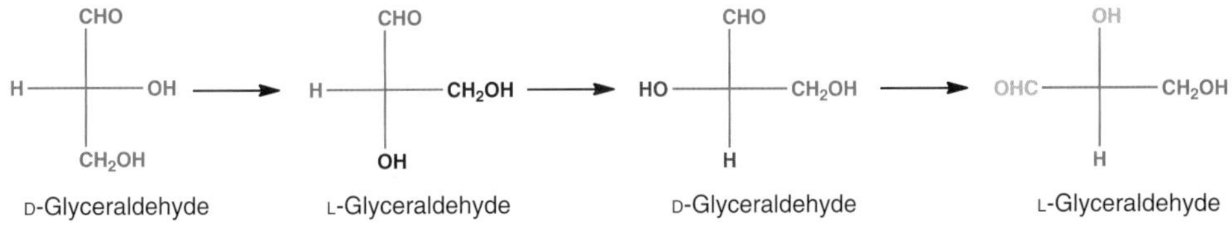

Table 3.2   Selected physical properties of the enantiomers and racemic mixture of ibuprofen

Molecule	Mol. wt. (g/mol)	Melting point (°C)	Aq. Solubility at pH 1.5 (mg/100 mL)	pK$_a$
(R)-Ibuprofen	206.28	52	9.5	4.43
(S)-Ibuprofen	206.28	52	9.5	4.43
Racemic ibuprofen (1:1 R/S)	206.28	76	4.6	4.43

Figure 3.27   The enantiomers of ibuprofen

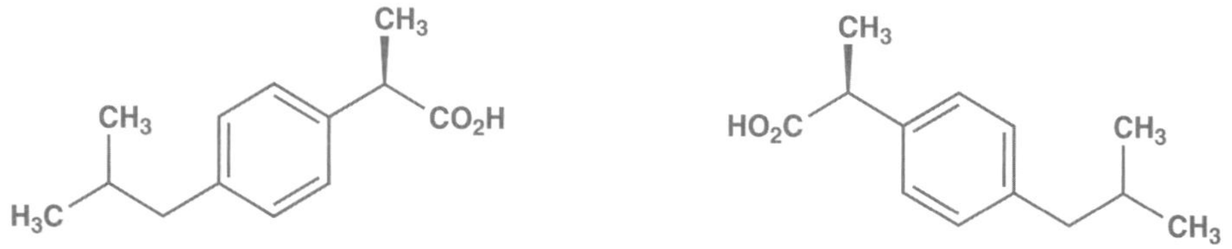

3. Pharmacokinetics: although the standard 400 mg dose contains only 200 mg of the active (S)-enantiomer, about 50–60% of the (R)-enantiomer is slowly converted to the active (S)-form, resulting in an overall total dose of 300–320 mg of (S)-ibuprofen being delivered.

Distinguishing properties of enantiomers

The properties of a pair of enantiomers only differ in:

•   the way each enantiomer interacts with plane-polarized light (PPL);

•   the way in which each enantiomer reacts or interacts with another chiral species.

Because biological molecules are chiral, this latter difference is most relevant to us in the world of pharmaceutical science and it helps to explain the 'thalidomide disaster' (see Box 3.1).

Interaction with plane-polarized light

Light from the sun, or from a normal light bulb, radiates out from the source in all directions and planes. Plane-polarized light has been passed through a filter which only allows light to pass through in the plane of the filter (see Figure 3.28). This is the principle upon which polarized sunglasses and car windscreens are based; the filter cuts the glare that arises from bright sunlight.

In 1815, Jean Baptiste Biot discovered that plane-polarized light could be rotated by some naturally occurring compounds. Many years later, the action was defined: the enantiomers of a compound rotate plane-polarized light by the same amount, but in opposite directions. One enantiomer rotates the light in a *clockwise* direction by X degrees, while the other enantiomer rotates the light *anticlockwise*, also by X degrees. An isomer that rotates plane-polarized light in a clockwise direction was classified as dextrorotatory (d), and an isomer that rotates plane-polarized light in an anticlockwise direction was labelled as laevorotatory (l); however, these lower-case letters were often confused with the Fischer nomenclature of D and L, so dextrorotatory is now labelled as (+) and laevorotatory as (−) (see Figure 3.29).

Figure 3.28 The origin of plane-polarized light

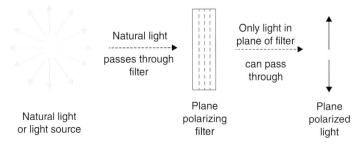

Natural light

passes through
filter

Only light in
plane of filter

can pass
through

Natural light
or light source

Plane
polarizing
filter

Plane
polarized
light

Figure 3.29 Dextrorotatory and laevorotatory illustrated

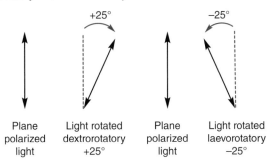

+25°

−25°

Plane
polarized
light

Light rotated
dextrorotatory
+25°

Plane
polarized
light

Light rotated
laevorotatory
−25°

Interaction with chiral molecules

The other property that distinguishes enantiomers is the way in which they interact with an-other chiral molecule; a chiral target molecule will often preferentially interact with one of a pair of enantiomers. There are many examples of this 'recognition' in our everyday life—perhaps not altogether surprising, given that we have already seen that our hands are chiral. The left-handed readers are at this point nodding sagely—we know all about this! Those of us who are left-handed will, at some stage, have struggled with a pair of scissors, a can opener, a golf club, or a corkscrew, which have been designed for a right-handed person.

The observed rotation of a solution of a mixture of isomers of known specific rotation can be used to calculate the % optical purity of the major component. A worked example is provided in the online resources, along with an example calculation using % concentration units (commonly used in pharmaceutical analysis).

Self-check 3.8

(a) Using the information about specific rotation, calculate the specific rotation of chloram-phenicol in ethanol at 27 °C, when a solution of 48.6 mg/mL gives an observed rotation of 0.904° using a cell of length 10 cm. (b) Calculate the observed rotation you would expect to see from a 50 mg/mL solution of (S)-naproxen in chloroform (cell length 1 dm).

Box 3.2

The enantiomers of a compound rotate plane-polarized light by the same amount, but in opposite directions.

A polarimeter, which incorporates two plane-polarizing filters, is used to measure the amount by which plane-polarized light is rotated; the observed rotation is given as a numerical value, either (+) or (−). However, the exact rotation measured by the polarimeter depends upon the concentration and the length of the sample container through which the light passes; the more molecules encountered by the light, the more it will be rotated. The standardized **specific rotation [α]** calculated using equation 3.1 takes concentration and path length into account, as well as temperature and the light source, which can also affect the observed rotation; the sodium D line is the usual source of light in a polarimeter.

It is usual to quote the concentration and solvent in parentheses after the $[\sigma]_D$ value.

$$[\alpha]_D = a\,/\,c.l \text{ at temperature T (°C)} \qquad \text{(eqn 3.1)}$$

Where $[\alpha]_D$ = specific rotation in degrees (using the D line from a sodium light source at 589 nm); a = observed rotation; c = concentration of sample solution (in g/mL); l = path length in dm.

For example, the observed rotation of a solution of (R)-ibuprofen (at 0.5 g/mL in ethanol) was found to be −28.8° at 25 °C using a polarimeter cell of length 10 cm. From these data, a = −28.8, c = 0.5 and l = 1 (10 cm = 1 dm), so

$$[\alpha]_D = -\,28.8\,/\,0.5 \times 1 = -\,57.6°\left(\text{ethanol},25°C\right)$$

This would usually be reported as $[\alpha]_D$ = −57.6° (c 0.5, EtOH), and from this we can deduce that the specific rotation of (S)-ibuprofen would be +57.6°.

Feet, like hands, are chiral; your left foot does not superimpose on your right foot. Socks, however, are (normally) achiral and we do not have to check each morning that we are putting the right sock on the right foot. Our feet interact with socks in much the same way as a chiral drug interacts with an achiral molecule, such as a solvent.

Not so with our shoes! From being a child, we have been taught that only one of our shoes will fit on the left foot and the other shoe will only fit on the right foot—indeed, getting it wrong is uncomfortable. Continuing the analogy, the chiral shoes recognize the chirality in our feet and each enantiomeric shoe interacts differently with our enantiomeric feet. This recognition feature is found extensively throughout nature, even down to the molecular level, where a chiral molecule, such as a receptor, recognizes the enantiomers of another chiral molecule, for example a drug, and usually selects (fits) one better than the other.

We experience selective recognition events daily, not only in the way biological molecules and pharmaceuticals interact in our cells, but also in the way external molecules affect us. For example, the olfactory and gustatory systems of smell and taste, respectively, rely on the way in which molecules interact with receptors in the nose and on the tongue. The enantiomers of some chiral molecules have an entirely different individual smell or taste, because each enantiomer binds to the chiral receptors in a different way. Two examples are carvone, a natural terpenoid, and tryptophan, a natural amino acid. (R)-Carvone smells (and tastes) of spearmint, while its (S)-enantiomer smells (and tastes) of caraway; L-tryptophan (the natural form found in proteins) has a bitter taste, but its unnatural enantiomer, D-tryptophan, tastes sweet, about thirty-five times sweeter than sucrose (sugar) (see Figure 3.30).

Box 3.3 Stereochemical nomenclature—make sure you know which is which!

Note that R and S correspond neither to D and L, nor to + or -. (Likewise, D and L do not correspond to + and -. It is important not to get these different assignment systems confused.) In the case of ibuprofen, we have (S)-(+)-ibuprofen and (R)-(-)-ibuprofen. The anti-inflammatory activity of the related molecule, naproxen, resides in the (S)-(+)-enantiomer, which has a specific rotation $[\alpha]_D$ of +66°, yet the $[\alpha]_D$ of (S)-naproxen sodium salt is -11°, showing that the exact structure of a molecule can have an acute effect upon its physical properties. Both naproxen and naproxen sodium are used clinically as analgesics.

The solvent in which a compound is dissolved can also have a profound effect upon the specific rotation; the example of (–)-ephedrine can be found in the online resources.

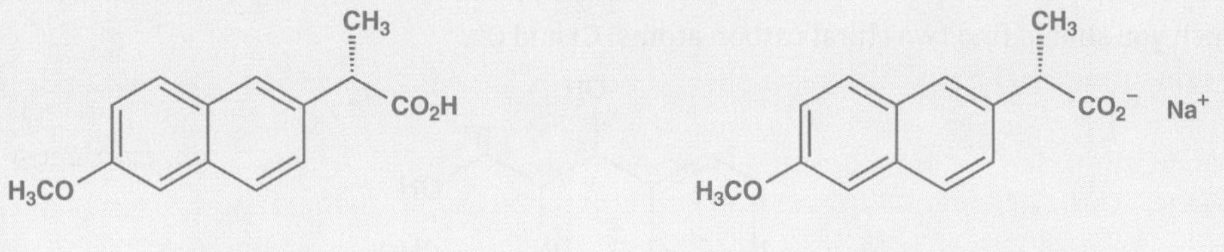

(S)-Naproxen
$[\alpha]_D = + 66°$ (CHCl$_3$)

(S)-Naproxen, sodium salt
$[\alpha]_D = - 11°$ (H$_2$O)

Figure 3.30   The enantiomers of carvone and tryptophan

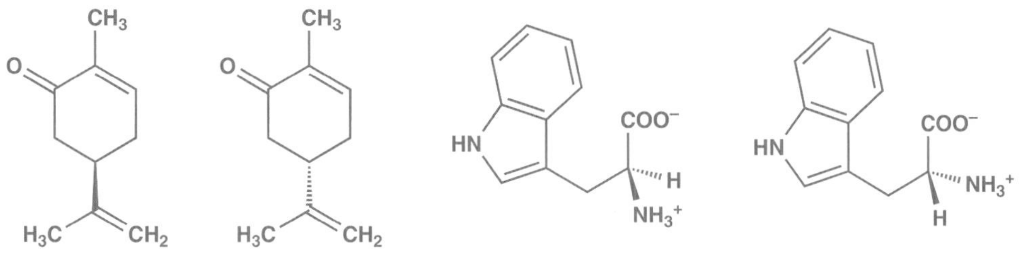

(R)-Carvone   (S)-Carvone   L-Tryptophan   D-Tryptophan

Self-check 3.9

The chirality of tryptophan has been given, as usual for amino acids, using the Fischer nomenclature—can you correctly assign each structure in Figure 3.30 as R or S?

Stereochemical consequences of two or more chiral centres

We saw in Chapter 1 that many pharmaceuticals have several chiral carbon atoms, and we now consider the effect of two or more chiral centres. We have already seen some examples of drugs with more than one chiral carbon in this chapter. In fact, chirality is hugely important in the worldwide multi-billion pound pharmaceutical market: more than 65% of newly approved drugs have at least one chiral centre; a large proportion of these have more than one, and about 40% of the pharmaceutical market consists of single enantiomers (single enantiomer drugs are marketed as the active enantiomer alone). Until recently, the three biggest sellers in the pharmaceutical world were all single enantiomer drugs: atorvastatin (used to lower blood cholesterol levels), esomeprazole (a 'proton pump inhibitor' used to treat gastric and duodenal ulcers), and clopidogrel (used in the prevention of atherothrombotic events).

The industrial-scale synthesis of one single enantiomer of a chiral drug, especially for those with more than one chiral centre, involves complex and challenging chemistry, which is generally reflected in their higher cost (see also Box 3.4).

Molecules with more than one chiral centre

For any molecule with n chiral carbon atoms, there are 2^n possible stereochemical isomers. We can see why when we consider an example. Chloramphenicol is a broad spectrum antibiotic, in which you should find two chiral carbon atoms: C1 and C2.

Chloramphenicol

If we draw out all of the possible stereoisomers, we find that there are four: (1R, 2R), (1S, 2S), (1S, 2R) and (1R, 2S), because each chiral carbon atom can take either R or S stereochemistry. The relationship between stereoisomers is illustrated in Figure 3.31: enantiomers are

Box 3.4   Chiral switching

When a patent on a drug expires there is no longer any legal protection, allowing anyone to make a generic form and sell it for the same indications. 'Chiral switching' is a term used to describe the actions of the pharmaceutical industry when this happens. The original company repatents the drug in its enantiomerically pure form, giving the owners another term of many years exclusivity. To reregister the active enantiomer, the company has to prove that it has therapeutic advantages over the racemic form, which is sometimes more difficult than it sounds! In the case of ofloxacin, a fluoroquinolone antibacterial agent, the greater aqueous solubility of the (S)-enantiomer resulted in an increased antibacterial action of 8–125 times better than the racemate, depending upon the target bacterial species, and the added bonus of decreased toxicity, resulting in the approval of a patent for levofloxacin.

Figure 3.31 The four possible stereoisomers of chloramphenicol

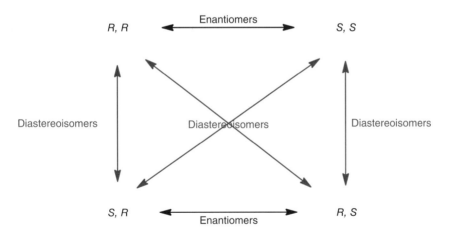

non-superimposable mirror images and diastereoisomers are non-superimposable, non-mirror image stereoisomers. The term 'diastereoisomer' is often written as 'diastereomer'.

The antibacterial activity resides in only one of these stereoisomers: the (1R, 2R) isomer, which tells us that the stereochemistry makes a big difference to the biological activity. We will look at this phenomenon in more detail when we look at properties of diastereoisomers. Some limitations to the use of chloramphenicol are outlined in Box 3.5.

For any molecule with n chiral carbon atoms, there are 2^n possible stereochemical isomers.

Box 3.5 Chloramphenicol

Chloramphenicol is a broad spectrum antibiotic with valuable activity against both Gram positive and Gram negative bacteria, used mostly for the topical treatment of bacterial infections, but used systemically sometimes to treat life-threatening infections, such as meningitis caused by *Haemophilus influenzae*. It acts to inhibit bacterial protein synthesis, but is not entirely selective for the bacterial process. Careful monitoring of blood levels is required to avoid adverse events, such as aplastic anaemia and 'grey baby syndrome', caused by its inhibition of mammalian mitochondrial protein synthesis, particularly in bone marrow cells, when used at high concentrations. When used systemically, it is given as the succinate ester (a prodrug) since chloramphenicol itself has a very low water solubility.

Molecules with two identical chiral carbon atoms

Consider the example of DMSA, **dim**ercapto**s**uccinic **a**cid, which has two chiral carbon atoms. Having read the previous section, you would probably expect there to be four stereoisomers of DMSA, and yet there are only three. To find out why, we need to draw out all of the possible structures (see Figure 3.32).

As before, there is a pair of enantiomers, the *R,R* and *S,S* pair, but the *R,S* and *S,R* pair are identical to each other. We can see why if we rotate the whole *S,R* stereoisomer through 180° as it becomes the mirror image *R,S* form, indicating that it is superimposable (see Figure 3.33); this is the same structure drawn in different ways. It is called the *meso-form.*

A *meso*-form results when a molecule with two or more chiral carbon atoms has identical substituents on the chiral carbon atoms and a mirror plane through the centre of the molecule.

Meso-DMSA can be used medically to reduce the toxic effects of ingested heavy metal ions, such as lead, mercury, arsenic and cadmium. The two thiol (SH) groups must be co-planar to complex

Figure 3.32 The three possible stereoisomers of dimercaptosuccinic acid (DMSA)

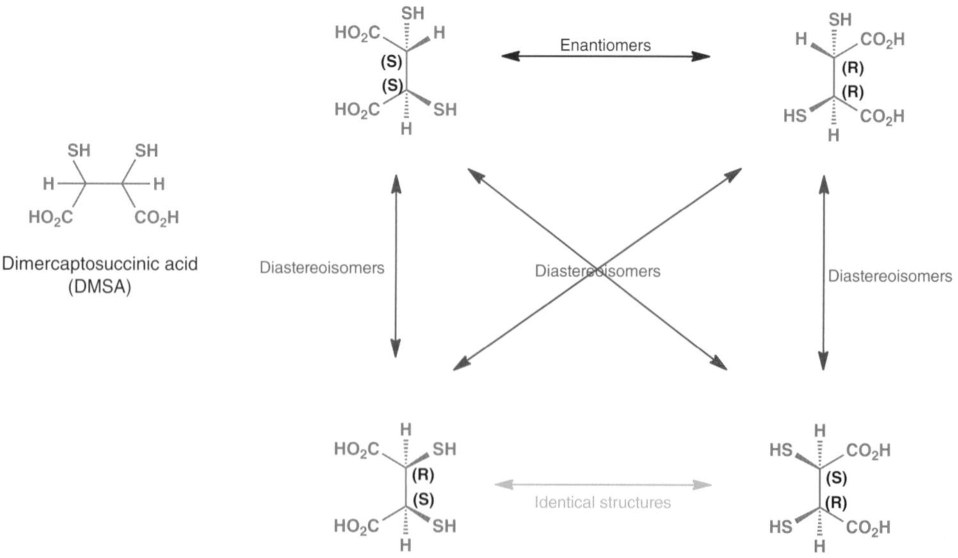

Figure 3.33 The *meso*-form of DMSA has a mirror plane through the middle of the structure

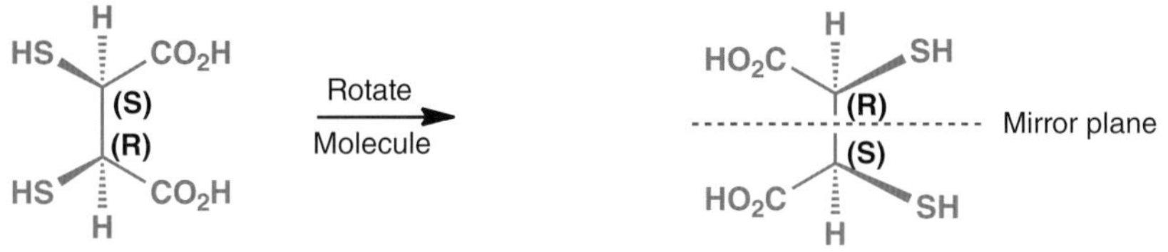

with (chelate) the metal ion, illustrated for lead (Pb^{2+}). Lead poisoning leads to irreversible central nervous system (CNS) damage in children at a concentration of $20-25$ mg Pb^{2+}/100 mL blood.

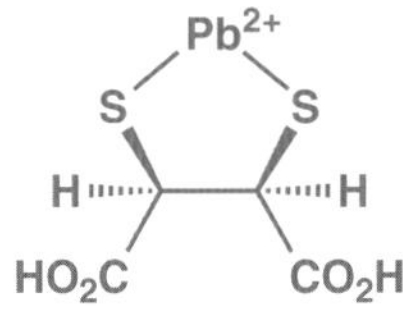

Properties of diastereoisomers

Pairs of enantiomers have identical physical and chemical properties, with the two exceptions noted before (interactions with plane-polarized light and with other chiral species). However, diastereosiomers often have very different physical properties despite having similar chemical properties (owing to having the same functional groups).

In the 1920s, two compounds were isolated from the Chinese herb Ma Huang; you have just met these compounds in Self Check 3.10. One, named ephedrine, is a potent bronchodilator. Pseudoephedrine, a nasal decongestant, was originally thought to be unrelated to ephedrine, because its physical and pharmacological properties are quite different (see Table 3.3), but it was later found to be a diastereoisomer. These compounds are related to amphetamine and are banned substances in sport.

The diastereoisomeric relationship of ephedrine to pseudoephedrine, with different physical properties, allows them to be separated fairly easily. Amines are often more easily crystallized as salts; in the 1920s, when the properties of these compounds were being studied, it was

---

Self-check 3.10

Study the structures of ephedrine and pseudoephedrine. They both have a long history of use in Traditional Chinese Medicine, sourced from the herb Ma Huang (*Ephedra sinica*), and are also components of the British National Formulary (BNF). Assign the stereochemistry of each chiral carbon and decide on the relationship of the two molecules: are they identical, enantiomers or diastereoisomers?

Ephedrine

Pseudoephedrine

Table 3.3 Selected properties of the stereoisomers of ephedrine

Stereoisomer	Alternative name	$[\alpha]_D$ (25 °C) (free amine* in EtOH)	Melting point of free amine (°C)	Source; pharmaco-logical activity
1R,2R-ephedrine	(–)-pseudoephedrine	–52	119	Not naturally occurring; inactive
1S,2S-ephedrine	(+)-pseudoephedrine	⁺52	119	Natural plant metabolite; sympathomimetic, nasal decongestant
Racemic pseudoephedrine	(±)-pseudoephedrine	0	118	Synthetic product; minimal activity
1R,2S-ephedrine	(–)-ephedrine	–6.3	35–40	Natural plant metabolite; anti-asthmatic, potent bronchodilator
1S,2R-ephedrine	(+)-ephedrine	⁺6.3	35–40	Not naturally occurring; inactive
Racemic ephedrine	(±)-ephedrine	0	76–78	Synthetic product; minimal activity

*The specific rotation values of the hydrochloride salts are different to those of the free amines; likewise, other salts of the amines, such as sulfate salts, also have different specific rotation values.

discovered that they could be separated by crystallization from water. The salt formed from the acid–base reaction of (–)-ephedrine with oxalic acid is poorly soluble in cold water, whereas (+)-pseudoephedrine oxalate is very soluble in cold water.

❯ You will find similar information about tartaric acid, along with Self-Check questions, in the online resources which accompany this book.

Separation of stereoisomers: the resolution of enantiomers

Enantiomers cannot be readily separated because of their identical physical properties, but they *can* be separated if converted into diastereoisomers with *different* physical properties. The process of separating enantiomers through the preparation of appropriate diastereoisomeric derivatives is called **resolution** and is a classical method of separation.

To convert an enantiomeric (R, S) pair into diastereoisomers, we can react them with a *single enantiomer* of another chiral molecule (e.g. an S enantiomer) to form a diastereoisomeric pair—the (R, S)-diastereoisomer and the (S, S)-diastereoisomer. We now have diastereoisomers with different physical properties, allowing their separation. For example, to resolve the enantiomers of ibuprofen, which has a carboxylic acid group, the racemic mixture can be reacted with one enantiomer of a chiral base, such as (S)-phenylethylamine to form the diastereoisomeric salts, the (R)-acid:(S)-base and the (S)-acid:(S)-base. The (S, S)-diastereoisomer is poorly soluble in aqueous solution and can be separated by filtration from the mixture, leaving the relatively pure (R, S)-diastereoisomer in solution (see Figure 3.34).

Once the diastereoisomers are in separate vessels, they can be acidified to release the ibuprofen carboxylic acid enantiomers as poorly soluble solids. The chiral base can also be recovered. The chiral molecule used to prepare a diastereoisomeric pair for resolution often comes from a natural source, and there are quite a number to choose from, including sugars and amino acids. These molecules make up a group often referred to as the 'chiral pool'—easily accessible chiral molecules of high enantiomeric purity.

Figure 3.34 Separation of ibuprofen enantiomers through the formation of diastereoisomeric salts

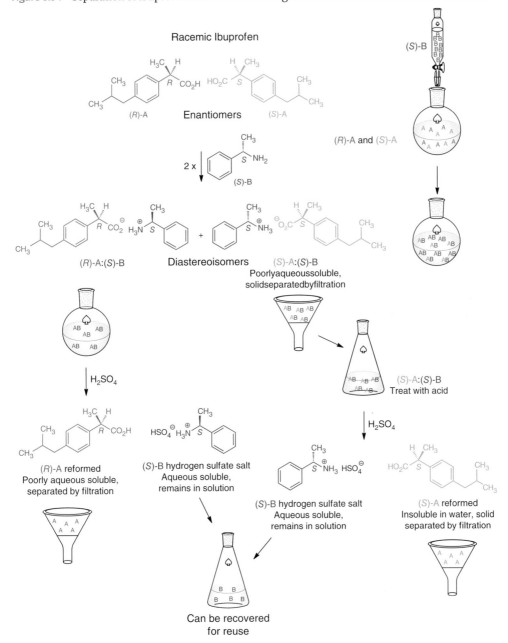

Drugs which can exist as optical isomers are increasingly being required to be tested and supplied as single enantiomers. If the synthesis of the drug produces a racemic mixture, as is often the case, the enantiomers can be separated (resolved) by formation of diastereoisomers; however, chiral synthesis resulting in the pure active isomer is preferred over wasting 50% of the material.

Case study 3.1 Stereochemistry, warfarin and pharmacogenetics

Warfarin is widely used as an anticoagulant—to prevent a patient's blood from clotting too easily. Without this treatment, some patients are at risk of thrombosis (a blood clot). If a thrombosis forms in a heart blood vessel, it could cause a heart attack.

Warfarin

Warfarin acts by inhibiting vitamin K epoxide reductase cofactor subunit 1 (VKORC1), an essential enzyme in blood clotting. Unusually, the enantiomers of warfarin have similar activity on the target enzyme (VKORC1). Their metabolism is, however, very different. The (R)-enantiomer is metabolized by at least three different cytochrome P_{450} (CYP) enzymes and is quickly removed from circulation and excreted. The (S)-enantiomer, by contrast, is metabolized by only one enzyme, called CYP 2C9; (S)-warfarin is mostly responsible for the anticoagulant effect.

Approximately 10% of people have a small change in the gene encoding CYP 2C9 and produce an almost inactive form of the enzyme. Another small group have extra copies of the CYP 2C9 gene and produce more CYP 2C9 than usual.

Patient variability in response to a drug caused by genetic differences is called pharmacogenetics.

Because of these pharmacogenetic variations, the dose of warfarin has to be identified for each patient individually and varies from 3 to 9 mg per day. You may hear pharmacists and doctors talking about the INR—international normalized ratio—of a patient taking warfarin. The INR is used to determine how quickly a patient's blood coagulates (or clots). Generally, for patients taking warfarin, an INR range of 2.5–3.5 is recommended.

Reflection questions

1. Identify the chiral carbon in warfarin. Draw each stereoisomer and assign each structure as R or S stereochemistry.

2. Why do you think the enantiomers are metabolized by different enzymes?

3. What will be the effect on a patient receiving warfarin if they produce an inactive form of CYP 2C9, or if they produce more CYP 2C9 than usual?

For answers, visit the online resources which accompany this textbook.

3.5 **PROTEIN FOLDING DISEASES**

So far, we have explained how the shape of molecules is very important, especially in pharmacy, and we have used common drugs, including tamoxifen, morphine and donepezil, to illustrate this point. Molecular shape also has an impact upon the function of large macromolecules found in our bodies and, to help illustrate our point, we will use proteins as an example.

Proteins are made up of amino acids, linked together by peptide (or amide) bonds. In our bodies, chains of amino acids are folded into three-dimensional shapes to form proteins; this 3D shape is essential to allow a protein to exert a specific function. In some cases, however, proteins can 'mis-fold', which changes their 3D shape and ultimately leads to a change, or even a loss, of their function. The mis-folding of proteins can, therefore, lead to the development of disease. Examples of protein folding diseases include bovine spongiform encephalopathy (or 'Mad Cow' disease), Creutzfeldt–Jacob disease (the human equivalent of Mad Cow disease), Alzheimer's disease, cystic fibrosis and even some cancers.

❯ You can read more about protein folding in Chapter 10, 'Proteins and enzymes'.

You can read more about protein folding in Chapter 10, 'Proteins and enzymes'.

CHAPTER SUMMARY

- Constitutional isomers (also called structural isomers) contain the same atoms but bonded together in different ways.
- Conformational isomers are different shapes adopted by the same molecule arising because of rotation about σ bonds.
- Conformational isomerism allows a molecule to adopt the most favourable shape for interaction with an enzyme or receptor.
- The conformation adopted by cyclohexane rings can be particularly important.
- Stereoisomers have the same connectivity of atoms but arranged differently in space. They include geometrical isomers and optical isomers.
- Geometrical isomers are compounds which differ from each other in the arrangement of groups with respect to a double bond, ring or other rigid structure and are identified as either *Z* or *E* isomers.
- Optical isomers are related as object to non-superimposable mirror image. They are also known as enantiomers and are adentified as either *R* or *S*.
- Optical isomerism arises as a result of the presence of one or more chiral atoms.
- Enantiomers interact differently with other chiral molecules such as enzymes and receptors, often resulting in preferential interaction with one enantiomer.
- Drugs which exist as enantiomers are often marketed as a 50:50 mixture of the two enantiomers, although, increasingly, single enantiomers are marketed as a result of regulatory requirements.
- New chiral drugs are now often marketed as the single active enantiomer, even when they are made synthetically (chiral natural products usually exist as single enantiomers);

93

however, there are still many examples of new racemic drugs. In some cases, the inactive forms cause no major adverse effects and, in others, the inactive form can cause serious adverse effects or can even augment the action of the therapeutically active enantiomer. The FDA and MHRA both require evidence that a mixture of stereoisomers has no adverse effects and, through these more careful considerations of stereochemistry and its influences upon interactions with human biochemistry, we can feel more confident that another thalidomide-type disaster will not occur.

As the 'expert on medicines', pharmacists have a crucial role to play in understanding how stereochemistry affects drug action, identifying potential problems, responding to changes, and supporting other healthcare professionals in executing their roles. Medicinal chemists contribute to the design and synthesis of chiral drugs, and pharmacologists evaluate and rationalize their biological actions; together the pharmaceutical science team ensure that each patient is treated by the safest and most effective medicine. We hope this chapter has helped you to achieve a sound understanding, not only of stereochemistry but of all forms of isomerism, which you can build upon as you progress through your studies.

FURTHER READING

Cahn, R.S., Ingold, C.K., and Prelog, V. 'Specification of molecular chirality', *Angewandte Chemie Int. Ed. Engl.* 1966, 5:385–415.

For more about the involvement of stereochemistry in drug design:

Nogrady, T. and Weaver, D. F. *Medicinal Chemistry: A Molecular and Biochemical Approach*, 3rd edn. Oxford University Press, 2005.

Provides an overview of the properties of drug molecules and the nature of drug-receptor interactions.

Self-check

For the answers to the Self-Check questions in Chapter 3, visit the online resources which accompany this textbook.

PROPERTIES OF ALIPHATIC HYDROCARBONS

Andrew J. Hall

In Chapter 2 you learnt about the ways in which atoms are bonded together and the remarkable ability of carbon to form bonds with other carbon atoms. This means that molecules can be produced that have short or long chains, or more complicated arrangements of carbon atoms. Hydrocarbons are compounds made solely of carbon and hydrogen atoms, in which each carbon forms four covalent bonds.

Hydrocarbons are extremely important in our everyday lives. They are a source of energy to heat and light our homes, and power our vehicles, and they provide us with many of the plastic items we use. Hydrocarbons are also abundant in nature—for example, as flavours or fragrances produced by plants, as insect pheromones, and as natural rubber and lipids.

In this chapter we will explore the properties of the **aliphatic** hydrocarbons: the **alkanes**, **alkenes** and **alkynes**. In Chapter 2 you saw that the types of bonds formed between atoms affect the shape of the molecules formed. Further, the differences in strength between the first (σ) bond and second/third (π) carbon–carbon bonds enable us to anticipate the different reactivity of the different classes of aliphatic hydrocarbon.

As we proceed, you will learn how to name aliphatic hydrocarbons and discover their physical properties. You will also learn where they come from, how they are made and how they react. You should come to realize the importance of aliphatic hydrocarbons in pharmaceutical and biological systems.

The properties of the aromatic hydrocarbons are altogether another story and will be covered in Chapter 7, Introduction to aromatic chemistry'.

Learning objectives

Having read this chapter you are expected to be able to:

- name any given hydrocarbon following the rules that chemists use
- relate the physical properties of aliphatic hydrocarbons to their behaviour
- give examples of the reactions of aliphatic hydrocarbons
- give examples of the importance of aliphatic hydrocarbons in pharmacy.

4.1 NOMENCLATURE

Before we go any further, we need to sort out how we name organic compounds. This is a little like learning a foreign language and is absolutely necessary for you to be able to navigate your way through the world of organic chemistry.

Alkanes

The best place to start is with the alkanes, as their names form the basis for naming the majority of organic molecules. These molecules contain *only* single bonds between the carbons and hydrogens.

Straight-chain alkanes

In straight-chain alkanes, the carbons form a continuous, non-branched chain. The first four members of the series are methane, ethane, propane and butane (see Figure 4.1).

You should notice that the alkanes have the general formula C_nH_{2n+2}, where n is a whole number, and that, as the series continues, the next member differs from the previous one by a $-CH_2-$ unit. Such a family of molecules is called a homologous series. Beyond butane, Latin or Greek prefixes are used for the number of carbons in the chain, followed by the 'ane' suffix. The series continues with pentane (C_5), hexane (C_6), heptane (C_7), octane (C_8), nonane (C_9), decane (C_{10}), undecane (C_{11}), dodecane (C_{12}) etc.

Branched-chain alkanes

Alkanes with more than three carbons can have branched chains. A hydrogen atom from a carbon in the middle of the chain is replaced by an alkyl group. For example, two possible structures fit the formula C_4H_{10}, the linear butane molecule, and its branched isomer, isobutane (2-methylpropane). As the number of carbon atoms increases, so does the number of isomers. While there are just three isomers of pentane C_5H_{12}, (see Figure 4.2), there are seventy-five isomers of decane, $C_{10}H_{22}$, and more than 300,000 possible isomers of eicosane, $C_{20}H_{42}$!

Self-check 4.1

Complete Table 4.1 by drawing 'stick' structures (see Chapters 1 and 2) for ethane, propane and butane. Can you see why we do not normally draw a stick structure for methane?

Table 4.1   Structural representations of alkanes

Alkane	Structure	Stick Structure
Ethane	H_3C-CH_3	
Propane	H_3C CH_3	
Butane	H_3C CH_3	
Pentane	H_3C CH_3	

Figure 4.1 Straight-chain alkanes (note that these are drawn as projections for clarity)

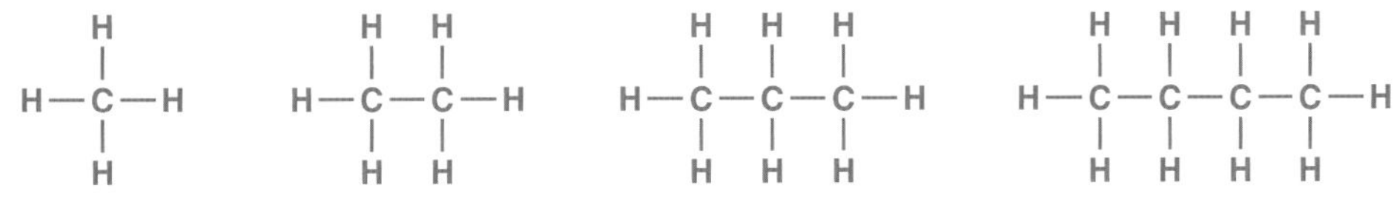

Methane CH$_4$ Ethane C$_2$H$_6$ Propane C$_3$H$_8$ Butane C$_4$H$_{10}$

Figure 4.2 Isomers of pentane

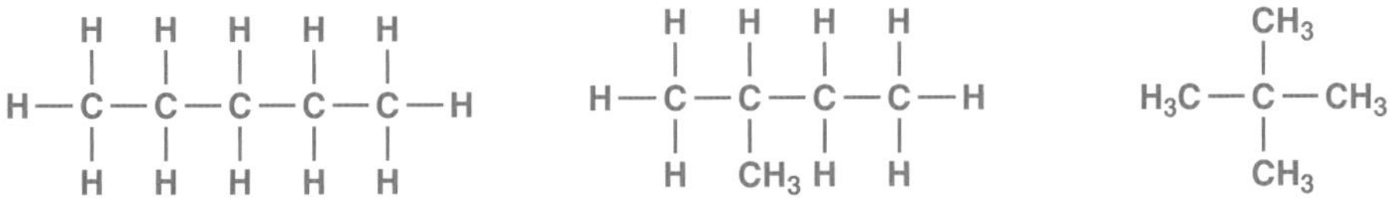

Pentane C$_5$H$_{12}$ 2-Methylbutane (isopentane) C$_5$H$_{12}$ 2,2-Dimethylpropane C$_5$H$_{12}$

In Figure 4.2, one of the isomers of pentane has also been given its common name (isopentane), but as we move to larger molecules with differing numbers of branches or, as you will see later, different functional groups, then we need a more systematic naming system to avoid confusion. The rules of this system are laid out below.

1. Identify the longest continuous carbon chain.

2. Identify the branching points on that chain and give the groups attached at these branching points names corresponding to the number of carbons they contain: methyl (one carbon), ethyl (two carbons), propyl (three carbons) and so on. Note that these are called alkyl groups.

3. Using the lowest numbers possible, number the carbon atoms on the longest chain to describe the positions of the branching groups.

4. Write the branches in alphabetical order.

5. If you find more than one branch with the same name, use the prefixes di-, tri-, tetra- etc.

The examples below should help you to visualize these rules.

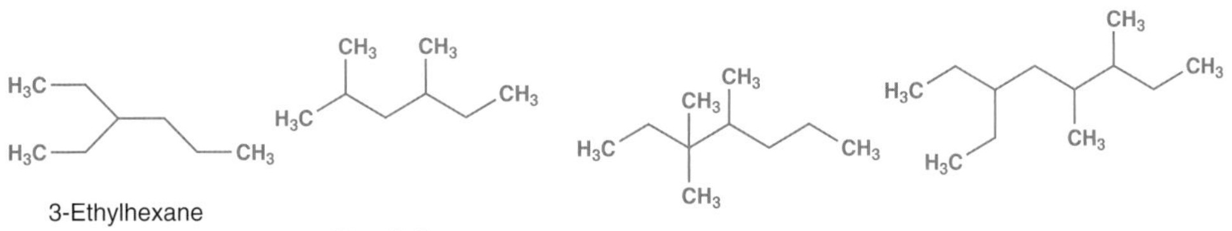

3-Ethylhexane

2,4-Dimethylhexane   3,3,4-Trimethylheptane   6-Ethyl-3,4-dimethyloctane

Self-check 4.2

Draw structures for decane and eicosane (just the straight chain forms).

Draw structures for 2-methylhexane, 3-ethyl-4-methylhexane, 3-ethyl-2,5-dimethylheptane and 3,5-diethyl-2,8-dimethyldecane, then name the compounds shown below.

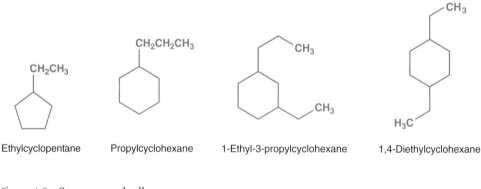

Cycloalkanes

Not all alkanes contain a straight or branched chain of carbon atoms. Cycloalkanes have their carbon atoms arranged in a ring. As a result, a cycloalkane has two fewer hydrogen atoms compared with the acyclic alkane with the same number of carbons, leading to a general formula of C_nH_{2n} for cycloalkanes. Some common cycloalkanes are shown in Figure 4.3 in skeletal form, which is how they are usually drawn.

These molecules are named simply by inserting the prefix 'cyclo' before the name describing the number of carbons in the ring. The rules for naming cycloalkanes follow those used for their acyclic counterparts.

1. For cycloalkanes with an alkyl substituent, the ring is the parent hydrocarbon.

2. If the ring has more than one substituent, write them in alphabetical order and give position number 1 to the first substituent.

The examples below should help you to visualize these rules.

Ethylcyclopentane   Propylcyclohexane   1-Ethyl-3-propylcyclohexane   1,4-Diethylcyclohexane

Figure 4.3   Common cycloalkanes

Cyclopentane   Cyclohexane   Cycloheptane   Cyclooctane

Self-check 4.4

Draw skeletal structures for butylcyclobutane, 1,4-diethyl-cyclooctane and 1-ethyl-3-methyl-5-propylcyclohexane, then name the compounds shown below.

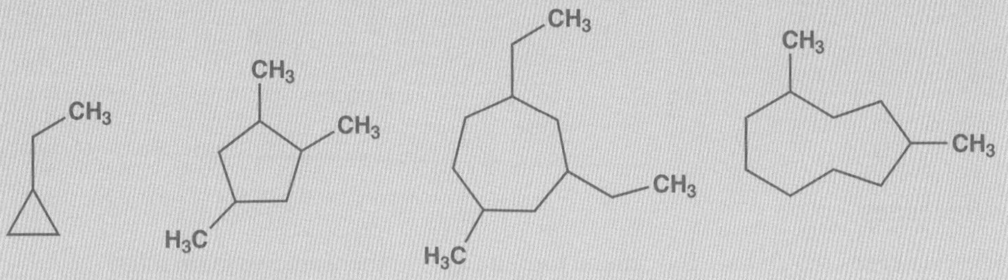

Alkenes

Alkenes, with the general formula C_nH_{2n} contain carbon–carbon double bonds (see Figure 4.4).

You get the systematic name for an alkene by replacing the 'ane' suffix at the end of the parent hydrocarbon's name with the suffix 'ene'. After this, we use the following rules:

1. Determine the longest continuous chain of carbon atoms containing the double bond.

2. Number the carbon atoms in the chain from the end nearest the double bond.

3. Pick the carbon with the lowest number to describe the position of the double bond.

4. If the chain has two double bonds, use the suffix 'diene'.

5. Place substituent names in front of the name of the longest continuous carbon chain.

6. List multiple substituents alphabetically, as before.

The examples below should help you to visualize these rules.

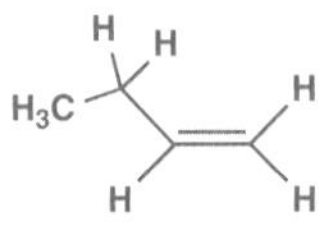

But-1-ene 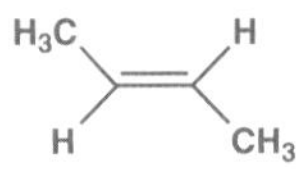   But-2-ene (*E* isomer) 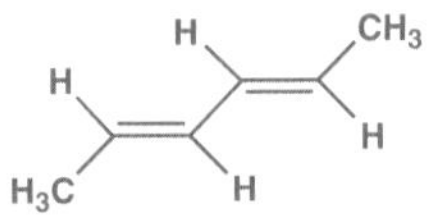   Hexa-2,4-diene (*E*, *E*-isomer) 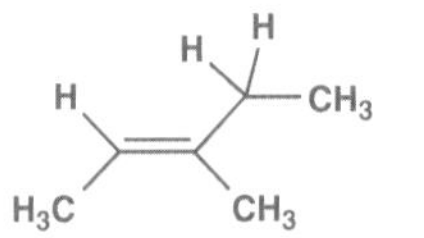   3-Methylpent-2-ene (*E*-isomer)

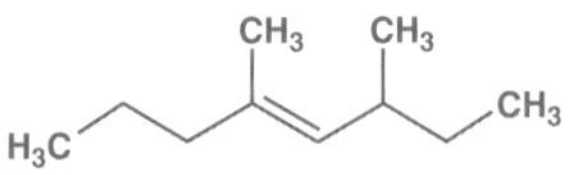

3, 5-Dimethyloct-4-ene (*E*-isomer)

(We will deal with the term *E*–isomer later.)

Figure 4.4   Common alkenes

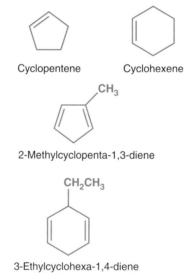

Ethene   Propene

Cycloalkenes

For cycloalkenes, which have the general formula C_nH_{2n-2}, there are two more rules:

1. The carbons in the double bond always take numbers 1 and 2, so such a molecule without substituents bears no numbers. The position of substituents takes the lowest number counting around the ring, bearing this in mind.

2. If the ring contains more than one double bond, numbers are used to define their positions.

   The examples below should help you to visualize these rules.

Cyclopentene   Cyclohexene

2-Methylcyclopenta-1,3-diene

3-Ethylcyclohexa-1,4-diene

Isomerism in alkenes

If we have an alkene with the structural formula, C_4H_8, there are three possible structural arrangements. However, there are in fact four isomers corresponding to this molecular formula, as there are two isomers of but-2-ene: the methyl groups can be on the same side of the planar double bond or on opposite sides of it (see Figure 4.5). These two arrangements are termed *cis* ('on the side') and *trans* ('across').

   As there is no free rotation around the carbon–carbon double bond, the two molecules have atoms oriented differently in space and are, therefore, physically and chemically different. They are geometric isomers. If one of the carbons in the double bond has two identical

Figure 4.5   Isomerism in alkenes

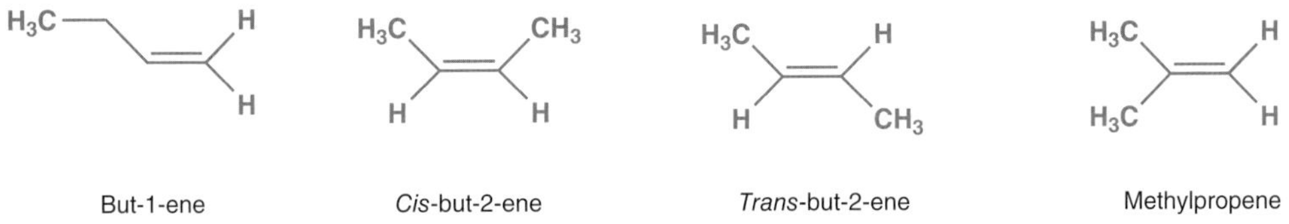

But-1-ene   Cis-but-2-ene   Trans-but-2-ene   Methylpropene

Figure 4.6   Interconversion between *cis* and *trans*-isomers

Heat or light

Cis-hex-2-ene   Trans-hex-2-ene

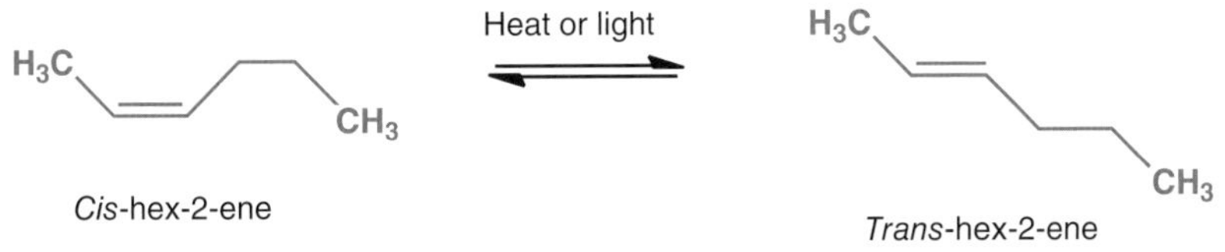

substituents, then there is only one possible structure for the compound and so there are no *cis* and *trans*-isomers (see Figure 4.5).

Interconversion between *cis* and *trans*-isomers is possible, but only if the molecule absorbs enough energy, in the form of heat or light, to cause the π-bond to break (see Figure 4.6). Once this bond has broken, free rotation around the remaining σ-bond can occur.

One important example of this sort of interconversion is the light-catalysed conversion of *cis*-retinal to *trans*-retinal, which is the central chemistry required in vision (See Figure 4.7). This is discussed in more detail in Chapter 1.

If each of the carbon atoms in the double bond has only one substituent, then we can use the *cis/trans*-nomenclature. However, this falls down when the number of substituents increases, e.g. 1-bromo-2-chloropropene. We need a new naming system to differentiate these two molecules—it is called the *E,Z* system (see Figure 4.8).

This system is described in detail in Chapter 3, but it is sufficiently important that we will briefly revisit it here. We first assign priorities (following the Cahn–Ingold–Prelog convention) to the substituents on the carbons of the double bond. If the higher-priority groups are on the same side, then we have the *Z*-isomer (from the German *zusammen* meaning 'together'). If the higher priority-groups are on opposite sides, we have the *E*-isomer (from the German *entgegen* meaning 'opposite'). Note that this nomenclature can be used for *all* alkenes, not just those with three or four substituents.

Figure 4.7   The conversion of *cis*-retinal imine to *trans*-retinal imine in vision

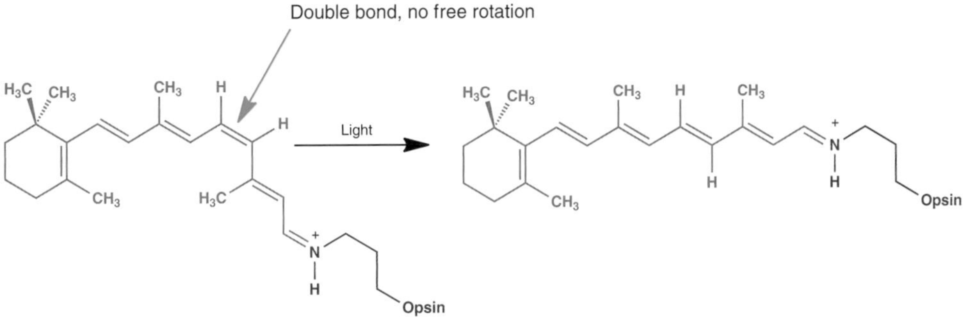

Double bond, no free rotation

Light

Figure 4.8   The E, Z system for naming molecules

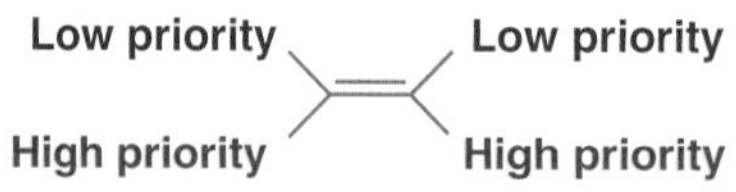

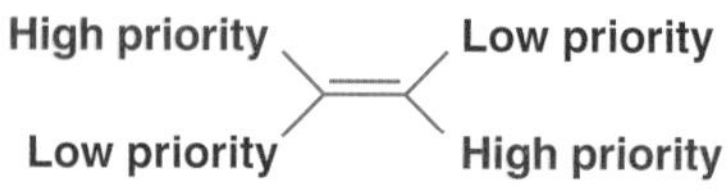

Z isomer

E isomer

> A more detailed discussion of the Cahn–Ingold–Prelog convention is given in Chapter 3, 'Stereochemistry and drug action'.

Priorities are determined by the atomic numbers of the atoms bonded directly to the carbons of the double bond. The greater the atomic number, the higher the priority. If two groups start with the same atom, we move to the next atom attached to the 'tied' atoms. The final 'rule' in this system concerns the case where the atom attached to a carbon of the double bond is doubly bonded to another atom. The priority system treats it as if it were bonded to two of these atoms (see Figure 4.9).

Figure 4.9   Examples of E, Z nomenclature

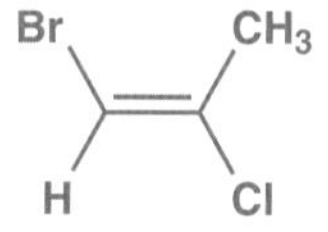

(E)-1-bromo-2-chloropropene

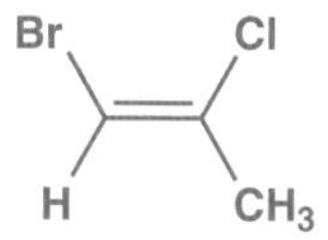

(Z)-1-bromo-2-chloropropene

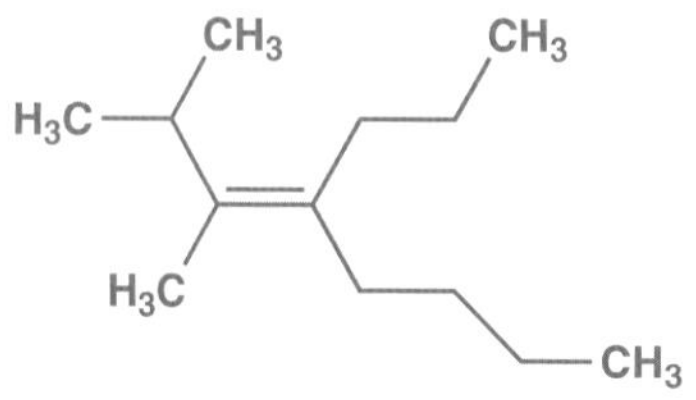

(E)-2,3-dimethyl-4-propyloct-3-ene

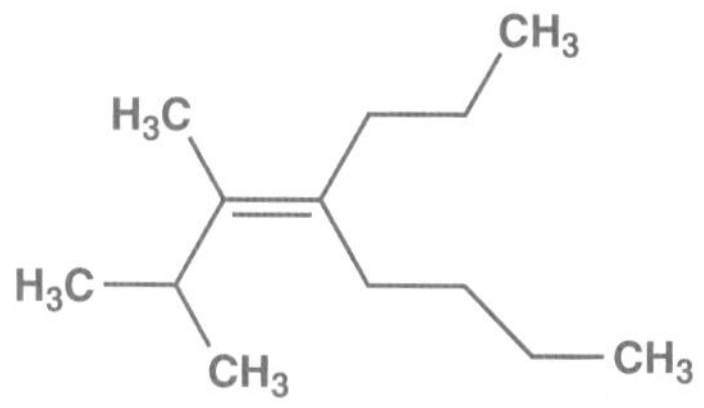

(Z)-2,3-dimethyl-4-propyloct-3-ene

Self-check 4.5

Draw structures for the E- and Z- isomers of 1-chloro-3-ethylhept-3-ene and 2-bromopent-2-ene, then identify the isomers below.

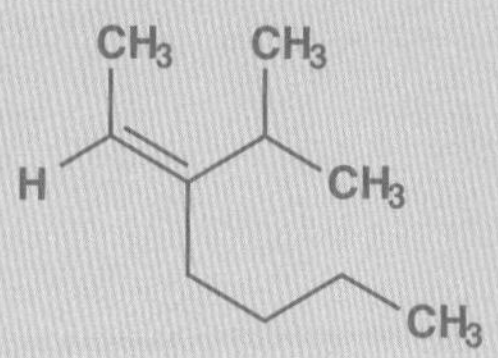

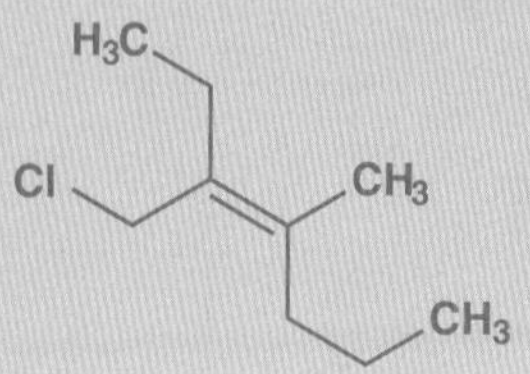

Alkenes can exhibit geometrical isomerism. Geometric isomers have different physical, chemical and biological properties.

> A more detailed guide to alkene stereochemistry and nomenclature is given in Chapter 3, 'Stereochemistry and drug action'.

Alkynes

To obtain the systematic name of an alkyne, we take the alkane name and substitute the 'ane' ending with 'yne'. Again, the longest continuous chain containing the carbon–carbon triple bond is numbered to give the alkyne functional group the lowest possible number.

The triple bond can be within the chain (internal alkynes) or at the end of the chain (terminal alkynes). In some circumstances, counting along the chain from either direction can lead to the alkyne having the same number. In such a case, the correct systematic name is the one where the substituents carry the lowest numbers. See the examples 1–bromo–5–methylhex–3–yne and 2–bromo–3–chlorooct–4–yne.

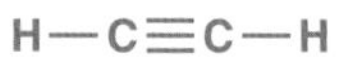

H—C≡C—H

Ethyne (acetylene)

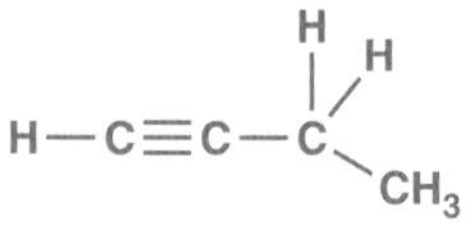

$H—C≡C—C\overset{\displaystyle H}{\underset{\displaystyle CH_3}{|}}H$

But-1-yne

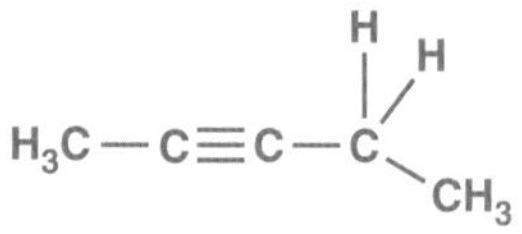

$H_3C—C≡C—C\overset{\displaystyle H}{\underset{\displaystyle CH_3}{|}}H$

Pent-2-yne

$H_3C—C≡C—C$ with CH₃ and C—CH₃ (H H)

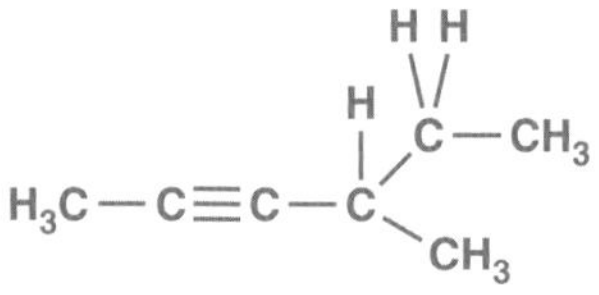

4-Methylhex-2-yne

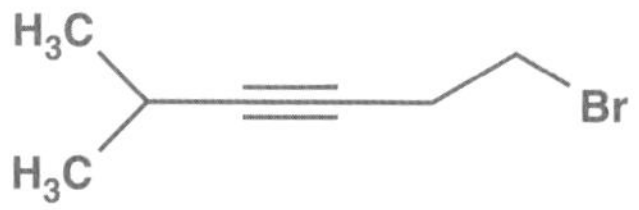

1-Bromo-5-methylhex-3-yne

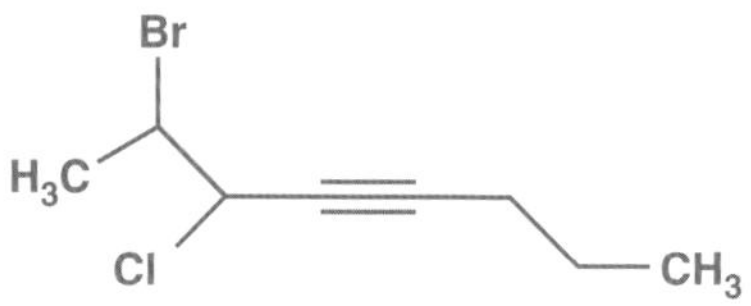

2-Bromo-3-chlorooct-4-yne

Self-check 4.6

Draw structures for 4-methoxyhex-2-yne and but-3-yn-2-ol, then name the structures below.

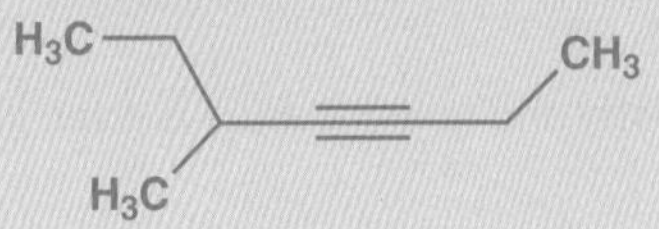

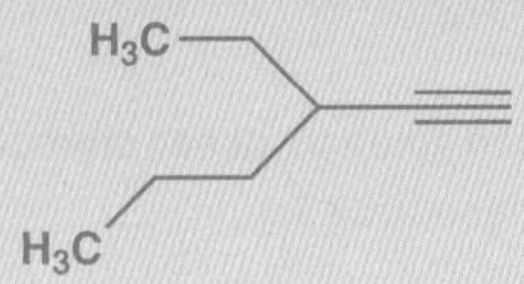

Alkanes, alkenes, and alkynes can exist as straight-chain, branched-chain or cyclic structures.

4.2 PHYSICAL PROPERTIES OF ALIPHATIC HYDROCARBONS

In this section we will examine the properties that are responsible for the physical characteristics of the aliphatic hydrocarbons. These properties include their intermolecular forces, their polarity (or rather lack of it) and, perhaps surprisingly, their acidity.

Boiling and melting points

The small difference between the electronegativities of carbon and hydrogen means that the bond between them is only very weakly polar—and the aliphatic hydrocarbons themselves are non-polar. The only intermolecular forces holding one molecule in contact with another are weak van der Waals' forces. This helps to explain why smaller alkanes, alkenes and alkynes are very volatile; it takes little energy to overcome the interactions between molecules.

As the molecular weight increases, so does the size of the molecules. This leads to greater contact between molecules and a consequent increase in the van der Waals' forces between them. This is why the boiling points increase as each series progresses, as shown in Table 4.2.

Chain branching causes a decrease in the area of contact. So, if two alkanes have the same molecular weight, the more highly branched one will have the lower boiling point. Alkynes have stronger van der Waals' interactions than alkenes and, consequently, higher boiling points, because of their more linear structures.

The melting points of aliphatic hydrocarbons also increase with size, but in a less regular manner. Under standard conditions, alkanes with 1–4 carbons are gases, from 5–17 carbons are liquids and from 18 carbons onwards are waxes and solids.

Solubility and density

As the hydrocarbons are non-polar, they tend to be very insoluble in water and other very polar solvents. Instead, they prefer to dissolve in non-polar solvents, such as benzene and diethyl ether. Thus, hydrocarbons can be described as hydrophobic (literally 'water-hating') or lipophilic (literally, 'fat loving'). The lipophilicity of hydrocarbon groups is especially important when considering how drug molecules get distributed in

Table 4.2 Physical properties of selected aliphatic hydrocarbons

	Number of carbons	Name	Boiling point (°C)	Melting point (°C)	Density at 25 °C (g/mL)
Alkanes	1	methane	−167.7	−182.5	−
	2	ethane	−88.6	−183.3	−
	3	propane	−42.1	−187.7	−
	4	butane	−0.5	−138.3	0.579 (20 °C)
	5	pentane	36.1	−129.8	0.626
	6	hexane	68.7	−95.3	0.659
Cycloalkanes	3	cyclopropane	−33	−128	−
	4	cyclobutane	12.5	−91	−
	5	cyclopentane	49	−94	0.751
	6	cyclohexane	80.7	4–7	0.779
	7	cycloheptane	118.5	−12	0.811
	8	cyclooctane	151	10–13	0.834
Alkenes	2	ethene	−103.7	−169	−
	3	propene	−47.6	−185	−
	4	but-1-ene	−6.1	−138	−
	4	*cis*-but-2-ene	3.7	−139	−
	4	*trans*-but-2-ene	0.9	−105	−
	5	pent-1-ene	30.2	−165	0.641
	5	*cis*-pent-2-ene	36	−180	0.65
	5	*trans*-pent-2-ene	37	−135	0.649
Alkynes	2	ethyne	−84	−	−
	3	propyne	−23.2	−102.7	−
	4	but-1-yne	8.1	−125.7	−
	4	but-2-yne	27.0	−32	0.691
	5	pent-1-yne	40.2	−105	0.691
	5	pent-2-yne	57	−109	0.71

the human body after administration; it also impacts on their mode of action, as we see in Box 4.1.

The hydrocarbons are less dense than water, meaning that they float on the surface of water, as seen to disastrous effect during the various oil spills that have occurred around the world.

Box 4.1   Polyene macrolide antibiotics

Polyene macrolide antibiotics play a major role in the treatment of systematic and topical fungal infections. Their lipophilic structure enables them to insert into fungal cell membranes, making them 'leaky'. This leads to the loss of small molecules from the cells, which eventually die.

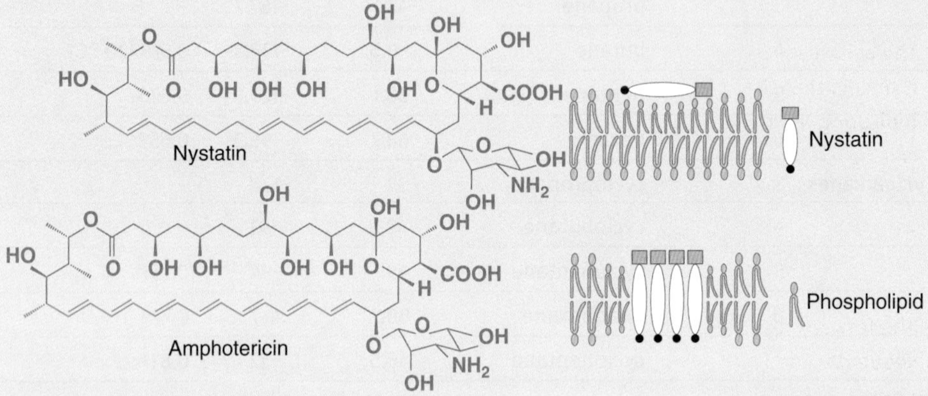

Nystatin

Amphotericin

Nystatin

Phospholipid

Typical examples are nystatin, used to treat topical *Candida* infections, and Amphotericin, which is also used to treat systemic infections. The latter drug suffers from toxicity issues, such as lowering of blood pressure and even kidney damage, but it remains the drug of choice for the treatment of life threatening fungal infections.

Acidity of aliphatic hydrocarbons

Of all the species you will encounter in organic chemistry, alkanes are without doubt the weakest Brønsted acids. In fact, they are so weakly acidic that it is difficult to measure just how acidic they are! In general, their pK_a values are very high. For example, the pK_a of ethane is greater than 50 (see Box 4.2).

Moving to alkenes, there is an increase in the s-character of the carbon–hydrogen bond. (Remember that the carbon of the double bond is sp^2 hybridized (33% 's') rather than sp^3 hybridized (25% 's') as in alkanes.) This increased s-character leads to an increase in acidity. For example, the pK_a of ethene is estimated to be 44, meaning that it is at least six orders of magnitude more acidic than ethane.

$$H_3C-CH_3 \qquad\qquad H_2C=CH_2$$

Ethane   Ethene (ethylene)

pKa > 50   pKa = 44

$$HC\equiv CH$$

Ethyne (acetylene)

pKa = 25

> ### Box 4.2 What is pK$_a$?
>
> You are probably rather surprised to find out that pK$_a$ can be defined for a hydrocarbon or that a proton can dissociate from a C–H bond! Let us take a step back to define what pK$_a$ actually represents. The general reaction of an acid with water is:
>
> $$HA + H_2O \rightleftharpoons H_3O^+ \quad K_a = \frac{[H_3O^+][A^-]}{[HA]} \quad pK_a = -\log_{10} K_a$$
>
> The acid dissociation constant, K$_a$, indicates the relative strength of the acid. If K$_a$ is large, it means that the reaction tends to the right-hand side (the forward reaction is favoured), indicating a strong acid. Given the relationship of pK$_a$ to K$_a$, this means that a strong acid will have a low pK$_a$ value.
>
> Let us take methane as an example of a typical hydrocarbon. The dissociation reaction would be:
>
> $$CH_4 + H_2O \rightleftharpoons H_3O^+ + H_3C^-$$
>
> The forward reaction is not very favourable as the methyl anion, H$_3$C$^-$, is very reactive. Consequently, the back reaction (which favours the reactants) happens to a greater extent. This means that K$_a$ will be very small and, consequently, the pK$_a$ will be very large, which is indeed the case.

In terminal alkynes, the s-character of the carbon–hydrogen bond is further increased (to 50%), leading to another increase in acidity. The pK$_a$ of acetylene (ethyne) is 25. This means that it is 10^{19} times stronger as an acid than ethene. The relative acidity of terminal alkynes is useful in the synthesis of higher alkynes, as you will see in Section 4.5 'Alkynes—preparation and reactions'.

A word of caution: although we refer to the terminal alkyne proton as acidic, this is only a relative term. While terminal alkynes are more acidic than other hydrocarbons, they are still very weak acids. To put this into perspective, compare the pK$_a$ value of ethyne to that of water (15.7), itself a very weak acid, and to acetic (ethanoic) acid (4.7), and hydrochloric acid (-7)!

4.3 ALKANES—PREPARATION AND CHEMICAL PROPERTIES

Alkanes are saturated hydrocarbons and are generally quite unreactive. Combustion of alkanes is, however, a very important reaction.

Isolation and preparation of alkanes

Alkanes are obtained primarily from fossil fuels. Natural gas contains 60–90% methane, the first molecule in the alkane series, with smaller amounts of other small alkanes such as ethane, propane and butane. Crude oil is a mixture of alkanes and cycloalkanes (together with aromatic hydrocarbons). Untreated, this would not be useful, but fractional distillation allows separation of the compounds into groups (fractions) of similar chain length.

Most industrial chemicals, including plastics and pharmaceuticals, originate from the alkanes obtained from crude oil. Small alkanes are obtained from the less useful long-chain alkanes by a process called 'cracking'. Cracking can be achieved thermally by heating the alkanes at high temperatures, thus generating smaller alkanes and small alkenes. Catalytic cracking involves heating the alkanes in the presence of a silica–alumina catalyst, leading to shorter alkanes suitable for use in petrol. In another type of process, catalytic reforming, linear alkanes are broken down and then reassembled into branched alkanes. The process can be used to convert low-grade petrol (low octane number) into higher grades.

Reactions of alkanes

Alkanes are exceptionally stable substances. They do not react with ionic or polar substances and they are resistant to the action of acids and bases. There is little surprise, then, that one of the earlier names for these compounds was 'paraffins', from the Latin for 'little affinity'. The alkanes are saturated molecules; other atoms cannot (easily) add to them. Consequently, alkanes exhibit little chemical reactivity.

Combustion of alkanes

One important reaction of alkanes is combustion—that is, they burn in a plentiful supply of oxygen. This is an oxidative process and follows a free-radical mechanism. The products of this reaction are water and the greenhouse gas carbon dioxide. This is a very exothermic reaction, which explains the use of alkanes as fuels. For example, the change in enthalpy (ΔH) for the combustion of methane is -890 kJ mol^{-1}. Each additional $-CH_2-$ group adds $630-670$ kJ mol^{-1} to the energy released.

$$CH_4(g) + 2O_2(g) \rightarrow CO_2(g) + 2H_2O(l)$$
$$C_{11}H_{24}(g) + 17O_2(g) \rightarrow 11CO_2(g) + 12H_2O(l)$$

The lower alkanes are efficiently oxidized, but heavier alkanes can burn with a sooty flame. This is because there is insufficient oxygen to convert all the alkane to CO_2 (complete combustion), leading to the formation of some carbon and some carbon monoxide (incomplete combustion).

Alkanes and alkyl groups are also oxidized in the body by metabolizing enzymes. These enzymes act to render the lipophilic alkane more hydrophilic and suitable for excretion, as discussed in Section 4.6, 'Hydrocarbons in pharmacy'.

Halogenation of alkanes

Another major reaction of alkanes is halogenation, which occurs very rapidly in the presence of ultraviolet (UV) light, following a free-radical mechanism. The amounts of halogen and alkane present determine what products are formed. For example, the chlorination of methane can lead to chloromethane, dichloromethane, trichloromethane (chloroform) and tetrachloromethane (carbon tetrachloride).

With higher alkanes, mixtures of different isomers are generally formed. The relative amounts of each isomer formed are related to the stability of the free radicals involved in the reaction. In the example below, 2-chlorobutane is the major product because it is formed via a more stable secondary radical (see Scheme 4.1).

These reactions produce mixtures of isomers and mixtures of products with different degrees of substitution, so they are not very suitable for the preparation of alkyl halides in the laboratory. They are used on an industrial scale, however, when it is economically worthwhile to separate the individual compounds.

> You will learn more free-radical processes and about radical stability in Section 4.4, 'Alkenes'.

Scheme 4.1

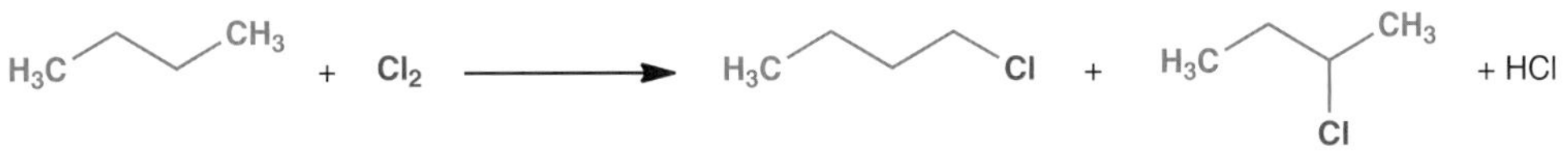

Butane   + Cl_2 1-Chlorobutane 29%   +   2-Chlorobutane 71%   + HCl

> Compared to other hydrocarbons, alkanes are relatively unreactive. They burn, but do very little else.

4.4 ALKENES—PREPARATION AND CHEMICAL PROPERTIES

In this section we will examine the preparation and reactions of alkenes. Unlike alkanes, in the previous section, alkenes undergo a wide range of reactions, largely because of the presence of the π bond.

Isolation and preparation of alkenes

As mentioned earlier, smaller alkenes are obtained from the cracking of alkanes. On an industrial scale, alkenes are also prepared by the dehydrogenation of alkanes (literally, the removal of hydrogens). As these methods tend to produce mixtures of compounds, they are not well suited for synthesizing alkenes in the laboratory where a particular target product may be sought.

Preparation by elimination reactions

There are a number of methods for producing alkenes in the laboratory, the most common being the elimination of HX (X = halogen atom) from alkyl halides or the elimination of water from alcohols. Alkenes can also be prepared via the hydrogenation of alkynes, as you will see later in this chapter, and using the Wittig reaction (you can find details of this reaction in an organic chemistry textbook).

> The elimination reactions of alkyl halides and alcohols are described in more detail in Chapter 5, 'Alcohols, phenols, ethers, organic halogen compounds, and amines'.

Dehydrohalogenation (elimination of HX) can take place via either an E1 or an E2 mechanistic pathway. (The numbers '1' and '2' indicate how many species are involved in the reaction's rate-limiting step—the step that determines how quickly the reaction proceeds. The E1 pathway is a two-step reaction where one species is involved in the rate-limiting step; the E2 pathway is a one-step reaction where two species are involved in the rate-limiting step.)

The E2 (Elimination Type 2) pathway is more useful for synthetic purposes because competing reactions are less important. It requires the use of a moderately strong base, for example KOH, and, sometimes, heat. This mechanism is concerted—there is no formation of an intermediate carbocation (hence it is a one-step reaction). Instead, the movement of electrons represented by the two curly arrows take place at the same time. Unhindered haloalkanes undergo

Figure 4.10 (A) E2 elimination mechanism (B) E1 elimination mechanism

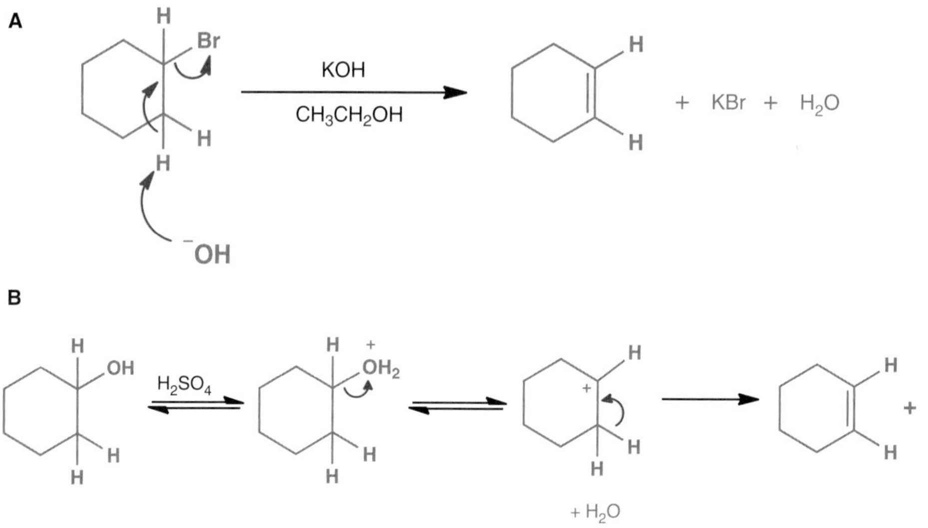

this reaction more readily than haloalkanes in which the approach of the base is hindered by bulky groups (see Figure 4.10).

The dehydration of alcohols requires the presence of an acid catalyst, commonly sulfuric acid; sometimes, the reaction mixture must also be heated. The reaction proceeds by an E1 mechanism, with the acid protonating the hydroxyl group, converting it to a good leaving group. Water leaves and the intermediate carbocation is formed (this is the first step). Loss of a proton (step two) then gives the alkene (see Figure 4.10B).

The reaction is an equilibrium reaction and the equilibrium constant is not particularly high. To ensure the forward reaction is favoured, one of the products needs to be removed from the mixture. Commonly, the alkene product has a lower boiling point than either water or the starting alcohol and can be distilled out of the mixture as it is formed.

E1 reactions are favoured according to the following series: tertiary alcohol favoured more than secondary; secondary alcohol favoured more than primary. This is because the intermediate carbocation is stabilized by σ-**conjugation**. Sigma conjugation occurs when electron density in a C–H or C–C bond interacts with a region of low electron density (in this case, an empty p-orbital) and helps to stabilize it. A tertiary carbocation is stabilized by three interactions at any particular time, a secondary carbocation is stabilized by two, and a primary carbocation by a single interaction.

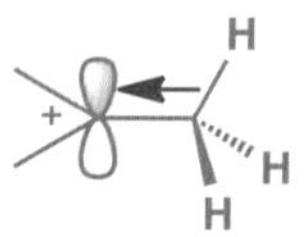

> We will meet sigma conjugation again later in this chapter and in Chapter 7, 'Introduction to aromatic chemistry'.

Box 4.3 Alkenes in nature

Alkenes have many important roles in biology and are therefore quite abundant in nature. Even the simplest alkene, ethene (also known as ethylene) is vital; it is a plant hormone that controls various stages of plant growth, including seed germination and fruit ripening.

The two enantiomers of the alkene limonene have different aromas: the (+)-isomer is responsible for the smell of oranges, while the (−)-isomer smells more of lemon (though less generous noses may say turpentine!). α-phellandrene can be found in the oil of eucalyptus.

(+)-Limonene   (−)-Limonene   (−)-α-phellandrene

Source: Koala: David Coleman; Oranges: Mark Mason

Pheromones are chemical substances released by insects that can be detected by other insects of the same species. Many of the sex and alarm pheromones of insects are alkenes. For example, bombykol and multifidene are the sex pheromones of the silk moth and brown algae, respectively.

Bombykol
(10E, 12Z)-hexadeca-10,12-dien-1-ol

Multifidene

Relative stabilities and reactivities of alkenes

Almost all the hydrocarbons that we will discuss are stable, almost indefinitely, at room temperature. Alkenes do not generally decompose spontaneously! However, some alkenes are more readily formed than others (their ground state energy is lower) and these tend also to be less reactive than other alkenes.

When chemists wish to prepare alkenes, they often find that the major product is the most stable alkene. Many reaction pathways allow for the rearrangement of carbon–carbon double bonds to the most stable isomer. Therefore, it is useful to know how the structure of an alkene relates to its relative stability.

An alkene with alkyl groups attached to the sp^2 carbons is more stable than one with only hydrogens attached. Indeed, the greater the number of alkyl groups, the more stable the alkene. Evidence for these differences in stability can be obtained from heats of hydrogenation for isomeric alkenes, exemplified using 3-methylbut-1-ene and 2-methyl-2-butene (see Figure 4.11).

The trisubstituted isomer is more stable by 14 kJ mol^{-1}. That alkyl groups have this stabilizing effect on alkenes has been summarized as Zaitsev's rule:

More substituted double bonds are usually more stable.

The alkyl groups stabilize the alkene as they are able to donate electron density, via σ-conjugation to the π-bond. This leads to an extended molecular orbital that stabilizes the system. In addition, the alkene will be more stable (less reactive) if bulky substituents are situated as far apart in space as possible. In alkenes, sp²-hybridized carbon atoms separate the substituents by 120° (compared to 109.5° for sp³-hybridized carbons in alkanes), acting to relieve steric effects.

> You will encounter similar effects in Chapter 7, 'Introduction to aromatic chemistry'.

As you have seen in the nomenclature section, alkenes can exist as geometric isomers, either *cis* or *trans*. Which of these is more stable? Let us take *cis*-pent-2-ene and *trans*-pent-2-ene as an example. Both molecules have two alkyl groups—a methyl and an ethyl group—bonded to the sp² carbons, so Zaitsev's rule cannot help us here. We need to look at how the molecules are arranged spatially. The *cis*-isomer has the alkyl substituents close together in space, leading to steric strain. In the *trans*-isomer, the two substituents are much further apart and so this is the more stable of the two isomers. Evidence from the heats of hydrogenation points to *trans*-pent-2-ene being more stable than the *cis*-isomer by 4 kJ mol⁻¹.

Reactions of alkenes

Like alkanes, alkenes burn in a plentiful supply of oxygen, forming carbon dioxide and water. As with alkane combustion, lots of heat energy is given off. For the combustion of ethene (ethylene), shown below, ΔH = –1410 kJ mol⁻¹

$$C_2H_4(g) + 3O_2(g) \rightarrow 2CO_2(g) + 2H_2O(l)$$

However, this is where the similarity in their reactivity ends. Alkenes have their own set of reactions, similar to one another but different from the reactions of alkanes. There is little mystery in this. Recall the structure of alkenes. You should remember that they are planar molecules with a region of electron density above and below the plane of the carbon–carbon double bond. This is due to the π-bond formed between the unhybridized p orbitals of each carbon atom. The π electrons are relatively loosely held and are attracted to electrophiles (electron-loving species). Thus, the first step in alkene reactions is the addition of an electrophile (E) to one of the sp² carbons; this is followed by addition of a nucleophile (Nu⁻) to the remaining sp² carbon. The overall result is the breaking of the π-bond and the formation of two new σ-bonds, which is energetically favourable. This characteristic reaction of alkenes is called an electrophilic addition reaction, as the first species to add is the electrophile (see Scheme 4.2).

Figure 4.11 The heats of hydrogenation for isomeric alkenes

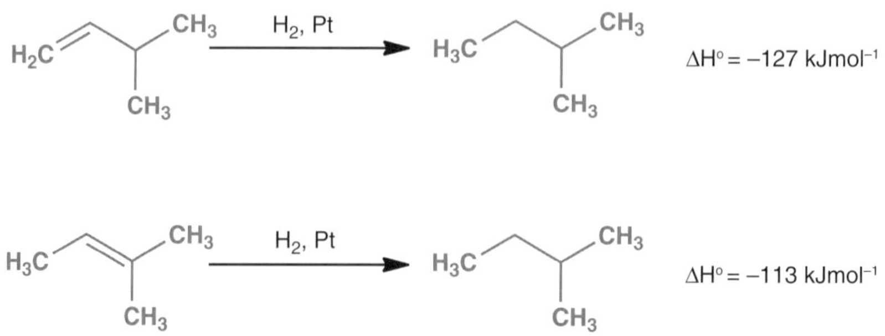

Scheme 4.2

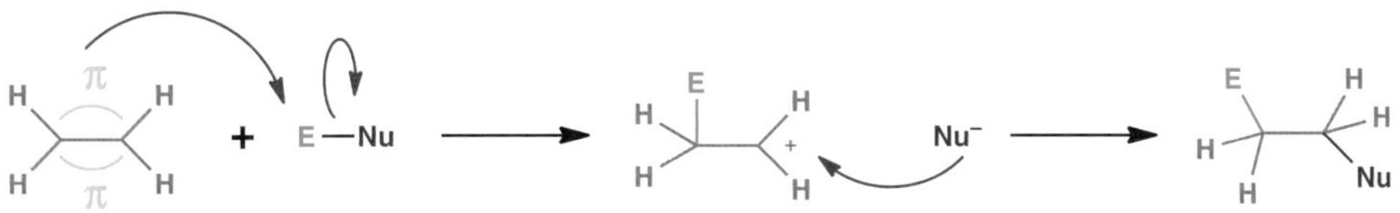

Alkenes also undergo electrophilic addition reactions mediated by free radicals. These are especially important in the synthesis of a variety of everyday polymers, such as polystyrene and poly(methyl methacrylate) [Plexiglas®]. We will return to polymers later in this chapter.

Addition of hydrogen halides to alkenes

Alkenes engage in electrophilic addition reactions with hydrogen halides (HX), where the proton from the hydrogen halide acts as the electrophile, adding first, and the halide ion is the nucleophile which adds in the second step. The first step is slow and determines the overall reaction rate (see Scheme 4.3).

If the sp^2 carbons in the alkene bear the same substituents, as shown, the product of the reaction is easy to predict. Whichever carbon the electrophile adds to in the first step, the same product will be formed. This is not the case when the sp^2 carbons are not identically substituted. Let us take the addition of HCl to 2-methylpropene as an example. There are two possible products, and we need to consider the intermediate in the reaction, the carbocation, and its stability, to determine which one forms. The most stable carbocation is the one fastest to form—and it is the carbocation that determines the final product (see Figure 4.12).

The only product formed in this reaction is 2-chloro-2-methylpropane (*tert*-butyl chloride), as the intermediate *tert*-butyl cation is more stable than the isobutyl cation involved in the alternative pathway. The relative order of stability for carbocations is tertiary > secondary > primary (see Scheme 4.4). Once again, σ-conjugation is at work. Alkyl groups are able to stabilize the positive charge, because overlap between the adjacent sigma bonds and the empty p-orbital spreads the positive charge and stabilizes it. (Some books call this effect 'hyperconjugation', but 'sigma conjugation' is more descriptive.)

These electrophilic addition reactions are **regioselective** (see Figure 4.13). This term is applied to any reaction where two (or more) isomers are produced, but one predominates. Note

Scheme 4.3

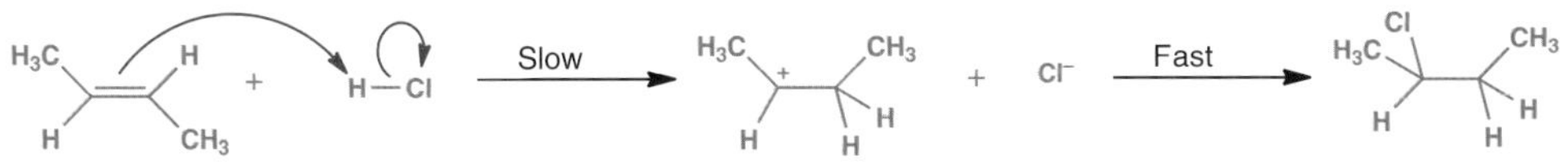

Scheme 4.4

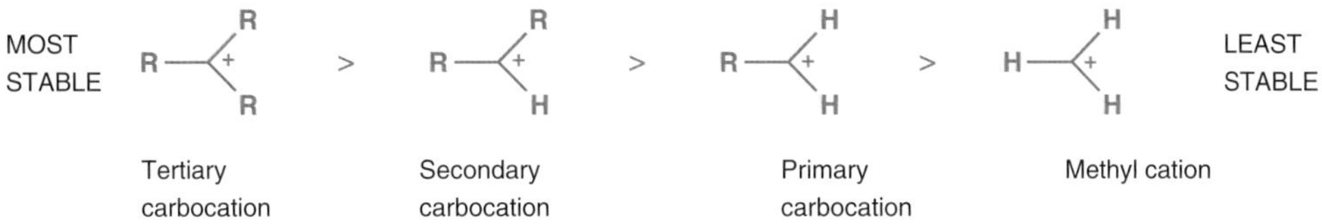

MOST STABLE							LEAST STABLE
Tertiary carbocation		Secondary carbocation		Primary carbocation		Methyl cation	

Figure 4.12 Addition of HCl to 2-methylpropene

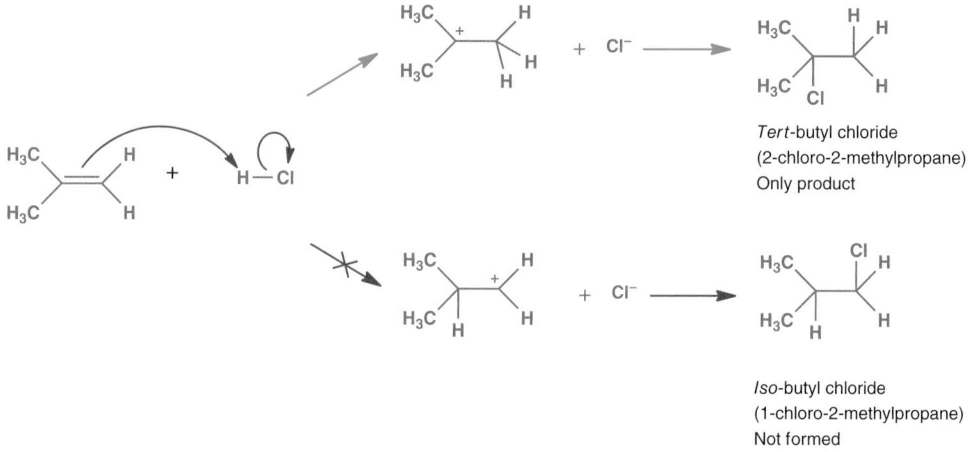

H_3C
H
Cl^-
Cl
Tert-butyl chloride
(2-chloro-2-methylpropane)
Only product
Iso-butyl chloride
(1-chloro-2-methylpropane)
Not formed

that, in many cases, the minor isomer is actually undetectable, but the reaction is still regioselective because the mechanism allows a second isomer to be formed in principle.

When pent-2-ene is reacted with HBr, the reaction is not regioselective, as a secondary carbocation is the intermediate in the pathway to each of the products, 2-bromo- or 3-bromopentane (see Scheme 4.5).

A general rule for determining the products of such reactions is as follows:

The proton of an acid (H–X) adds to the carbon in the double bond that already has the most hydrogens.

Figure 4.13 An example of regioselectivity in electrophilic addition

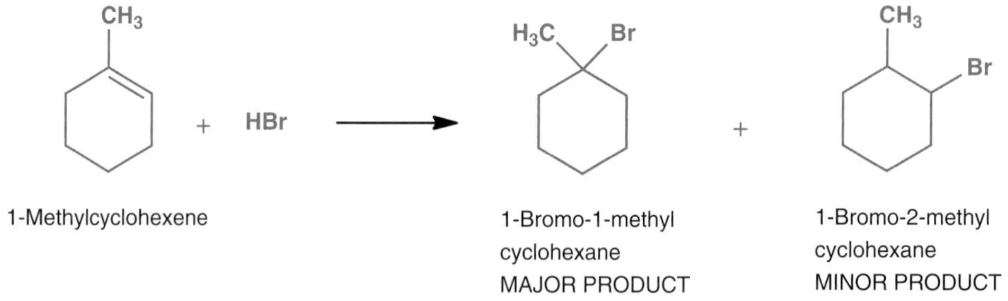

CH_3
HBr
H_3C
Br
1-Methylcyclohexene
1-Bromo-1-methyl cyclohexane
MAJOR PRODUCT
1-Bromo-2-methyl cyclohexane
MINOR PRODUCT

Scheme 4.5

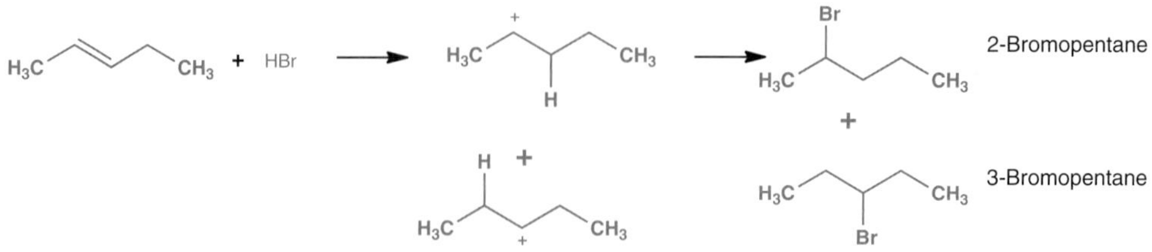

H_3C
CH_3
HBr
H
Br
2-Bromopentane
3-Bromopentane

Box 4.4 Vladimir Vasilyevich Markovnikov

Vladimir Vasilyevich Markovnikov (1837–1904) was born in Nizhny Novgorod and studied at Kazan University. Although initially an economist, he changed to chemistry. After graduating, he worked at the Universities of Kazan and Saint Petersburg. Later, he was a professor of chemistry at Kazan, Odessa and Moscow Universities.

Although best known for 'Markovnikov's rule', he also contributed to organic chemistry by synthesizing rings containing four and seven carbons, thus disproving the idea that carbon could form only five- and six-membered rings.

This is often referred to as Markovnikov's rule, after the Russian scientist who was the first to recognize this phenomenon (see Box 4.4). A more modern and general take on Markovnikov's rule is:

In an electrophilic addition to an alkene, the electrophile (E^+) adds in such a way as to form the most stable intermediate.

This second definition is the more useful.

❯ Markovnikov's rule is discussed in more detail in Chapter 2, 'Organic structure and bonding'.

Addition of HBr to alkenes in the presence of peroxides

HBr can add to alkenes to give so-called anti-Markovnikov products. This type of addition proceeds via the free-radical pathway shown in Figure 4.14. In this case, it is the stability of the radical intermediate that determines which product is formed. Free radical stabilities run in the same order as the carbocation stabilities shown in Scheme 4.4, and for the same reasons.

Figure 4.14 An example of a free-radical reaction pathway

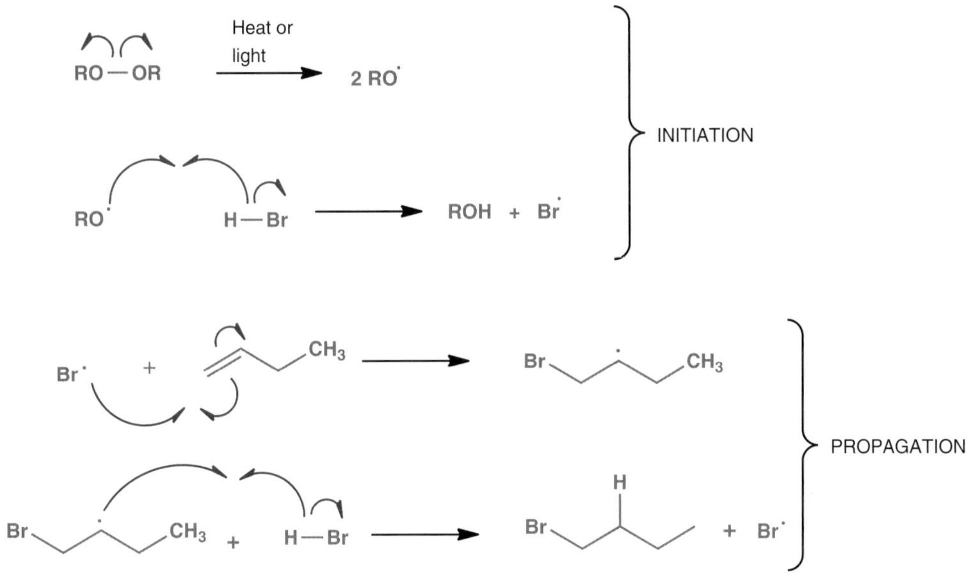

Self-check 4.7

What would be the major products, A, B and C, from the reactions shown?

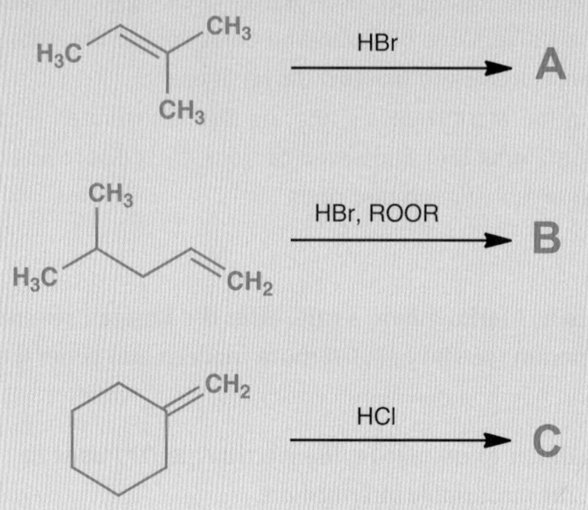

Note that in the reaction pathway in Figure 4.14 it is the bromine radical which first attacks the double bond. The radical intermediate then takes a proton from HBr to give the product. The mechanism has three distinct phases—initiation, propagation and termination, the first two of which are shown in the reaction scheme. Polymers can also be formed by free-radical reactions, as we shall see later.

Termination involves the reaction of two radicals to give a product which cannot propagate the chain reaction further. Only HBr has the correct bond energy to undergo this free-radical reaction. The HCl bond is too strong, while HI tends to break down to form ions rather than free radicals.

Addition of water and alcohols to alkenes

The O−H bond in water is strong, so water is only a very weak acid and is unable to react with an alkene as an electrophile. Therefore, the addition of water to an alkene (hydration) requires some assistance in the form of an acid catalyst, most often sulfuric acid (H_2SO_4). The presence of the acid now provides the reaction with an electrophile, namely H^+ (as H_3O^+) (see Scheme 4.6).

The product of the hydration of an alkene is an alcohol, and the mechanism for its formation is shown in Scheme 4.7. Note that the Markovnikov product is formed.

As you might expect, alcohols react with alkenes in much the same way as water. Again, a strong acid catalyst is required and the products of such reactions are ethers. As you can see in Scheme 4.8, the mechanism is very similar to that for hydration.

Scheme 4.6

$$H_2SO_4 + H_2O \rightleftharpoons HSO_3^- + H_3\overset{+}{O}$$

Hydronium ion

Scheme 4.7

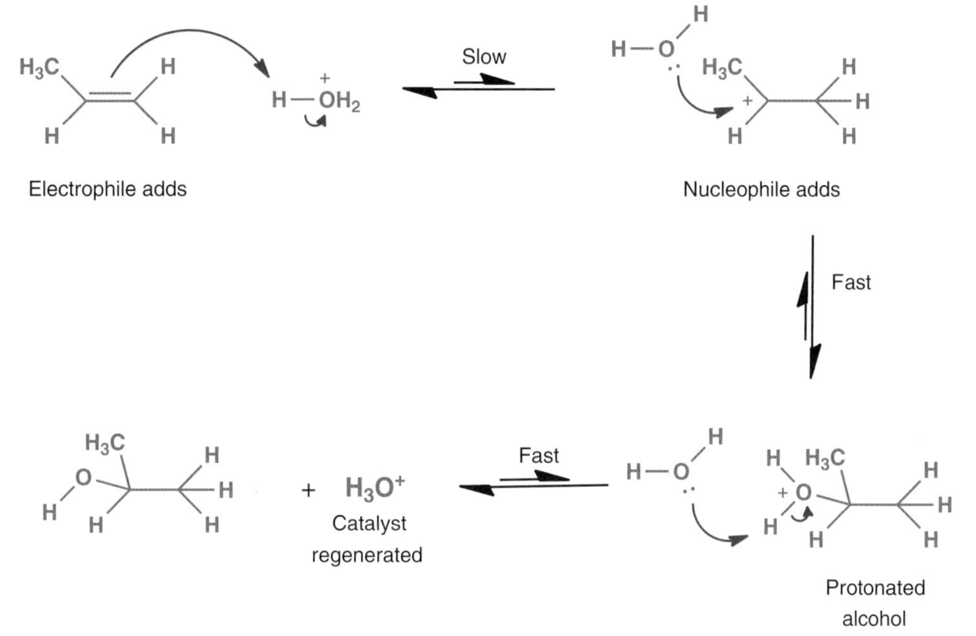

Electrophile adds

Slow

Nucleophile adds

Fast

Protonated
alcohol

Fast

+ H_3O^+

Catalyst
regenerated

Scheme 4.8

Electrophile adds

Slow

Nucleophile adds

Fast

Protonated ether

Fast

Catalyst
regenerated

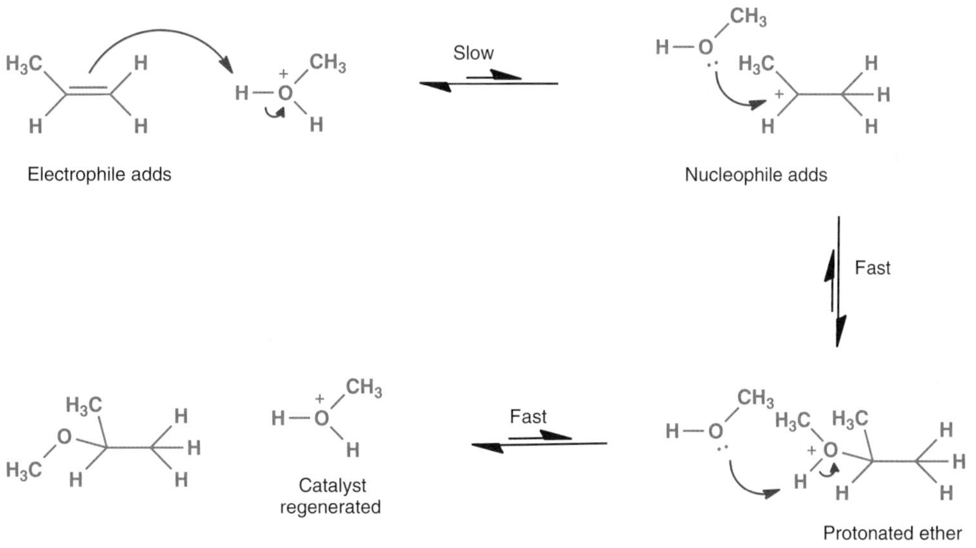

Addition of halogens to alkenes

Chlorine (Cl_2), bromine (Br_2) and sometimes iodine (I_2), add across the alkene carbon–carbon double bond to form **vicinal dihalides**. Indeed, the decolorization of bromine solution is used as a test for the presence of alkenes.

A carbocation mechanism would lead to a mixture of *syn*- and *anti*- addition, but halogenation always involves *anti*-addition. (*Syn* addition refers to addition on the same side of

Self-check 4.8

What alkenes could be used as starting materials to make the compounds A, B, C, and D? What other reagents would be required?

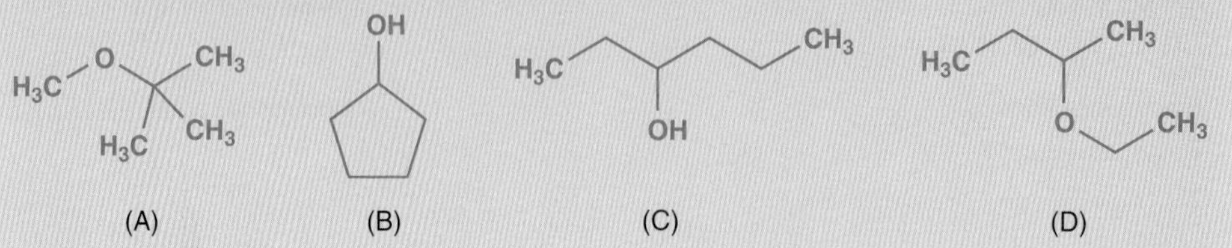

(A) (B) (C) (D)

Self-check 4.9

Draw the products of the reaction of chlorine with 2-methylpropene and 3-methylbut-1-ene.

the double bond; *anti*-addition describes addition to opposite sides of the double bond.) The π electrons of the double bond attack to give a cationic intermediate and a bromide ion. The intermediate is not a simple carbocation, but something called a cyclic halonium ion (here a bromonium ion), which is more stable. The bromide ion then attacks the cation from the rear, leading to the vicinal dibromide product (see Scheme 4.9).

Addition of hydrogen to alkenes (reduction)

The addition of hydrogen to an alkene can be achieved in the presence of precious-metal catalysts, such as palladium or platinum. This process is called **catalytic hydrogenation** and leads to the production of an alkane. The metals are usually in a finely divided state and are adsorbed onto activated charcoal.

While the overall hydrogenation reaction is highly exothermic, it does not occur in the absence of an appropriate catalyst. Rather than lowering the high activation energy of the original reaction (an energy barrier in the reaction pathway which must be overcome), the catalyst provides an alternative pathway (see Figure 4.15). Remember that a catalyst increases the rate of a reaction without itself changing or becoming part of the product.

Scheme 4.9

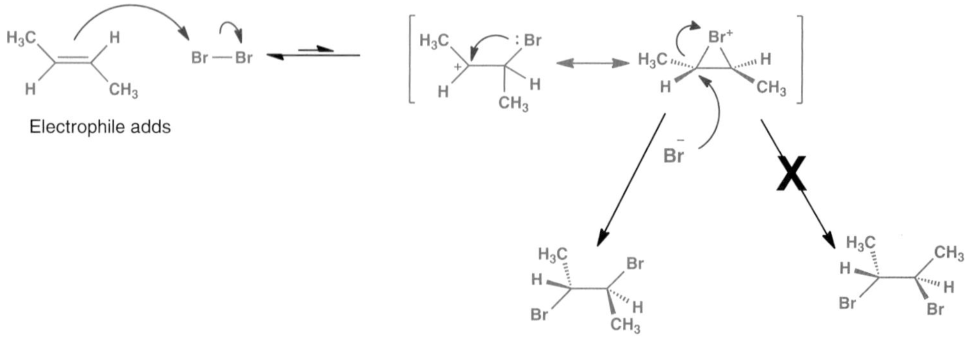

Electrophile adds

James is 32 and, because of his family history, is at risk of developing coronary heart disease. His GP has advised him to take statins to reduce his blood cholesterol levels but he does not want to take a drug that he will have to take for the rest of his life. Does he have any alternative ways of reducing his cholesterol levels?

Reflection questions

1. Would modifying his diet help to reduce his blood cholesterol levels?

2. What are *trans*-fats?

For answers, visit the online resources which accompany this textbook.

A full picture of the mechanism for such reactions does not yet exist, but it is known that both the alkene and the hydrogen must be adsorbed to the metal surface and that all the bond breaking and making events happen on that surface. Because the two hydrogens add from the solid surface, they add with *syn* (same side) stereochemistry. After formation, the alkane diffuses away from the surface as it is less strongly adsorbed.

Oxidation of alkenes

Alkenes are susceptible to combustion, typically to carbon dioxide and water, but also to a number of other oxidative reactions that introduce oxygen into molecules. These reactions include epoxidation, hydroxylation and oxidative cleavage.

Epoxides are three-membered cyclic ethers. They are useful synthetic intermediates and can be produced by reacting alkenes with peroxy acids. The reaction mechanism is a one-step concerted process, with several bonds breaking and forming at the same time. This means that there is no chance for rearrangement during the reaction and that the stereochemistry in the starting alkene is preserved in the epoxide (see Scheme 4.10).

The epoxides are generally stable and can be isolated. However, the presence of aqueous acid leads to protonation and then attack of the protonated epoxide by water to give a *trans*-1,2-diol (a glycol). There is no need to isolate the epoxide, and performing the reaction in aqueous peroxy acid leads directly to the diol product (see Scheme 4.11).

To form a *cis*-1,2-diol from an alkene, different reagents are required. Hydroxylation reactions are performed by reacting an alkene with either catalytic quantities of osmium tetroxide in the presence of hydrogen peroxide, or with cold, dilute aqueous potassium permanganate.

Figure 4.15 Hydrogenation of an alkene

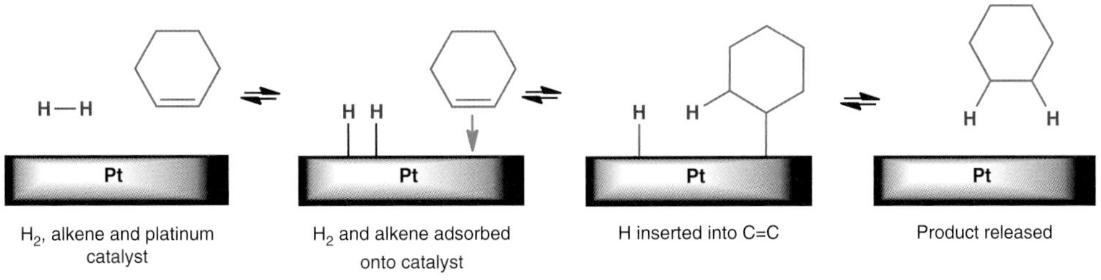

H₂, alkene and platinum catalyst / H₂ and alkene adsorbed onto catalyst / H inserted into C=C / Product released

119

Scheme 4.10

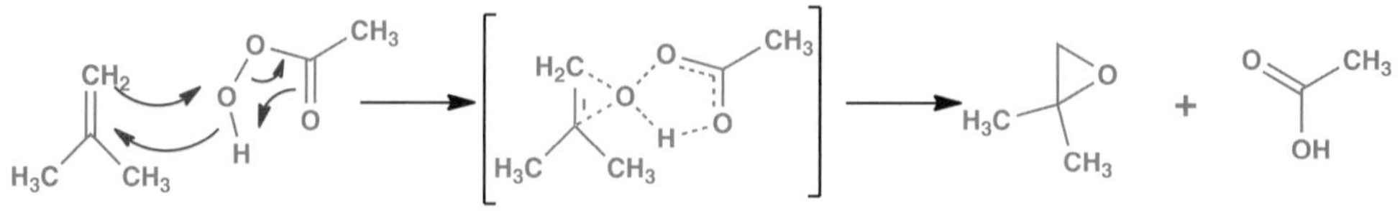

Scheme 4.11

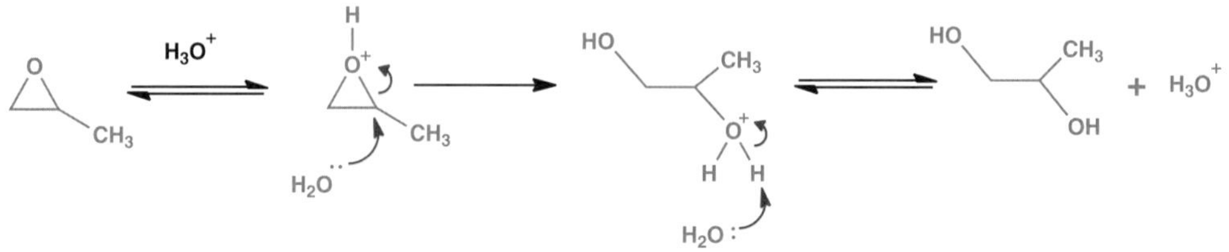

The former gives higher yields, but osmium tetroxide is expensive, volatile and highly toxic. In both cases, the two C–O bonds are formed simultaneously through esters (osmate or manganate), meaning that they add to the same face of the double bond and give the *cis*-diol.

> For more information about epoxides and glycols, see Chapter 5, 'Alcohols, phenols, ethers, organic halogen compounds, and amines'.

Oxidative cleavage can be achieved using warm or acidic solutions of potassium permanganate, leading to ketones and aldehydes. Any aldehydes formed are quickly oxidized to carboxylic acids (see Scheme 4.12).

Ozone is also capable of cleaving carbon–carbon double bonds. It is a milder oxidizing agent than permanganate and allows for isolation of both the ketones and aldehydes produced (see Scheme 4.13).

Scheme 4.12

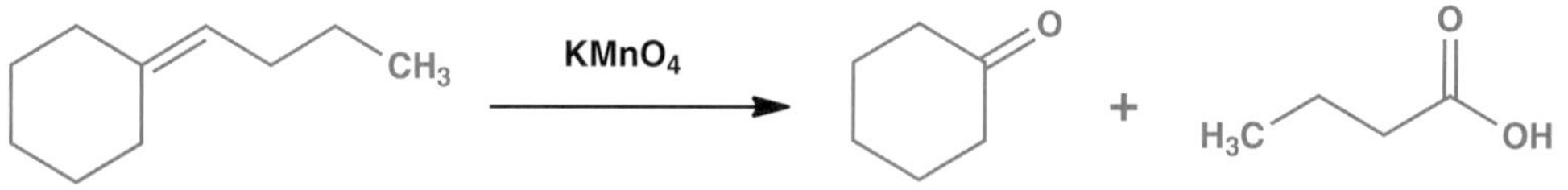

Scheme 4.13

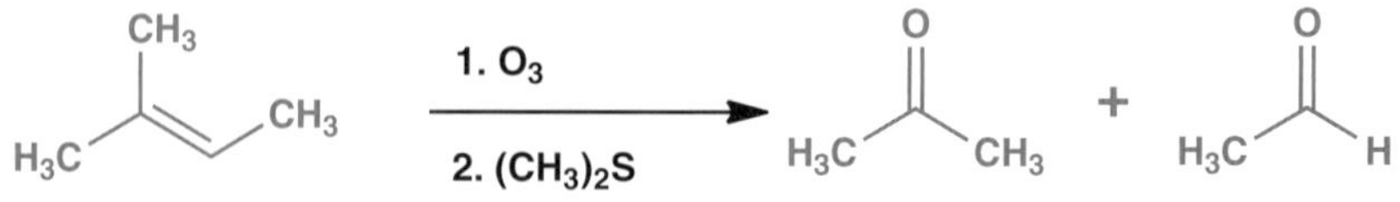

> Because of the presence of the π bond, alkenes are very reactive. The type of reaction they undergo is electrophilic addition.

Synthetic polymers

We encounter polymers (from the Greek for 'many things') every day of our lives, generally without giving them a second thought. You may have spent the early years of your life in disposable nappies. The absorbent material in these products is the sodium salt of poly(acrylic acid), which can absorb up to 200–300 times its mass in water! As a student, could you really imagine being without food wrap, Superglue, plastic bottles and synthetic fibres? One day you may benefit from artificial joints. All of these are made from polymers. Some common polymers that will have touched your lives are shown in Table 4.3.

Many important polymers (though by no means all) are prepared from substituted alkenes. These are termed chain-growth polymers due to the mechanism of their formation. Table 4.3 provides a small selection and should bring home to you the importance of these compounds.

So what is a polymer? Well, essentially, it is a large molecule (macromolecule) made by linking together smaller repeating units called **monomers** in a process called polymerization. The most common method for making polymers from alkenes is free-radical polymerization. You have seen earlier in the chapter that radical reactions have three distinct steps: initiation, propagation and termination.

Table 4.3   Some common vinyl polymers

Monomer	Repeat unit	Name	Uses
$H_2C{=}CH_2$	$-[CH_2-CH_2]-$	polyethene polyethylene	films, toys, bottles, plastic bags
$H_2C{=}CHCl$	$-[CH_2-CH]-$ with Cl	poly(vinyl chloride) (PVC)	flooring, pipes, window surrounds, 'squeeze' bottles
$H_2C{=}C$ with H and phenyl group	$-[CH_2-CH]-$ with phenyl group	poly(styrene)	toys, egg cartons, packaging, hot drink cups
$H_2C{=}C$ with CH_3 and $-OCH_3$, O	$-[CH_2-CH]-$ with $COCH_3$, O	poly(methyl methacrylate) (perspex, plexiglas)	skylights, signs, lighting fixtures, solar panels
$F_2C{=}CF_2$	$-[CF_2-CF_2]-$	poly(tetrafluoroethylene) (Teflon)	non-stick surfaces, cable insulation
$H_2C{=}CHCOOH$	$-[CH_2-CH]-$ with COH, O	poly(acrylic acid)	disposable nappies

Figure 4.16 Initiation, propagation and termination in radical polymerization

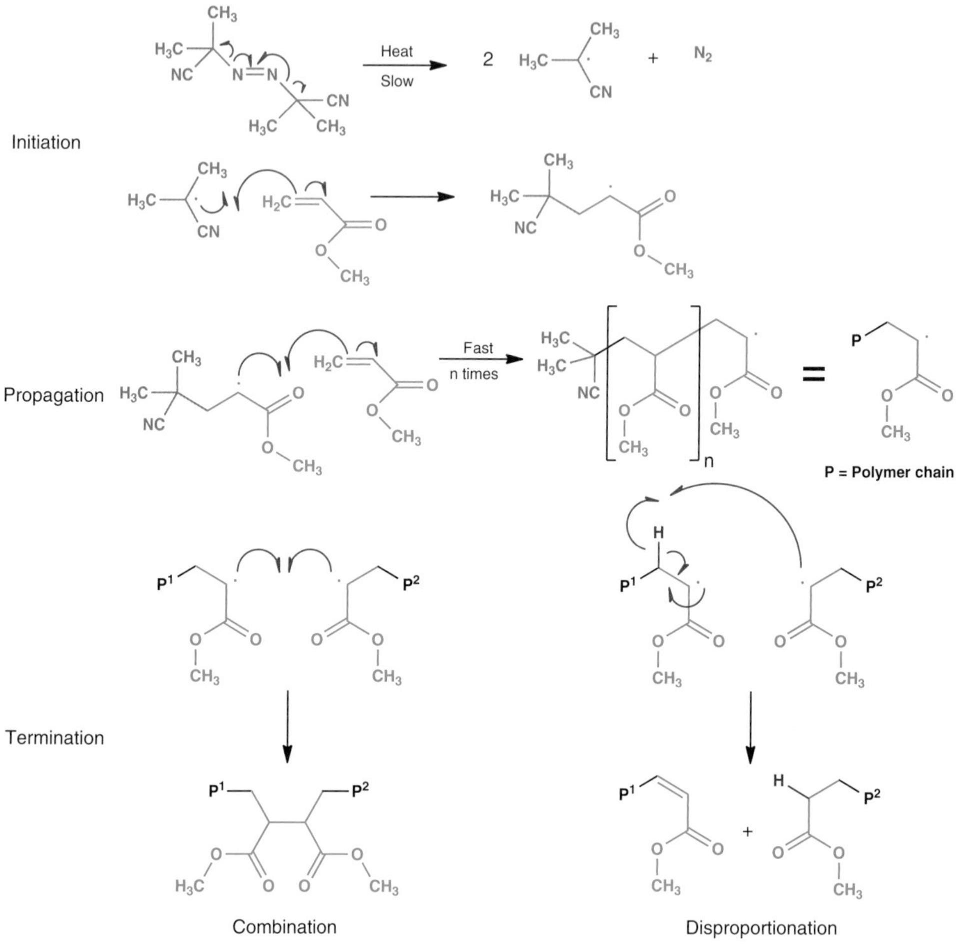

Initiation

Propagation

Termination

P = Polymer chain

Combination

Disproportionation

In radical polymerization, the initiation process is actually two steps—one to create the radicals and the second to form the radical that will propagate the chain reaction. The radical is an electrophile and thus adds to the carbon bearing the greater number of hydrogen atoms. Once the radical is formed, it adds to another monomer molecule, creating another radical and propagating the chain reaction (see Figure 4.16).

Destruction of the propagating site stops the chain reaction, and this can happen in a number of ways. Two major pathways are (i) the combination of two free radicals and (ii) the disproportionation of two free radicals. Look at Figure 4.16, and note that the disproportionation reaction leads to an alkene, from which further initiation can occur, and a 'dead' chain (the alkane on the right). The third major pathway (not shown) is through reaction of the propagating chain with impurities.

4.5 ALKYNES—PREPARATION AND REACTIONS

In this section we will deal with the reactions of alkynes. As you might expect, these reactions are very similar to those of alkenes, because of the presence of two π bonds. However, you need to be aware of some significant differences.

Preparation of alkynes

Alkynes are much more reactive than alkanes and alkenes. This means that they are much rarer, and are normally synthesized in the laboratory rather than being isolated from natural sources (see, however, Box 4.5).

Acetylide ions as synthetic intermediates

As mentioned in Section 4.2, the proton of a terminal alkyne is *relatively* acidic. Thus, a strong base may abstract this proton to give an acetylide ion. The acetylide ion is a very useful synthetic intermediate.

The formation of carbon–carbon bonds is extremely important in organic chemistry and acetylide ions allow chemists to perform such reactions. For example, reaction of an unhindered alkyl halide with an acetylide ion leads to formation of a carbon–carbon bond to give a larger internal alkyne (see Scheme 4.14).

This alkylation reaction is a bimolecular nucleophilic substitution (S_N2), the mechanism of which is well understood. The negatively charged acetylide anion attacks the carbon bearing the halide, which carries a partial positive charge, kicking out the bromide ion. These reactions are very useful, as they allow terminal alkynes to be turned into internal alkynes of any length we choose, simply by picking the right alkyl halide (see Scheme 4.15).

Acetylide ions also react with carbonyl groups, as found in aldehydes and ketones (see Chapter 6), to give alcohols, after protonation of the alkoxide ion initially formed (see Scheme 4.16).

Box 4.5 Alkynes in medicines

Alkynes are not as prevalent in nature as alkenes, but some plants use them to protect against disease or predators. An example is capillin, which shows fungicidal activity and is produced by the oriental wormwood plant. The alkyne functional group is also rare in drugs, the most common example being 17-ethynyl estradiol (ethinylestradiol), a common ingredient in birth control tablets.

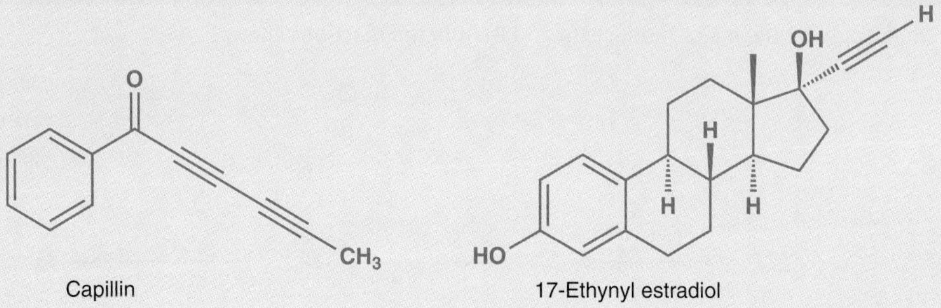

Capillin

17-Ethynyl estradiol

Scheme 4.14

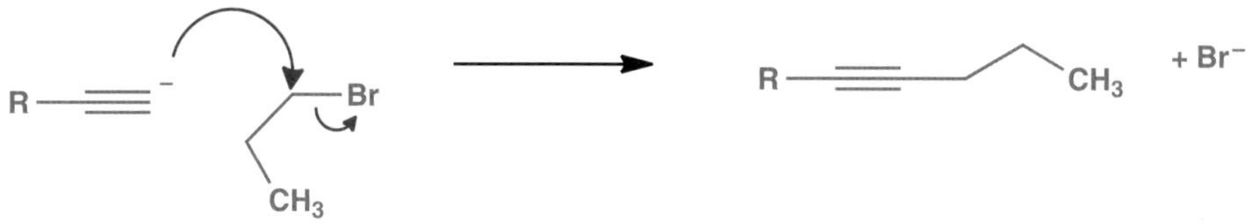

Scheme 4.15

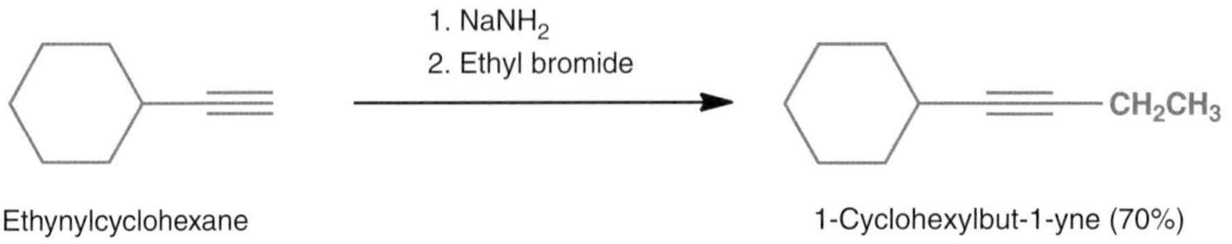
1. NaNH2
2. Ethyl bromide
CH2CH3
Ethynylcyclohexane
1-Cyclohexylbut-1-yne (70%)

Scheme 4.16

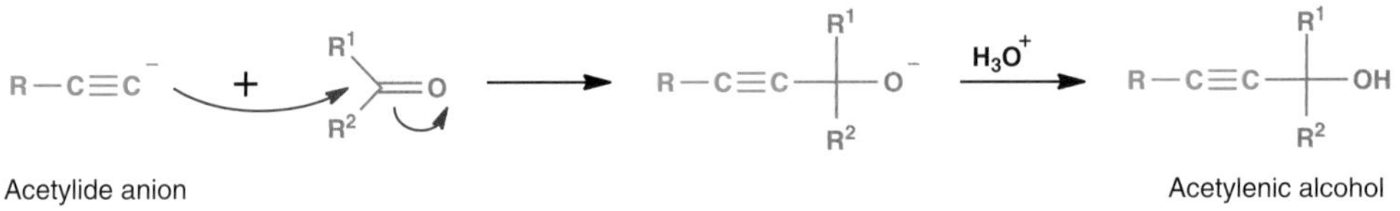
R—C≡C
R1
R2
H3O+
OH
Acetylide anion
Acetylenic alcohol

Addition to formaldehyde gives a primary (1°) alcohol, while addition to higher aldehydes gives secondary (2°) alcohols (see Scheme 4.17). Finally, addition of acetylide ions to ketones furnishes us with tertiary (3°) alcohols.

The preparation of alkynes using elimination reactions

It is possible, in some cases, to prepare alkynes through a double dehydrohalogenation of **vicinal** or **geminal** dihalides. The first loss of HX gives a vinyl halide, which can lose a second HX molecule under extremely basic conditions (see Scheme 4.18).

High temperatures are also required, and these rather brutal conditions can lead to side reactions, which lower the yield. The use of KOH tends to give the most stable internal alkyne, as shown in Scheme 4.19.

Self-check 4.10

What would be the major products (A and B) from the reactions shown?

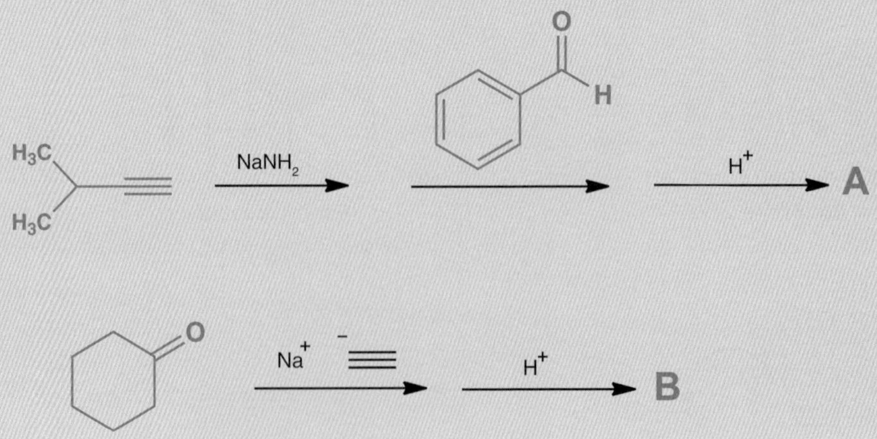
H3C
H3C
NaNH2
H
H+
A
Na+
H+
B

Scheme 4.17

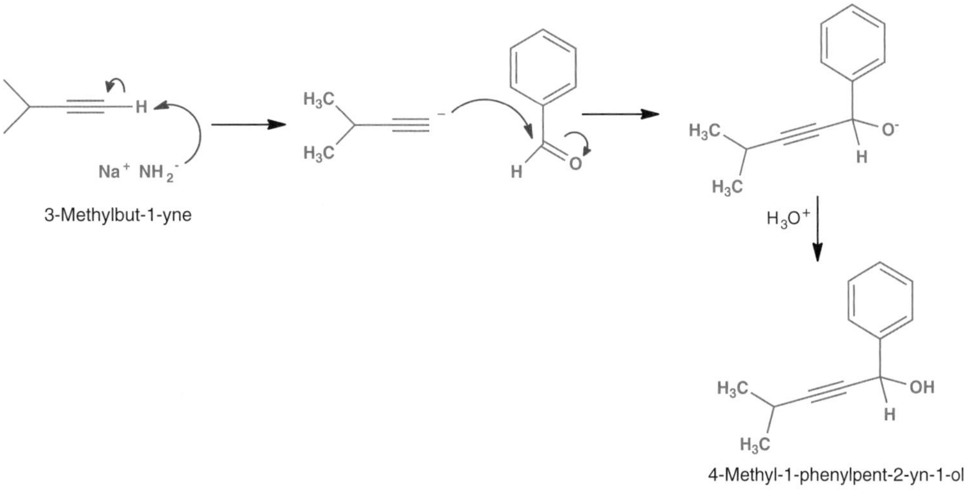
H
Na$^+$ NH$_2^-$
3-Methylbut-1-yne
H$_3$C
H$_3$C
H
O
H$_3$C
H$_3$C
O$^-$
H
H$_3$O$^+$
H$_3$C
H$_3$C
OH
H
4-Methyl-1-phenylpent-2-yn-1-ol

Scheme 4.18

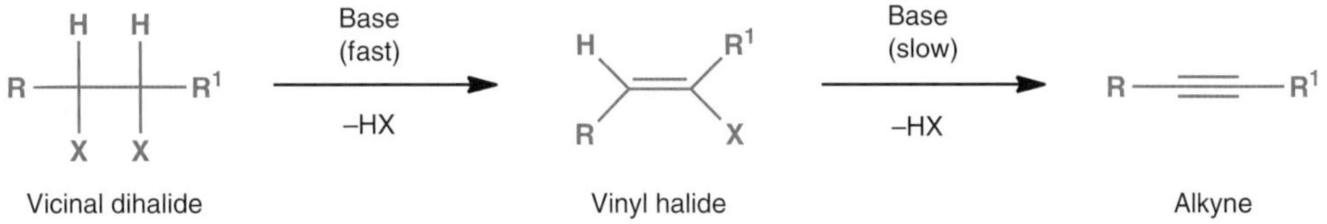
H H
R
R^1
X X
Vicinal dihalide
Base
(fast)
–HX
H
R^1
R
X
Vinyl halide
Base
(slow)
–HX
R
R^1
Alkyne

Scheme 4.19

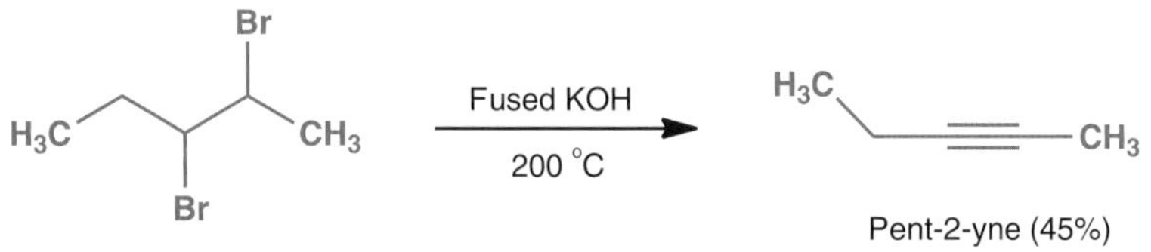
Br
H$_3$C
CH$_3$
Br
Fused KOH
200 °C
H$_3$C
CH$_3$
Pent-2-yne (45%)

Box 4.6 Synthesis of ethchlorvynol

The synthesis of ethchlorvynol—a drug used to cause drowsiness and induce sleep—involves the addition of acetylide ion to a carbonyl group. The non-polar nature of the drug enhances its distribution into the fatty tissue of the central nervous system.

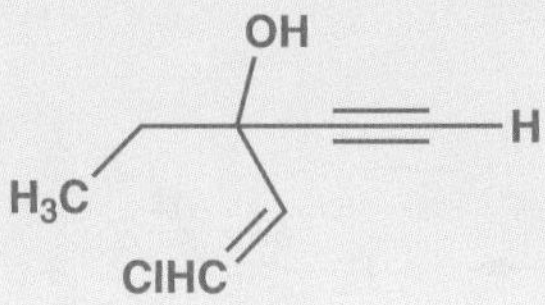
OH
H
H$_3$C
ClHC

Reactions of alkynes

The carbon–carbon triple bond in an alkyne is made up of one σ and two π-bonds. These π-bonds are perpendicular to both the plane of the σ-bond and to each other.

This leads to areas of high electron density both above and below, and in front and at the back of the σ-bond. Because of the shape of these π-bonds, they blend to form a cylinder of electron density which encircles the σ-bond. This makes alkynes electron rich and, therefore, they behave as nucleophiles. Consequently, the reaction profile of alkynes is very similar to that of alkenes — that is, they typically undergo addition reactions across the carbon–carbon triple bond.

Before we consider these addition reactions, we should mention the combustion of alkynes. In air, alkynes burn with a luminous, smoky flame. When they are combined with pure oxygen, the mixtures are explosive and are used in welding (for example, in oxyacetylene torches). The reaction is extremely exothermic ($\Delta H = -1300$ kJ mol^{-1}) and temperatures reach around 3,000 °C (Figure 4.17). Acetylene (ethyne) undergoes complete combustion under these conditions.

$$2C_2H_2(g) + 5O_2(g) \rightarrow 4CO_2(g) + 2H_2O(l)$$

Addition of hydrogen halides and halogens to alkynes

Moving to the addition reactions, let us first consider the addition of hydrogen halides (HX). The mechanism of these reactions is the same as for addition to alkenes. The first, slow step is the breaking of a relatively weak π-bond. The second step, the reaction of the carbocation intermediate with the negatively charged halide anion, is rapid (see Scheme 4.20).

For terminal alkynes, the proton adds to the sp carbon bearing the hydrogen, as this leads to the more stable secondary carbocation. For example, the addition of HBr to pent-1-yne leads only to the Markovnikov product, 2-bromopent-1-ene. In the presence of excess HX, a second addition occurs, again following Markovnikov's rule.

When excess HX is added to internal alkynes, where the sp carbons bear different groups, two products are formed. This is because H$^+$ can add with equal ease to either carbon of the triple bond in the first step of the reaction, as shown for the addition of excess HBr to pent-2-yne in Scheme 4.21.

In the presence of excess HBr, the alkene products of Scheme 4.21 react to give two geminal dihalides: 2,2-dibromopentane and 3,3-dibromopentane (see Scheme 4.22). This happens as the second molecule of HBr generally adds with the same orientation as the first.

Addition of HBr to symmetrical alkynes (internal alkynes bearing the same substituents) is much less complex. Reaction of an excess of HBr with hex-3-yne leads only to 3,3-dibromohexane.

Halogens add to alkynes in the same way as to alkenes, generally yielding mixtures of *cis* and *trans*-isomers. In the presence of excess halogen, a second addition reaction can occur to give the tetrahaloalkane (see Scheme 4.23).

Scheme 4.20

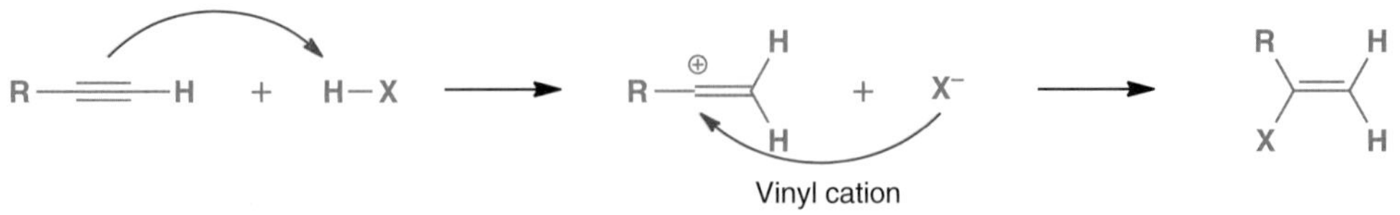

Vinyl cation

Scheme 4.21

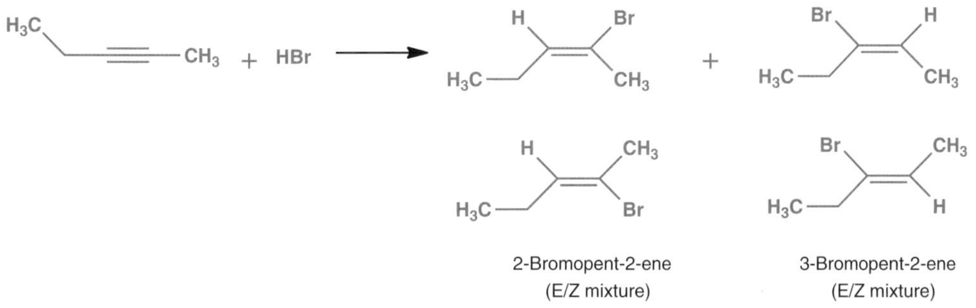

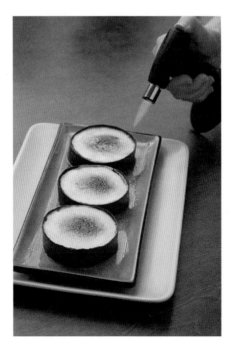

2-Bromopent-2-ene
(E/Z mixture)

3-Bromopent-2-ene
(E/Z mixture)

Scheme 4.22

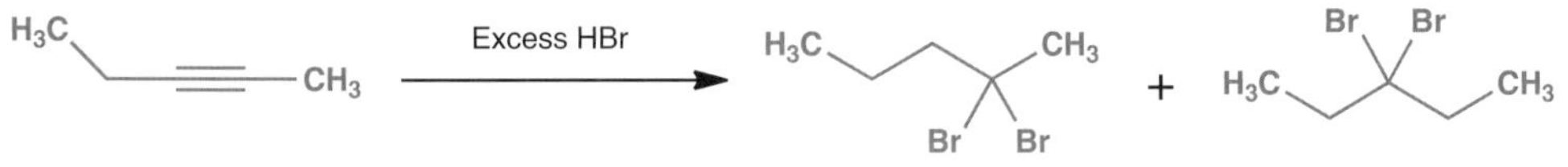

Excess HBr

Scheme 4.23

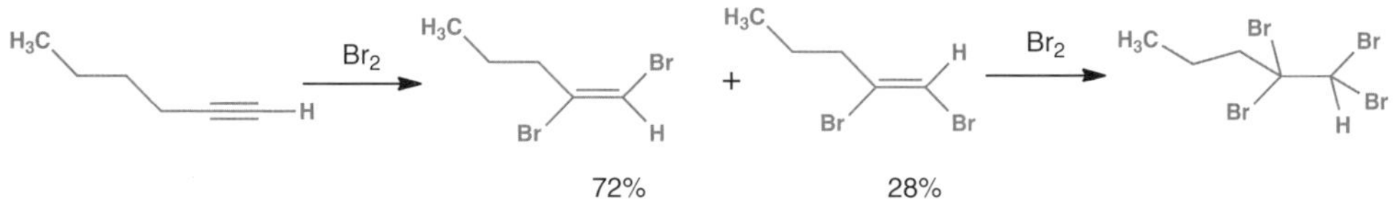

Br₂

72%   28%

Br₂

Figure 4.17 Using an oxyacetylene torch to make crème brulee. The high temperatures create the perfect crisp top! *Source*: crème brulee blow torch. Istock File #20895116
iStock.com/skodonnell

Self-check 4.11

Draw the mechanism for the reaction of excess HBr to hex-3-yne.

Self-check 4.12

Draw the products of the following reactions.
1. But-1-yne +HBr (1 equivalent)
2. 4-Methylhex-2-yne +HCl (1 equivalent)
3. 2-Bromo-but-1-ene +HCl (excess)
4. Oct-4-yne +HBr (excess)
5. Oct-2-yne +HCl (excess)

Addition of water to alkynes

Acid–catalysed addition of water (hydration) to alkynes is also seen, as with alkenes. The initial products of these reactions are **enols**, which rearrange immediately to give ketones (see Chapter 6). The enol and ketone differ only in the location of the double bond and are termed keto–enol tautomers. **Tautomers** are isomers that are in rapid equilibrium. The more stable isomer predominates, and this is usually the ketone (see Scheme 4.24).

With symmetrical, internal alkynes, a single product results. Hydration of an internal alkyne bearing different substituents on the *sp* carbons may lead to the formation of two products.

Terminal alkynes are less reactive towards the addition of water than their internal alkyne relatives. However, they can be hydrated if mercuric acid (Hg⁺) is added to the acidic medium. The mercuric acid acts as a catalyst to increase the rate of the reaction (see Scheme 4.25).

Scheme 4.24

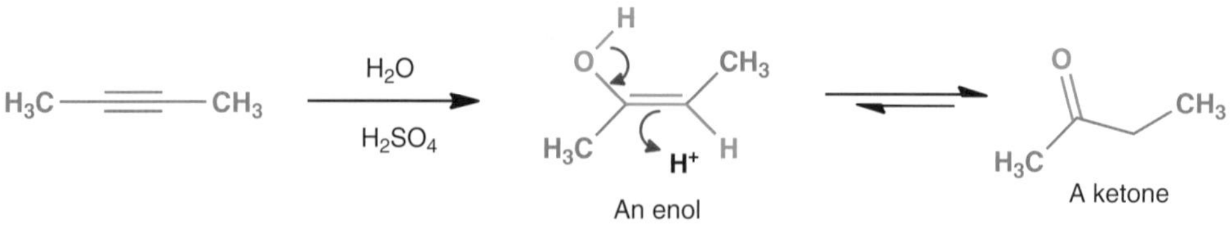

An enol

A ketone

Scheme 4.25

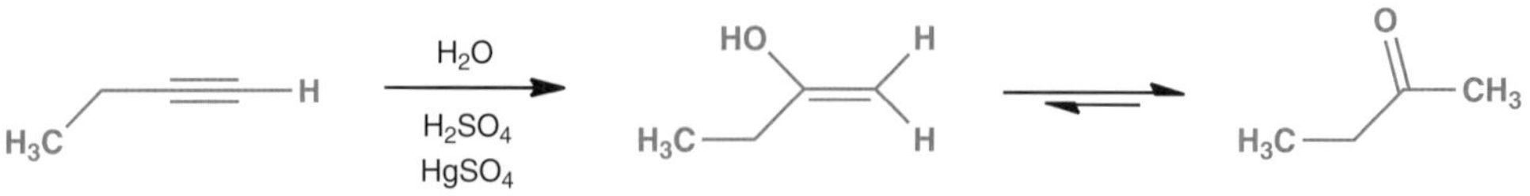

Self-check 4.13

What is the product of the hydration of hex-3-yne? There are two possible products of the reaction of pent-2-yne with water/acid. What are they?

Addition of hydrogen to alkynes (reduction)

Hydrogen adds across the alkyne triple bond in the presence of a metal catalyst, typically palladium or platinum, much as with alkenes. The initial product of this hydrogenation is an alkene, but it is difficult to halt the reaction at this point. The efficiency of the catalysts used means that hydrogen will tend to add across the double bond of the alkene formed. Thus, an alkane is generally the result of such a reaction (see Scheme 4.26).

To limit the hydrogenation reaction and allow the preparation of alkenes from alkynes, a 'poisoned' or partially deactivated catalyst is used (see Scheme 4.27). The most common of these is Lindlar's catalyst, which can be prepared by treating the conventional palladium catalyst with, for example, lead acetate or quinoline.

The hydrogens add to the same side of the triple bond—this is termed *cis* (syn) addition—to give a *cis*-alkene. *Trans* (anti) addition of hydrogen to an alkyne, to give a *trans*-alkene, is achieved by reacting the alkyne with either sodium or lithium in liquid ammonia, generally at −78 °C. The reaction proceeds via a radical mechanism.

Oxidation of alkynes

The addition of cold, aqueous potassium permanganate to an internal alkyne under near-neutral conditions leads to the formation of an σ-diketone. The reaction is actually a double hydroxylation of each of the π bonds of the alkyne, followed by the loss of two molecules of water (see Scheme 4.28).

Under the same conditions, terminal alkynes yield keto-acids, probably via keto-aldehydes which are further oxidized (see Scheme 4.29).

Scheme 4.26

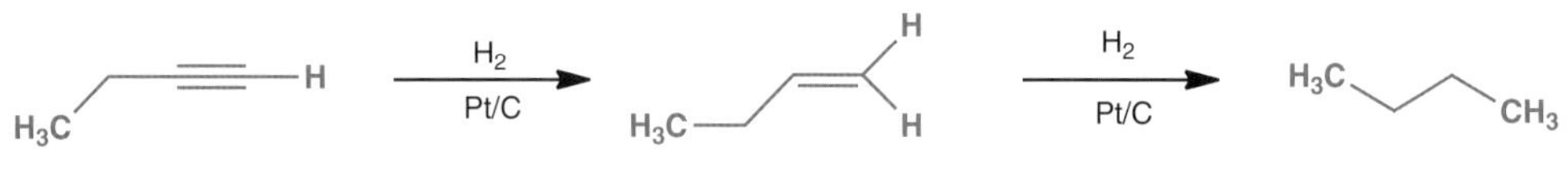

Scheme 4.27

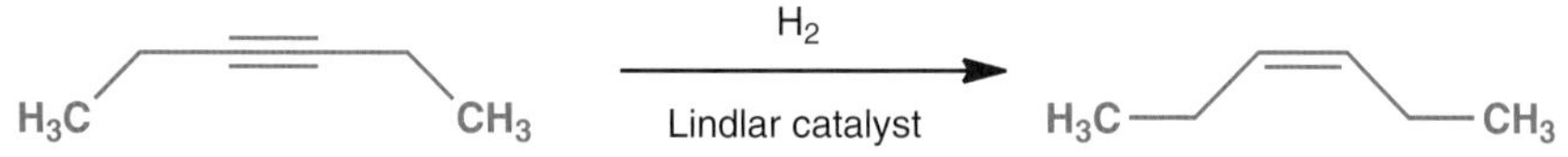

Scheme 4.28

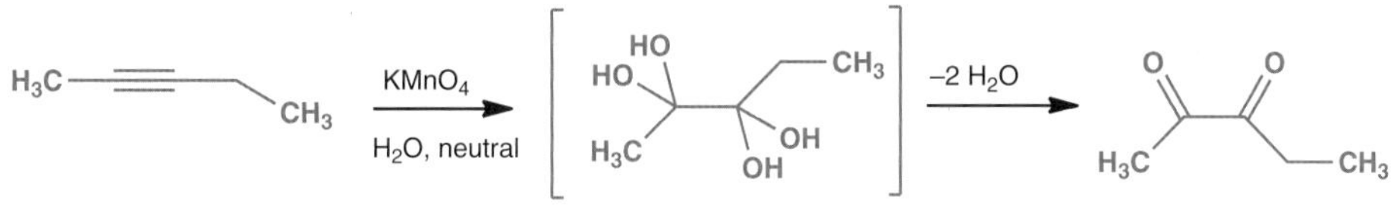

Scheme 4.29

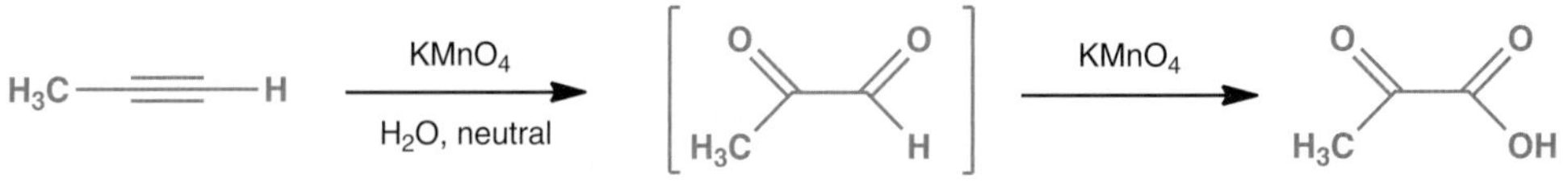

The product in Scheme 4.29 is pyruvic acid, the anion of which (pyruvate) is a key compound in several metabolic pathways. In the laboratory, this reaction is reasonably straightforward, even if the conditions are a little harsh, while nature has to work quite hard to prepare this molecule. In the body, 2 moles of pyruvic acid are made from 1 mole of D-glucose through the process called 'glycolysis'. This involves a lengthy series of enzyme-catalysed reactions.

> More details about glycolysis can be found in Chapter 11, 'Carbohydrates and carbohydrate metabolism'.

When an internal alkyne is treated with warm or basic potassium permanganate, the diketone is oxidatively cleaved to give carboxylic acid salts. These are converted to the free acid by adding dilute mineral acid, for example HCl (see Scheme 4.30).

The cleavage of a terminal alkyne gives a carboxylate ion and the formate ion. The latter is further oxidized to carbonate which, after protonation, yields carbonic acid. Under the aqueous conditions used, carbonic acid decomposes to water and carbon dioxide. You will see that this gives us a carboxylic acid that is one carbon shorter than the alkyne we started with (see Scheme 4.31).

Alkynes also undergo ozonolysis, i.e. the addition of ozone, O_3. Hydrolysis of the addition product cleaves the triple bond to give two carboxylic acids. For example, under these conditions 2-pentyne gives acetic (ethanoic) and propionic acids, while 1-pentyne gives butanoic and formic (methanoic) acids. Thus, the method can be used analytically, to determine the position of the carbon–carbon triple bond.

Scheme 4.30

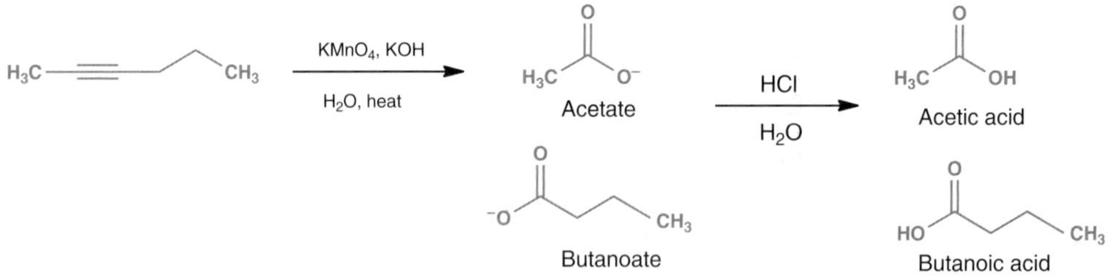

Scheme 4.31

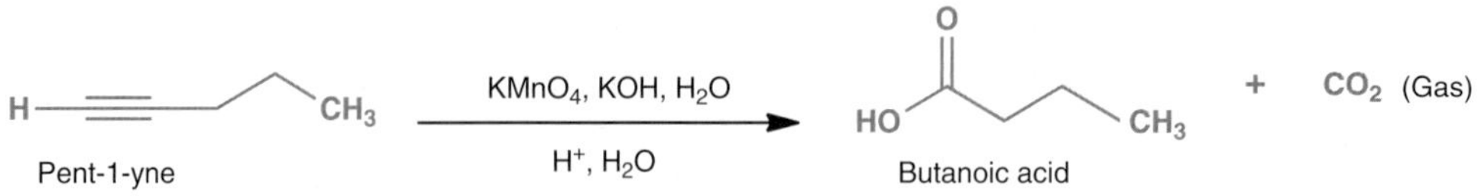

🔑 Alkynes, like alkenes, also undergo electrophilic addition reactions. Generally, but not always, two molecules of reactant are added.

4.6 HYDROCARBONS IN PHARMACY

In this section we will show how hydrocarbons may be used in pharmacy as drugs, excipients and biologically important molecules.

Active pharmaceutical ingredients (APIs)

No common APIs consist only of aliphatic hydrocarbons, although 'liquid paraffin' is still used occasionally as a laxative, especially in a veterinary setting. The limited use of aliphatic hydrocarbons stems from their lack of polarity: the interactions of drugs with receptors are normally polar. However, hydrophobic groups are very important in drugs—they help drugs cross membranes, so aliphatic hydrocarbons can play a role here. An alkyl chain can also contribute conformational flexibility; longer chains give more conformational flexibility.

An example of the effect of a hydrocarbon chain on drug action comes from the barbiturate family of hypnotic drugs. The parent compound, barbituric acid, has no hypnotic properties, but such properties can be introduced by the addition of substituents at the 5-position. The length and degree of branching in these chains influences both how potent a particular barbiturate is and also its duration of action. For example, secobarbital is slightly more potent than pentobarbital owing to a single extra carbon in one of the 5-substituents. Addition of a methyl group to one of the ring nitrogen atoms leads to methohexital. This compound shows a rapid onset and short duration of action, but also increased levels of side-effects. Generally, any modification that causes an increase in lipophilicity in this series leads to an increase in potency and rate of onset, but also increased excretion and a reduction in the duration of action.

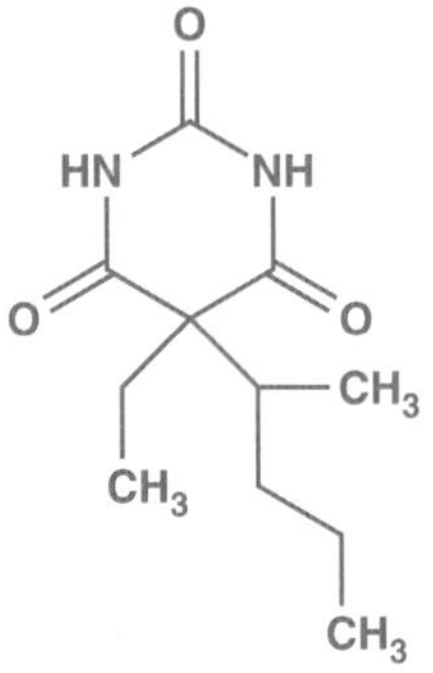

Pentobarbital

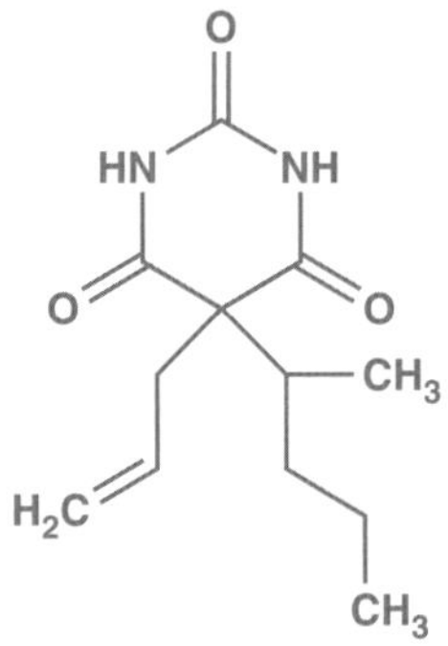

Secobarbital

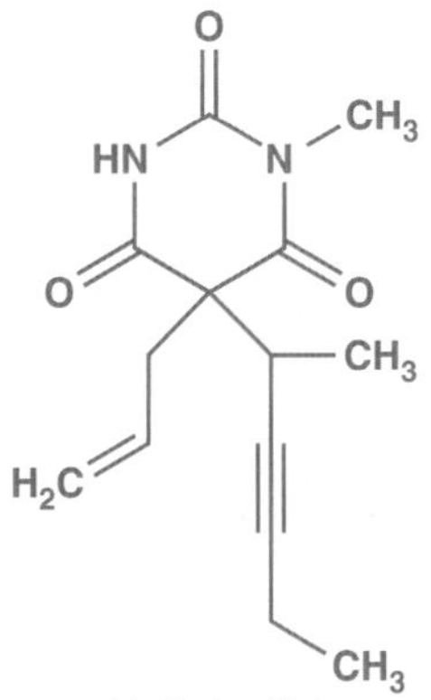

Methohexital

These two cases are examples of the kind of **structure–activity relationship studies** that are generally part of the modern drug discovery process. You will meet this topic in later stages of your pharmacy studies.

> More information about drug discovery processes can be found in Chapter 13, 'Origins of drug molecules'.

Stability of medicines

When considering the stability of a medicinal product, it is not only the active pharmaceutical ingredient (API) or 'drug' that we need to think about. Most of the mass of a tablet actually comes from other ingredients, called 'excipients'. These play diverse roles and include fillers, binding agents, lubricants, plasticizers, antioxidants, colouring and flavouring agents. In topical formulations, oils of various types are used, e.g. fatty acids, triglycerides and 'soft' paraffin (petroleum jelly).

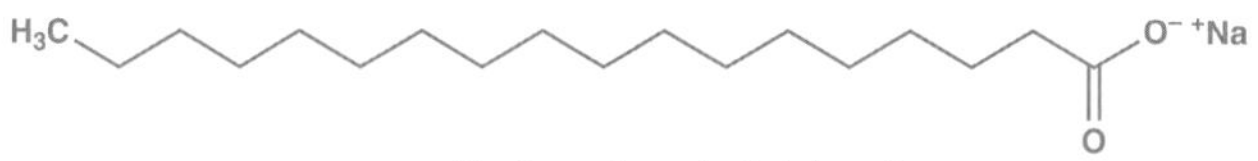

Sodium stearate (lubricant)

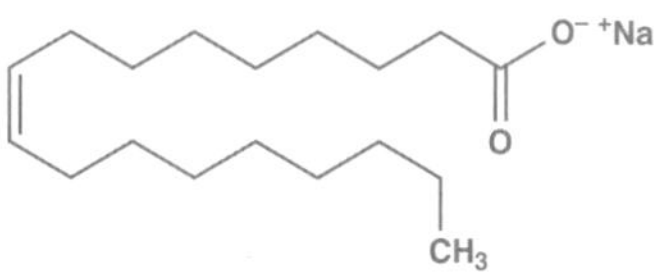

Sodium oleate (lubricant)

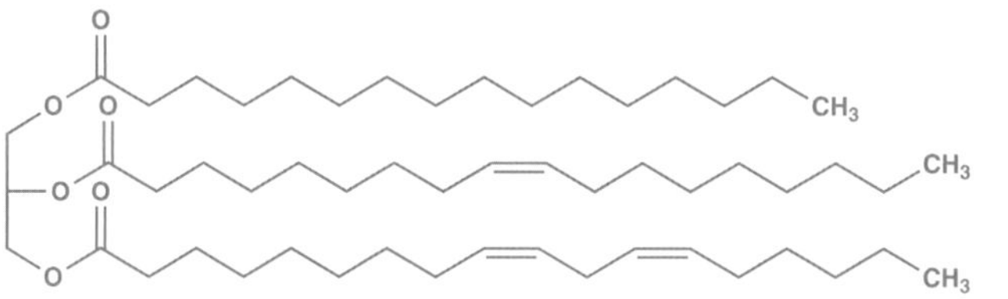

A mixed triglyceride formed from glycerol and three fatty acids (top to bottom): palmitic, oleic and linoleic acids

Many excipients contain hydrocarbons. The primary route through which the hydrocarbon chain degrades is through oxidation. As you saw earlier, there are many ways in which to oxidize hydrocarbons but, in terms of the stability of medicines, the most interesting is spontaneous oxidation in air at ambient temperatures.

Oxygen, although a diradical, is not a good initiator of the process, but light (and especially ultraviolet light) has sufficient energy to initiate oxidation reactions. Among aliphatic hydrocarbons, the most susceptible compounds are those with allylic groups, because the formation of an allylic radical is favoured. Allylic radicals are stabilized by resonance and so are more stable than the tertiary alkyl radicals you saw earlier.

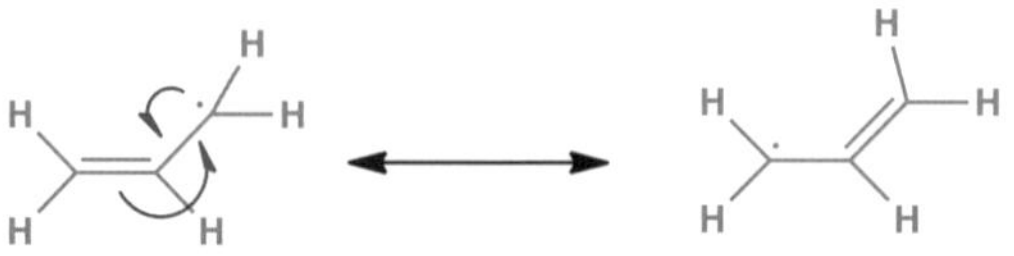

The oxidation of alkenes in unsaturated fatty acids causes fats and oils to taste and smell rancid. The oxidation of linoleic acid is shown in Figure 4.18, as an example.

Figure 4.18 The oxidation of linoleic acid

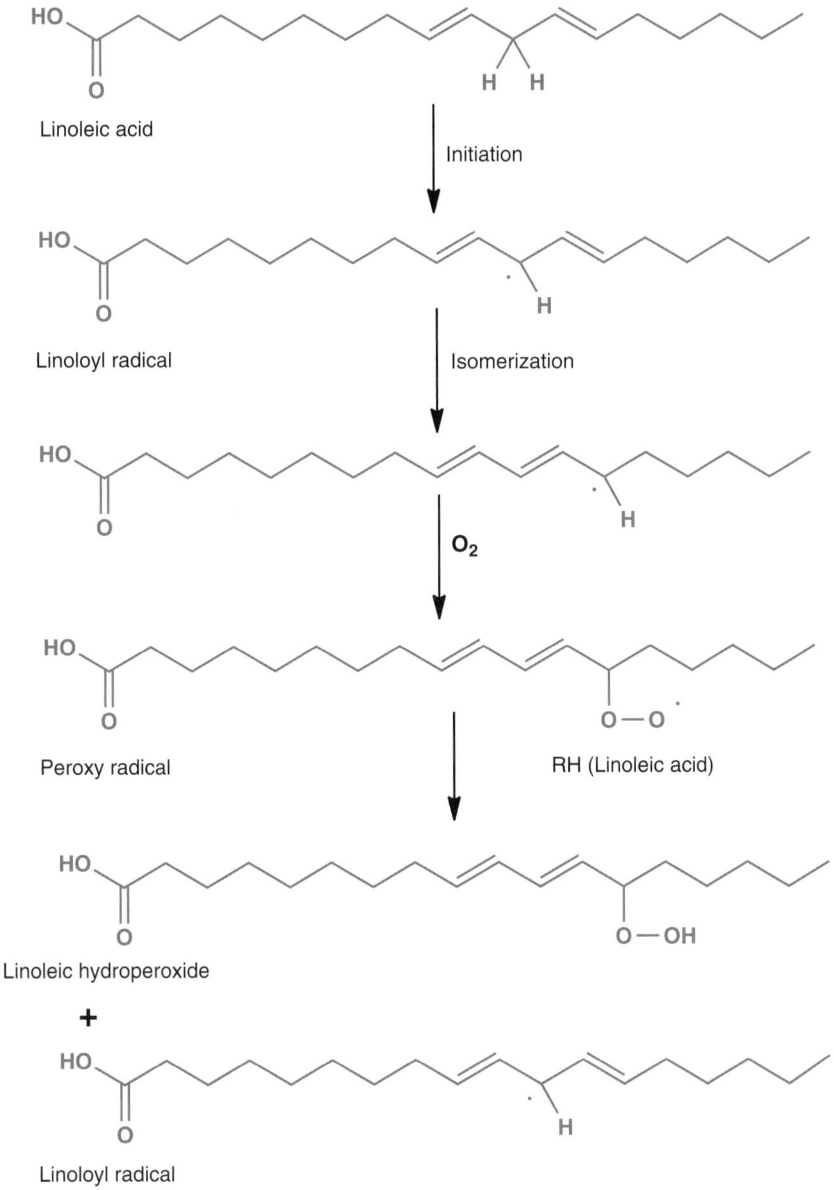

Linoleic acid

Initiation

Linoloyl radical

Isomerization

O_2

Peroxy radical

RH (Linoleic acid)

Linoleic hydroperoxide

+

Linoloyl radical

The hydroperoxide formed in Figure 4.18 can decompose via a number of pathways to give carboxylic acids, acid aldehydes and aldehydes. It is the aldehydic compounds in particular, e.g. 2-nonenal, that lead to the bad smell of oxidized fats.

Linoleic acid is one of the essential fatty acids required by humans. The body cannot make it and so we get it from our diet, e.g. from vegetable oils. As well as being a cell membrane component, metabolism of linoleic acid in the body generates arachidonic acid and, subsequently, prostaglandins, which are essential to the contraction of smooth muscle.

Absorption, distribution, metabolism and excretion (ADME)

The presence of lipophilic hydrocarbon groups in drugs affects each of these processes. While a wider discussion is beyond the scope of this chapter, we will briefly consider the ADME of hydrocarbons.

> You will find more detailed information on ADME in Chapter 14, 'Absorption, distribution, metabolism and excretion'.

Most drugs are taken orally, at least in the UK. This means that the drug must dissolve in the gastrointestinal tract, an aqueous environment, before it can be absorbed. The presence of hydrocarbon chains in a drug molecule will lower its water solubility; lipophilic groups such as these are, however, necessary for a drug molecule to cross cell membranes, e.g. in the small intestine, and to enter into the systemic circulation. The distribution of a drug within the body depends on its lipophilicity and on its affinity for different environments within the body, such as tissue and plasma proteins.

Pharmaceuticals are, in evolutionary terms, rather recent. Our bodies recognize drugs as foreign substances (xenobiotics) which need to be disposed of, generally in our urine or faeces. However, most drugs need to be altered such that they become more water soluble before this can happen. The body, most especially the liver, has a wide range of enzymes which are capable of performing such reactions. These enzymes have evolved to deal with all manner of endogenous compounds and xenobiotics and are also capable of metabolizing drug substances.

Alkyl groups are mostly inert to metabolism, meaning that such groups are often excreted from the body unchanged. However, there are some occasions when alkyl groups are reactive. For example, hydroxylation (addition of OH) can occur at terminal (omega, ω) methyl groups and at the ($\omega-1$) position (the carbon next to the end) through the action of mixed-function oxidases. Further metabolic reactions can lead to the generation of carbonyl compounds and to shortening of the carbon chain. As shown for the non-steroidal anti-inflammatory drug ibuprofen, oxidation can occur at either position, leading to either the alcohol (OH) metabolite or, after a second oxidation, the carboxylic acid (COOH) metabolite (see Scheme 4.32). Neither of these metabolites shows any pharmacological activity, which illustrates how important the lipophilic side chain is for the activity of ibuprofen.

The alkene components of drugs and other substances are oxidized to epoxides by cytochrome P450 enzymes, found mainly in the human liver. Epoxides are rather reactive species and are easily hydrolysed by enzymes called epoxide hydrolases, to give diols. The change from alkene to diol greatly increases the aqueous solubility of the substance and the likelihood of its excretion from the body. This is illustrated by the metabolism of carbemazepine, an anticonvulsant and mood stabilizing drug, as shown in Scheme 4.33. While thirty-three different

Scheme 4.32

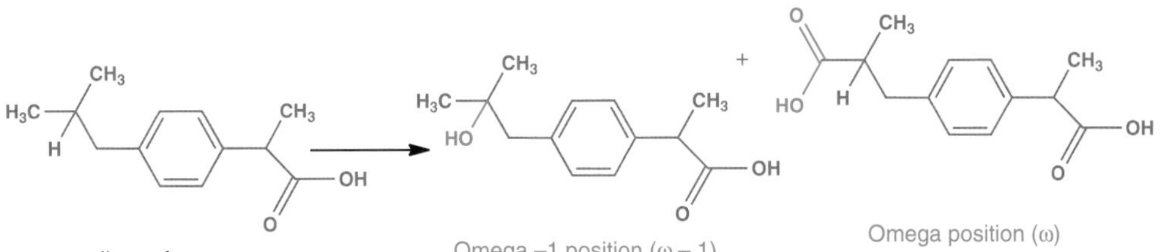

Ibuprofen

Omega −1 position (ω − 1)

Omega position (ω)

Scheme 4.33

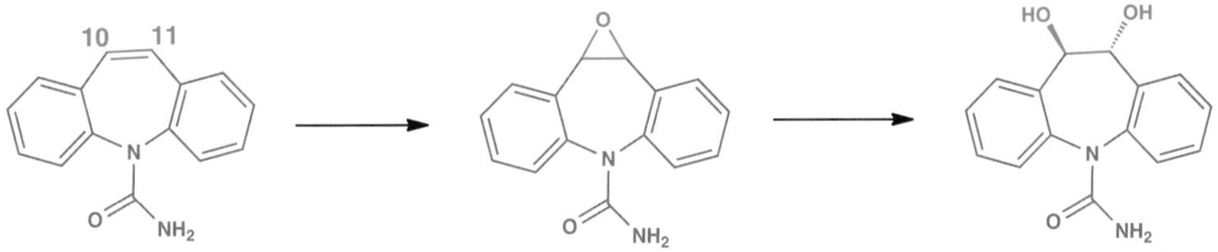

10   11

Carbamazepine

metabolites of carbamazepine have been identified, the pathway shown predominates. The epoxide metabolite shows anticonvulsant activity comparable to that of carbamazepine. The diol metabolite is excreted either unchanged or in a conjugated form. The diol itself accounts for 30% of carbamazepine metabolites found in a patient's urine.

There are other important metabolic pathways for alkenes, and these include hydration, peroxidation and reduction.

Like alkenes, alkynes are oxidized readily, and usually much more quickly. The products of these oxidations depend upon which carbon of the alkyne is attacked. Attack at a terminal alkyne carbon leads to a carboxylic acid metabolite (via a very reactive substance called a ketene), while attack at the internal alkyne carbon causes the compound to become permanently attached to the enzyme performing the oxidation, inactivating it irreversibly. This latter mechanism has been proposed as one pathway in the metabolism of drugs such as the female contraceptive, ethinylestradiol (17-α).

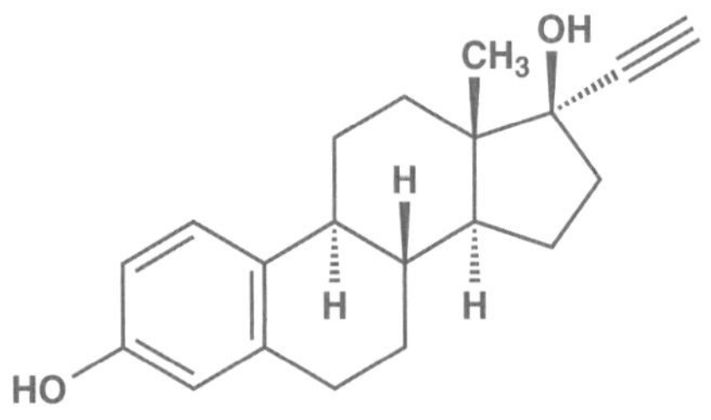

17 α-ethinylestradiol

135

CHAPTER SUMMARY

This chapter contains information on the more important physical properties of the aliphatic hydrocarbons and their chemical reactivity. You should now understand:

- Alkanes, alkenes and alkynes can exist as straight-chain, branched-chain and cyclic structures.

- Alkenes can exhibit geometrical isomerism.

- Alkanes are relatively unreactive.

- Alkenes are very reactive because of the presence of the π bond. They undergo electrophilic addition.

- Alkynes also undergo electrophilic addition reactions.

- Aliphatic hydrocarbons can be found throughout pharmacy as features in drugs, excipients and in biologically important molecules.

FURTHER READING

There is an enormous number of organic chemistry texts available. The list below contains some personal favourites! The internet also contains a number of decent sites. Those below may be trusted, but you should always exercise some care when looking for information on a topic for the first time. Gathering information from more than one source is always a good idea.

Baird, C. *Chemistry in your Life*, 2nd edn. W. H. Freeman, 2006.

http://www.organic-chemistry.org

http://www.chemguide.co.uk/orgmenu.html

http://www.chemtube3d.com

http://www.periodicvideos.com

Bruice, P. *Essential Organic Chemistry Global Edition*, Pearson, 2016.

Clayden, J., Greeves, N., and Warren, S. *Organic Chemistry*, 2nd edn. Oxford University Press, 2012.

Wade, L.G. *Organic Chemistry*, 9th edn. Pearson, 2017.

Self-check

For the answers to the Self-Check questions in Chapter 4, visit the online resources which accompany this textbook.

ALCOHOLS, PHENOLS, ETHERS, ORGANIC HALOGEN COMPOUNDS, AND AMINES

Chris Rostron

In this chapter we consider a number of **functional groups**. You will be familiar with oxygen (O_2) in the air that you breathe and as a component of water (H_2O), but oxygen atoms are also found in many molecules as parts of functional groups. Functional groups are made, changed and destroyed in chemical reactions.

Oxygen's value as a component of functional groups stems from its high **electronegativity**, which means that it strongly attracts electrons. As a consequence, it often has a direct and important role in chemical reactions. In the periodic table, oxygen is flanked by nitrogen and fluorine. These too are electronegative elements: nitrogen is somewhat less electronegative than oxygen, but fluorine is the most electronegative element of all. The other halogens, chlorine, bromine and iodine, are also electronegative. Because of the electronegativities of these elements, their functional groups tend to take part in a range of similar chemical reactions, and we therefore discuss selected functional groups containing these elements in this chapter.

The hydroxyl group (–OH) is probably the most biologically significant functional group considered so far, as it is one of the most widely occurring in nature, being present in carbohydrates, proteins and nucleic acids. The properties of carbohydrates, for example, are essentially a combination of hydroxyl (OH) chemistry and the chemistry of aldehydes and ketones. Equally important is the amine functional group (NH_2). This group also occurs widely in nature, often in its protonated form ($-NH_3^+$); it is found in proteins, enzymes and nucleic acids. The amine group is also present in many drugs, often having a vital role in the interaction of the drug with a receptor. Halogens, although rarely found in nature, are often found in drugs because they can have a profound influence on distribution of a molecule throughout the body.

In this chapter we study hydroxyl-containing compounds, ethers, amines and halogen-containing compounds, before turning to the carbonyl group (C=O) in the next chapter.

Learning objectives

Having read this chapter you are expected to be able to:

- identify the differences between the primary, secondary and tertiary alcohols and amines
- recognize how the presence of a functional group influences the physical properties of molecules
- recognize how the presence of a functional group influences the chemical properties of molecules
- explain the biological and pharmaceutical significance of these physical and chemical properties.

5.1 THE HYDROXYL GROUP

The hydroxyl group (−OH) needs very little introduction. People with no background in science are usually aware that water is H_2O or H−OH. Those who have studied chemistry at school are often aware that ethanol (ethyl alcohol) is C_2H_5OH, and many will also have realized that the sugar (sucrose) molecule contains hydroxyl groups. The hydroxyl group features in the molecules of everyday life, and every day we encounter more hydroxyl groups than we could ever realize or count.

Some important terminology

Before considering the properties of the OH group, we must introduce some important terminology. There are two pieces of terminology associated with the OH group, which must not be confused. The first of these refers to the number of OH groups present in a molecule. Monohydric, dihydric and trihydric molecules contain one, two and three OH groups, respectively. Often dihydric and trihydric alcohols are referred to as polyhydric alcohols. They have pharmaceutical and biological significance, and we will return to these later in this chapter.

The second type of terminology relates to the type of carbon to which the OH group is attached. These different OH groups are referred to as primary (1°), secondary (2°) and tertiary (3°).

Self-check 5.1

Identify the following alcohols as primary, secondary or tertiary: methanol, propan-1-ol, butan-2-ol, 2-methylpropan-2-ol, cyclohexanol. (Hint: Draw the structures in full before attempting to answer.)

Self-check 5.2

Find the structure of hydrocortisone, a widely used steroid drug. Identify the OH groups in its structure as primary, secondary or tertiary.

Figure 5.1 General structures of primary, secondary and tertiary alcohols

Primary   Secondary   Tertiary

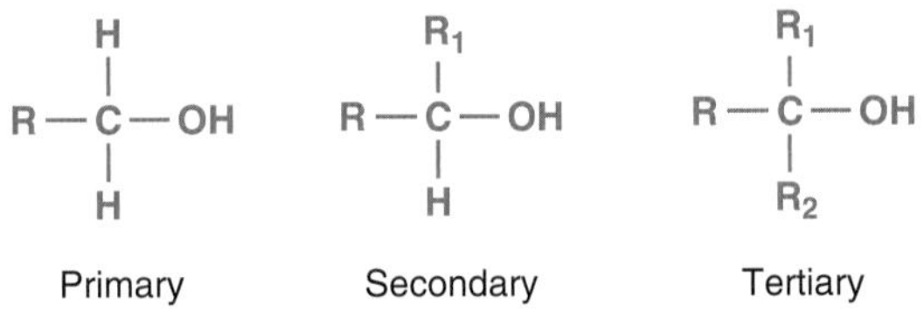

Figure 5.1 shows how a primary alcohol has two hydrogens and a single carbon on the carbon to which the OH group is attached, a secondary alcohol has one hydrogen and two carbons, and a tertiary alcohol has no hydrogens and three carbons attached. This is an important distinction because the three types of OH group have different physical properties, react at different rates and sometimes even undergo different reactions.

Physical properties of alcohols

The physical properties of alcohols are quite different from those of the hydrocarbons considered in the preceding chapter. The hydroxyl group has a profound influence on boiling point and solubility; these properties in turn affect drug action and drug metabolism.

Boiling points

Methane and butane are, as we know from Chapter 4, gases at room temperature, but the equivalent alcohols, methanol and butan-1-ol, are liquids. Table 5.1 shows how the simpler alcohols are low-boiling-point liquids, but the boiling points increase quite quickly with increasing molecular mass.

What is responsible for this difference between alcohols and hydrocarbons? The answer lies in the ability of alcohols to form **hydrogen bonds**, which dominate the physical properties of alcohols. Hydrogen bonds are stronger intermolecular forces than **van der Waals interactions** or **dipole–dipole interactions**. Consequently, the boiling points of alcohols are higher than those of hydrocarbons (which experience van der Waals intermolecular forces but do not form hydrogen bonds) and halogenated hydrocarbons (which experience dipole–dipole intermolecular forces but also lack hydrogen bonds).

If the hydrocarbon chain to which the OH group is attached is branched, the boiling point is lowered. Secondary and tertiary alcohols have boiling points lower than primary alcohols with the same molecular mass, because their branched structures interfere with the formation of intermolecular hydrogen bonds. Table 5.1 shows the boiling points of some representative alcohols, which illustrate these points.

Table 5.1 Boiling points of selected alcohols

Examples of alcohols	Boiling point °C
Methanol (primary)	65
Butan-1-ol (primary)	118
Decan-1-ol (primary)	233
Butan-2-ol (secondary)	100
2-Methylpropan-2-ol (tertiary)	83

Self-check 5.3

Explain why propane boils at –45 °C, whereas propan-1-ol boils at 97 °C.

> Look at Chapter 2, 'Organic structure and bonding', to remind yourself about intermolecular forces.

Solubility

Unlike hydrocarbons, simple alcohols are generally soluble in water. This property is also explained by the ability of hydroxyl groups to take part in hydrogen bonds. The smaller alcohols are totally soluble in water (miscible with water)—a property that permits the preparation of screen wash, alcoholic handwash and, of course, alcoholic beverages. Table 5.2 shows how water solubility decreases with increasing size of the hydrocarbon chain, because larger hydrocarbon chains interfere with the hydrogen bond formation.

As the length of the hydrocarbon chain increases, an interesting property of long-chain alcohols begins to emerge. At one end of the chain there is a water-soluble OH group; the rest of the molecule is a water-insoluble hydrocarbon chain. Such a molecule will accumulate at an oil–water interface, with the OH group residing in the water phase and the hydrocarbon chain in the oil phase. Molecules with both water-soluble and water-insoluble portions are called amphipathic molecules, and can be used as emulsifying agents. Emulsifying agents can be used to make water-insoluble and water-soluble substances mix (see Figure 5.2). The water-insoluble molecules cluster into tiny droplets, which are coated by the amphipathic molecules. The hydrocarbon portion of each amphipathic molecule interacts with the water-insoluble molecules inside the droplet, while their OH groups interact with the water molecules surrounding the droplet.

Table 5.2   Water solubilities of selected alcohols at 20 °C

Examples of alcohols	Solubility in g/100 g
Methanol	Completely miscible
Butan-1-ol	7.9
Hexan-1-ol	0.6

Figure 5.2   Formation of an oil-in-water emulsion

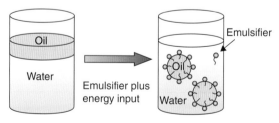

🔑 The ability to form hydrogen bonds dominates the physical properties of alcohols, both in terms of boiling points and water solubility.

The influence of hydroxyl groups on drug metabolism

The human body makes good use of the increased water solubility brought about by the presence of an OH group. One of the key transformations brought about by the xenobiotic-metabolizing enzymes in the liver is the introduction of an OH group into a molecule. These transformations increase the water solubility of the molecule, making it more easily excreted from the body by the kidney. An example of this process can be seen in Figure 5.3. Diazepam is an anxiolytic drug (a drug used to treat anxiety) with a very long duration of action. One of its metabolites is temazepam, which is formed from diazepam by the introduction of an OH group. Temazepam is also used as a drug in its own right when a shorter duration of action is required. The shorter duration of action of temazepam is due to its increased water solubility, and hence more rapid excretion, as a result of the presence of the OH group.

> See Chapter 1, 'The importance of pharmaceutical chemistry', and Chapter 14, 'Absorption, distribution, metabolism and excretion', for more information about drug metabolism.

Chemical properties of OH-containing compounds

The polarity of the C−O−H functional group (see Figure 5.4) allows the formation of the hydrogen bonds that so profoundly influence the physical properties of hydroxyl compounds. This polarity also plays a significant role in determining the chemical properties of OH-containing

Figure 5.3   Metabolic transformation of diazepam

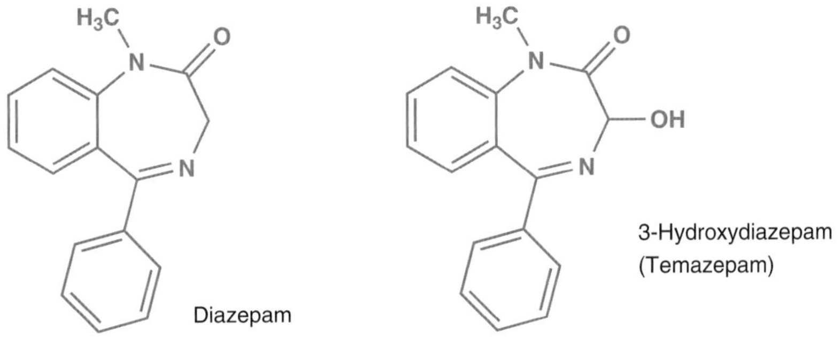

Diazepam

3-Hydroxydiazepam
(Temazepam)

Figure 5.4   Partial polarization of the C−O−H group

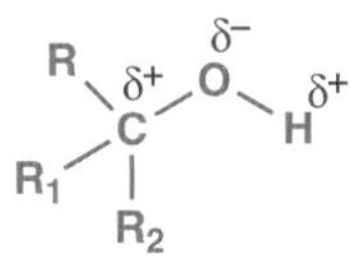

compounds: both the C–O bond and the O–H bond are readily broken in chemical reactions because of the partial polarization of these bonds.

Breaking the C–O bond

The δ+ charge on the carbon of the C–O bond (see Figure 5.4) makes this carbon susceptible to nucleophilic attack, leading to substitution reactions. As described in Chapter 2, however, nucleophilic substitution is often in competition with an elimination reaction. Nucleophilic substitution of alcohols (or their derivatives) is largely of synthetic significance, whereas the competing elimination reaction—the removal of water (dehydration)—is a very important reaction in biological systems as well as in the laboratory.

Elimination reaction of alcohols—dehydration

In the laboratory, dehydration can be achieved by the action of heat on an alcohol, but is usually assisted by the use of a catalyst. A strong acid, such as sulfuric acid, is a good example of a catalyst in the elimination of water from an alcohol (see Figure 5.5). We have encountered this reaction in Chapter 4, because it is a method of preparing alkenes.

As can be seen in Figure 5.5, this dehydration reaction involves the formation of a carbocation. The relative stabilities of carbocations formed from the different types of alcohols determine the rate of the dehydration reaction. A tertiary alcohol will dehydrate more readily because the reaction involves the formation of a relatively stable tertiary carbocation (see Box 5.1).

> Revise the stability of carbocations in Chapter 4, 'Properties of aliphatic hydrocarbons'.

Sometimes dehydration reactions in the laboratory can give rise to unexpected alkene products because of rearrangement of the intermediate carbocation. In the human body, however,

Figure 5.5 Dehydration reaction scheme

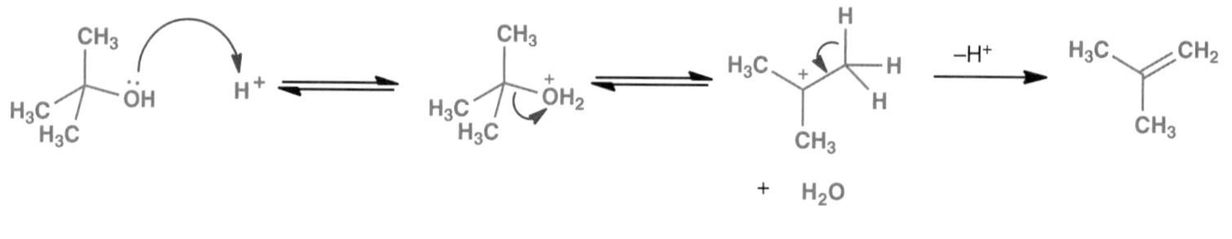

$+ \quad H_2O$

Self-check 5.5

What is the name of the product of the dehydration reaction in Figure 5.5?

Box 5.1 Relative reaction conditions for dehydration of alcohols

The rate-determining step in the acid-catalysed dehydration of alcohols is the formation of an intermediate carbocation. The relative ease with which the dehydration takes place mirrors the ease of formation of the carbocation, which in turn mirrors the stability of the carbocation: 3° > 2° > 1°. Therefore, tertiary alcohols are most readily dehydrated (5% H_2SO_4 at 50 °C), followed by secondary alcohols (75% H_2SO_4 at 100 °C), and primary alcohols are very difficult to dehydrate (95% H_2SO_4 at 170 °C).

Self-check 5.6

Which of the following alcohols would you expect to undergo dehydration in acid most readily: butan-2-ol, butan-1-ol, 2-methylbutan-2-ol?

Figure 5.6   An example of biological dehydration

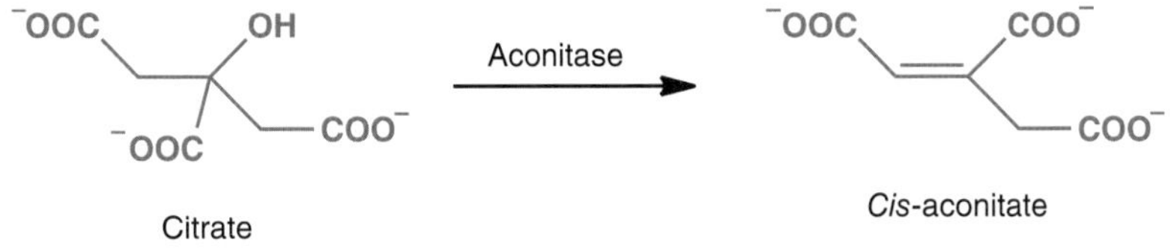

Citrate

Cis-aconitate

dehydration reactions are catalysed by enzymes and so just one specific product is formed (see Figure 5.6).

> We encountered aconitase, which converts citrate to isocitrate, in Chapter 1, 'The importance of pharmaceutical chemistry'. Figure 5.6 shows the intermediate in this reaction: *cis*-aconitate.

Substitution reactions of alcohols

If a secondary or tertiary alcohol is treated with acid in the presence of a nucleophile, the intermediate carbocation may react with the nucleophile, rather than losing a proton. In this case there is a substitution reaction, rather than an elimination reaction (see Scheme 5.1).

The formation of the carbocation is once again the slow step, so the ease of acid-catalysed substitution is once again in the order 3° > 2° > 1°. This reaction is known as an S_N1 reaction: substitution nucleophilic, type 1. We will meet S_N2 reactions later in this chapter.

Breaking the O–H bond

Two reactions of biological and pharmaceutical significance involve the O–H bond being broken. The first of these is esterification, which we explore in detail in the next chapter. The other reaction is oxidation. Chemically, oxidation is achieved by reacting an alcohol with an oxidizing agent (typically potassium permanganate or potassium dichromate) in the presence of acid.

Figure 5.7 shows how this oxidation reaction is one in which the three types of alcohol behave differently.

- primary alcohols are oxidized to aldehydes
- secondary alcohols are oxidized to ketones
- tertiary alcohols are not oxidized at all

Scheme 5.1

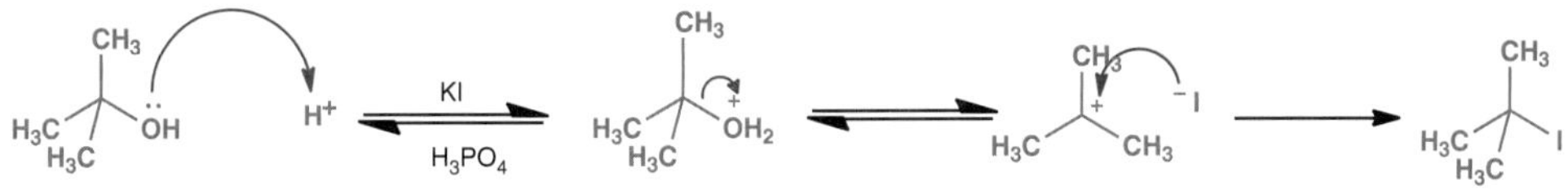

Figure 5.7 Oxidation of alcohols

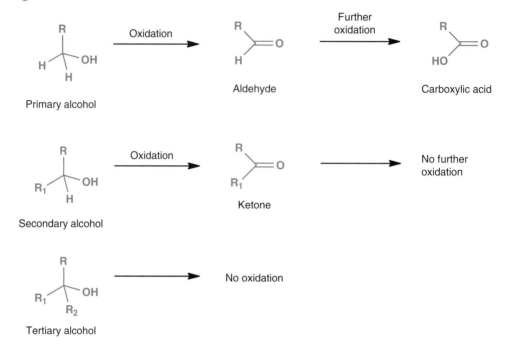

Primary alcohol → Oxidation → Aldehyde → Further oxidation → Carboxylic acid

Secondary alcohol → Oxidation → Ketone → No further oxidation

Tertiary alcohol → No oxidation

> Aldehydes and ketones are both types of carbonyl compound; carbonyl compounds are discussed in Chapter 6.

Biological oxidation follows the same pattern as the chemical oxidation described previously. Ethanol (R = CH_3 in Figure 5.7) is an example of a primary alcohol, and is oxidized in the body to an aldehyde (acetaldehyde or ethanal). The enzyme involved is alcohol dehydrogenase. Of course, when something is oxidized (the alcohol), something else must be reduced. In this case, as with so many biological oxidations, the compound that is reduced is nicotinamide adenine dinucleotide (NAD)⁺. This molecule is referred to as a co-enzyme—it operates in conjunction with the enzyme catalysing the oxidation.

> More details on biological oxidation can be found in Chapter 1, 'The importance of pharmaceutical chemistry', and Chapter 11, 'Carbohydrates and carbohydrate metabolism'.

Low-molecular-weight secondary alcohols are oxidized biologically to ketones by the same enzyme (alcohol dehydrogenase). For example, propan-2-ol (isopropyl alcohol, IPA, see Box 5.2) is oxidized to the ketone, propan-2-one (acetone). Acetone cannot be oxidized further and, being volatile and water-soluble, can be excreted via the lungs or in the urine.

Self-check 5.7

Why is IPA used in antiseptic wipes, rather than ethanol?

Case study 5.1

Ana had been to the Freshers' party the previous evening and was now feeling quite poorly—she had a hangover! Initially at the party she had felt a little lonely because she did not really know anyone. Eventually a third year student started chatting to her and he bought her a couple of drinks. After these she felt more relaxed and soon she was enjoying herself on the dance floor and chatting to all sorts of people.

The drinks continued to flow, and after a short while Ana started to feel a little unsteady on her feet. Fortunately one of her flat mates decided to take Ana back to her flat before any more damage was done. The next thing Ana knew was the following morning when she woke up feeling quite ill. She knew she had a hangover, but as it was the first time she did not know what to do. She decided to ring her older sister Su for advice. Su was not particularly sympathetic and said there was very little that could be done. She knew that one of the reasons for feeling bad was that alcohol had been metabolized to acetaldehyde, which is the molecule primarily responsible for the hangover symptoms.

Ana said that she had had only a few drinks so why did she feel so bad? Su did not know, told her to take two paracetamol tablets, drink plenty of water and sleep it off—that had always worked for her. She also said she would not tell Mum.

Reflection questions

1. Why did Ana feel more relaxed after a couple of drinks?
2. Why did Ana start to feel unsteady on her feet after a few more drinks?
3. Why did Ana have such a bad hangover after having a relatively small amount to drink?

For answers, visit the online resources which accompany this textbook.

Box 5.2 Pharmaceutical use of IPA

Isopropyl alcohol (propan-2-ol, IPA) is used as a topical disinfectant. Various concentrations in water are used, ranging between 50 and 95%. Antiseptic wipes are often pieces of gauze or similar material impregnated with IPA.

Tertiary alcohols are not oxidized, chemically or biologically. When the liver metabolizes tertiary alcohols, it normally converts them to water–soluble esters such as sulfates and glucuronides, known as conjugates, which can be excreted in the urine.

Metabolic oxidation of primary and secondary alcohols takes place in the liver, as does the conjugation of tertiary alcohols. When a drug is administered orally it is normally absorbed

Self-check 5.8

Why are tertiary alcohols not oxidized? (Hint: Draw the structure of a tertiary alcohol, such as 2-methylpropan-2-ol.)

> **Self-check 5.9**
>
> What would be the oxidation products of the alcohols in Self-check 5.4?

🔑 Dehydration is a key reaction for alcohols, both chemically and biologically. Another key reaction is oxidation. In both of these reactions, it is important to recognize the differences between primary, secondary and tertiary alcohols.

from the gastrointestinal tract into the hepatic blood circulation, ensuring it passes through the liver before reaching the general circulation. This ensures that any metabolic oxidation or conjugation of the drug will take place before it reaches the general circulation. This process is referred to as 'first pass metabolism'. If a drug is rapidly inactivated by this process, consideration may have to be given to an alternative route of administration so that first pass metabolism can be avoided.

> Numerous examples of biological oxidation of alcohols in the citric acid cycle, and the β-oxidation of fatty acids, can be found in Chapter 11, 'Carbohydrates and carbohydrate metabolism', and Chapter 12, 'Lipids'.

5.2 POLYHYDRIC ALCOHOLS

We referred earlier in this chapter to polyhydric alcohols. These alcohols have certain properties that are useful in a variety of ways (see Box 5.3). Figure 5.8 shows some well-known polyhydric alcohols.

As you would expect, their numerous OH groups make small polyhydric alcohols miscible with water. In fact, they are so effective at forming hydrogen bonds with water molecules that they disrupt the normal ordered structure of water and depress its freezing point. That is why polyhydric alcohols, such as ethylene glycol (ethane-1,2-diol), are used as antifreeze in car radiators. Another property that arises from their highly effective hydrogen bonding to water is **hygroscopicity**. They form hydrogen bonds so effectively with water that they actually absorb water from the air.

You might expect the boiling points of polyhydric alcohols to be elevated relative to their monohydric counterparts, and you would again be right. The boiling point of propan-1-ol is 97 °C, but the boiling point of glycerol (propan-1,2,3-triol) is 290 °C. Ethanol has a boiling point of 78 °C, but ethylene glycol (ethane-1,2-diol) boils at 197.3 °C.

> Hydrogen bonds are also discussed in Chapter 2, 'Organic structure and bonding'.

Finally in this section, the different metabolic fates of simple polyhydric alcohols are of interest. Glycerol is metabolized, by oxidation, to glycerate, which is then converted to 3-phosphoglycerate—a component of the glycolytic pathway; 3-phosphoglycerate poses no problem to the body. On the other hand, ethylene glycol is metabolized by oxidation to oxalic acid.

This product is extremely toxic because it interferes with the functioning of the electron transport chain, a process which is vital to the operation of cells (see Figure 5.9).

Figure 5.8 Polyhydric alcohols and some of their uses

Source: Soap: Gareth Boden; Antifreeze: Jane Norton/istock; Cupcake: Chris Leachman/istock.

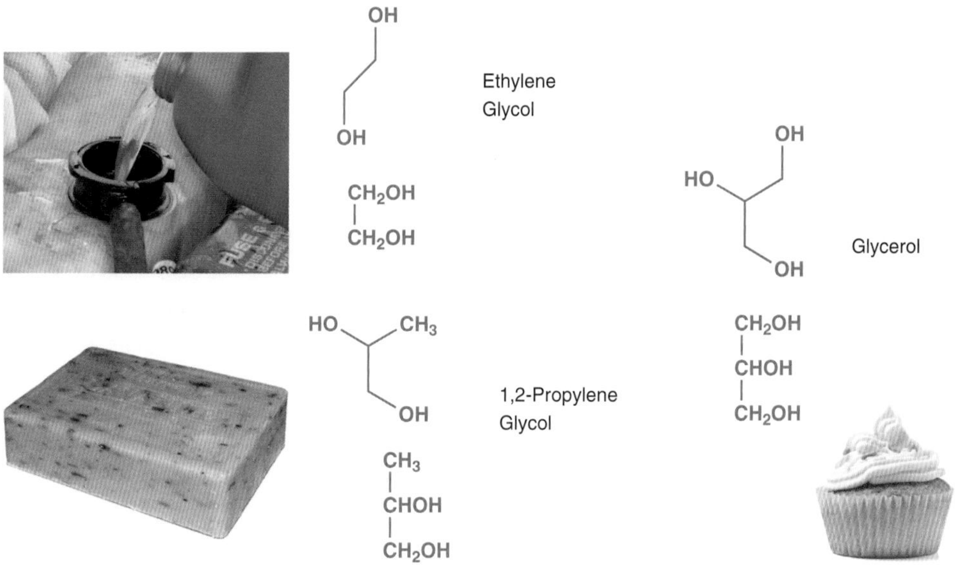

Ethylene Glycol

Glycerol

1,2-Propylene Glycol

Figure 5.9 Oxidation of some polyhydric alcohols in the body

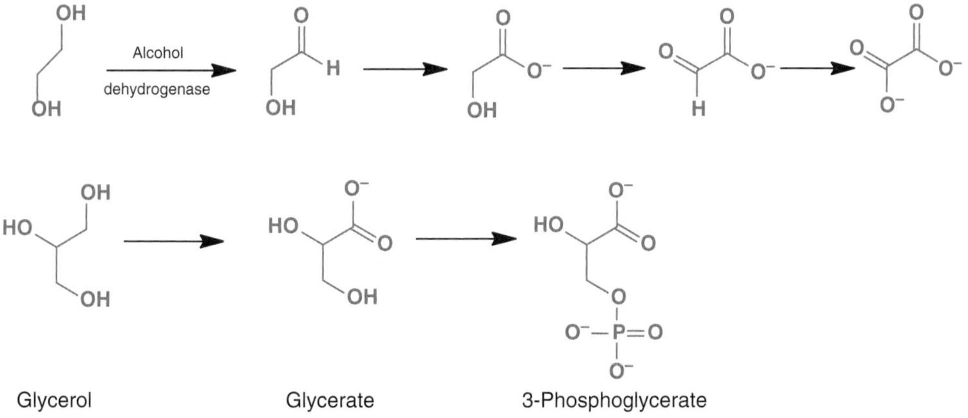

Glycerol   Glycerate   3-Phosphoglycerate

Self-check 5.10

Why might you add glycerol (also known as glycerine) as an ingredient when preparing icing for a cake?

> **Box 5.3 Pharmaceutical uses of glycerol**
>
> Glycerol is used in pharmaceutical products because it provides lubrication and has the ability to absorb water (it is a humectant). It is found in syrups, elixirs and pastilles used to treat coughs and sore throats, as well as in mouthwashes and skin care products. It is sometimes used as a binding agent in the preparation of tablets, and glycerol suppositories can be used to treat constipation.

> More details on glycolysis and the electron transport chain can be found in Chapter 11, 'Carbohydrates and carbohydrate metabolism'.

> **Box 5.4 Treating ethylene glycol poisoning**
>
> Strange as it may sound, one of the ways of treating ethylene glycol poisoning is by administering ethanol. Ethanol acts by competing with ethylene glycol for the enzyme, alcohol dehydrogenase. Ethanol has a much higher affinity than ethylene glycol for this enzyme (~100×) and effectively blocks the conversion of ethylene glycol to its toxic products.

5.3 PHENOLS

There is one more type of OH group that we need to consider: an OH group attached to an aromatic hydrocarbon ring, such as benzene. The aromatic ring dramatically changes the physical and chemical properties of the OH group; indeed, the differences are so great that this type of OH group is regarded as a different functional group and is given a different name. It is not an alcohol but a phenol.

The OH group attached to an aromatic ring is more polarized than in an alcohol, causing stronger intermolecular hydrogen bonds. You might expect this to have a significant effect on boiling/melting points and water solubility. However, the rest of the molecule is hydrocarbon in nature and the resulting properties are as a consequence of a balance between these two factors. Increasing the number of OH groups increases the melting point and water solubility, but increasing the hydrocarbon component dramatically reduces the water solubility (see Table 5.3).

Acidity of phenols

Unlike alcohols, which are not acidic (the pK_a of ethanol is about 16), phenols are weak acids (see Box 5.5). They are acidic enough to turn blue litmus paper red, and to react with sodium carbonate to yield carbon dioxide. The acidity of a phenol stems from the way that the hydrogen attached to the oxygen of the OH group is more easily lost as a proton (relative to an alcohol), with a pK_a of about 9.

Phenol   Phenolate

Table 5.3 Physical properties of some phenols

Molecule	Structure	Melting point (°C)	Water solubility (g L⁻¹)
Phenol	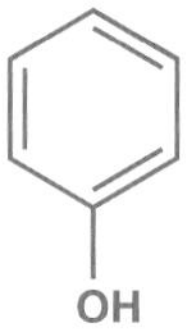	41	83
Benzene-1,3-diol	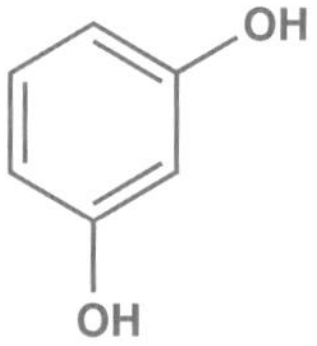	110	1100
Naphthalen-2-ol	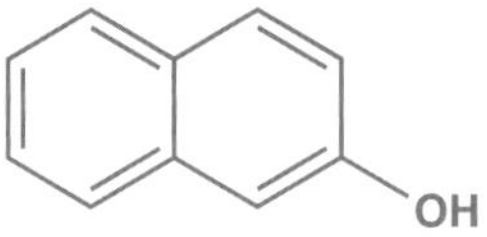	123	7

The ease with which a proton is lost depends upon the stability of the resulting anion: the more stable the anion, the more easily the proton will be lost. If the negative charge on the anion can be effectively delocalized (shared with other atoms), then the anion will be relatively stable. In phenols, the negative charge on the phenoxide anion can be delocalized into the aromatic ring as illustrated in Figure 5.10, hence the weak acidity observed.

Figure 5.10 Delocalization of the negative charge of phenolate anion

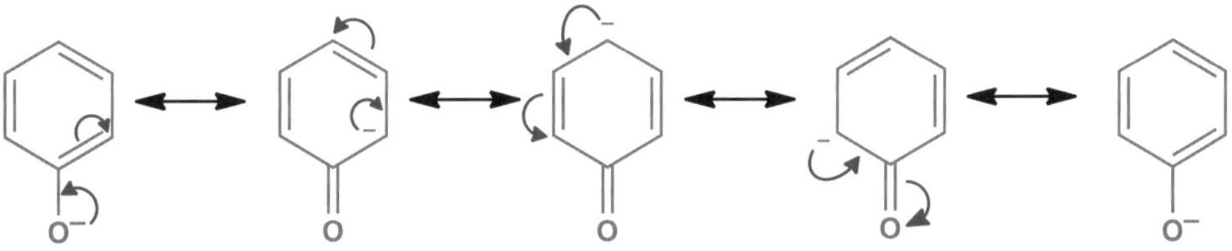

Phenolate

Self-check 5.11

The side-chain of the amino acid tyrosine is a phenol, with a pK_a of about 9. What percentage of tyrosine residues are ionized in the small intestine at pH 8?

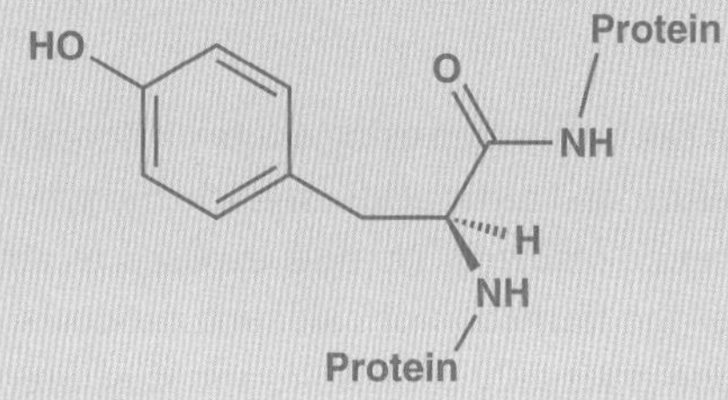

A tyrosine residue in a protein.

> **Box 5.5   The Henderson–Hasselbalch equation**
>
> The pK$_a$ of ethanol is about 16; this tells us that ethanol is half-ionized at pH 16. In other words, the following equilibrium reaction lies in the middle at pH 16: 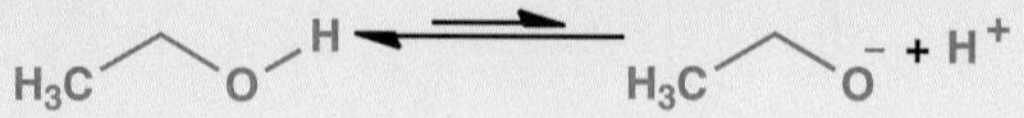
>
>
> The Henderson–Hasselbalch equation tells us that
>
> $$pH = pK_a + \log\frac{[A^-]}{HA}$$
>
> So at pH 7, $\log\dfrac{[A^-]}{HA}$ is $^-9$, so $\dfrac{[A^-]}{HA}$ is 10^9.
>
> So, at pH 7, just one molecule of ethanol per billion (10^{-9}) is ionized.

Scheme 5.2

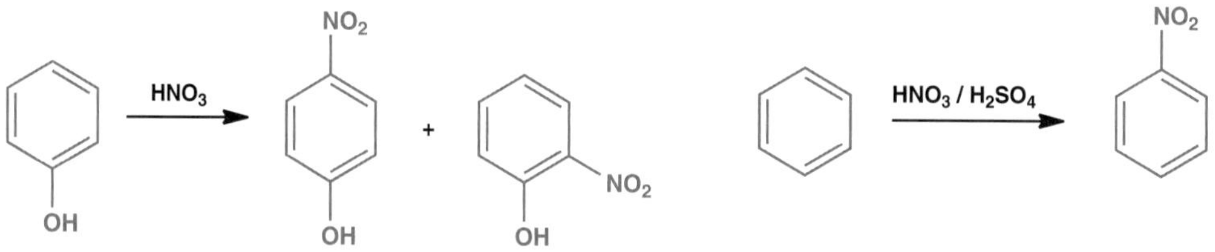

Such delocalization is not possible in alcohols and so they are not normally regarded as acidic (pK$_a$ ~ 16). You will see in Chapter 6 that the anion of a carboxylic acid is highly stabilized and hence they are more acidic even than phenols; their pK$_a$s are around 4.

Reactions of phenols

Because alcohols and phenols both possess the OH group, one might expect them to undergo similar reactions. However, whereas alcohols readily undergo nucleophilic substitutions and elimination reactions, phenols undergo neither. Phenyl carbonium ions are very difficult to form because of the geometry of the benzene ring, so S$_N$1 and elimination reactions are out of the question. The geometry also rules out S$_N$2 reactions (see the section on 'Chemical properties' of 'Haloalkanes and other organic halogen compounds' in this chapter). Instead, phenols undergo electrophilic aromatic substitution and do so very easily because the OH group is strongly ring-activating.

> See more about electrophilic aromatic substitution in Chapter 7, 'Introduction to aromatic chemistry'.

For example, phenol itself can be nitrated using dilute nitric acid, whereas benzene requires a mixture of concentrated sulfuric and nitric acids (see Scheme 5.2).

Phenols, like alcohols, can be oxidized. Phenols exposed to air for a period of time often become coloured because of the formation of oxidation products. The oxidation of benzene-1,4-diol to 1,4-benzoquinone is actually reversible, and this interconversion is an important biological reaction (see Figure 5.11).

Figure 5.11   Oxidation of benzene-1,4-diol, an example of oxidation of a phenol

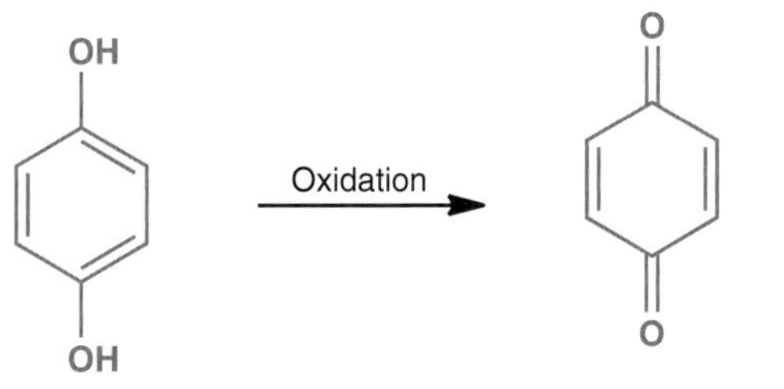

1,4-Dihydroxybenzene   1,4-Benzoquinone

Phenols as antioxidants

Phenols are useful as antioxidants, both pharmaceutically and biologically (see Box 5.6). They are known as **free radical scavengers**—that is, they mop up free radicals by reacting with them and rendering them unreactive. Figure 5.12 illustrates this reaction; look at this figure and

Figure 5.12   Reaction scheme for antioxidant activity of phenols

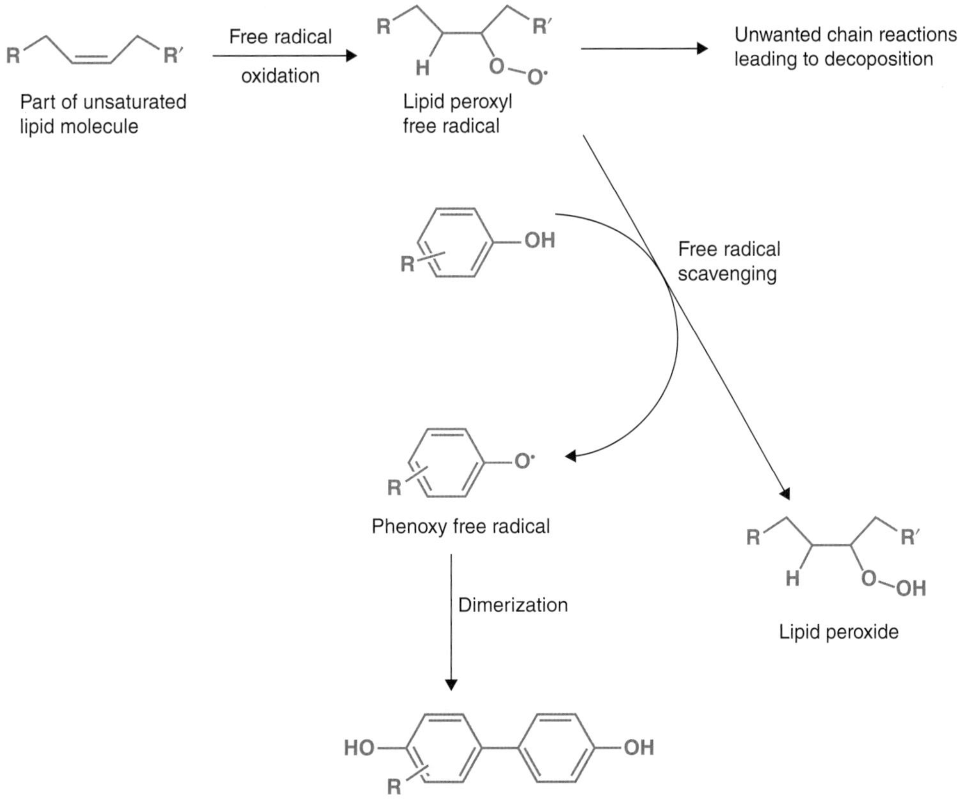

Self-check 5.12

Can you identify the most commonly occurring natural antioxidants?

Box 5.6 The biological problem of free radicals

Free radicals are highly reactive and can cause significant damage to biological structures. This damage is often associated with reactive oxygen species, such as superoxide (O_2^-) and the hydroxyl free radical (OH˙) and is referred to as oxidative stress. Oxidative stress can cause damage to cells by initiating chain reactions, such as lipid peroxidation or by oxidizing DNA or proteins. Damage to DNA, for example, can cause mutations, which may increase the risk of cancer. Because of the risk of damage, plants and animals possess a variety of antioxidants such as vitamins C and E. These compounds act as free radical scavengers like the phenolic antioxidants, which are now widely added to foodstuffs and pharmaceutical preparations.

> More information on free radical reactions can be found in Chapter 4, 'Properties of aliphatic hydrocarbons'.

Phenols are acidic and alcohols are not. Alcohols (but not phenols) can undergo nucleophilic and elimination reactions. Phenols can undergo electrophilic substitution reactions. Both functional groups can undergo oxidation reactions but the circumstances in which this happens are different.

notice how the hydrogen atom of the phenolic OH is transferred to the free radical species, thus neutralizing it. Of course, this also results in the formation of a phenolic free radical. This is not a problem, however, as phenolic free radicals have a great tendency to react with each other (**dimerize**) rather than with anything else. This dimerization inactivates the free radicals, rendering them harmless.

Nature also utilizes phenols as antioxidants; indeed, the antioxidant properties of phenols lies behind the proposed benefits to health of drinking small quantities of red wine, which contains polyphenol antioxidants (see Figure 5.13).

Figure 5.13   Tannic acid is present in red wine
Source: Wine: Photodisc.
Wine: Image by Maciej Szewczyk from Pixabay

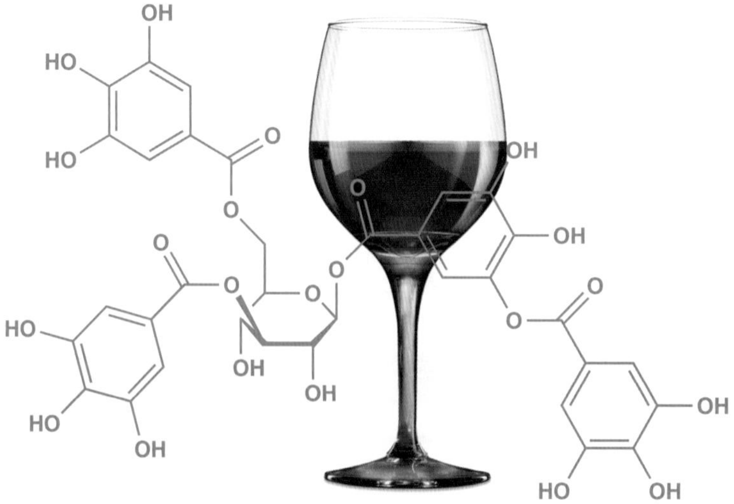

5.4 **ETHERS**

Ethers are formed by the replacement of the hydrogen of an alcohol OH group by an alkyl (hydrocarbon) group, which generates an −OR group. Figure 5.14 shows how an ether oxygen can be present in an open chain or as part of a cyclic structure.

The replacement of the hydrogen by an alkyl group results in significant changes to both the physical and chemical properties of ethers, when compared with alcohols.

Physical properties of ethers

Generally speaking, ethers have low boiling points and are immiscible with water (quite unlike alcohols). These differences arise because of the loss of intermolecular hydrogen bonding capacity as a result of there being no hydrogen attached directly to the oxygen. This loss, and the addition of the extra hydrocarbon component, results in the water insolubility.

Although they cannot form intermolecular hydrogen bonds, ethers can self-associate by dipole−dipole attraction. This self-association is not especially effective, because the two hydrocarbon groups attached to the oxygen often prevent molecules approaching each other closely. Ethers are, however, good solvents for a wide range of organic molecules. They are widely used as extraction solvents (see Box 5.7) because their volatility makes them easy to remove at the end of the extraction process. There are, however, disadvantages to their use. As one might expect, they are highly flammable and have a tendency to undergo free radical oxidation to generate peroxides, which are highly explosive (see the next section).

The volatility of ethers and their high affinity for lipid tissue also makes them effective general anaesthetics (see Box 5.8).

Figure 5.14   Some common ethers

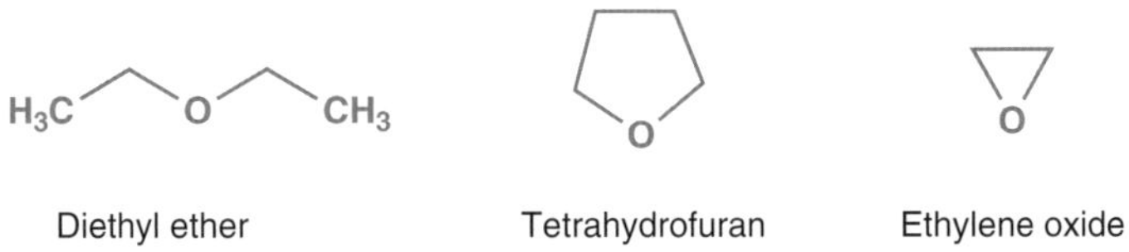

Diethyl ether   Tetrahydrofuran   Ethylene oxide

Box 5.7   Ether-water extraction

A hydrophobic compound can be extracted from water into ether. Ether is less dense than water, so forms a layer above the water. The water layer is easily removed, but, although water does not mix with ether, a small amount (1.5 g per 100 mL ether) does dissolve in the ether. Before evaporating the ether, it is necessary to remove the dissolved water (to dry the solvent), usually by mixing it with a solid drying agent, such as magnesium sulfate ($MgSO_4$), then filtering off the drying agent.

Self-check 5.13

Diethyl ether is widely used as a solvent in Northern Europe, but not in Australia. Why is this?

> ### Box 5.8   General anaesthetics
>
> Anaesthesia is required for three purposes—to achieve analgesia (pain relief), to cause loss of consciousness, and to bring about muscle relaxation. However, until the middle of the nineteenth century, when diethyl ether was first used in a surgical procedure, no general anaesthetics were used in surgery.
>
> A good inhalational anaesthetic should be highly volatile, lipid soluble, chemically stable and non-toxic. Diethyl ether fulfils most of these criteria but is dangerous to use because of its flammability. Nitrous oxide (laughing gas) and chloroform have been used in the past. However, these have all been superseded by halogenated compounds such as halothane and enflurane (see Figure 5.21).
>
> There is still considerable debate about the mechanism by which general anaesthetics bring about their action. A number of theories have been proposed over the years, but they are all variations on a basic theme—that general anaesthetics cause reversible changes in nerve cell membranes.

Chemical properties

Chemically, ethers are unreactive. They therefore bear more resemblance to saturated hydrocarbons than to alcohols. This lack of reactivity adds to their usefulness as organic solvents and general anaesthetics. However, their tendency to form **peroxides** renders their use potentially hazardous. The peroxides are formed by free radical reaction with oxygen, as illustrated in Figure 5.15.

In particular, this free radical reaction is catalysed by light, which explains the instruction that ethers should be stored 'in dark, well-filled bottles'. Use of well-filled bottles reduces the amount of oxygen available for reaction, and dark glass reduces entry of the ultraviolet component of light which initiates the free radical reaction.

Epoxides

Generally, cyclic ethers have similar chemical properties to those of acyclic ethers. Three-membered cyclic ethers (also called epoxides) are quite different, however. The structures of some epoxides are shown in Figure 5.16.

Epoxides (more rarely called oxiranes) are very reactive. This is because a three-membered ring is very strained and any reaction that will relieve that strain by breaking the ring is

> The replacement of the hydrogen of the OH group by an alkyl group renders both the physical and chemical properties of ethers significantly different from alcohols.

> ### Self-check 5.14
>
> Explain why propane boils at −45 °C, dimethyl ether boils at −23 °C and ethanol boils at 78 °C.

Figure 5.15   Peroxide formation from diethyl ether

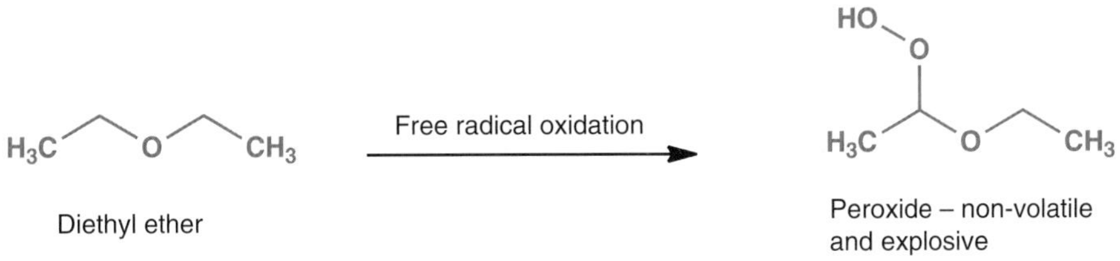

Diethyl ether

Free radical oxidation

Peroxide – non-volatile
and explosive

Figure 5.16   Oxiranes or epoxides

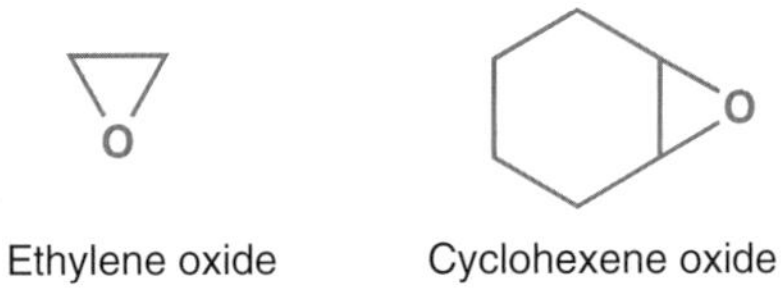

Ethylene oxide   Cyclohexene oxide

Whereas ethers are generally unreactive, small ring cyclic ethers, like ethylene oxide, are very reactive.

favoured. This reactivity is the basis for the use of ethylene oxide for cold gaseous sterilization, as explained in Box 5.9.

The reactivity of epoxides also causes problems within the body's xenobiotic metabolizing processes. The body finds aromatic hydrocarbons (present, for example, in cigarette smoke) difficult to metabolize and processes them by forming epoxides, which are extremely reactive. These epoxides can be considered to be **proximate carcinogens**. They remove a hydrogen radical from cellular constituents, becoming converted into a non-toxic hydroxyl compound in the process. However, the substrate from which the hydrogen was abstracted is now a very reactive species, and can cause further unwanted reactions within the cells. Nucleic acids are particularly susceptible to reaction with epoxides in this way, making epoxides potentially carcinogenic. This is described in more detail in Chapter 7 ('Metabolism and toxicity' section in 'Aromatic chemistry in the body').

Box 5.9   Cold gaseous sterilization

The usual method of sterilization (killing bacteria) employs heat and high pressure. However, some materials cannot be sterilized by this means because they are heat-sensitive. In these cases cold gaseous sterilization, employing ethylene oxide, can be used.

Ethylene oxide's reactivity ensures that the bacteria are killed, but there is a potential disadvantage in that it is so reactive that it may react with the material itself or its container. Also, it will not penetrate far below the surface of a material because of its reactivity. This means it can only be used for surface sterilization. Its reactivity also makes it highly toxic and so any remaining traces must be removed before the sterilized material can be used.

5.5 HALOALKANES AND OTHER ORGANIC HALOGEN COMPOUNDS

If you look for organic halogen compounds (organic compounds containing halogens) in an organic chemistry textbook, you will find almost a whole chapter devoted to two reaction types—nucleophilic substitution and elimination. These are reactions of haloalkanes and they have some relevance in pharmaceutical chemistry, but in fact there are other aspects of organic halogen compounds that are far more interesting from a pharmaceutical (see Figure 5.17) and biological point of view.

Nomenclature

This chapter is about functional groups, and when we talk about haloalkanes we mean the haloalkane functional group (also known as an alkyl halide). The distinction between a haloalkane functional group and a haloalkane molecule is not always made in organic chemistry textbooks; if chemists want to study substitution reactions at R−Cl then R might as well be an alkyl group (made up of sp^3 carbon and hydrogen only). However, complex drug molecules such as chlorambucil (see Box 5.10) also contain haloalkane functional groups. R is certainly not a simple alkyl group, but the haloalkane functional group behaves in a predictable way; indeed, the reactions of chlorambucil are not very different from those of 1-chloropropane.

Like alcohols, haloalkane compounds can be primary, secondary or tertiary, and they can also be mono- or polyhalogenated. The difference between mono- and polyhalogenations is perhaps less profound than the difference between mono- and polyhydroxylation, but the difference between primary, secondary and tertiary organic halogen compounds is important.

Physical properties

Halogens are very electronegative elements and so haloalkanes and other organic halogen compounds (sometimes called organohalogen compounds or organohalides) tend to self-associate by dipole−dipole attraction. Like ethers, these molecules are poorly soluble in water,

Figure 5.17   Some chlorine-containing drugs

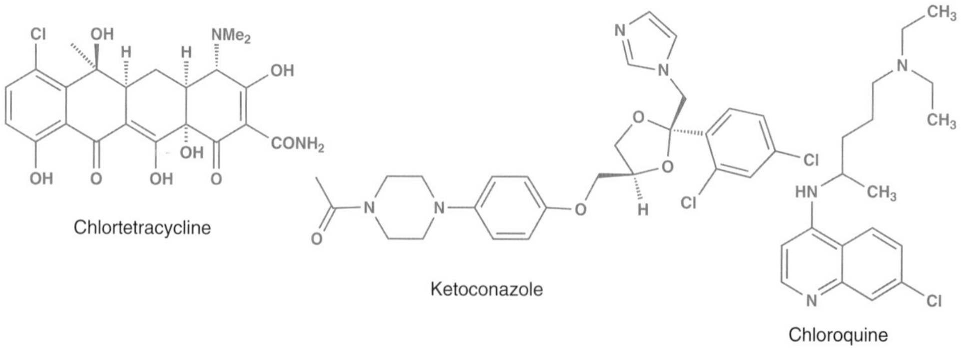

Chlortetracycline

Ketoconazole

Chloroquine

Self-check 5.15

The boiling point of methane (CH_4) is −164 °C. The boiling point of methanol is 65 °C. Estimate the boiling point of chloromethane (CH_3Cl).

Figure 5.18   Hydrogen bonds in an alkyl halide

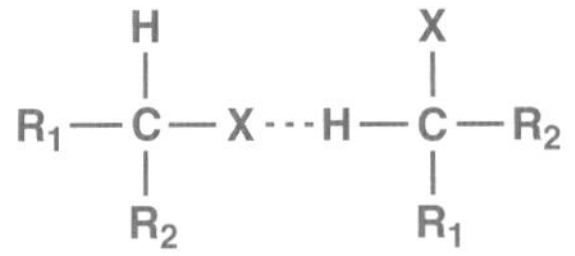

$$R_1 - \underset{\underset{R_2}{|}}{\overset{\overset{H}{|}}{C}} - X \cdots H - \underset{\underset{R_1}{|}}{\overset{\overset{X}{|}}{C}} - R_2$$

because they cannot readily form hydrogen bonds with water molecules. However, in a hydrophobic environment they *can* form hydrogen bonds (see Figure 5.18). These hydrogen bonds can be important in drug-receptor interactions, leading to prolonged retention of the drug at the receptor site. Consequently, halogen atoms are often introduced into the structure of potential drug molecules in an attempt to improve their biological activity.

These physical properties make many halogen compounds useful as solvents for a wide range of organic molecules. They have the added advantage over ethers in that they are largely non-flammable and are therefore safer to use. However, because of their high lipophilicity they easily cross lipid membranes and tissue boundaries and can accumulate in fatty tissues. This can give rise to toxicological problems, as discussed in the next section.

Chemical properties

As was stated previously, a key reaction of haloalkanes is nucleophilic substitution, as shown in Figure 5.19.

For an organic chemist the most interesting part of the molecule in Figure 5.19 is usually R. The nucleophile just modifies the structure R and may well be removed in the next reaction step. In the biological context, however, the nucleophile is an important biological molecule, such as DNA or a protein; halogen compounds are often referred to as alkylating agents, because they have the effect of alkylating (adding an alkyl group to) such biomolecules as described in Box 5.10.

Earlier in this chapter we talked briefly about S_N1 reactions in which a carbocation is an intermediate. The alkylation of biomolecules by organohalogen compounds more usually has the mechanism called S_N2. No carbocation is formed. Instead, the bond to the leaving group breaks at the same time as the bond to the nucleophile forms. Provided there is a good leaving group (such as a halide ion) and a good nucleophile (the $-SH$ of glutathione is a very good nucleophile, see Figure 5.20), extreme conditions of temperature and pH are not required. For a full description of an S_N2 mechanism you should consult an organic chemistry text book, such as Clayden et al. For our purposes it is important to note that the S_N2 mechanism proceeds best if the haloalkane is primary; the five-membered transition state is crowded and primary haloalkanes take up less space than their secondary and tertiary counterparts.

Because of the potential toxicity of these molecules, it is useful that the human body has a very effective mechanism for inactivating them. The detoxification process involves reaction (by S_N2 nucleophilic substitution) with glutathione, a tripeptide that possesses a SH (thiol)

157

Figure 5.19   Nucleophilic (S_N2) substitution of a halogen: general scheme

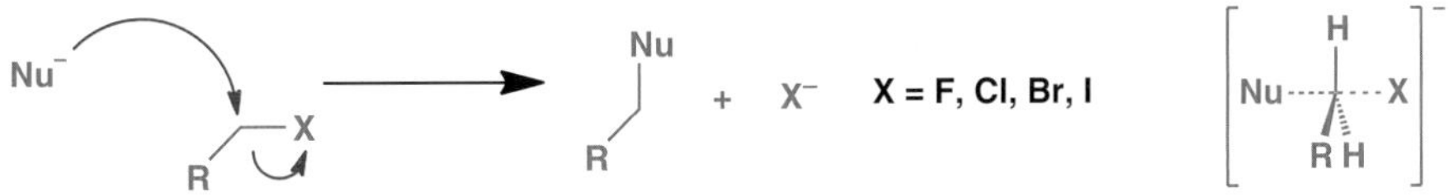

Nu⁻ ⟶ ... R—X ⟶ Nu—R + X⁻   X = F, Cl, Br, I

$$\left[Nu \cdots \underset{\underset{R\ H}{|}}{\overset{\overset{H}{|}}{C}} \cdots X \right]^{-}$$

5-membered transition state

Figure 5.20 S_N2 substitution of a chloride ion on chlorambucil by glutathione

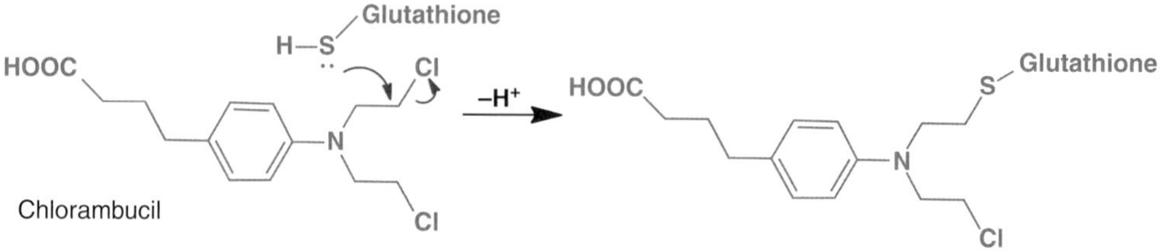

Box 5.10   Alkylating agents in cancer and cancer chemotherapy

Alkylating agents were first used as highly toxic chemical weapons during World War One. Their toxicity stems from the way they can alkylate the guanine bases of DNA, leading to potential gene mutations. They are therefore carcinogenic. However, more selective molecules have now been developed, to the extent that alkylating agents can now be used to treat certain cancers.

Alkylating agents react preferentially with cancer cells, which divide more rapidly than healthy cells. However, they remain toxic to normal cells and so cause severe side-effects, particularly in those tissues where cells are rapidly dividing, such as bone marrow and reproductive organs.

Alkylating agents used as drugs include chlorambucil and cyclophosphamide. Note that they are both primary organohalogen compounds.

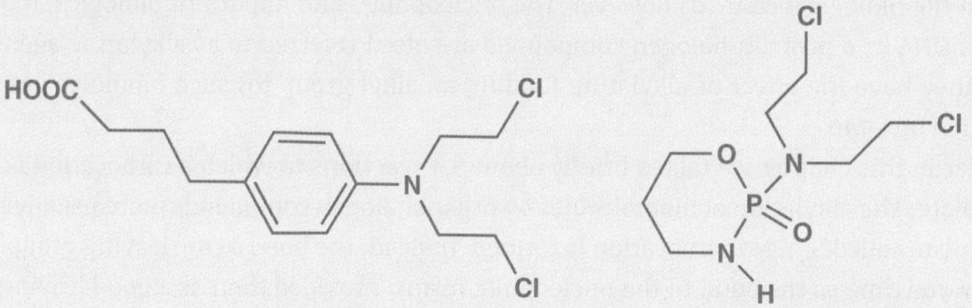

group. The SH group is an excellent nucleophile, so the halogen compounds react with glutathione in preference to other cellular constituents (see Figure 5.20).

5.6 AROMATIC HALOGEN COMPOUNDS

Aromatic halogen compounds have similar physical properties to haloalkanes for similar reasons. For example, chlorobenzene and 1-chlorohexane have similar boiling points (131 °C and 135 °C) above those of benzene and hexane (81 °C and 69 °C). The chemical properties are quite different, however.

Halogen atoms on aromatic rings cannot take part in nucleophilic substitution. This means that they are stable in the body and are much more common in drug molecules than haloalkanes. A halogen in an aromatic ring introduces subtle changes in polarity, which can be advantageous. Examples of halogenated aromatic drugs are the antibacterial agent chlortetra-cycline and the antifungal ketoconazole.

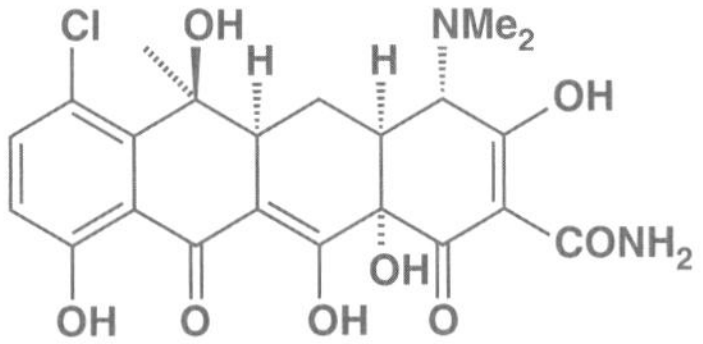

Chlortetracycline

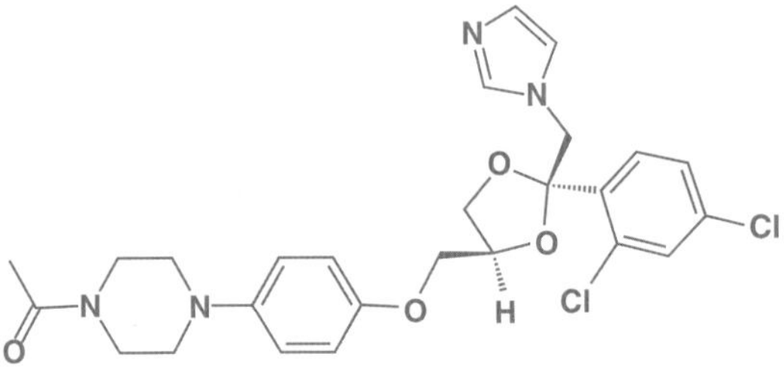

Ketoconazole

The lack of reactivity means that aromatic halogen compounds cannot be detoxified by glu-tathione. (This is explained in more detail in Chapter 7.) The lack of reactivity of some haloge-nated molecules (for example, DDT) has led to environmental problems, as explained in Box 5.11. (See Figure 5.21 for some halogenated environmental hazards).

5.7 POLYHALOGEN COMPOUNDS

Molecules possessing multiple halogen atoms have found a variety of uses—for example, as solvents, general anaesthetics, refrigerants and aerosol propellants (which are important com-ponents of some drug delivery devices such as the inhalers used for the treatment of asthma). The polyhalogen compounds that have been used for this purpose are known as CFCs (chloro-fluorocarbons) and two of these are shown in Figure 5.21. Nowadays, however, drug delivery devices are CFC-free. Why is this?

CFCs are good solvents, and are volatile, non-flammable and unreactive—properties that made them attractive in aerosols. Their lack of reactivity, however, caused an environmental problem when they were used widely in this context. While most organic chemicals are broken down in the lower atmosphere, CFCs accumulated in the upper atmosphere. This accumulation became problematic because the C-Cl bonds are broken under the influence of ultraviolet ra-diation from space, and the chlorine atoms (free radicals) that are formed damage the ozone layer, which protects the Earth from harmful ultraviolet radiation. Pharmaceutical and other aerosols now utilize other propellants and are often labelled 'CFC-free'.

Self-check 5.16

Two of the three molecules shown in Figure 5.21 have chiral centres. Which are they?

Organic halogen compounds possess properties that can be potentially useful (solvents, general anaesthetics), but they also have a potential for toxicity (alkylating agents, environmental problems).

Figure 5.21   Halogenated environmental toxins

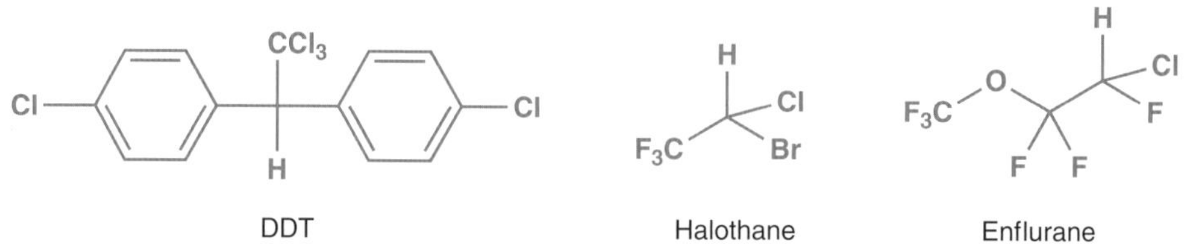

DDT   Halothane   Enflurane

Box 5.11   DDT

DDT is a highly effective insecticide. It was discovered in 1939 and was regarded as a significant scientific breakthrough. At the time, the stability of DDT was seen as one of its greatest benefits—it would remain active for longer. This, however, proved to be its undoing: DDT began to accumulate in the food chain wherever it was heavily used. DDT is highly lipid soluble and so accumulates in the fatty tissue of species at the top of the food chain (including humans), with potentially toxic effects. Subsequently it received a world-wide ban.

160

5.8 AMINES

A number of organic functional groups contain nitrogen (e.g. nitro, amide, nitrile), but one particularly important nitrogen-containing group is the amine group.

Nomenclature

Amines can be classified as primary (1°), secondary (2°) or tertiary (3°) in a manner similar, but not identical, to alcohols. A primary amine is derived from ammonia (NH_3) by replacement of one hydrogen atom with an alkyl group. Secondary amines have two hydrogens replaced by alkyl groups, and tertiary have all three hydrogens replaced by alkyl groups, as illustrated in Figure 5.22.

In addition to this classification, amines may be aliphatic (whereby the amine group is attached to an alkyl chain), aromatic (where the amine group is attached directly to an aromatic ring) or heterocyclic (where the nitrogen atom of the amine group is contained in a ring system).

Physical properties

Because of the presence of the electronegative nitrogen atom, amines are polar molecules. Primary and secondary amines can self-associate by hydrogen bonding, but tertiary amines cannot because they lack a hydrogen attached to nitrogen. Nitrogen is less electronegative than

Figure 5.22   Primary, secondary and tertiary amines

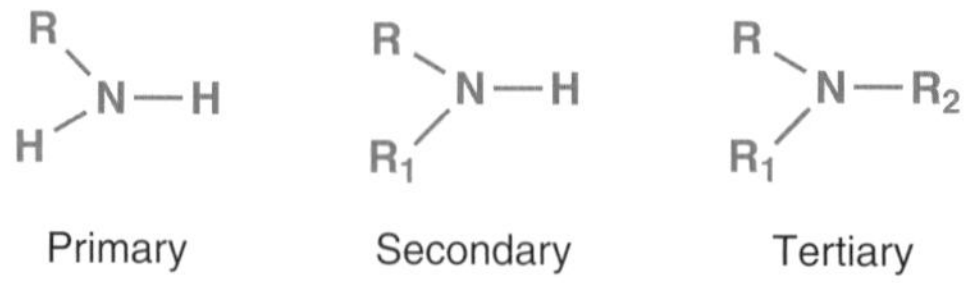

Primary   Secondary   Tertiary

oxygen so these hydrogen bonds are weaker than those in alcohols. Consequently, the boiling points of amines are lower than those of their corresponding alcohols: whereas methanol boils at 65 °C, methylamine is a gas (with a disgusting smell) with a boiling point of −6 °C.

Because of their ability to hydrogen bond to water molecules, amines are relatively water soluble.

Chemical properties

Amines are basic: they can accept a proton and become positively charged. The lone pair of electrons on the nitrogen acts as a nucleophile and reacts with a positively charged hydrogen ion. Reaction with an acid (a proton donor) will lead to the formation of a salt.

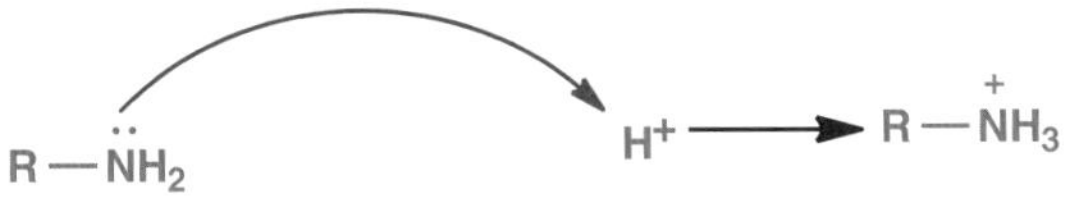

$$R-\ddot{N}H_2 \qquad H^+ \longrightarrow R-\overset{+}{N}H_3$$

Aliphatic amines are stronger bases than aromatic amines. We usually refer to the pK_a of the conjugate acid to illustrate this point. The conjugate acid of $R-NH_2$ is $R-NH_3^+$ (see below).

$$R-\overset{+}{N}H_3 \rightleftharpoons R-NH_2 \;+\; H^+$$

For aliphatic amines the dissociation shown above is 50% complete at pH 10, so the pK_a of the conjugate acid of an aliphatic amine is about 10.

It is very important to appreciate that because amines are bases they become more protonated at low pH (see Box 5.12).

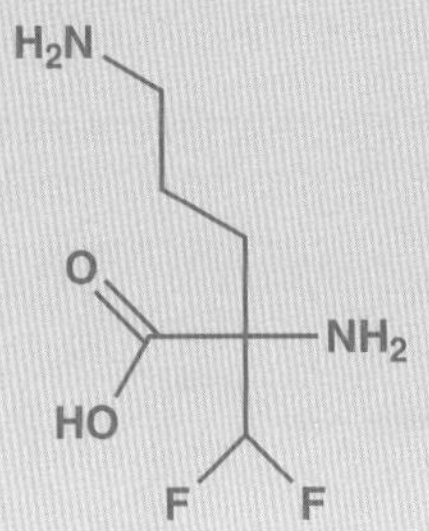

Box 5.12 pK$_a$s of bases

A K$_a$ represents an **acid dissociation constant** so a pK$_a$ tells you the pH at which an *acid* is half-dissociated. Therefore, strictly speaking, the pK$_a$ of an amine refers to the following reaction, where the amine is acting as an acid:

$$R-NH_2 \quad \rightleftharpoons \quad R-\overset{-}{N}H \quad + \quad H^+$$

When R = Ph, the pK$_a$ for this reaction is over 30! Because pK$_a$s of over 30 are not relevant in aqueous solution, biologists and pharmacists sometimes get a bit lazy and refer to the pK$_a$ of an amine, when they are really referring to the pK$_a$ of its conjugate acid.

You may find references to the pK$_b$ of an amine, especially in older books. The pK$_b$ of an amine refers to the dissociation of a base, and has a value that is approximately equal to 14 – pK$_a$ of the conjugate acid. The use of the pK$_b$ has the advantage that you do not have to keep saying 'of the conjugate acid'; the disadvantage is that strong bases have lower pK$_b$s and weak bases have higher pK$_b$s, which can be confusing; the use of pK$_b$ is much less common than it once was.

Aromatic amines are less basic than aliphatic amines and their conjugate acids have pK$_a$s of about 5. This means that they are generally protonated in the stomach at pH 2 (the equilibrium reaction, shown earlier in this section, lies to the left, favouring the conjugate acid), but exist in the unprotonated (free base) form in the intestine at pH 8 (the equilibrium reaction, on shown earlier in this section, lies to the right). Why do we see this difference between aliphatic and aromatic amines? The reason is that the lone pair of electrons on the amine nitrogen is delocalized into the aromatic ring and is less readily available to bind to a proton (see Figure 5.23); consequently, it acts as a weaker base. In aliphatic amines, the lone pair is not delocalized and so a proton can be accepted more readily.

Amines in drugs

Many drug molecules possess an amine group, which can be reacted with an acid to form a salt; the salt is generally more water-soluble than the original drug molecule. This can be useful; for example, you cannot inject a solid, so it is helpful to be able to **formulate** an insoluble amine as a soluble salt.

The amine group in a drug molecule is often a key binding point between a drug and a receptor site. Indeed, a number of the functional groups in this chapter have the capacity, if present in a drug molecule, to be involved in interactions between the drug and a receptor. The hydroxyl group, be it an alcohol or a phenol, may be involved in hydrogen bonding to the receptor. The

Figure 5.23   The delocalization of the electron pair of an aromatic amine

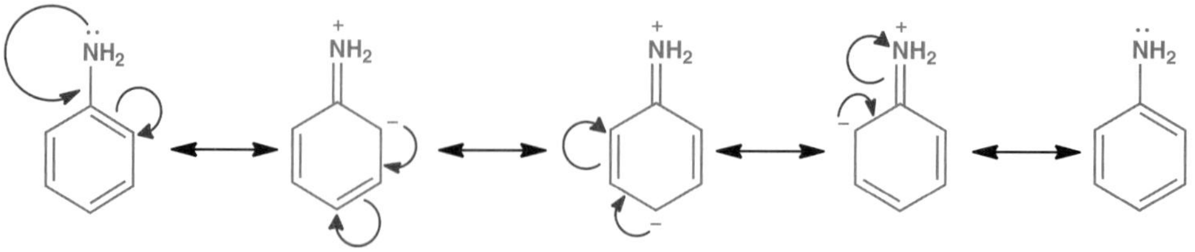

Figure 5.24   Oxidative deamination of an amino acid

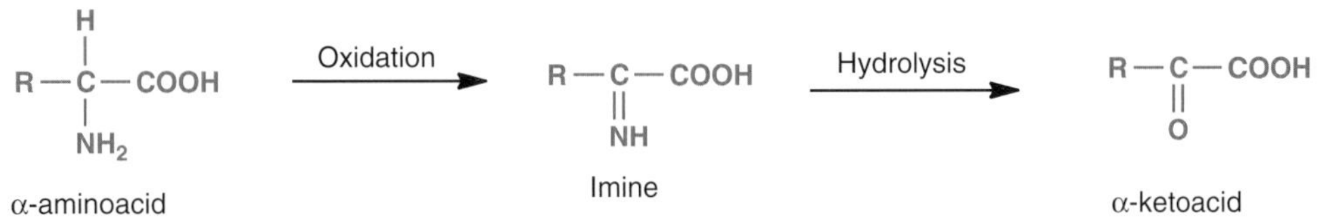

R—C—COOH with H and NH$_2$ substituents →(Oxidation)→ R—C—COOH with NH double bond →(Hydrolysis)→ R—C—COOH with O double bond

α-aminoacid   Imine   α-ketoacid

> The ability of amines to act as bases is an important property, particularly when the group is present in a drug molecule.

amine group, which is likely to be ionized at physiological pH, may be involved in an ionic interaction with an anionic site on the receptor. These are likely to be primary sites of interaction. An ether group may, if present, provide an additional electrostatic interaction.

Oxidation of amines

In the laboratory, the oxidation of amines is not a particularly important reaction. Biologically speaking, however, it is vital. The majority of energy-producing reactions in the cell involve molecules containing carbon, hydrogen and oxygen only (carbohydrates and fatty acids). Most of us take in more protein than we need, and excess amino acids are metabolized by removal of nitrogen so that they can join the citric acid cycle. The removal of nitrogen happens by a process known as oxidative deamination and is often carried out by monoamine oxidase enzymes, as illustrated in Figure 5.24.

Alkylation of amines

Amines are able to undergo numerous reactions in which they act as nucleophiles, and these reactions are important in the synthesis of drugs. Nucleophilic attack of amines on suitable carbonyl compounds leads to the formation of amides and is described in the next chapter. Amines can be alkylated by nucleophilic attack on haloalkanes. (Can you draw the mechanism?). Further reading about the reactions of amines can be found in Clayden et al.

5.9 QUATERNARY AMMONIUM COMPOUNDS

Tertiary amines are formed by progressive replacement of the hydrogens on nitrogen by alkyl groups. If a tertiary amine reacts with a halogenated hydrocarbon, a quaternary ammonium compound, such as that shown in Figure 5.25, is formed.

Quaternary ammonium compounds exhibit different properties from amines. Amines are basic, but quaternary ammonium compounds are neutral. Amines are relatively volatile, but quaternary ammonium compounds are solids. Quaternary ammonium compounds will dissolve in water, but not in organic solvents, unlike amines which dissolve in both. The reason for these

Figure 5.25   A quaternary ammonium salt

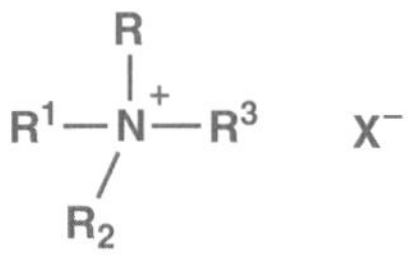

R^1—$\overset{\overset{\displaystyle R}{|}}{\underset{\underset{\displaystyle R_2}{/}}{N^+}}$—$R^3$ X^-

163

Self-check 5.19

Find an example of a quaternary ammonium compound that is used for the following purposes: (a) neurotransmitter, (b) topical antibacterial agent, (c) neuromuscular blocking agent.

changes is that quaternary ammonium compounds are ionic and so behave like ionic molecules, unlike the amines which are completely covalent molecules.

If one or more of the alkyl chains in quaternary ammonium compounds is a long alkyl chain
(C_{12}–C_{20}), then these molecules will concentrate at the oil–water interface and can act as detergents.
(They are known as cationic detergents, because of the positive charge on the nitrogen atom.) This
ability to concentrate at an oil–water interface is also responsible for the antibacterial activity
of some of these molecules. They penetrate the cell membrane of micro-organisms, particularly
those classified as Gram negative organisms. Because of their inability to cross lipid membranes,
they are only used as topical antibacterial agents (e.g. antibacterial swabs, throat lozenges).

CHAPTER SUMMARY

- The nature of the intermolecular forces of attraction is the major factor in determining
  the boiling points and water solubilities of molecules.
- Hydrogen bonding is a particularly important intermolecular force.
- Dehydration and oxidation are important reactions of alcohols, particularly from a bio-
  logical perspective.
- Although both possess an OH group, alcohols and phenols differ considerably in their
  physical and chemical properties.
- Small ring cyclic ethers are very reactive, unlike other types of ether.
- Organic halogen compounds have a wide range of potentially useful properties, but are
  also generally quite toxic.
- The basicity of amines is a very important property, both biologically and pharmaceutically.

FURTHER READING

Clayden, J., Greeves, N. and Warren, S. *Organic Chemistry*, 2nd edn. Oxford University Press, 2012.
  A student-friendly undergraduate textbook with an emphasis on clarity and understanding of the
  key concepts of organic chemistry.
Holum, J. R. *Organic and Biological Chemistry*. John Wiley and Sons, 1996.
  Emphasizes the functional groups that occur widely among the molecules of life.
McMurry, J. *Fundamentals of Organic Chemistry*, 7th edn. Cengage Learning, 2011.
  Another student-friendly organic chemistry textbook.

Self-check

For the answers to the Self-check questions in Chapter 5, visit the online resources which
accompany this textbook.

THE CARBONYL GROUP AND ITS CHEMISTRY

Matthew Ingram

This chapter considers the nature of the carbonyl group and the fantastic chemistry it can undergo. We can find this chemistry in lots of situations: in the body, in the environment, in manufacturing and, of course in pharmaceutical applications. Before reading this chapter, it is important that you are familiar with key concepts covered earlier in this book; these include nomenclature, acids and bases, electrophiles and nucleophiles. If you are unsure, we would recommend revisiting these before attempting to understand the materials in this chapter.

Learning objectives

Having read this chapter you are expected to be able to:

- distinguish between the different types of carbonyl compounds, draw their chemical structures and name simple derivatives
- predict simple reactions and their likely products
- understand how nature uses carbonyl chemistry
- understand how the medicinal chemist or pharmacist can manipulate different types of carbonyl compounds for a desired clinical outcome.

6.1 CARBONYL STRUCTURE AND NOMENCLATURE

At the heart of the chemistry of the carbonyl group is the carbonyl bond, a double bond comprising one σ and one π bond, which joins the carbon and the oxygen. The difference in electronegativity between the carbon and oxygen (with oxygen being strongly electronegative) means a dipole moment exists between the two atoms.

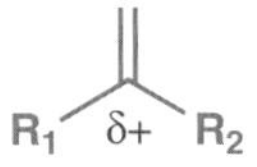

More details on this type of bonding can be found in Chapter 2, 'Organic structure and bonding'.

The carbonyl group is central to pharmaceutical chemistry and is present in many drug molecules and **excipients** that you may already be familiar with.

As you can see from Figure 6.1, the carbonyl group is present in many different types of compound. If we draw the carbonyl in the form:

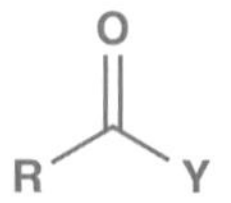

Self-check 6.1

Find the carbonyl group(s) in each of the molecules in Figure 6.1.

Self-check 6.2

Briefly explain the use of each of these carbonyl compounds in pharmacy.

Box 6.1 Phosphate esters

Table 6.1 shows that if we take an ester, such as ethyl acetate (ethyl ethanoate), we can replace one of the oxygens with sulfur or even selenium to give a thioester or a selenium ester. So we might expect to be able to replace the nitrogen of an amide by phosphorus (which is immediately below nitrogen in the periodic table). In fact, phosphate esters are based on the P=O group, not on the C=O group, because phosphorus has similar electronegativity to carbon and acts as an electrophile rather than as a leaving group. Phosphate esters are incredibly important in biochemistry and are considered in Chapter 9, and their chemistry is covered in detail in Chapter 8.

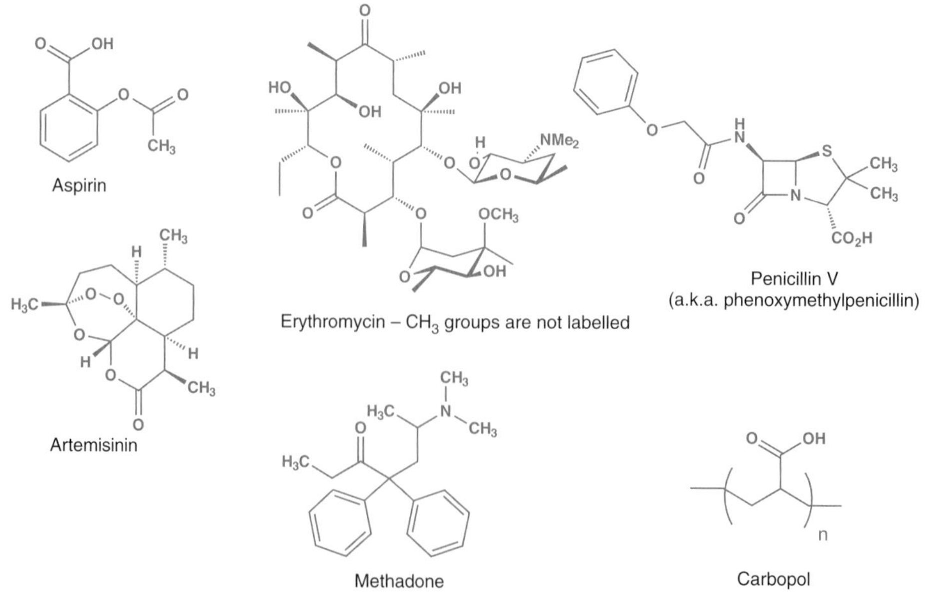

Figure 6.1 Common molecules in pharmaceutical chemistry that all contain the carbonyl functionality

then Y can be H, or C, or an electronegative element. In nature and in drug molecules, the position Y is very often occupied by O (as in aspirin) or N (as in penicillin) (see also Box 6.1). The family of carbonyl compounds is as shown in Table 6.1.

Table 6.1 Different types of carbonyl compound

Name	Name ending	Structure	Typical example with systematic name. Trivial names (where appropriate) are given in brackets
Aldehyde	-al	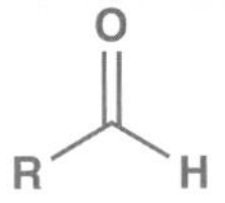 O‖ R–C–H	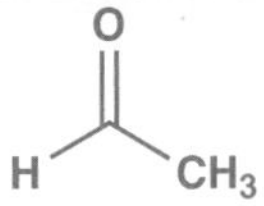 O‖ H–C–CH₃ Ethanal (acetaldehyde)
Ketone	-one	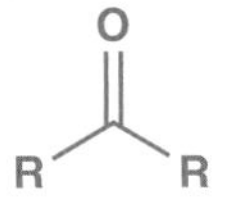 O‖ R–C–R	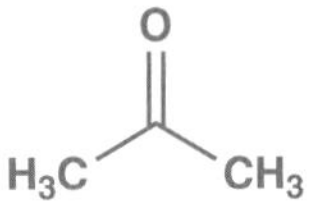 O‖ H₃C–C–CH₃ Propan-2-one (acetone)
Carboxylic acid	-oic acid	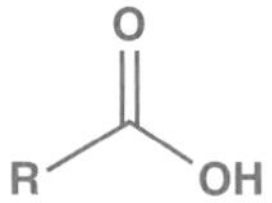 O‖ R–C–OH	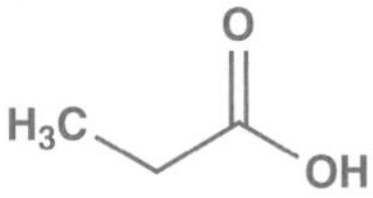 O‖ H₃C–CH₂–C–OH Propanoic acid
Acyl halide	-onyl chloride, bromide or iodide	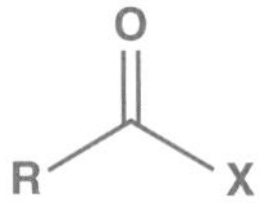 O‖ R–C–X	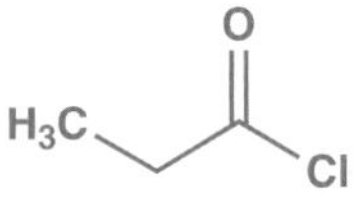 O‖ H₃C–CH₂–C–Cl Propanoyl chloride
Acid anhydride	-oic anhydride	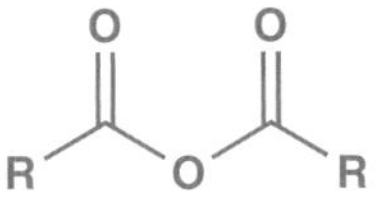 O‖ O‖ R–C–O–C–R	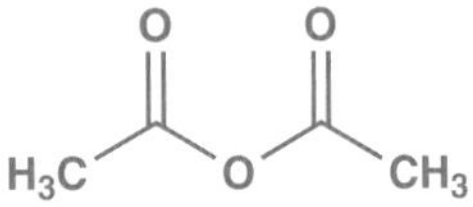 O‖ O‖ H₃C–C–O–C–CH₃ Ethanoic anhydride (acetic anhydride)
Ester	-oate	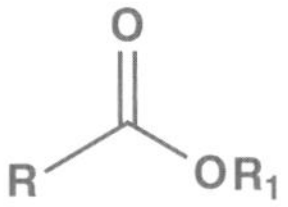 O‖ R–C–OR₁	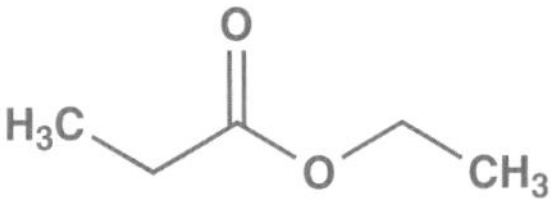 O‖ H₃C–CH₂–C–O–CH₃ Ethyl propanoate
Thioester	thioate	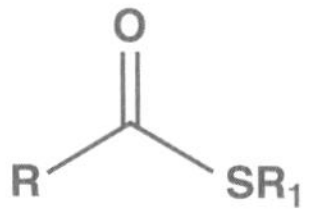 O‖ R–C–SR₁	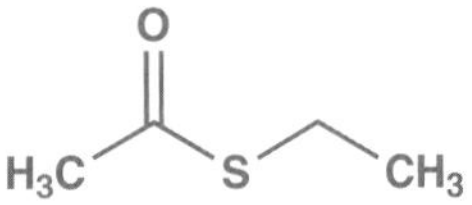 O‖ H₃C–C–S–CH₃ S-Ethyl ethanethioate (Ethyl thioacetate)
Amide	-amide	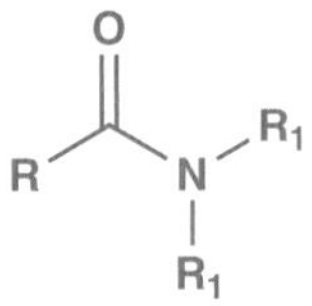 O‖ R–C–N(R₁)(R₁)	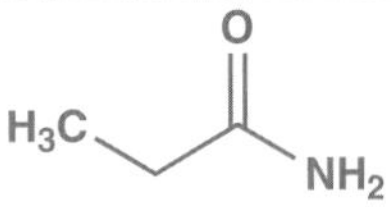 O‖ H₃C–CH₂–C–NH₂ Propanamide

Self-check 6.3

Name these compounds using the IUPAC system. Tip: Revise the nomenclature of alkenes in Chapter 4.

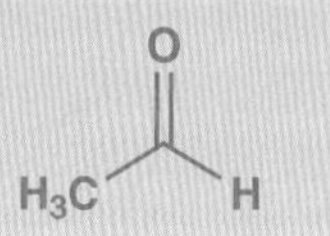

(A) 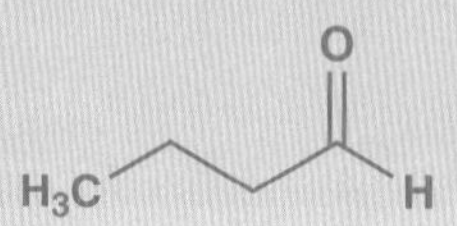 (B) 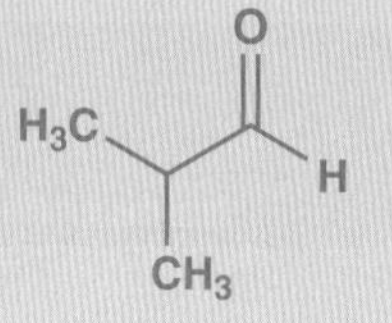 (C)

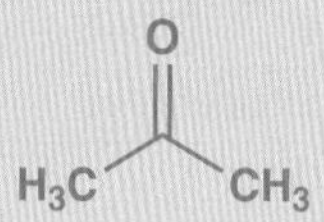

(D) 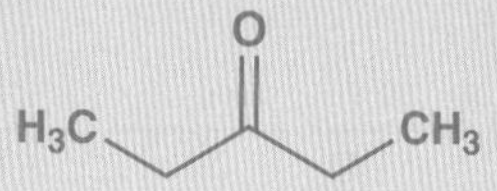 (E) 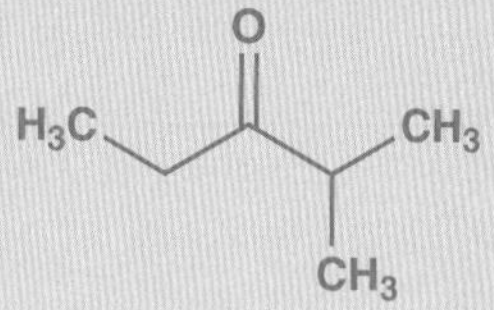 (F)

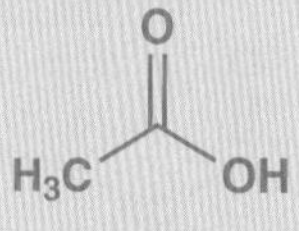

(G) 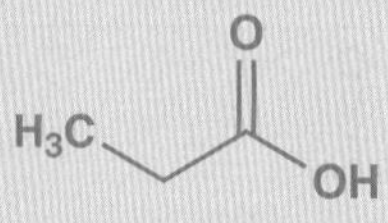 (H) 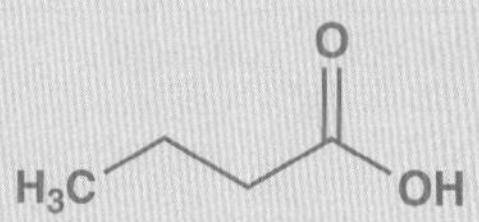 (I)

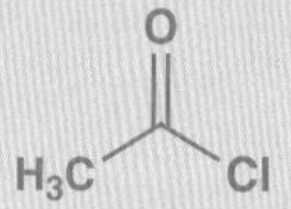

(J) 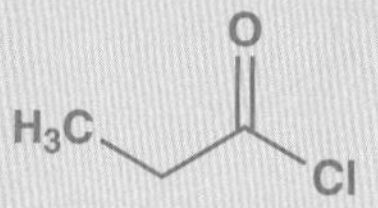 (K) 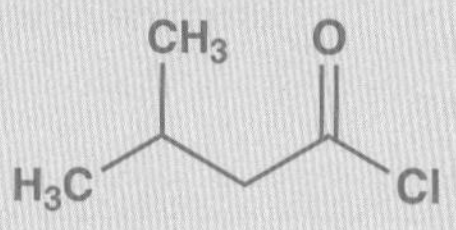 (L)

We need to be able to name these families of molecules using the IUPAC system. The names are made up from the prefix, which is described in Chapter 2, and the ending, which depends on the type of carbonyl compound. The name endings are given in Table 6.1.

In addition to the systematic names, there are common names that are still used and you will come across these during your studies and in your future careers. Figure 6.2 gives the common names for some important molecules that contain carbonyl groups.

The common names existed before the creation of the IUPAC system and are still widely used. For example, acetic acid is still the preferred name in the laboratory, and is even preferred by IUPAC over the systematic name. Sportsmen and women, as well as scientists and healthcare professionals, refer to (S)-2-hydroxypropanoic acid as L-lactic acid. Pharmacists need to be aware of both systems in order to bridge the gap between chemists, healthcare professionals and the general public.

> Common (trivial) names are discussed in Chapter 1, 'The importance of pharmaceutical chemistry'.

Self-check 6.4

Can you convert these names into structures?

1. Acetaldehyde (ethanal)

2. Pentanal

3. Octan-2-one

4. 3-Methylpentanoic acid

5. 2,2-Dimethylbutanedioic acid

6. Propanoic anhydride

7. Hexanoic acid

8. Butanal

9. Benzophenone (diphenyl ketone)

10. Acetyl chloride (ethanoyl chloride)

Figure 6.2   Some important carbonyl compounds and their trivial names

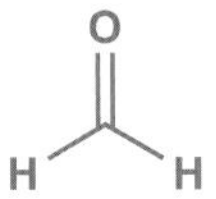

Formaldehyde 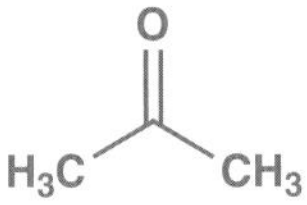   Acetone 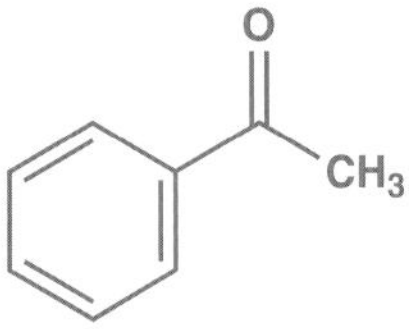   Acetophenone

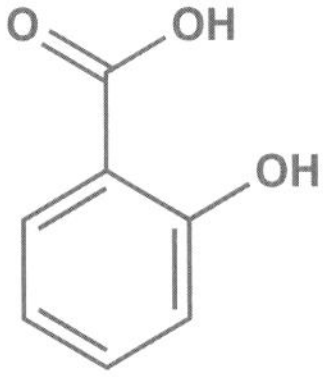

Salicylic acid 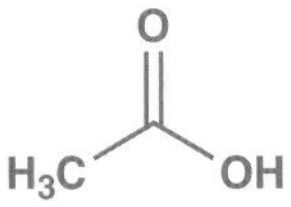   Acetic acid 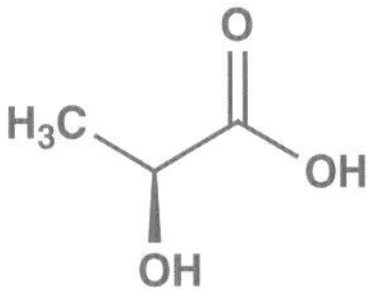   L-lactic acid

6.2 THE POWER OF THE CARBONYL GROUP

The central importance of carbon is discussed in Chapter 2. A moment's thought (or breathing) will remind you of the importance of oxygen. A functional group containing both carbon and oxygen is, therefore, likely to be important. Spend a moment trying to think of a drug *without* a carbonyl group, and a biochemical intermediate *without* a carbonyl group. This exercise should convince you that the carbonyl group holds a special place in pharmaceutical chemistry. It is, indeed, powerful!

Carbonyl groups and physical properties

Oxygen is **electronegative** and draws electron density away from the carbon, leaving the carbon with a δ+ charge and the oxygen with a δ− charge. This is described as a **chemical dipole moment** (see Figure 6.3).

Figure 6.3 The chemical dipole moment of a carbonyl group and its reactivity

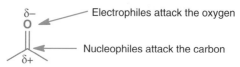

In aldehydes, ketones, acyl chlorides, acid anhydrides and esters, dipole–dipole attraction is the intermolecular force found between adjacent molecules and, thus, influences the boiling/melting points of these compounds. Because dipole–dipole attractions are relatively weak, these classes of carbonyl compounds are predominantly liquids with relatively low boiling points (see Table 6.2). With carboxylic acids and amides, however, the key intermolecular force is hydrogen bonding (see Figure 6.4). Hydrogen bonding is a much stronger intermolecular force than dipole–dipole attraction. Consequently, carboxylic acids and amides have higher boiling points—indeed, many are solids rather than liquids (see Table 6.2).

❯ More detail can be found on intermolecular interactions in Chapter 2, 'Organic structure and bonding'.

The ability to form hydrogen bonds also influences water solubility. Aldehydes, ketones and esters cannot form hydrogen bonds with each other, but they can act as hydrogen bond acceptors with water. Simple aldehydes and ketones, therefore, are readily soluble in water, but the solubility rapidly decreases with an increasing hydrocarbon component (see Table 6.3).

The increased hydrocarbon component already present in esters (RCOOR′) means that their water solubility is compromised from the start (because R′ is usually a hydrocarbon).

Carboxylic acids can interact with water as both a hydrogen bond acceptor and a donor, and so low molecular weight carboxylic acids are very soluble in water. Acids up to four carbons are completely miscible with water. This solubility, again, rapidly decreases with an increasing hydrocarbon component, so that hexanoic acid has only 1% water solubility.

Table 6.2 Boiling points of some C3 organic compounds

Compound	Boiling point (°C)
Propene	−47.4
Acetone	56.6
Ethyl acetate	77
Propanoic acid	141
Dimethylformamide (DMF)	153

Figure 6.4 Hydrogen bonding in propanoic acid. Dimers are formed, raising the boiling point, relative to propanone

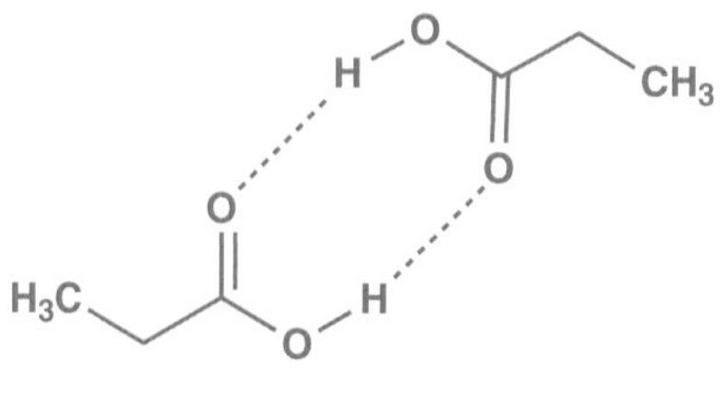

Table 6.3   Water solubility of carbonyl compounds

Compound	Water solubility (%)
Acetone	Completely miscible
Butan-2-one	25.6
Pentan-2-one	5.5
Hexan-2-one	1.6
Acetic acid	Completely miscible
Hexanoic acid	1.0
Dimethylformamide	Completely miscible

Amides exhibit similar solubility profiles because they, too, can form effective hydrogen bonds with water. We do not have to worry about the water solubility of acid anhydrides and acyl chlorides because they react with water (see later in this chapter).

Why do carbonyls undergo useful reactions?

Aspirin is a pain-killer that has been used for well over 100 years, and it actually contains two carbonyl groups. The reaction that forms aspirin is reviewed several times in this book, particularly in Chapter 7. However, for now let us celebrate the coming together of two carbonyl containing compounds.

In Figure 6.5, salicylic acid, which already has one carbonyl group, acquires another. The hydroxyl function of salicylic acid reacts with acetic anhydride (ethanoic anhydride) and is acetylated, to give an acetate ester. The transfer of acyl ($CH_3C=O$) groups from one molecule to another is also important in biological systems. For example, food enters the citric acid cycle in the form of acetyl coenzyme A; the acetyl group is transferred to oxaloacetate to give citrate. However, anhydrides are very reactive and are incompatible with biological systems, so nature uses alternative carbonyl compounds, typically thioesters, for acyl transfer in cells.

> ❯ Further details on the citric acid cycle can be found in Chapter 11, 'Carbohydrates and carbohydrate metabolism'.

If we understand why carbonyl compounds behave as they do, we should be able to predict how they will react with other molecules and how they might react in a biological situation.

171

Figure 6.5   The synthesis of aspirin from acetic anhydride and salicylic acid

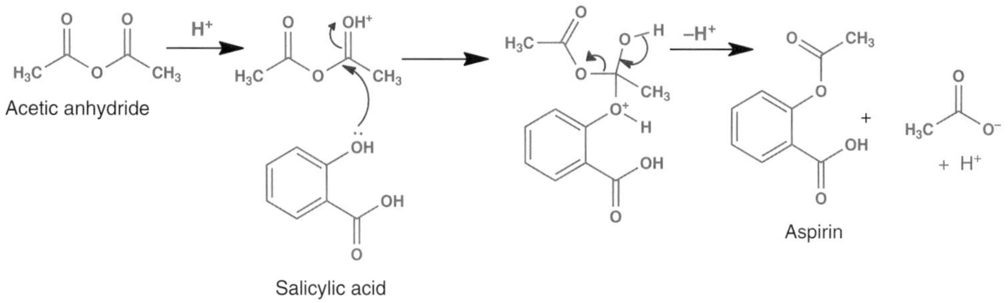

It's all in the electrons: the power of electronegativity

From a thermodynamic point of view, the carbonyl group is very stable. The presence of carbonyls in drugs and in nature therefore comes as no surprise. This thermodynamic stability does not, however, prevent carbonyls from taking part in reactions; this is something they do rather eagerly. However, the endpoint of a reaction involving a carbonyl is very often another carbonyl. As we read further through this chapter we will come to understand why this is.

If we examine Figure 6.3 again we can see how the dipole moment influences the reactivity of carbonyl compounds. Electrophiles (such as H^+) seek out areas of high electron density (the oxygen), whereas nucleophiles (such as amines) are attracted to areas of low electron density (the carbon).

Carbonyls are subject to nucleophilic attack

In practice, the chemistry of carbonyl groups is dominated by nucleophilic attack on carbon, as shown in Figure 6.6. Nucleophiles may either be negatively charged or neutral, and Table 6.4 shows some examples.

The action of the nucleophile on the carbonyl group gives us an intermediate in which the π bond breaks and the carbon is single-bonded to four species. The four bonds arrange themselves to be as far apart as possible, and the intermediate is tetrahedral.

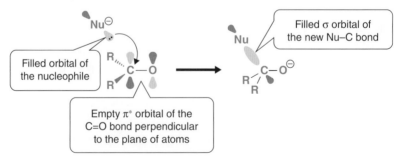

Tetrahedral intermediate

> For more about tetrahedral carbon atoms see Chapter 2, 'Organic structure and bonding'.

Table 6.4   Some nucleophiles capable of reacting with carbonyl groups

Examples of negative nucleophiles	Examples of neutral nucleophiles
HO^-	H_2O
RO^-	H_3N
R_3C^-	ROH
NC^-	RNH_2

Figure 6.6   Nucleophilic attack on the carbonyl group. Redrawn with permission from Burrows et al. (2009) Chemistry³, OUP

Filled orbital of the nucleophile

Filled σ orbital of the new Nu–C bond

Empty π* orbital of the C=O bond perpendicular to the plane of atoms

The fate of the tetrahedral intermediate is determined by the best **leaving group**. Let us consider what happens when:

- Nu is a good leaving group (better than Y)
- Y is a good leaving group (better than Nu)
- neither Nu nor Y is a good leaving group

> For a detailed description of leaving groups, see Section 6.3, 'Reactions of carbonyl compounds—nucleophilic attack on carbon'.

Nu is a good leaving group

If Nu is a good leaving group, it simply leaves at the end of the reaction. In other words, the reaction simply reverses (see Scheme 6.1).

Cl⁻ is an example of a good leaving group, and you cannot make acyl chlorides by treating another carbonyl compound with chloride ion. Similarly, acetate is a good leaving group (see the synthesis of aspirin, Figure 6.5), and you cannot make acid anhydrides by attacking another carbonyl with an acetate ion.

An everyday example is shown in Figure 6.7. Chloride ion, a good leaving group, does not react with acetic acid. So, for example, the chloride ions in salt do not react with acetic acid in vinegar, because Cl⁻ is a good leaving group. If they did, an acyl chloride would be generated—not something you would want with your chips! If you eat chips with salt and vinegar too often, you might get fat from the fried food, or you might get hypertension from the salt, or you might get tooth decay from the acid, but otherwise it is perfectly safe.

Scheme 6.1

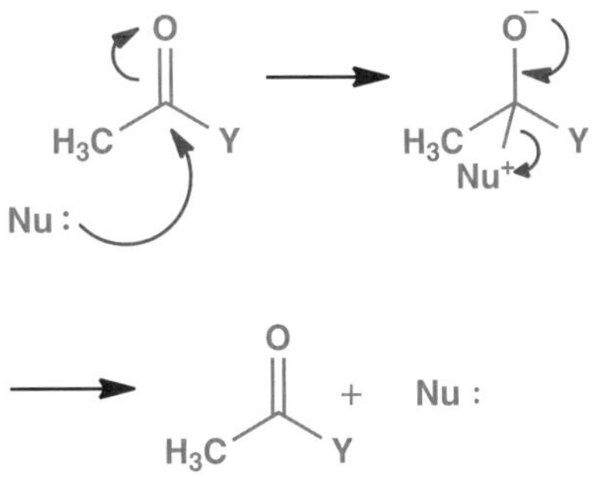

Figure 6.7 Lack of reaction of Cl⁻ with acetic acid: there is no reaction between the salt and vinegar on your chips
Source: Viktor Fischer.

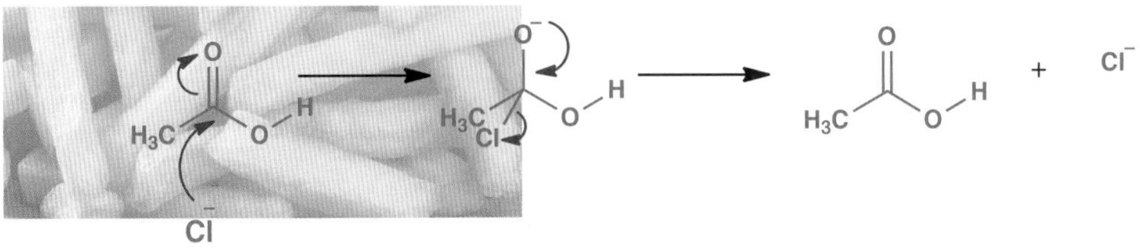

Y is a good leaving group

If Y is a good leaving group, Y leaves at the end of the reaction (see Scheme 6.2). This behaviour leads us to some very important reactions of carbonyl compounds:

- formation of esters from carboxylic acids
- hydrolysis of esters to carboxylic acids
- formation of esters from acyl chlorides (acid chlorides) or acid anhydrides (acyl anhydrides)
- formation of amides from acyl chlorides or acid anhydrides
- hydrolysis of amides

These reactions will be discussed in Section 6.3, 'Reactions of carbonyl compounds—nucleophilic attack on carbon'.

Neither Y nor Nu is a good leaving group

Aldehydes and ketones do not have good leaving groups. When a nucleophile attacks an aldehyde or ketone, the carbonyl π-bond breaks and does not reform (see Scheme 6.3). There are three major classes of reaction of this type:

- addition of water or alcohols to give hemiacetals and acetals
- addition of the equivalent of H⁻, a reduction reaction
- addition of a R_3C^- equivalent; formation of a C–C bond

These are discussed in Section 6.3 too.

Scheme 6.2

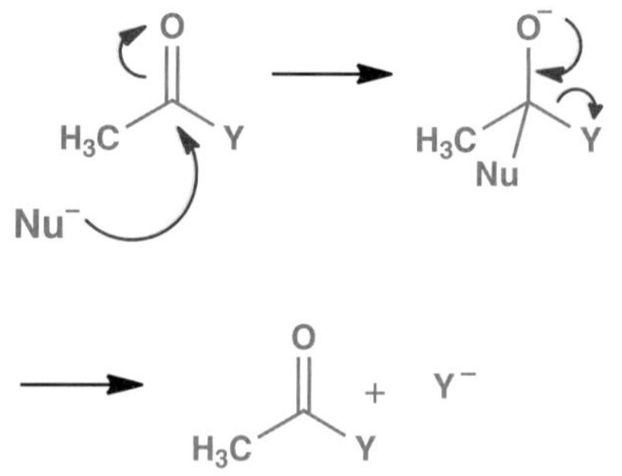

Scheme 6.3

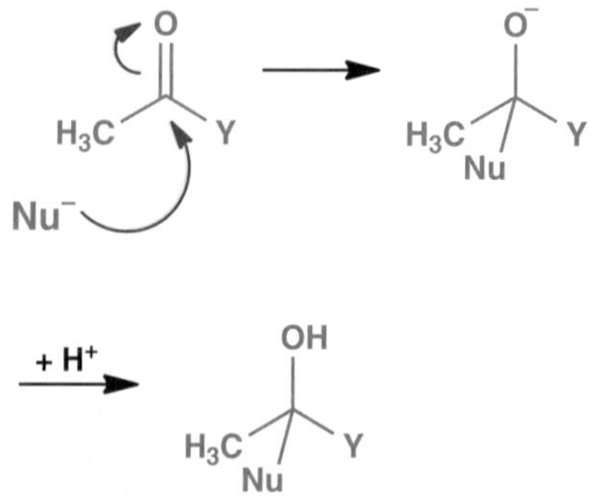

6.3 REACTIONS OF CARBONYL COMPOUNDS— NUCLEOPHILIC ATTACK ON CARBON

The most important reactions of carbonyl compounds involve attack of the carbon with the δ+ charge by a nucleophile. This section describes reactions of this type which have significant pharmaceutical and biological relevance.

Making carbonyls reactive

Many carbonyl compounds are stable. Acetone can be used as a solvent because it dissolves reactants without itself reacting. The 'best before' date on a bottle of vinegar (dilute acetic acid) is months after you buy it. Many of the proteins in your body (which are polyamides) are metabolized only very slowly. To make carbonyl compounds react, we often need to add an acid or base catalyst to boost the reactivity (see Figure 6.8).

By adding acid we can build up the positive charge at the carbon of the carbonyl group. This type of catalysis has been used in carbonyl chemistry extensively. You may have come across this simple reaction, the Fischer esterification, in your pre-university courses.

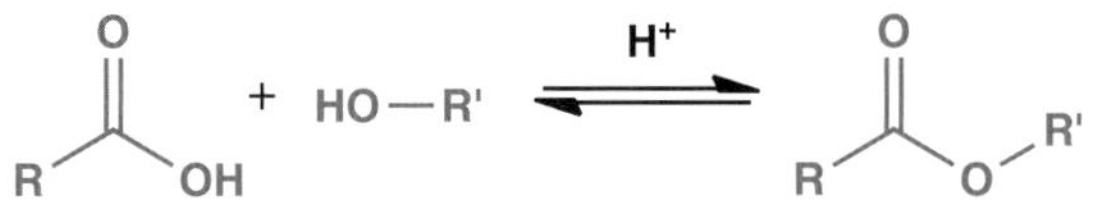

The Fischer synthesis of esters—an example of acid catalysis

In the first step of the reaction, acid catalysis makes the carbonyl more reactive. This activation of the carbonyl group then allows nucleophilic attack by the alcohol, forming a tetrahedral intermediate. Protonation of the oxygen from the acid (pink), and deprotonation of the oxygen from the alcohol, (green) makes the hydroxyl group a good leaving group (see Scheme 6.4).

All of these steps are reversible. All other things being equal, this reaction will give a mixture of ester and carboxylic acid. This reaction is often used to illustrate Le Chatelier's principle:

> *If a chemical system at equilibrium experiences a change in concentration, temperature, volume, or partial pressure, then the equilibrium shifts to counteract the imposed change and a new equilibrium is established.*

The position of equilibrium may be driven to the right (that is, towards completion of the reaction) by adding a large excess of alcohol (normally by using the alcohol as a solvent) or by removing water from the reaction mixture.

Acid + alcohol gives you an ester+water.

Figure 6.8   Activation of a carbonyl by an acid catalyst

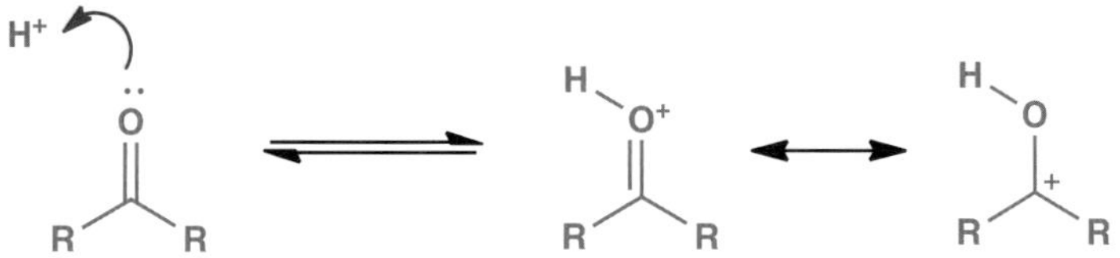

Scheme 6.4

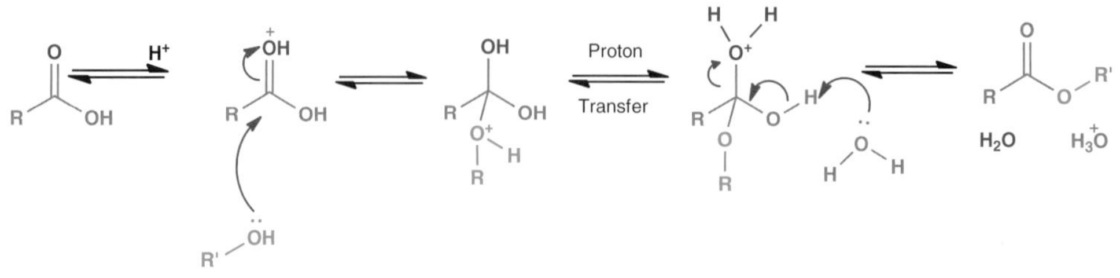

The problem with the Fischer esterification is that it does not normally go to completion. Because all the reactions are in equilibrium, the final ester needs to be purified from a complex mixture of starting materials and products. For small- and medium-scale synthesis, we generally use more sophisticated reagents and organic solvents, which are discussed below.

Equilibrium reactions of carbonyl compounds are, however, very important in pharmacy. The body makes extensive use of equilibrium reactions, at low temperature and in aqueous solution.

Base-catalysed hydrolysis of esters

We have already encountered esters as pro-drugs, in Chapter 1. Because esters are generally more hydrophobic than the corresponding alcohols, they can be used to enable drugs to cross membranes and reach their sites of action. They then need to be hydrolysed to obtain the active drug. The bloodstream is sufficiently alkaline to hydrolyse many esters (pH 7.4 does support some base-catalysed reactions!). In addition, the bloodstream contains many esterases, which catalyse ester hydrolysis. Figure 6.9A shows the hydrolysis of aspirin in basic conditions.

The hydroxide ion attacks the carbonyl group to give a tetrahedral intermediate, and when the carbonyl is reformed, salicylate leaves. Now, in this case, loss of salicylate is preferred compared with the alternative loss of hydroxide, because salicylate is a better leaving group.

The hydrolysis of erythromycin A acetate proceeds by the same mechanism (see Figure 6.9B), but now the intermediate loses the erythromycin ion, which is not really a better leaving group than a hydroxide.

> For more details on esters as pro-drugs, see Chapter 1, 'The importance of pharmaceutical chemistry'.

Self-check 6.5

Why is salicylate a better leaving group than hydroxide? (Note: you should draw the structures and mechanisms—this becomes much easier with practice.)

Self-check 6.6

The hydrolysis of erythromycin A acetate is, however, favoured. Look at the final products and see if you can work out why. (Hint: what will the basic solution do to the molecule coloured green?)

Figure 6.9 Hydrolysis of (A) aspirin and (B) erythromycin A acetate in base (Note that the terminal methyl groups in erythromycin are not drawn in)

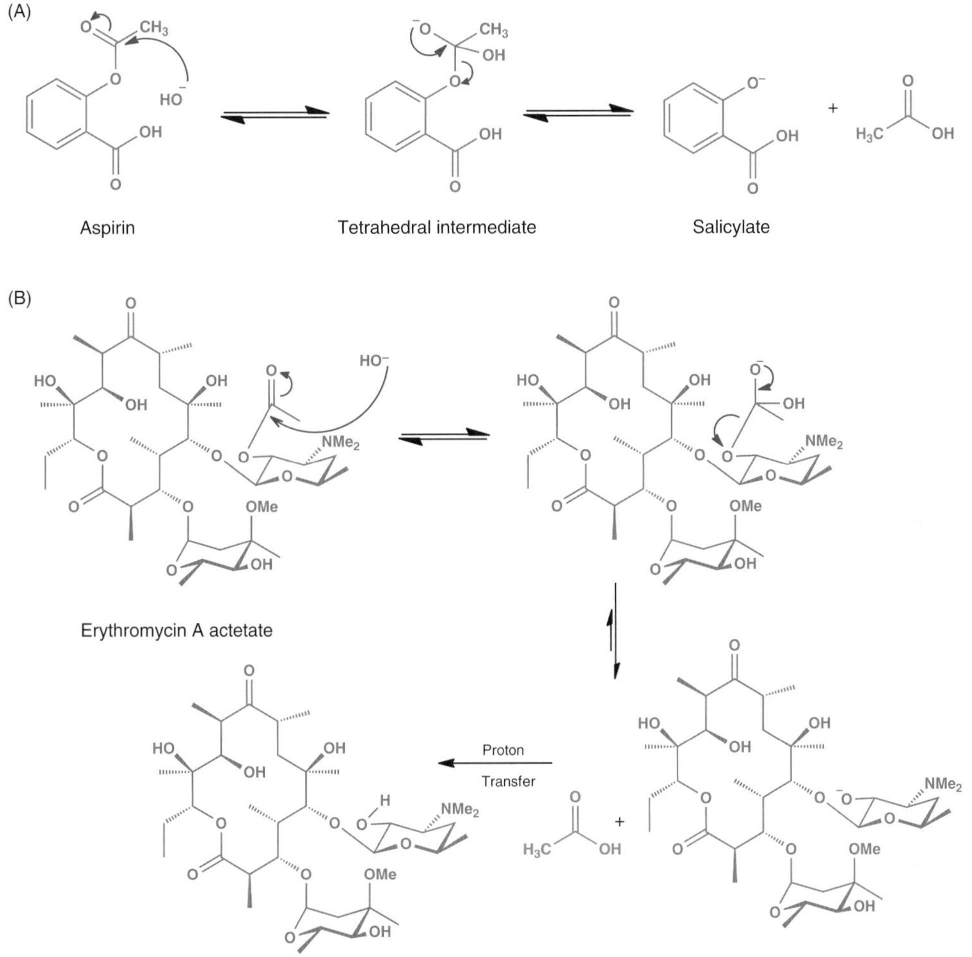

(A)

Aspirin   Tetrahedral intermediate   Salicylate

(B)

Erythromycin A actetate

Proton
Transfer

Interconversion of carbonyl compounds

The Fischer esterification is an example of the conversion of one type of carbonyl compound into another—namely, a carboxylic acid into an ester. Protonation (acid catalysis) means that the leaving group is HY, rather than Y^-. The hydrolysis of an ester in basic conditions is the reverse interconversion: an ester is converted to a carboxylic acid. Both of these reactions, and the other reactions described in this section, are *substitution* reactions during which Nu substitutes for Y^- (see Scheme 6.5).

The interconversion of carbonyl compounds is extraordinarily important, both in pharmaceutical chemistry and in the body. You have already seen numerous examples of the interconversion of carboxylic acids and esters. There is a clear order of reactivity among the various carbonyl compounds, as illustrated by their reactivity towards water (see Scheme 6.6).

Acetyl chloride (ethanoyl chloride) reacts violently with water to form acetic acid and HCl. Acetic anhydride reacts rapidly with water at neutral pH. Esters, such as ethyl acetate, do not react (ethyl acetate mixes poorly with water and forms a layer on top of the water layer).

Scheme 6.5

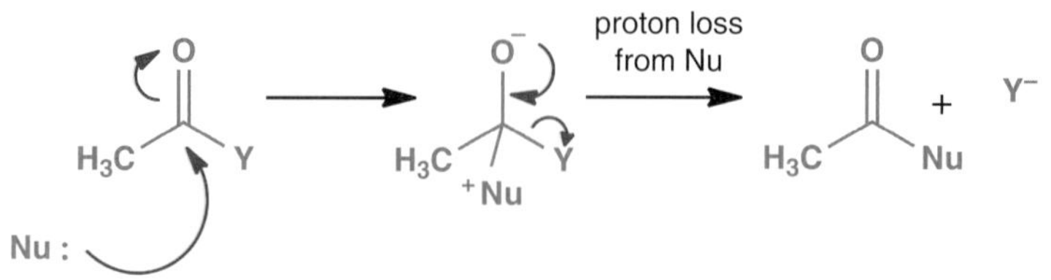

Scheme 6.6

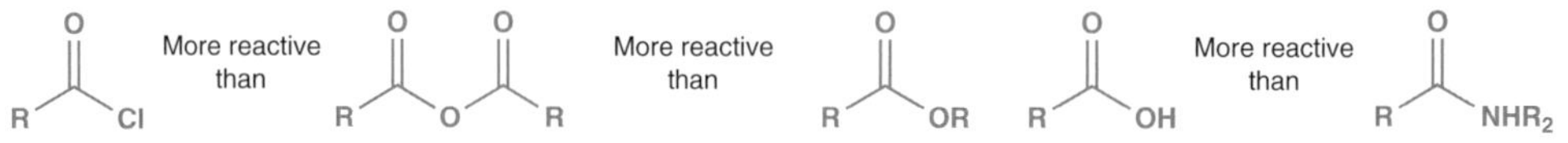

Acetic acid just dissolves quietly in water, and with a few trace flavourings, you put it on chips. Finally, the amide bond is a very strong bond, which is why your hair does not fall out in the rain.

What makes a good leaving group?

The order of reactivity of carbonyls depends upon the stability of the leaving group. Cl^- is an excellent leaving group, $RCOO^-$ is pretty good, HO^- and RO^- are poor, and NR_2^- is terrible. Good leaving groups are groups that do not require protonation to stabilize them. Put another way, their conjugate acids have low pK_a values. So the pK_a of HCl is -7 and Cl^- is a very good leaving group. The pK_a of RCOOH is about $4.5-5$, making acetate a good leaving group. By contrast, H_2O and ROH have pK_a values around $15-16$; HO^- and RO^- are poor leaving groups. Finally, the pK_a value for RNHR′ is typically $30-40$ and $RN-R'$ is not a leaving group at all. Acid anhydrides and acyl chlorides are too reactive to be found in nature, but they are very useful synthetic intermediates.

Synthesis of esters from acyl chlorides

An example of the usefulness of acyl chlorides is in the preparation of diacetylmorphine, also known as diamorphine, or heroin. Esterification is often used to make a drug more lipid-soluble, enabling it to cross membranes more readily, and so helping it to reach its cellular target. Diamorphine is used for palliative care in end-stage terminal disease. When the diacetate is given as an injection, the increased lipid solubility increases the potency and means less drug needs to be used to achieve the analgesic effect.

Self-check 6.7

What is the main constituent of hair? Why is the strength of the amide bond important to the stability of hair?

Self-check 6.8

Thioesters and thioacids, such as thioacetic acid, are seldom used in synthetic chemistry, but nature makes enormous use of them. Where would you expect thioesters to come in the order of reactivity described above?

Figure 6.10 Synthesis of diamorphine from morphine

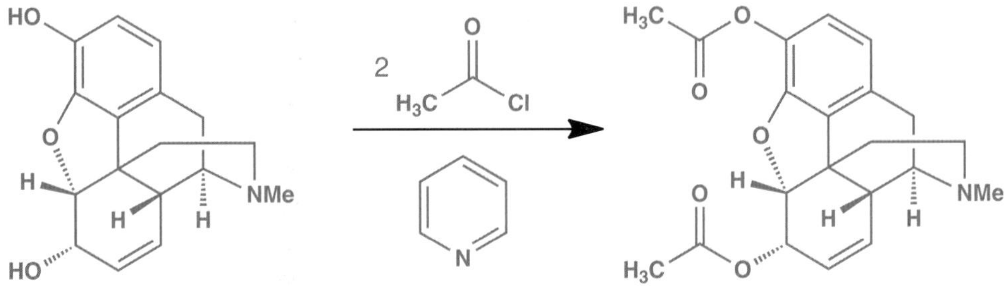

Self-check 6.9

Draw a simple mechanism for the formation of diamorphine from morphine. Note that pyridine is able to drive the reaction by reacting with the HCl produced as a by-product.

You can draw chemical structures in various different orientations, without them being wrong. (The acetyl groups in Figure 6.11 are drawn in different orientations from Figure 6.10 for convenience.)

In Figure 6.10 we have introduced the acetyl groups using two equivalents of acetyl chloride (ethanoyl chloride). The hydroxyl groups of morphine act as nucleophiles and the weakly basic pyridine acts as both catalyst and solvent.

The complete mechanism, shown in Figure 6.11, demonstrates how pyridine acts as a catalyst. It is a very advanced mechanism for introductory pharmacy students, and in an examination you would be very likely to get full marks if you drew the morphine hydroxyl groups attacking acetyl chloride directly. Pyridine acts as a catalyst because it is both a good nucleophile and a good leaving group.

Synthesis of amides from acyl chlorides

Acyl chlorides can also be used to make amides. If you look in the BNF, you will see that there are many penicillins used clinically, and for each successful penicillin there are many more that were synthesized, but proved to be unsuccessful in a clinical context. Unsuccessful drugs may be inactive; or active but toxic; or active, non-toxic but no better than existing drugs; or active, non-toxic, with some unique properties but simply too expensive to bring to market.

The various penicillins available are manufactured from the fungal product 6-aminopenicillanic acid. This compound has negligible antibacterial activity, but when it is treated with a suitable acyl chloride, a penicillin molecule is produced, as shown in Figure 6.12.

Meticillin and oxacillin are just two examples of the plethora of penicillins that can be made from acyl chlorides. Both have activity against the most common penicillin-resistant bacteria, and are used to treat serious infections.

Figure 6.11 Complete mechanism of synthesis of diamorphine from morphine

Diamorphine

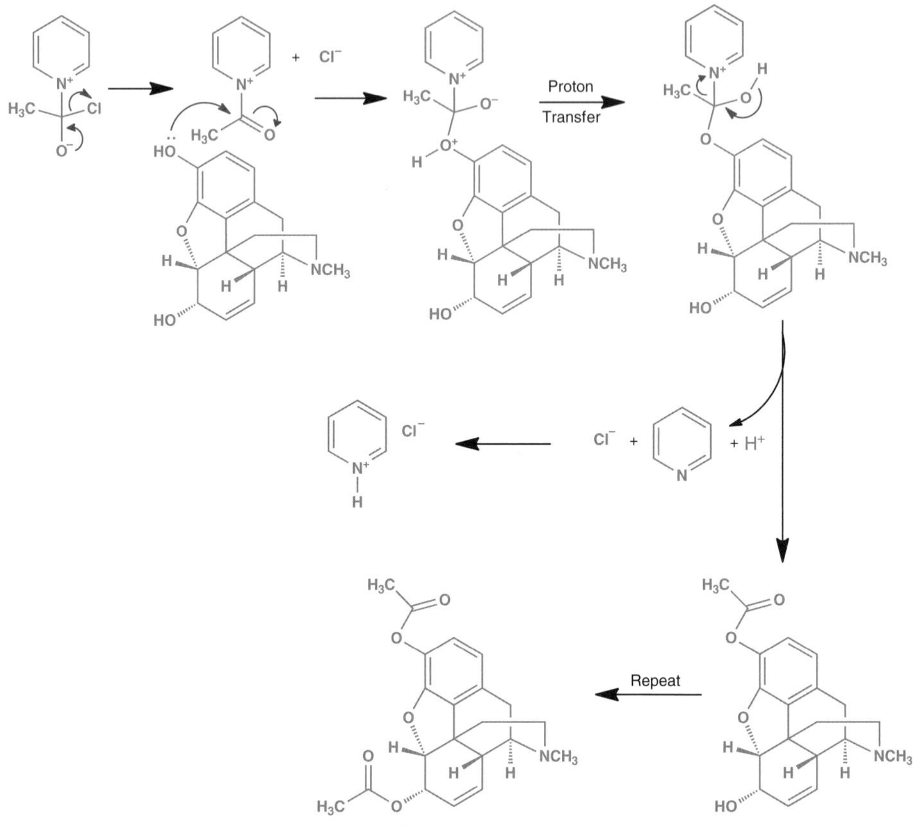

Self-check 6.10

Find the new amide bonds in meticillin and oxacillin.

Synthesis of esters and amides from acid anhydrides

Acid anhydrides are less reactive than acyl chlorides, but are normally reactive enough for the synthesis of esters and amides. The most readily available acid anhydride is acetic anhydride (ethanoic anhydride), and this reagent can be used to synthesize diamorphine from morphine, or erythromycin A acetate from erythromycin A. Probably its most familiar use is in the synthesis of aspirin from salicylic acid, as shown in Figure 6.5.

When it is used to prepare esters, acetic anhydride is used in strictly non-aqueous conditions because water competes effectively with salicylic acid or morphine for acetic anhydride. Acetic anhydride can, however, be used in aqueous solution at pH 9–11 to prepare amides. For example, in studies of protein structure and abundance, it can be very useful to modify one type of amino acid residue, as explained in Box 6.2. Lysine is the only amino acid with a primary amine side chain, and it is the only residue modified by acetic anhydride in aqueous solution (see Figure 6.13).

> Further details on amino acids can be found in Chapter 10, 'Proteins' and enzymes.

Figure 6.12 Synthesis of penicillins from 6–aminopenicillanic acid and acyl chlorides

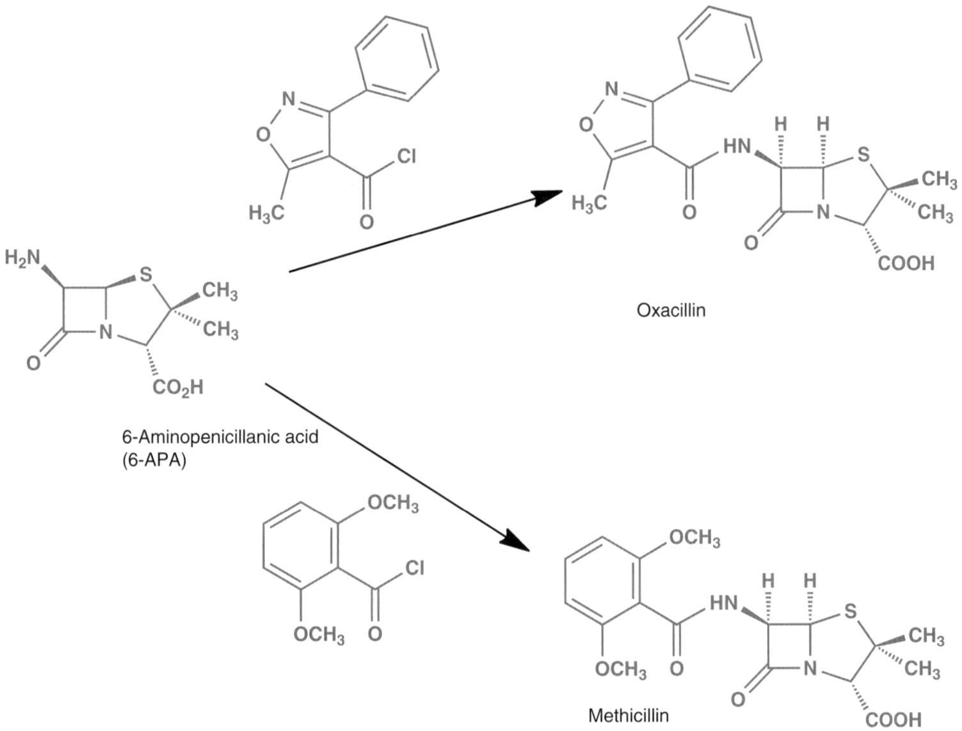

6-Aminopenicillanic acid
(6-APA)

Oxacillin

Methicillin

Figure 6.13 The conversion of a lysine side chain to an amide using acetic anhydride

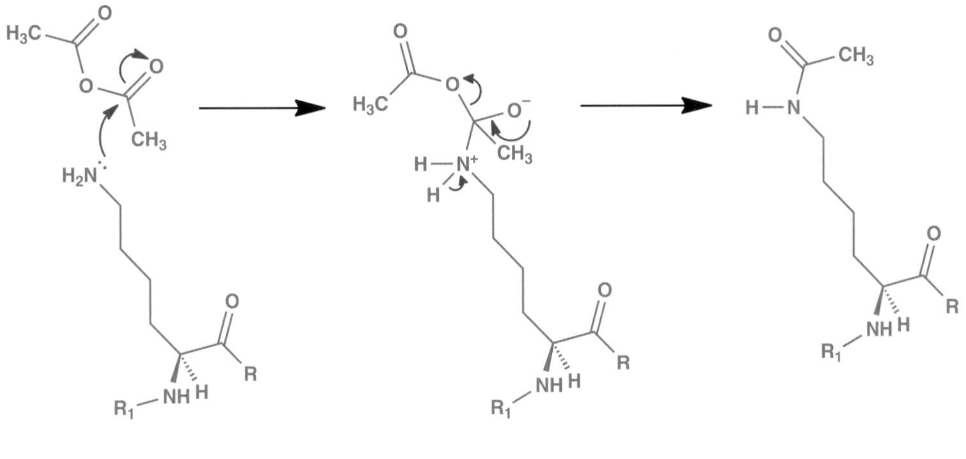

Lysine in a protein or peptide

Meticillin Self-check 6.11

There is an alternative method of making penicillins from 6-aminopenicillanic acid. Use a specialist database, such as PubMed (www.ncbi.nlm.nih.gov) to find it.

Box 6.2 Derivatizing proteins for structural determination

The digestive enzyme trypsin cleaves proteins adjacent to the most basic amino acids, arginine and lysine. The resulting peptides can be analysed by mass spectrometry. Some proteins, however, are very rich in basic residues and trypsin cleavage is inefficient where there are clusters of arginines and lysines. Treatment with acetic anhydride converts the basic amine side chain of lysine to a neutral amide, and trypsin does not cleave adjacent to the modified lysine residue. This results in more efficient reactions at arginine only.

Lysine is an essential amino acid. Mammals cannot manufacture it and require it in food. The protein in grains, such as wheat, are low in lysine, so lysine deficiency can occur in vegetarians, and there is some evidence that lysine deficiency can cause clinical anxiety. Milk, cheese, peas and beans are all rich in lysine, however, so a varied vegetarian diet should not lead to lysine deficiency.

How do you make acyl chlorides and anhydrides?

We have discussed making useful ester and amide drugs from acyl chlorides, but this raises the question: how do we make the reactive carbonyls—acyl chlorides and anhydrides?

Acyl chlorides are not made by simple substitution at other carbonyls because the chloride ion does not react with the carboxylic acid to give an acyl chloride. To make an acyl chloride requires treatment of a carboxylic acid with thionyl chloride ($SOCl_2$) or a similar reagent. Figure 6.14 shows the overall reaction (A) and the mechanism (B).

Again, Le Chatelier's principle is at work. Thionyl chloride is a liquid; it is added to the carboxylic acid, usually in a 'dry' solvent—that is, a solvent from which all traces of water have been removed. SO_2 and HCl are gases that diffuse away from the reaction mixture, so the reaction cannot reverse. The acyl chloride forms quite rapidly at room temperature. Because acyl chlorides are very reactive (and smelly) they are very often used without isolation or purification. For example, numerous esters of the antibiotic erythromycin have been made in this way (see Figure 6.15).

› More information on the esters of erythromycin can be found in Chapter 1, 'The importance of pharmaceutical chemistry'.

Figure 6.14 The reaction of thionyl chloride with a carboxylic acid to produce an acyl chloride (A) overall reaction (B) mechanism

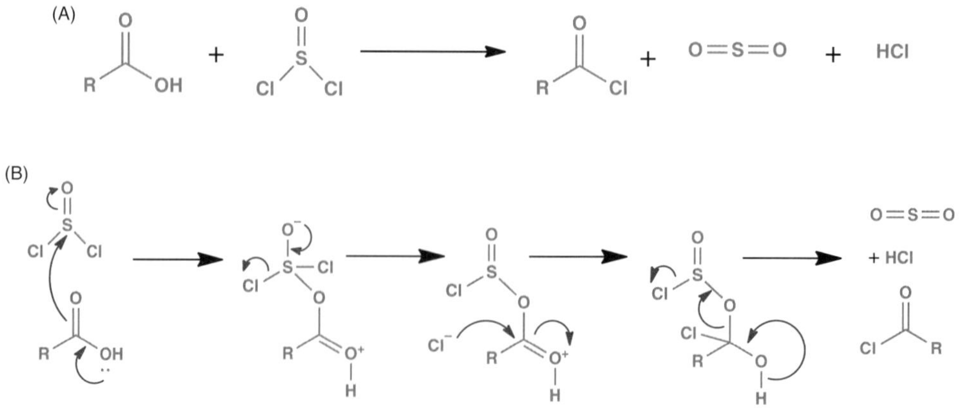

Self-check 6.12

There are five hydroxyl groups in erythromycin, three of them secondary, two tertiary (see Figure 6.15). You have learnt in Chapter 5 that secondary hydroxyl groups are more reactive than tertiary hydroxyl groups. Now look back at the role of pyridine in the esterification of morphine and see if you can work out why the hydroxyl coloured in red in erythromycin is the only one to be esterified at room temperature if no catalyst is added.

Figure 6.15 The synthesis of esters of erythromycin A

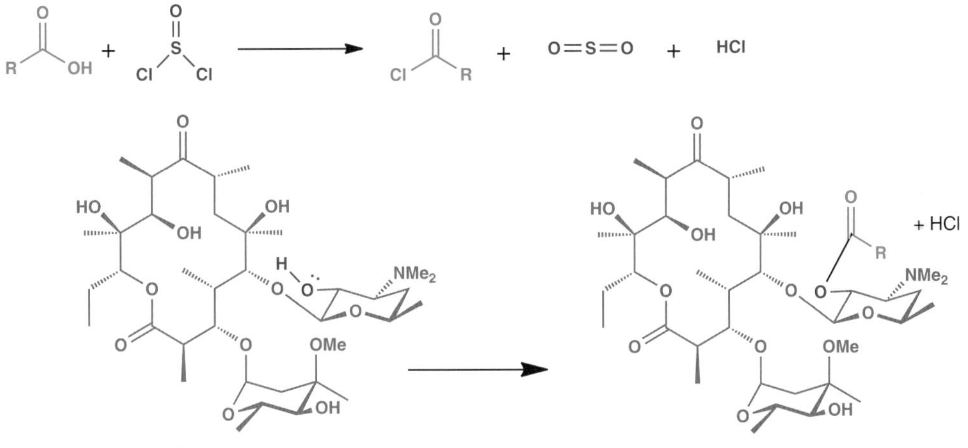

Erythromycin A

Erythromycin A ester

Synthesis of acid anhydrides

In the laboratory it is generally much easier to make acyl chlorides than acid anhydrides. If you need the anhydride (because the acyl chloride is unstable or too reactive to work with) you treat the corresponding carboxylic acid with a drying agent, such as phosphorus pentachloride, and distil the anhydride, leaving the drying agent in the reaction flask, Figure 6.16. This may need to be repeated to ensure complete reaction.

Aldehydes and ketones: What can you do without a good leaving group?

Aldehydes and ketones do not have good leaving groups. Neither hydrogen nor carbon readily accommodates a negative charge, so these compounds cannot undergo the substitution reactions we have seen previously. We have lost the ability to exchange groups and so our only option is to add groups, leading to nucleophilic addition (see Figure 6.17).

Figure 6.16 Synthesis of trifluoroacetic anhydride by dehydration of trifluoroacetic acid

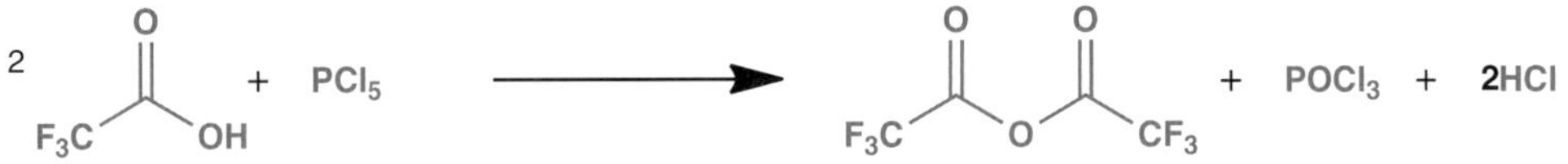

Self-check 6.13

Predict the products of the following reactions giving both their names and their structures.

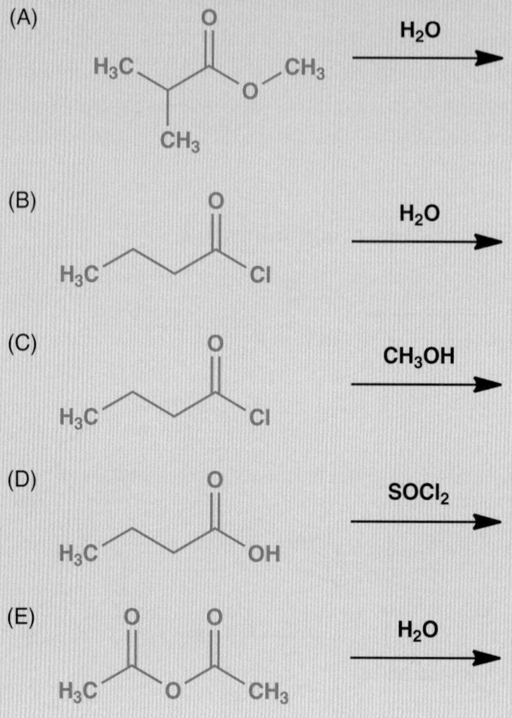

(A)

H₃C — CH(CH₃) — C(=O) — O — CH₃ $\xrightarrow{H_2O}$

(B)

H₃C — CH₂ — C(=O) — Cl $\xrightarrow{H_2O}$

(C)

H₃C — CH₂ — C(=O) — Cl $\xrightarrow{CH_3OH}$

(D)

H₃C — CH₂ — CH₂ — C(=O) — OH $\xrightarrow{SOCl_2}$

(E)

H₃C — C(=O) — O — C(=O) — CH₃ $\xrightarrow{H_2O}$

Figure 6.17 Mechanism of addition to aldehydes (R' = H) and ketones. The nucleophile may be either a neutral or negatively charged species

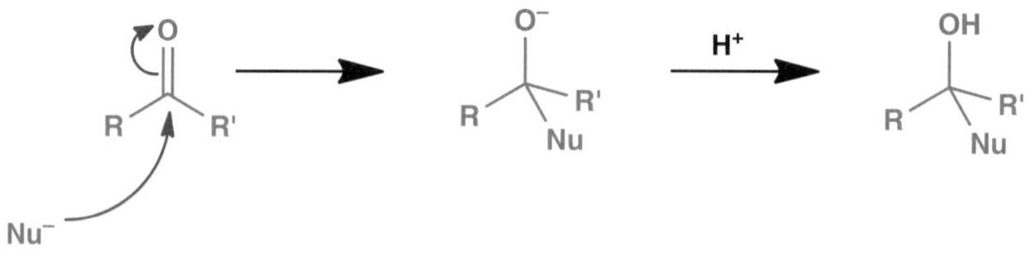

Here we are concerned with three situations (see Figure 6.18 for examples):

- when Nu is an oxygen nucleophile, leading to hemiacetals
- when Nu⁻ is a hydrogen nucleophile, leading to reduction reactions
- when Nu⁻ is a carbon nucleophile, enabling us to form carbon–carbon bonds.

Figure 6.18   Common transformations of aldehydes and ketones

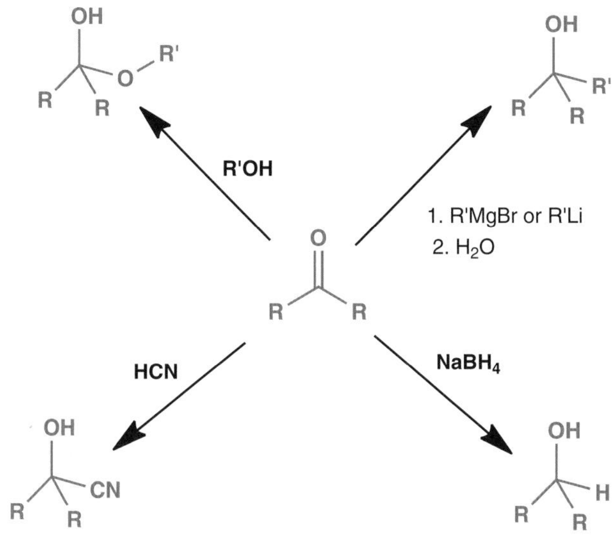

Formation of acetals and hemiacetals

If you add an aldehyde to an alcohol, an equilibrium is set up between the aldehyde and the addition product, known as a hemiacetal (see Figure 6.19). A hemiacetal is characterized by a carbon bonded to OH, OR^2, R and either H or R^1.

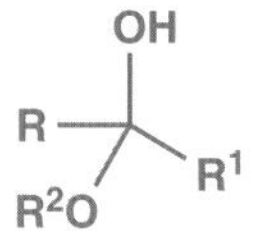

Hemiacetal

The hemiacetal cannot normally be isolated, but we know that it is there because certain forms of spectroscopy, such as infrared and NMR spectroscopy, can detect hemiacetals in solution.

Human beings are absolutely dependent on a group of hemiacetals known as sugars (see Figure 6.20). Sugars are internal hemiacetals—the aldehyde and the alcohol are in the same molecule—and they are more stable than hemiacetals formed from two different molecules.

Figure 6.19   Formation of a hemiacetal from acetaldehyde (ethanal) and ethanol

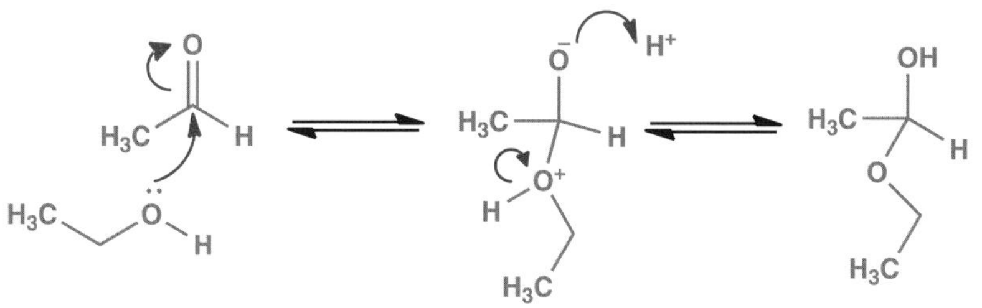

More details on sugars and carbohydrates can be found in Chapter 11, 'Carbohydrates and carbohydrate metabolism'.

Self-check 6.14

Can you think of an important sugar that normally exists as a hemiketal? (Hint: your sugar bowl might be a source of inspiration.)

Ketones can also undergo reactions with alcohols in the same way. The products are also known as hemiacetals, although you can use the term 'hemiketal' if you prefer. (IUPAC considers hemiketals to be a sub-class of hemiacetals.)

Aldehydes and ketones can react with alcohols under acid catalysis to produce acetals, as shown in Figure 6.21. Acetals have the general structure shown here, and are characterized by a carbon bonded to OR^2, OR^2, R and either H or R^1.

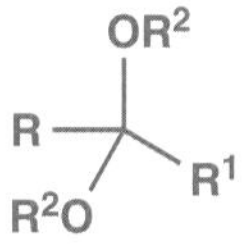

Acetal

Organic chemists love this mechanism (see Figure 6.21) because it illustrates lots of important points—for example, that the electrophile is always a protonated carbonyl (an oxonium ion). Pharmacy students are more likely to ask 'What is it for?'

Acetals:

- can be used as **protecting groups** in the synthesis of drugs and other molecules
- are found in carbohydrates in all life forms
- are found in drugs, for example, the aminoglycoside antibiotics.

Figure 6.20 Some important hemiacetals: ribose is found in RNA and in ATP; deoxyribose is found in DNA; glucose is the entry point of glycolysis, the metabolic pathway that enables us to derive energy from food

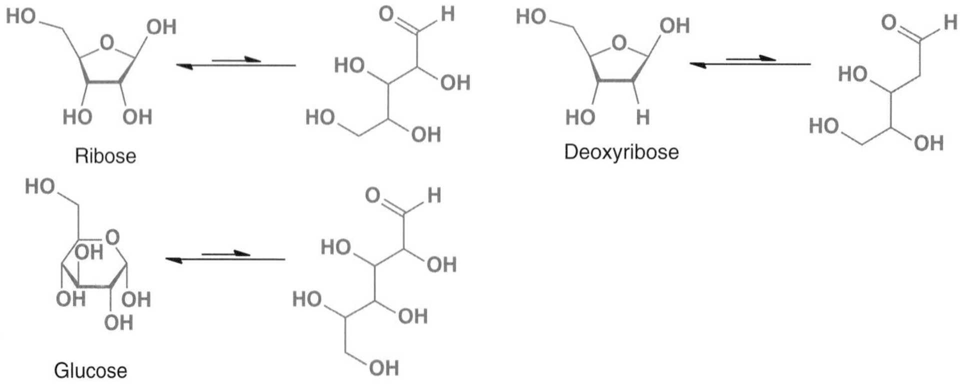

Figure 6.21 Formation of an acetal by reaction of an alcohol and a ketone under acid catalysis

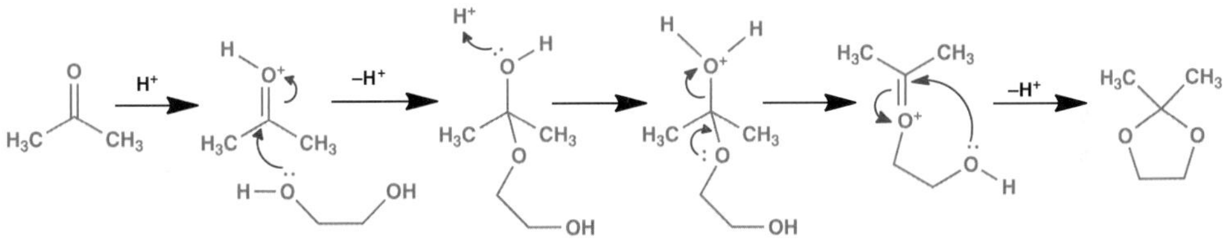

Self-check 6.15

Find the acetal functions in the glucose polymer and in streptomycin, and label them.

Self-check 6.16

There is an unmodified carbonyl in streptomycin. What is it?

If you wanted to modify the carboxylic acid functional group of the pain-killer ketoprofen, but preserve the ketone, you might need to protect the ketone, as shown in Figure 6.22(A). Figure 6.22 also shows some important acetals found in nature. Figure 6.22(B) shows a polymer of glucose. This type of polymer is found in food stores, starch in plants and glycogen in animals. Figure 6.22(C) shows streptomycin, an aminoglycoside antibiotic. It has two acetal functions, connecting the sugar rings.

> More information on carbohydrates, including glucose polymers, can be found in Chapter 11, 'Carbohydrates and carbohydrate metabolism'.

Reduction of aldehydes and ketones

In order to reduce an aldehyde or a ketone to the corresponding alcohol, we have to add the equivalent of H$^-$. Hydride (H$^-$) is a hopeless nucleophile; it acts only as a base and normally abstracts a proton from a carbonyl compound to give H$_2$. To make H$^-$ into a good nucleophile, we make it bigger and spread the negative charge over several hydrogens.

Typically, the hydride equivalents that we use are sodium borohydride (NaBH$_4$) or lithium aluminium hydride (LiAlH$_4$). Sodium borohydride is a mild reducing agent; it is easy to use and is compatible with water or alcohols in the solvent. Lithium aluminium hydride will reduce even the most stubborn ketones (indeed, it reduces esters to alcohols) but must be used in very dry (water-free) solvents. Figure 6.23 shows how sodium borohydride is used to reduce a ketone to an alcohol, a key step in the synthesis of duloxetine. Duloxetine is an antidepressant, used to treat major depressive disorder.

One very good way of finding new drugs is to make small modifications to old drugs (that is, to make analogues of the old drugs). With very complex molecules, the number of analogues that can be produced is often severely restricted by the chemistry.

Figure 6.22 Acetals in pharmacy: (A) use of an acetal protecting group. Note the reagent LiAlH$_4$. This reagent would react with the ketone, which needs to be protected; (B) a polymer of glucose units; (C) streptomycin

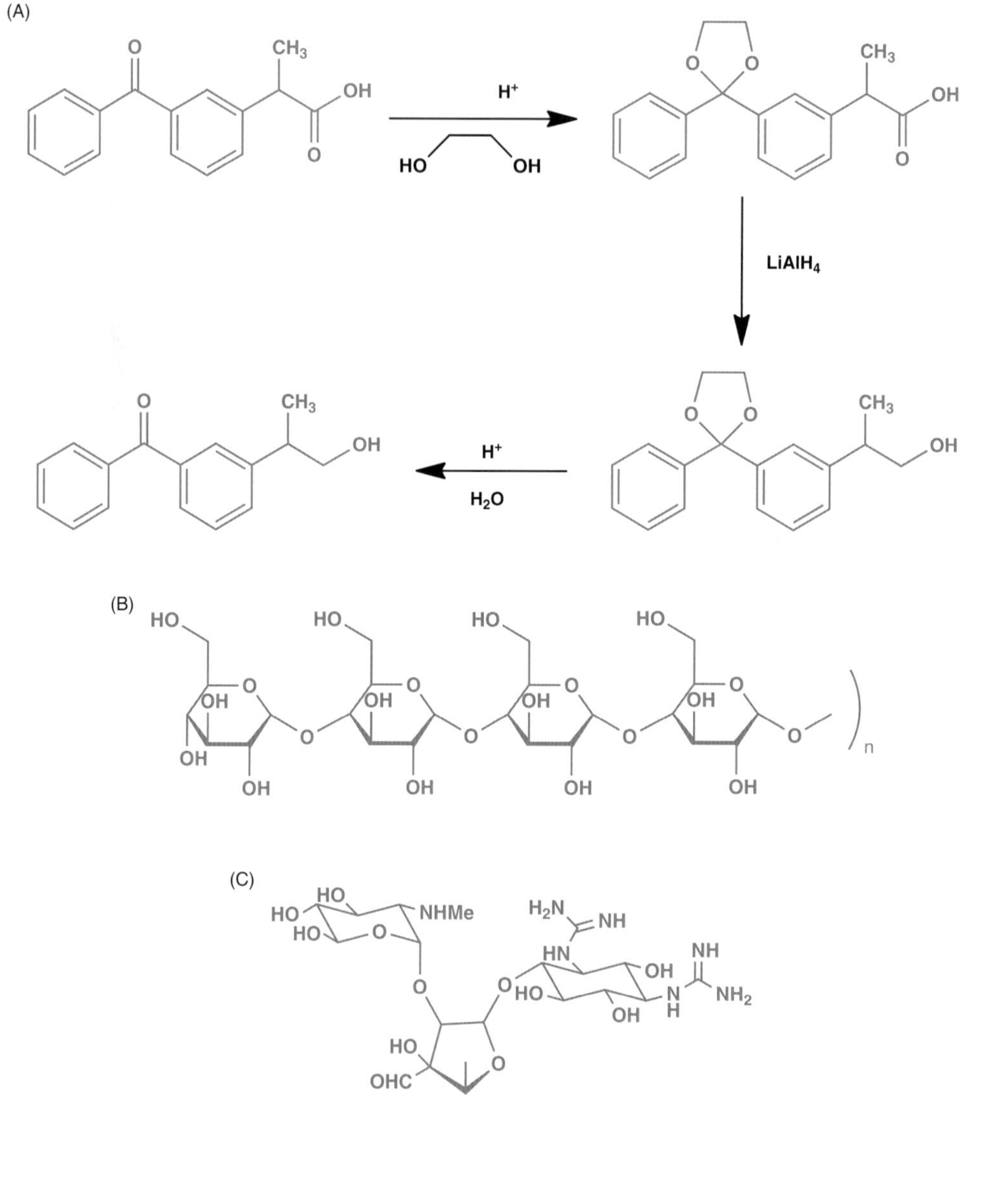

(A)

(B)

(C)

Self-check 6.17

See if you can draw the mechanism for the reduction of an ester to an alcohol by lithium aluminium hydride. (Hint: you have seen two mechanisms—interconversion and addition—for the reaction of carbonyls with nucleophiles and you will need both of them.)

Figure 6.23 Reduction of a ketone to an alcohol using sodium borohydride. This is an important step in the synthesis of duloxetine

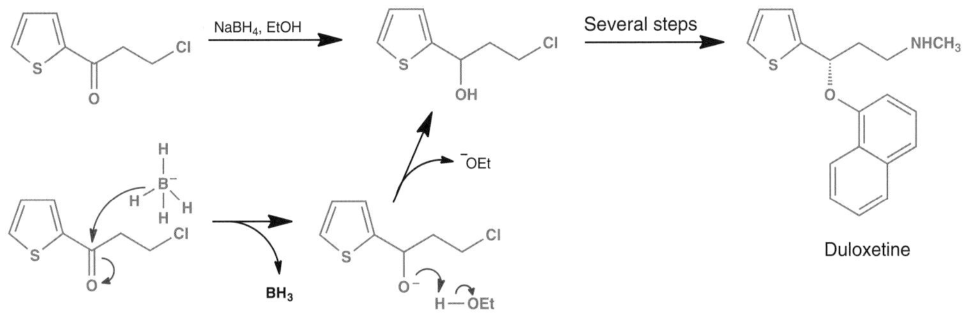

Duloxetine

Self-check 6.18

It is very dangerous to use a carbon dioxide fire extinguisher if lithium aluminium hydride is present. Why?

You might have expected the reaction featured in Self-Check 6.19 to produce a mixture of 9S- and 9R-dihydroerythromycin. Erythromycin, however, has eighteen chiral centres, so the mixture would be of diastereomers, not of enantiomers. The other chiral centres have a profound influence on the course of the reaction, and in practice the 9R-compound cannot be detected.

> Enantiomers and diastereomers are covered in more detail in Chapter 3, 'Stereochemistry and drug action'.

Self-check 6.19

Lots of analogues of erythromycin (most of them unsuccessful) have been made over the years, and 9-S-dihydroerythromycin is one of them. What reagent would you use to make this compound from erythromycin?

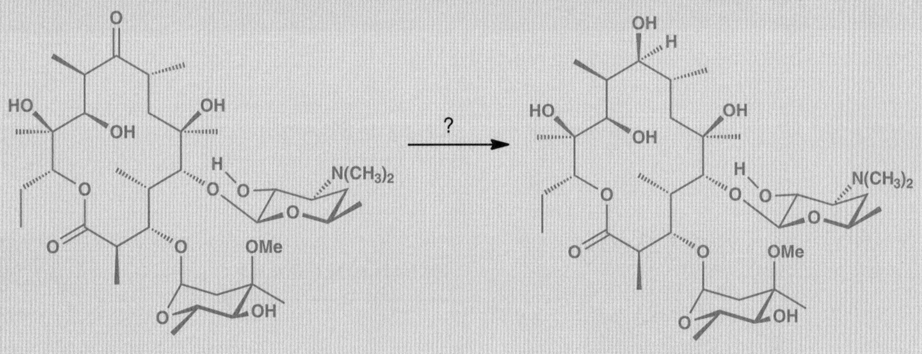

Erythromycin A

9S-Dihydroerythromycin A

Formation of carbon–carbon bonds

Pre-university courses often include the action of cyanide on ketones and aldehydes to give cyanohydrins. This reaction does form a carbon–carbon bond but the reaction is rather limited; it is frustrating that only a single carbon can be added. More importantly, however, huge amounts of safety legislation now surround the use of cyanide, and this reaction is only permitted if there is an exceptionally good reason for it. Fortunately, there are better ways of making carbon–carbon bonds.

To make a carbon–carbon bond, one carbon (usually an alkyl or aryl group) needs to support a negative charge. Carbocations (carbons supporting positive charges) are explored in Chapters 4 and 5, and should be familiar, but we now require the equivalent of C⁻. To make carbon carry a negative charge, we add it to a less electronegative element, typically a metal. Lithium, zinc and magnesium are common choices. The mechanisms of action are also closely similar, so we will consider the reactions of organomagnesium compounds, known as Grignard reagents, as a representative example.

A Grignard reagent (Grignard was a French chemist who published this reaction in 1900) is made by the treatment of an alkyl halide with magnesium in an inert solvent. The Grignard reagent is then equivalent to C^-, because magnesium is less electronegative than carbon. A typical Grignard reagent, derived from bromoethane, can be drawn in full like this:

Here is the type of reaction it can undergo (Scheme 6.7).

Now this really is a fantastic reaction. If you can make carbon–carbon bonds, you can make almost anything.

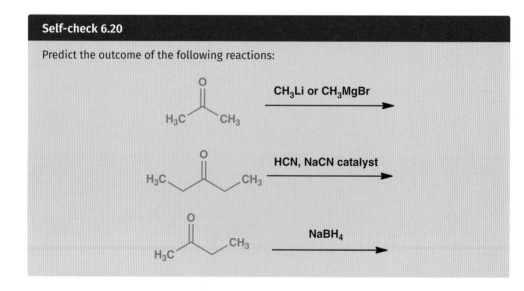

Self-check 6.20

Predict the outcome of the following reactions:

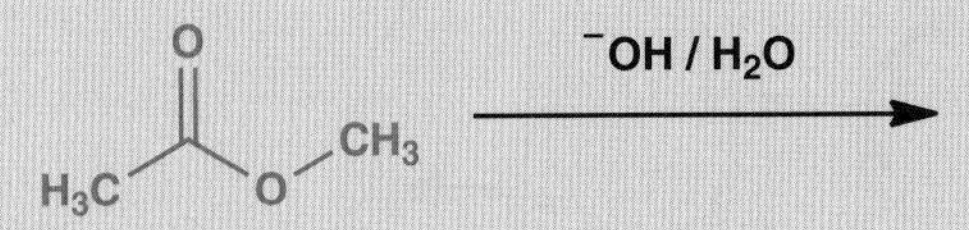

Carboxylic acids and derivatives are able to undergo substitution reactions. Aldehydes and ketones possess functional groups that cannot act as leaving groups so any product must be an addition product.

Scheme 6.7

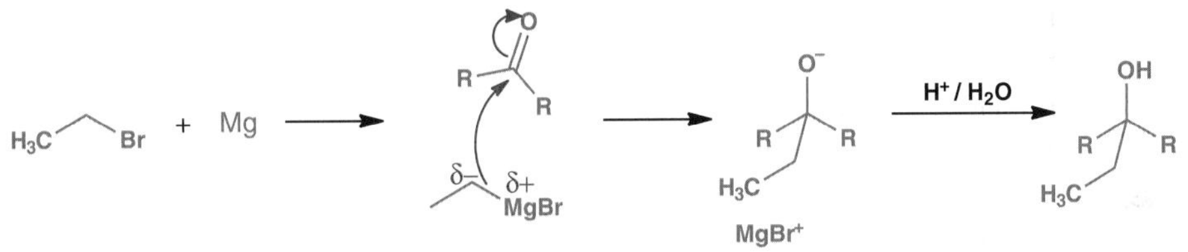

6.4 α-SUBSTITUTION REACTIONS

A third major type of carbonyl reaction is the α-substitution reaction, which occurs at the position next to (or 'α' to) the carbonyl group. H⁺ is removed from this position and is substituted by another atom or group. These reactions not only have a place in medicinal and organic chemistry but are also prevalent in biochemical processes. Let us consider the overall factors that can bring about these reactions.

Keto-enol tautomerism

In the presence of acid, a carbonyl with an α-hydrogen is able to undergo an equilibrium reaction, known as keto-enol tautomerism. The enol tautomer is only present in very low concentrations, and its formation occurs very slowly under neutral conditions but, as we have learnt from other areas of reactivity, the presence of either an acid or a base can be a game changer in terms of chemical reactivity (see Scheme 6.8).

> For more about keto-enol tautomerism, see Chapter 4, 'Properties of aliphatic hydrocarbons'.

Scheme 6.8

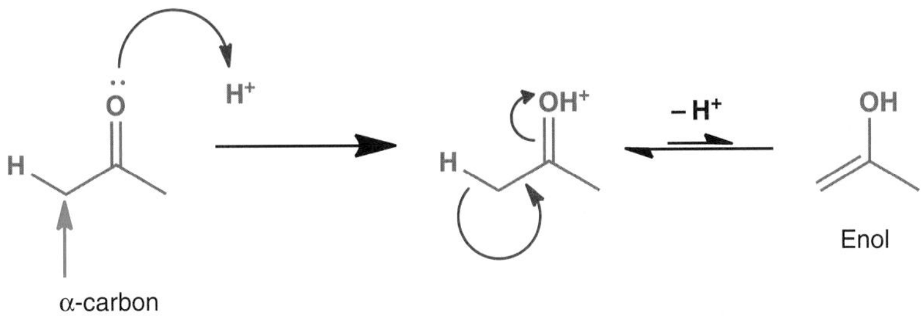

Scheme 6.9

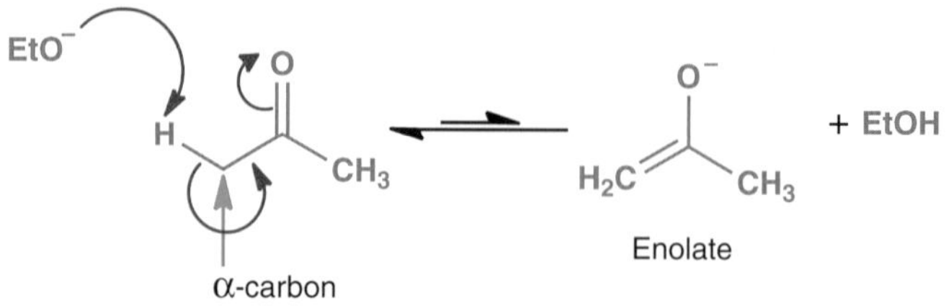

α-carbon

Enolate

In the enol form of a carbonyl, the α-carbon takes part in a π-bond, and is therefore able to act as a nucleophile, a C⁻ equivalent. Something similar occurs in base, with an enolate rather than an enol being formed (see Scheme 6.9).

Sodium ethoxide (made by dissolving sodium in ethanol) is a suitable base for catalysing keto-enol tautomerism.

The ability to form enols or enolates makes the σ-hydrogen relatively acidic; it has a pK_a of about 19. ('Relatively' in this context means relative to an alkene with a pK_a of 44; it is still nothing like as acidic as acetic acid, pK_a 4.7.) There are plenty of strong bases capable of removing a proton from the σ-carbon of a carbonyl compound, enabling it to act as a nucleophile.

> pK_a is discussed in more detail in Chapter 4, 'Properties of aliphatic hydrocarbons'.

Reactions in which the carbonyl is the nucleophile

When a carbonyl forms an enol or an enolate, it acquires the ability to act as a nucleophile; in order to form a double bond, the α-carbon loses a proton, and the π-electrons can now react with an electrophile. We have met several electrophiles so far in this book, and many of them can react with enols or enolates. We will now consider some of the most useful of these reactions.

Halogenation

Halogenation is one of the most useful α-substitution reactions of carbonyls, because the α-halocarbonyls formed in these reactions are excellent synthetic intermediates. Let us start by considering the bromination of acetone (propanone), which is shown in Figure 6.24.

Figure 6.24   The monobromination of acetone (propanone)

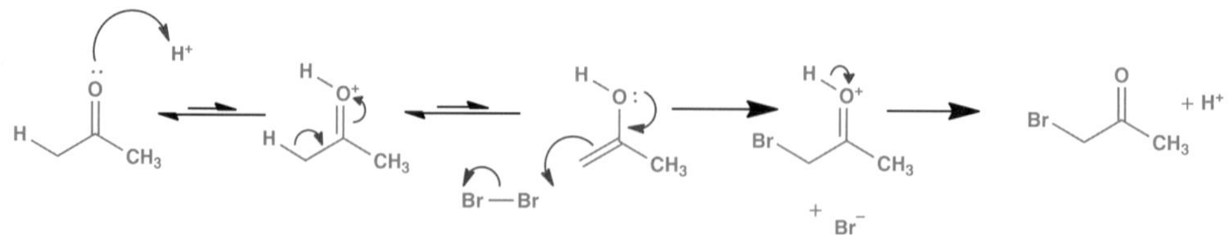

Self-check 6.21

If acetone is treated with two equivalents of bromine in acid conditions, what would you expect the product to be?

Self-check 6.22

Draw a mechanism for the acid-catalysed bromination of 1-tetralone.

The reaction is initially very slow in neutral conditions, but eventually speeds up because HBr is generated in the reaction and can act as a catalyst. It is more usual to add some acid (such as acetic acid) to the reaction mixture at the outset.

The electronegative bromine in bromopropanone makes enol formation more difficult, so if one equivalent of bromine is used to brominate acetone, the product is almost exclusively bromopropanone. As a consequence, this reaction is considered to be very 'clean'.

Benazepril is an ACE (angiotensin converting enzyme) inhibitor used to treat high blood pressure. Its synthesis starts with 1-tetralone, which looks rather unpromising (see Figure 6.25). However, monobromination allows the position α to the carbonyl to be built upon. After several synthetic steps, a large group (almost half the molecule) is built onto the α-carbon, resulting in a very profitable drug.

The halogenation of carbonyls in base is rather different as shown in Scheme 6.10.

The first bromination proceeds in a similar way to the acid-catalysed reaction (though note that the OH⁻ is consumed; it is not strictly a catalyst). The hydrogens coloured green are now,

Scheme 6.10

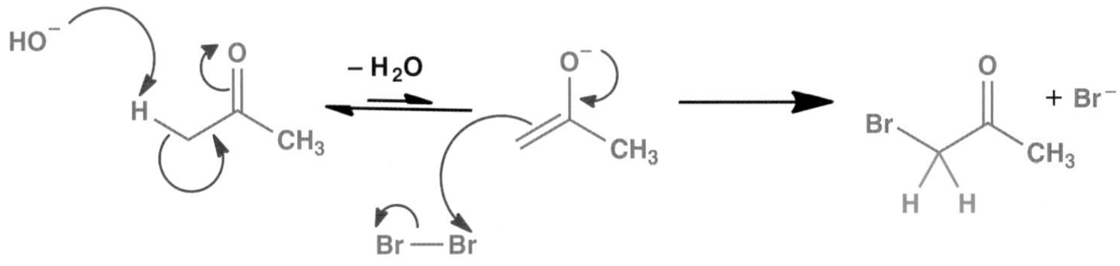

Figure 6.25 The synthesis of benazepril. The part of the molecule that replaces the bromine is coloured in purple. If the rest of this synthesis (such as the ring expansion or the separation of enantiomers) interests you, you can find it in *The Art of Drug Synthesis*, ed. Johnson and Li, Wiley, 2007, p. 150

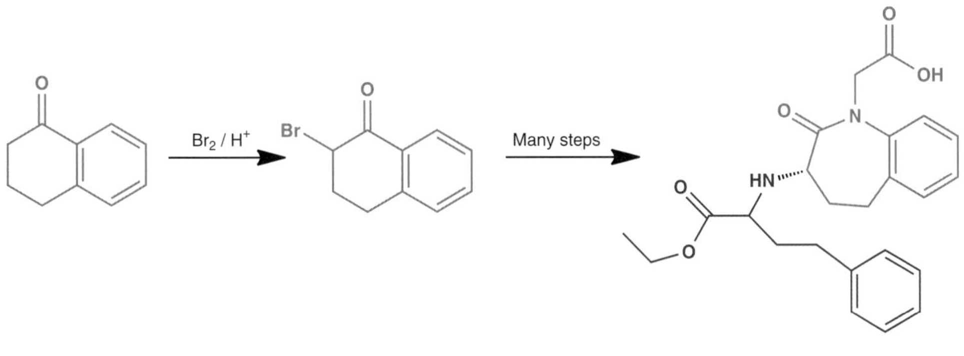

Benazepril

Scheme 6.11

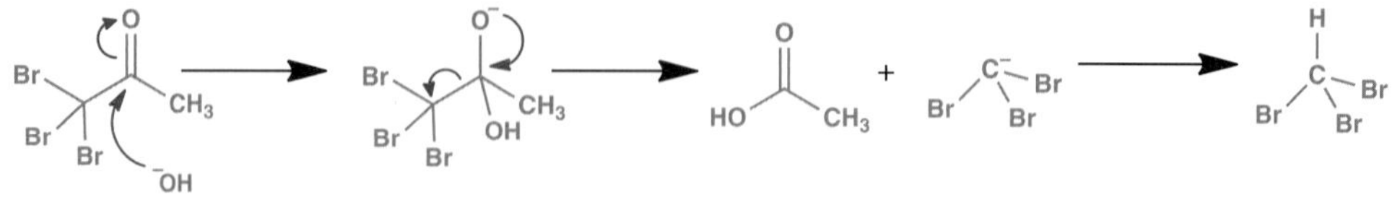

Self-check 6.23

What happens if you treat 1-tetralone with iodine and sodium hydroxide? Draw the mechanism.

however, relatively acidic. The enolate generated from bromopropanone is stabilized by the electron-withdrawing bromine. The second bromination is faster than the first, and the third is faster again.

And now, Br—C—Br is actually a better leaving group than OH⁻, so the reaction shown in Scheme 6.11 occurs.

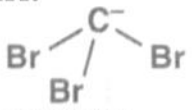

When iodine is used in place of bromine, we get the so-called 'iodoform' reaction. Iodoform, CHI_3, is pale yellow and insoluble in water. A methyl ketone gives iodoform on treatment with sodium hydroxide and iodine; other ketones do not. So if you want to test for a methyl ketone you can simply conduct an iodoform test rather than investing half a million pounds in an NMR spectrometer.

The aldol reaction

Enols and enolates are nucleophiles, but their parent carbonyl compounds are electrophiles. If you add just a tiny amount of base to an aldehyde or ketone, a small amount of enolate forms and this nucleophile reacts with a carbonyl molecule. The reaction of acetaldehyde with base is shown in Figure 6.26. This reaction is known as an aldol reaction because the historical name for the product (3-hydroxybutanal) was aldol.

Aldehydes, ketones and carboxylic acid derivatives can all undergo aldol reactions provided they have at least one α-hydrogen. The important step is the formation of the enolate ion, which can then act as a nucleophile and form a new carbon–carbon bond.

Aldol products can rather easily lose water as shown in Figure 6.27, especially if too much base is added. This is why the aldol reaction is sometimes termed the aldol condensation. (Loss of water or another small molecule=condensation).

Figure 6.26 The aldol reaction of acetaldehyde. Note that a new carbon–carbon bond is formed (shown in black)

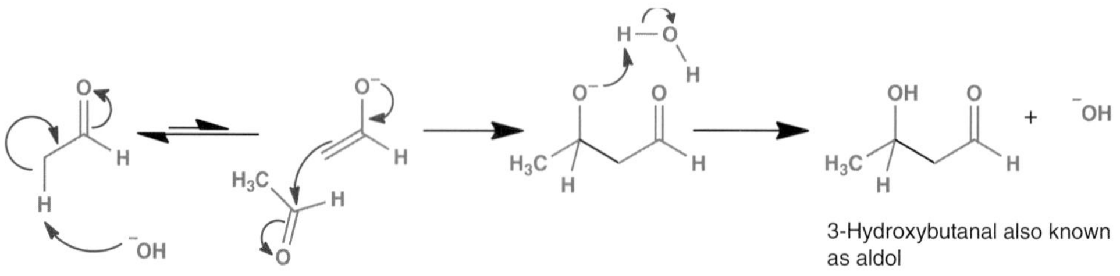

3-Hydroxybutanal also known as aldol

Figure 6.27 Loss of water from an aldol product to give an unsaturated aldehyde

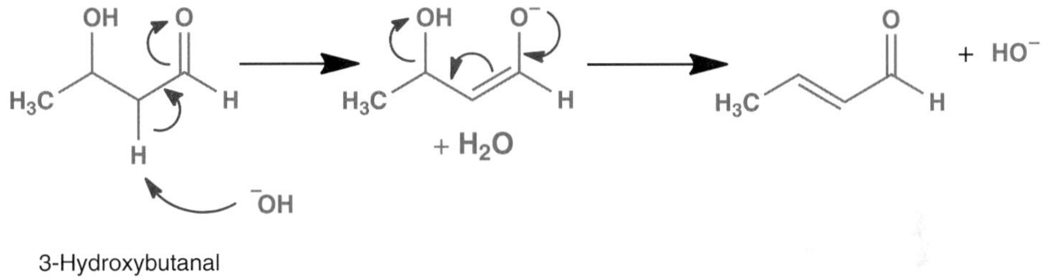

3-Hydroxybutanal

Self-check 6.24

Draw a mechanism for the aldol reaction of acetone (propanone).

The Claisen condensation

The Claisen condensation is a close relative of the aldol reaction; however, esters—rather than aldehydes or ketones—are the reactants. The overall reaction is shown in Scheme 6.12.

Let us explore it step-by-step, starting with the enolate ion (see Scheme 6.13).

Now we have formed our nucleophile (the enolate) we can seek out an electrophile, which is, of course, the carbonyl of another ester molecule (see Scheme 6.14).

A tetrahedral intermediate is formed, with the new bond shown in black. Actually it is quite easy to forget the new bond when you draw the intermediate. Try counting the carbons when you draw intermediates, or use colours as above. If all else fails, draw out the complete structures with all the carbons and hydrogens; this is not wrong, remember, just a bit laborious.

Finally, the tetrahedral intermediate loses EtO⁻ (see Scheme 6.15).

Scheme 6.12

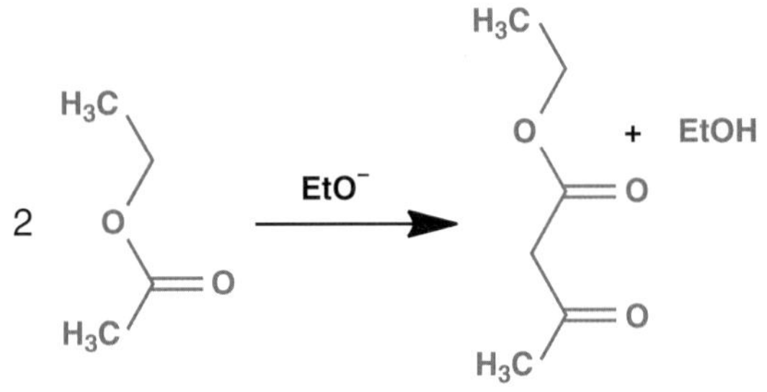

Scheme 6.13

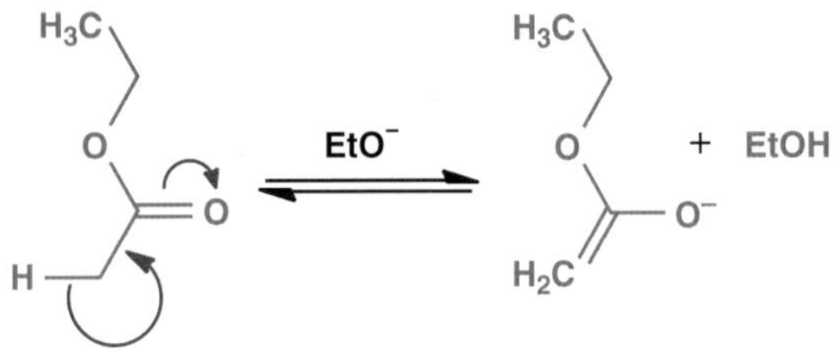

Scheme 6.14

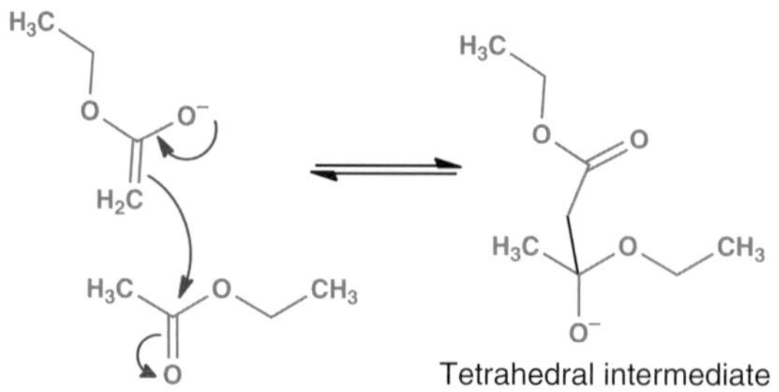

Tetrahedral intermediate

Scheme 6.15

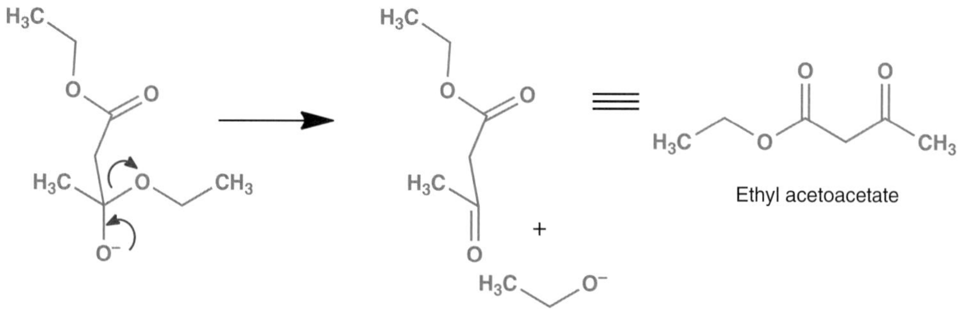

Ethyl acetoacetate

Reading most textbooks, it is easy to imagine that other people (teachers and fellow students) draw their structures perfectly, with nice bond angles, every time. They do not. At the end of a complex mechanism, you may well have a dreadful-looking structure like the one in the middle of the scheme. If so, just redraw it, as shown.

The entire Claisen reaction scheme is summarized in Figure 6.28.

Figure 6.28   The Claisen condensation in full

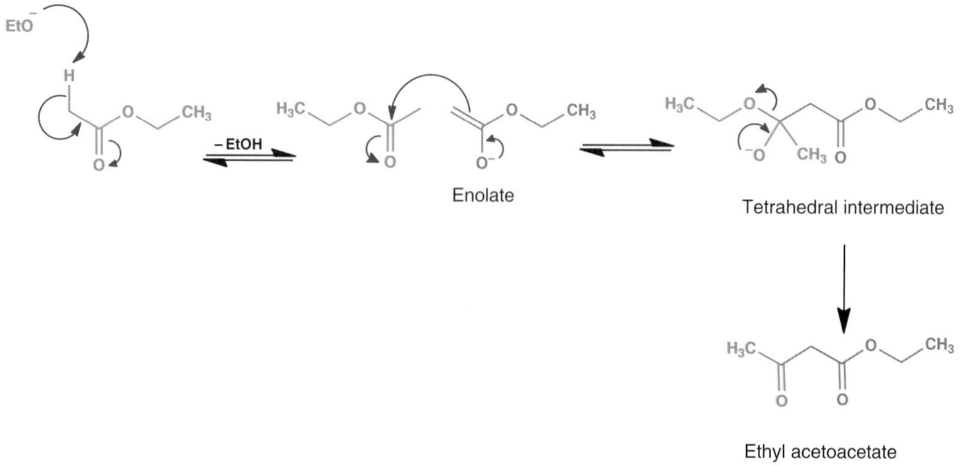

Enolate

Tetrahedral intermediate

Ethyl acetoacetate

Aldol and Claisen reactions: summary

Aldol	Claisen
Aldehyde or ketone	Ester
↓	↓
Enolate ion	Enolate ion
↓	↓
Tetrahedral product	Tetrahedral intermediate
	↓
	Product (ketoester)

The aldol and Claisen reactions in focus

Aldol and Claisen reactions are used in the synthesis of drugs, but they are normally limited to cases where the mechanism and hence the reaction products are unambiguous. The problem is that a molecule like butanone has five σ-hydrogens. An initial deprotonation may take place at carbon-1 or carbon-3—but even after this reaction four σ-hydrogens remain. A complex mixture of products is likely to be formed.

Elzasonan was a promising antidepressant that was withdrawn after phase II clinical trials. The final stages in the synthesis involved an aldol condensation reaction of a benzaldehyde derivative with a thiamorpholine (see Figure 6.29).

This reaction works well because only one of the two carbonyls can form an enolate, and it can only form *one* enolate (there are hydrogens on only one side of the C=O function). In the laboratory, the aldol and Claisen reactions are quite limited because mixtures of products are often formed. Nevertheless, a great many drugs are made by Claisen condensations, and all are natural products known as polyketides.

Polyketide synthesis—Claisen-type reactions in biology

Polyketides are made by plants, fungi and bacteria, and consist of acetate or propionate units (or sometimes other simple carboxylic acid derivatives), which are polymerized using Claisen-type reactions. Many of these compounds have biological activity. The polyketides include the drugs mentioned previously—erythromycin, nystatin and tetracycline—but they also include environmental toxins such as the aflatoxins.

Self-check 6.25

Consider the effect of adding base to a mixture of acetone and butanone. How many aldol products can you draw?

Figure 6.29 The synthesis of elzasonan

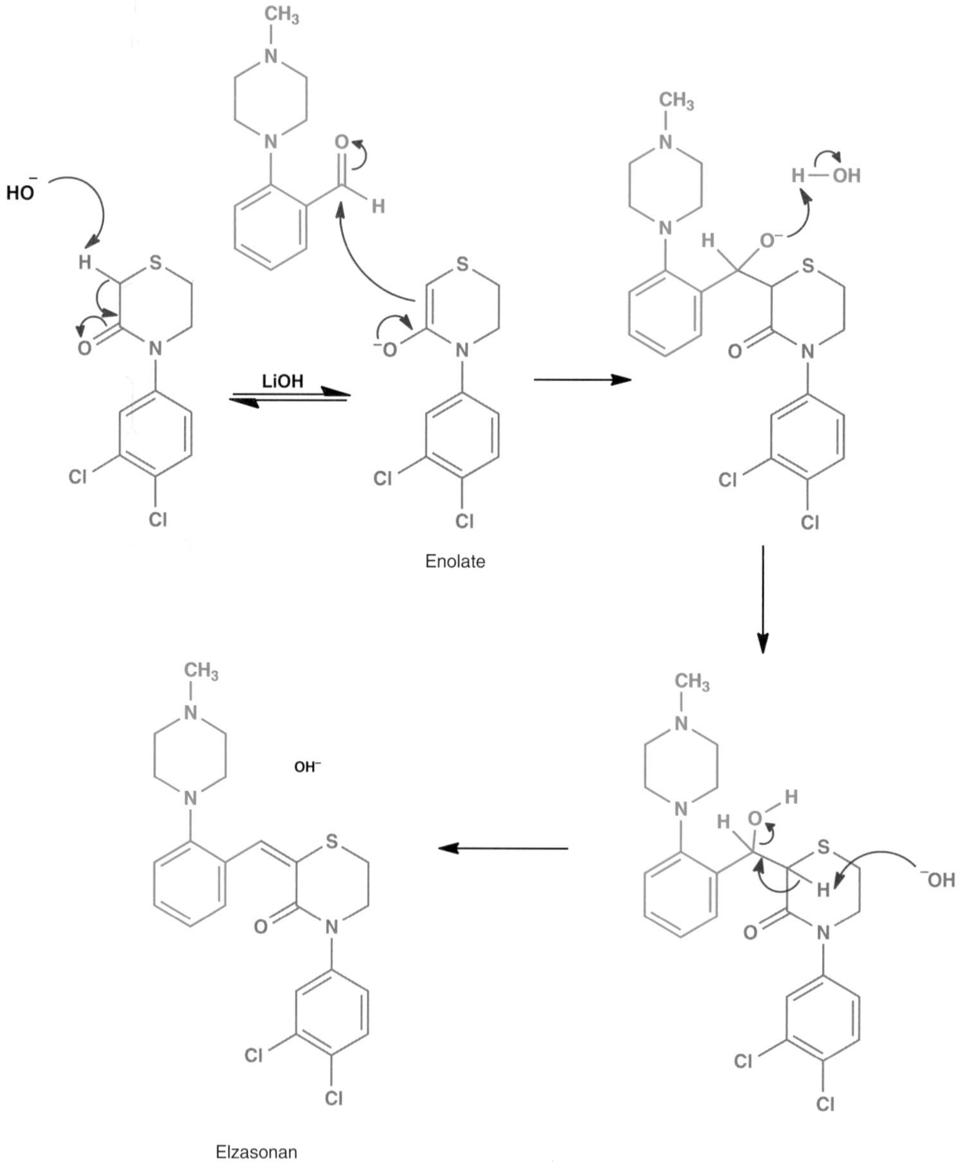

Enolate

Elzasonan

The biosyntheses (that is the syntheses by biological systems) of polyketides are dependent on huge multi-enzyme complexes. The multi-enzyme complex that synthesizes the lactone ring of erythromycin is made up of over 20 subunits; these 20 proteins act together to catalyse Claisen-like reactions. Strip away the sugars and the hydroxyl group at carbon-12 from erythromycin A and you get erythronolide B, the portion of the antibiotic made on the multi-enzyme complex called a polyketide synthase. Erythronolide B is made by joining seven propanoate (3-carbon) units together. Figure 6.30 shows how the first two units are joined together.

Propanoate (the starter unit in pink) is bound to the enzyme using a thioester bond. As we have seen previously, thioesters are electrophiles, whose reactivity is intermediate between that of esters and acid anhydrides. Using thioesters is biology's way of making an active species.

Figure 6.30 (A) Erythromycin A, (B) Erythronolide B stick structure and (C) Erythronolide B with methyl groups marked—you can see how seven three-carbon units make up this structure; (D) the first stage in the biosynthesis of erythronolide B—a Claisen-type reaction

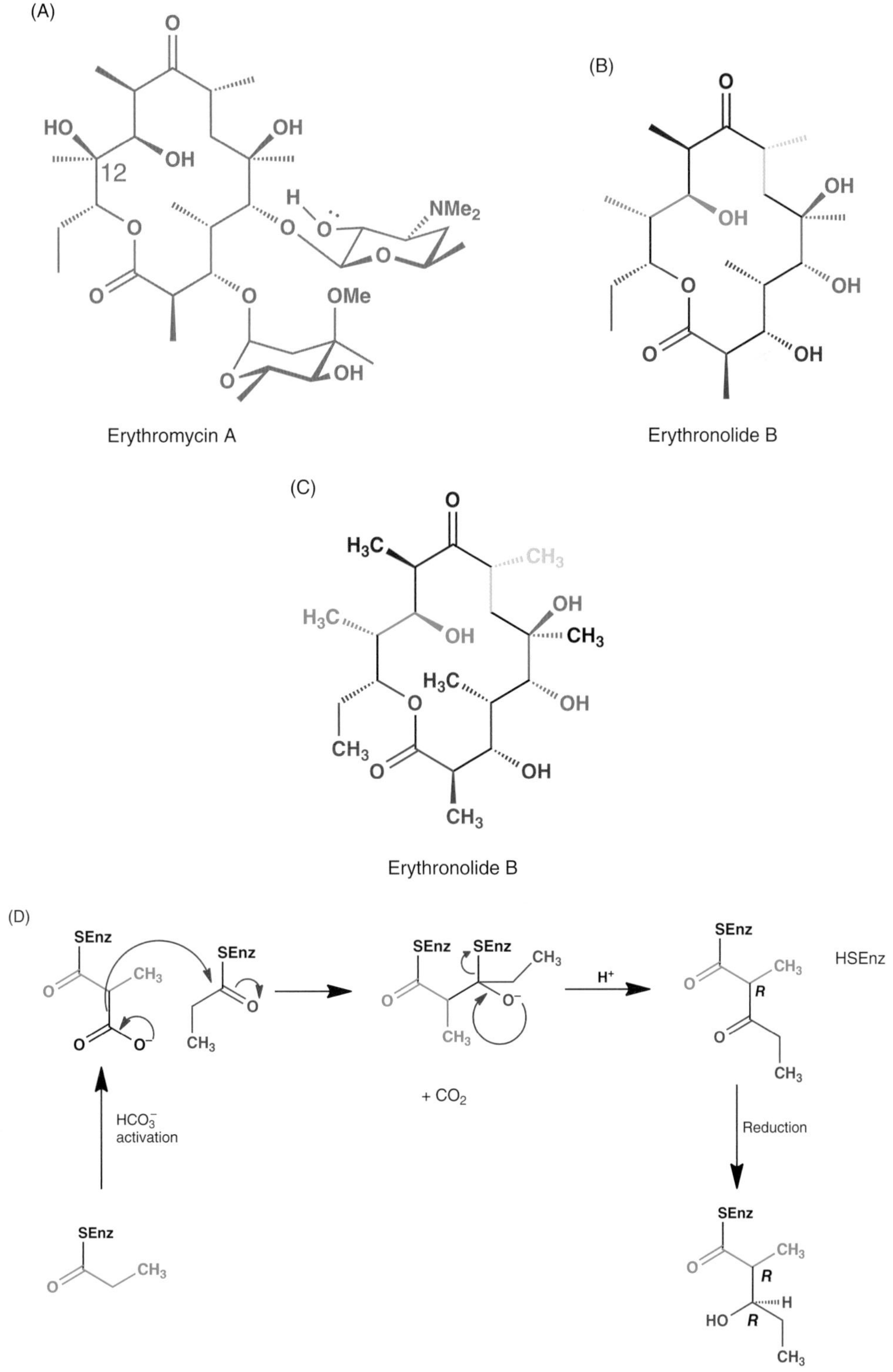

(A) Erythromycin A

(B) Erythronolide B

(C) Erythronolide B

(D)

Self-check 6.26

Draw the mechanism for the reaction of the next propanoate unit (the blue one) to the growing erythronolide molecule. Notice that there is no reduction step.

Self-check 6.27

Can you see how the completed chain cyclizes to give enzyme-free erythronolide B?

The pink starter unit is poised to react with a second molecule of propanoate (in dark green), which will act as the nucleophile. The soil bacterium that makes erythromycin does not add an acid or base catalyst. Instead, it activates propanoate as a nucleophile by replacing a proton with a carboxylic acid functional group to give methyl malonate.

With a carbonyl on either side, the central carbon is now a very reactive nucleophile; it reacts with the starter unit with loss of carbon dioxide to give an enzyme-bound thioester, made up from two propanoate units. A chiral centre is produced in this reaction, and it has R-stereochemistry.

Finally, there is a reduction involving nature's reducing agent **NADPH**, to give the alcohol with R-stereochemistry.

A further five propanoate units are added to complete the erythronolide molecule. Each addition is both regiospecific (the reactants go to the right place) and stereospecific (only one stereoisomer is formed). Nature has spent millions of years evolving enzymes that carry out very clean Claisen-like reactions.

6.5 CARBONYLS IN THE BODY

So far we have looked at the potential of the carbonyl group to be transformed. We have seen how the powerful acyl chlorides and acid anhydrides are the most reactive amongst this useful family. Acyl chlorides and acid anhydrides, however, have no place in the body. They react violently with water and with many other nucleophiles. So which carbonyls *are* of value in biological systems?

Natural carbonyl compounds: the importance of thioesters

Thioesters are very versatile compounds. During the biosynthesis of polyketides they serve as both nucleophiles and electrophiles in Claisen-like reactions; as such, they behave as nature's equivalent of esters. Their intermediate reactivity also enables them to act as nature's equivalent of acid anhydrides.

Coenzyme A (see Figure 6.31) is readily acylated (often with an acetyl group) to give a thioester, which can be used in acyl transfer reactions.

Thioesters are less reactive than acid anhydrides, so they can be used in biological systems, but they are more reactive than esters, and much more reactive than amides.

Figure 6.31 Formation of acyl CoA from coenzyme A. When R=CH$_3$, the molecule is acetyl CoA

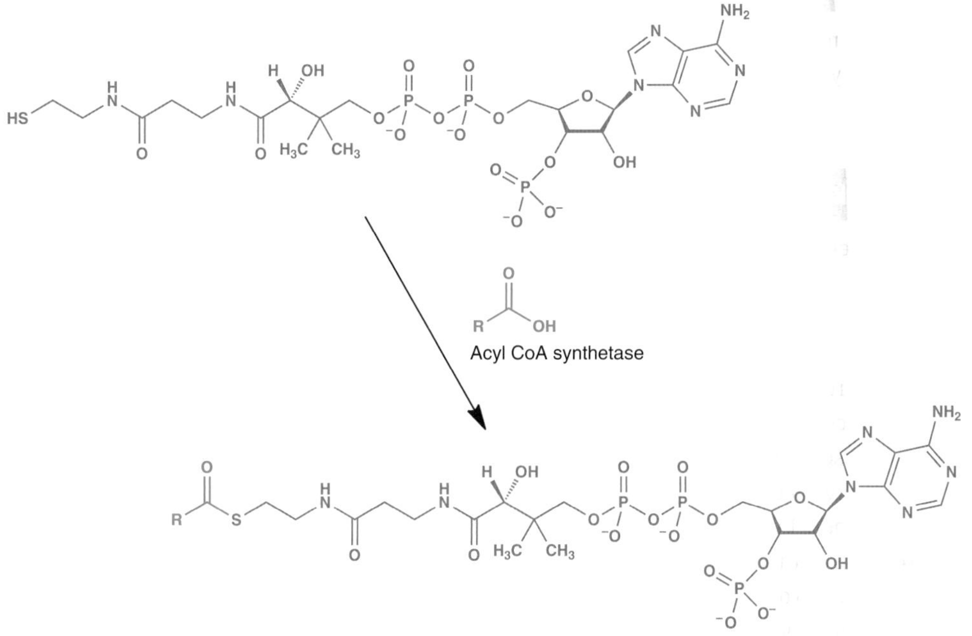

Acyl CoA synthetase

Figure 6.32 The synthesis of N-acetylglucosamine from glucosamine and acetyl CoA. Note the abbreviation for coenzyme A—you would not normally draw out the whole molecule in a mechanism!

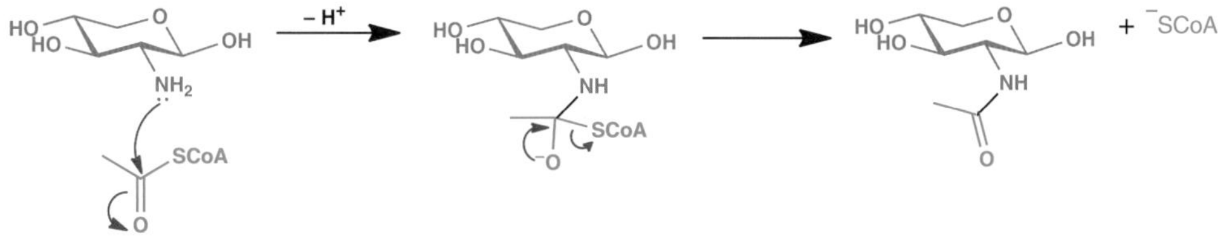

An example of how nature uses these powerful thioesters is in the synthesis of N-acetylglucosamine. This sugar is used in many biochemical processes, and is a component of bacterial cell walls. Here it is synthesized by an aminolysis reaction between glucosamine and acetyl CoA (see Figure 6.32).

6.6 CARBONYLS IN DRUGS—OPPORTUNITIES AND PROBLEMS

We have seen throughout this book, and especially in this chapter, that many drugs contain carbonyls. We have also seen that carbonyls can be reactive. This means that their presence in drugs is often vital but can lead to problems. We have already discussed many of the opportunities and problems of carbonyl chemistry in pharmacy. Here are two specific examples.

Drug storage—aspirin

Acetyl salicylic acid is stable enough to be compressed into a tablet and used as a pharmaceutical. But would you advise storing aspirin tablets in a bathroom cabinet for a long time? We have seen hydrolysis of esters in base in Figure 6.9, but Figure 6.33 shows how esters can also be hydrolysed in acid, in a reversal of the Fischer ester synthesis. So aspirin, which is an acidic molecule, can react with moisture to be converted back to salicyclic acid, so it would not be a good idea to leave a bottle of aspirin tablets in the bathroom cabinet!

It used to be common to smell vinegar on old aspirin tablets. Now, however, aspirin is often coated to enhance its stability. Of course, aspirin works in the body as a pro-drug. In the intestine, it is converted to salicylic acid by base-catalysed hydrolysis.

Proteins and other amides

A visit to your hairdresser should convince you that it is difficult to break amide bonds. Hair is made of protein, and protein is made of amino acids linked by amide bonds (known as peptide bonds when they are found in proteins). Hair can be straightened, curled, bleached and

Figure 6.33 The acid-catalysed hydrolysis of aspirin

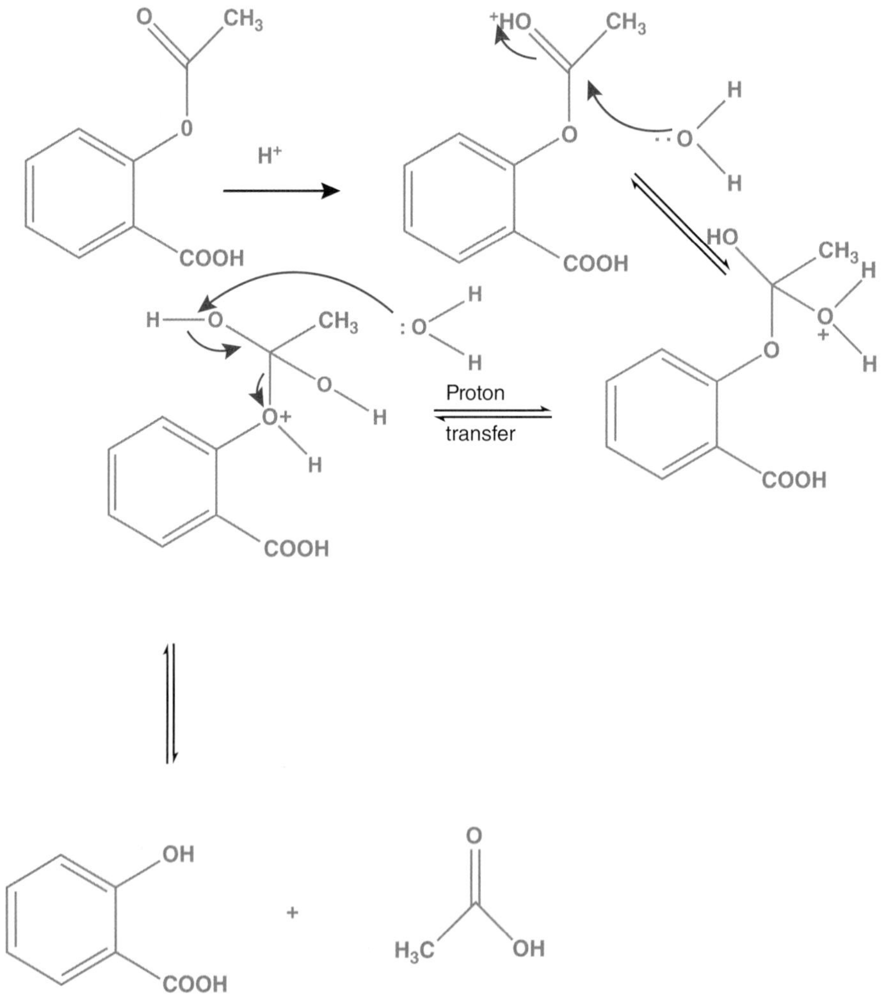

dyed, but the amide bonds remain intact. Hairdressers have to study biology and are often very knowledgeable about protein chemistry.

Similarly if you boil an egg, the protein coagulates and solidifies, but the peptide bonds do not break. This raises questions about nutrition! You can boil, scramble, fry or bake eggs and the protein remains intact, so how does egg work as a nutrient?

The answer is that our digestive tracts are full of enzymes that catalyse the hydrolysis of peptide bonds. Pepsin in the stomach cleaves peptide bonds adjacent to aromatic residues; trypsin in the intestine cleaves peptide bonds adjacent to basic residues; carboxypeptidase cleaves peptide bonds at one end of a protein, and so on. Because of these enzymes, proteins are processed very efficiently. Each individual enzyme is, however, quite specific, which means that some amide bonds are able to evade all these enzymes.

Consider meticillin, for example.

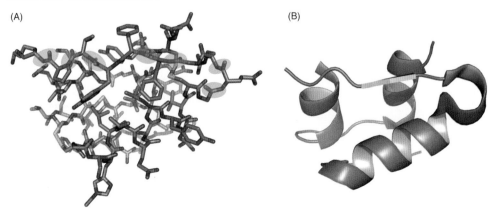

This molecule contains two amide bonds. The β-lactam bond is rather reactive for an amide. This is because amide carbons, like all sp^2 carbons, prefer bond angles of 120°, but the four-membered ring constrains the β-lactam bond to a 90° bond angle. Despite this reactivity, both the green and the pink amide bonds escape attack by digestive enzymes and so methicillin can be delivered orally.

It is a different story with insulin, a medicine required daily by patients with Type 1 diabetes. Diabetics have to inject themselves regularly with insulin. Despite modern 'pens', it would be much more convenient to take the drug orally. Unfortunately, the enzymes in the digestive tract recognize insulin as food (see Figure 6.34).

Figure 6.34   Insulin—a small protein with many peptide (amide) bonds. (A) A structure highlighting the amide bonds; (B) ribbon structure showing the secondary structure of insulin
Source: life-enhancement.com.

(A) (B)

The hydrolysis of a peptide bond proceeds by nucleophilic attack on the carbonyl as described in Section 6.3. For the tetrahedral intermediate to lose an amine rather than water requires a complex enzymic mechanism (see Figure 6.35). In the laboratory, amide bonds can be cleaved by heating at boiling point in 6 M acid.

ACE inhibitors

A very important class of drugs in use today are the ACE (angiotensin converting enzyme) inhibitors. ACE catalyses the hydrolysis of a specific peptide bond. By doing this, it converts angiotensin I to angiotensin II. Angiotensin II is a potent vasoconstrictor, which causes high blood pressure and related conditions when present in excess.

ACE inhibitors are currently used in the treatment of hypertension. They work by stopping the production of angiotensin II from angiotensin I by the zinc-containing ACE (see Figure 6.36). The first drug in this family was captopril. It was proposed that it binds at the active site of ACE, with the S⁻ of the drug interacting with Zn^{2+} in the enzyme and oxygens in both carbonyl groups also involved in binding. These oxygens (whether charged or not) are able to act as hydrogen bond acceptors.

> Hydrogen bonds are discussed in more detail in Chapter 2, 'Organic structure and bonding'.

Captopril is a relatively simple molecule (count the chiral centres and calculate the molecular weight) and many analogues of this compound have been synthesized. A particular motivation

Case study 6.1

A patient who suffers from diabetes comes into the pharmacy with a prescription for 'Ketostix®'. He asks what they are for and how do they work.

Reflection questions
1. What is the reason for diabetes patients using 'Ketostix®'?
2. How do 'Ketostix®' work?

For answers, visit the online resources which accompany this textbook.

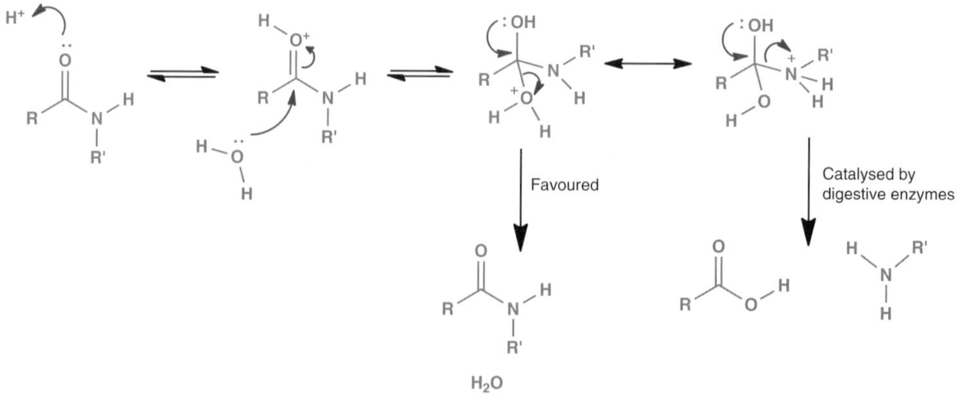

Figure 6.35 The action of digestive enzymes in cleaving peptide bonds

has been to improve the **bioavailability**. Captopril needs to be taken two or three times per day, yet for long-term therapy it is far preferable to have a drug that is taken just once per day. In addition, captopril has a nasty taste due to the sulfur in the molecule.

Further studies led to the development of enalaprilat. However, as is often the case with drug development, there was one step forward and one step back. Enalaprilat was not orally active and was only suitable for use as an injectable. The scientists at Merck were not deterred by this, however; they esterified enalaprilat to give enalapril. Enalapril is an inactive pro-drug; for the ACE inhibitor activity to take effect the ethyl ester is hydrolysed back to enalaprilat after the pro-drug has passed through the gut wall and entered the blood stream. Truly fantastic carbonyl chemistry: a carbonyl compound has been converted to another to make a drug that is suitable for oral delivery, then metabolism has converted it back to the active form to save lives (see Figure 6.37).

Figure 6.36 (A) Conversion of angiotensin I to angiotensin II by angiotensin converting enzyme; (B) Ionized form of captopril

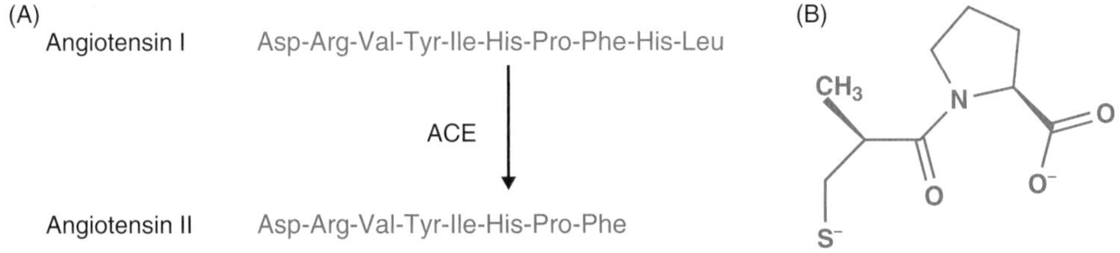

(A)
Angiotensin I   Asp-Arg-Val-Tyr-Ile-His-Pro-Phe-His-Leu

ACE

Angiotensin II   Asp-Arg-Val-Tyr-Ile-His-Pro-Phe

(B)

Figure 6.37 Conversion of the pro-drug enalapril to the active drug enalaprilat

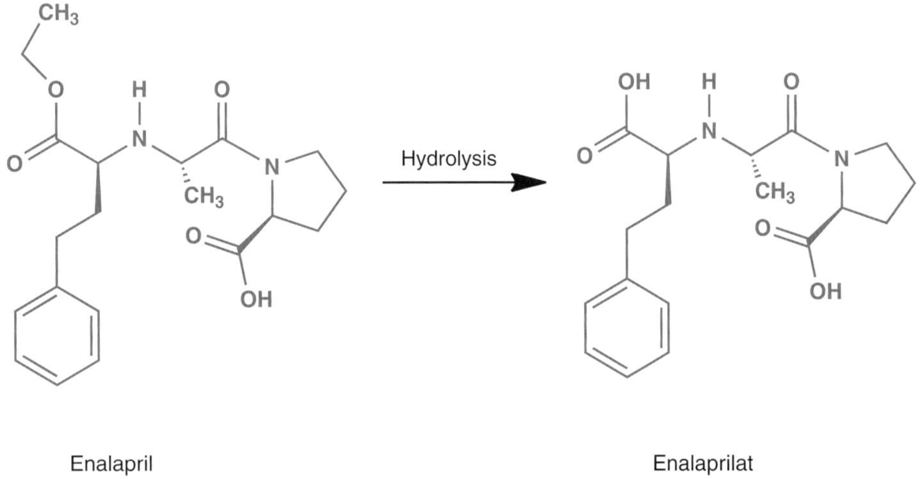

Enalapril   Hydrolysis   Enalaprilat

205

Self-check 6.28

Draw a mechanism for the conversion of enalapril to enalaprilat. Hint: when drawing mechanisms in assessments, it is usually acceptable to refer to most of the molecule as 'R' and to focus on the important functional groups!

CHAPTER SUMMARY

- The chemistry of the carbonyl group arises from the difference in electronegativity between carbon and oxygen.

- The carbonyl group is present in many important pharmaceutical and biochemical compounds and is the component of a number of key functional groups.

- Carbonyl groups undergo nucleophilic attack at the carbon atom.

- The outcome of nucleophilic attack at the carbon atom of carbonyl compounds is dependent on the nature of the leaving group.

- Aldehydes and ketones undergo addition reactions.

- Carbonyl groups can, if appropriately structured, undergo α-substitution reactions.

- Aldon and Claisen condensation reactions are important synthetic and biosynthetic reactions.

FURTHER READING

In the 1970s, Stuart Warren wrote a ground-breaking book entitled *The Chemistry of the Carbonyl Group*, which you may be able to find in your university library. The fact that a whole textbook could be written about it illustrates just how fantastic carbonyl chemistry is.

Further information on aspirin can be found on the following website: http://www.aspirin.com

self-check

For the answers to the Self-Check questions in Chapter 6, visit the online resources which accompany this textbook.

INTRODUCTION TO AROMATIC CHEMISTRY

Mike Southern

What do aspirin, paracetamol, salbutamol and chloramphenicol have in common? You might know that they are all synthetic drugs, but additionally they are members of a class of organic molecules known as aromatic compounds. The chemistry of aromatic compounds started with the discovery of benzene (the basic unit of aromatic chemistry) by Michael Faraday in 1825. The precise structure of benzene was elusive and it was not until 1865 that the correct structure was first described by Kekulé. The importance of aromatic chemistry cannot be overstated; it was the driving force behind the dyestuff industry in the mid- to late 1800s, and that was the start of the chemical industry we know today. In the intervening years we will see that aromatic compounds have been adopted by the pharmaceutical industry and feature heavily in lists of the best-selling drugs.

Learning Outcomes

Having read this chapter you are expected to be able to:

- appreciate the importance of aromatic compounds to the drug industry

- describe the structure of benzene and other aromatic hydrocarbons

- predict how benzene and its derivatives react with electrophiles in electrophilic aromatic substitution reactions

- describe key points in the synthesis of paracetamol and aspirin from phenol

- show awareness of the influence that some aromatic compounds have in the body and the role they play either as endogenous compounds or as drugs

- provide an overview of how the body metabolizes aromatic compounds, how this can deactivate drugs and sometimes form compounds that are hazardous to health.

7.1 WHAT IS AROMATIC CHEMISTRY?

Aromatic compounds were initially identified by their characteristic odour. Many of these early compounds were derivatives of benzene, and we will focus on the chemistry of benzene and its derivatives in this chapter. However, there is much more to aromatic chemistry than smell, and the term 'aromatic' has now been extended to cover a wide range of molecules, many of which have little detectable odour.

Benzene is a volatile liquid that has a boiling point of 80 °C, a melting point of 5.5 °C, a density of 0.874 g mL^{-1} and a molecular formula of C_6H_6. The structure of benzene was the topic of considerable debate until Kekulé described the currently accepted structure in 1865. Some of the early proposed structures, including Kekulé's, are shown in Figure 7.1. The structure is an average of the two rapidly interconverting forms shown, and this accounts for the structural observations described.

Benzene is a planar molecule in which all the carbon–carbon bond lengths are equal at 1.39 **Angstroms** (Å) (a value between the C–C single bond length of 1.48 Å and the C–C double bond length of 1.34 Å). The σ-bond framework of benzene consists of a planar six-membered ring in which each carbon is sp^2 hybridized. This leaves a single electron in a p-orbital on each C atom of the six-membered ring; these orbitals and electrons combine to form the characteristic π-cloud shown in Figure 7.2. The π-system of benzene (and other aromatic molecules) dominates their chemistry and reactivity. The electrons of the π-system are delocalized; they can take part in resonance or conjugation.

> Aspects of delocalization are discussed in Chapter 2, 'Organic structure and bonding', and Chapter 5 'Alcohols, phenols, ethers, organic halogen compounds, and amines'.

A common representation of benzene is shown in Figure 7.3. The circle within the six-membered ring represents the π-system. While this representation is structurally satisfactory because it illustrates that the six π electrons are delocalized across the six carbon atoms of the ring, it is not, however, amenable to mechanistic aspects of aromatic chemistry. In order to predict reaction pathways and plan sensible syntheses we must understand the mechanisms of aromatic chemistry—and to do this we must employ the single- and double-bonded model shown in Figure 7.3.

Figure 7.1   Proposed structures of benzene

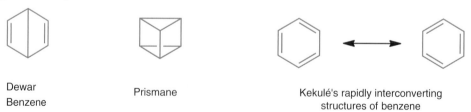

Dewar
Benzene

Prismane

Kekulé's rapidly interconverting
structures of benzene

Early representations of benzene that have
subsequently been synthesized
–but behave nothing like benzene itself

Figure 7.2   The σ- and π-bonding of benzene

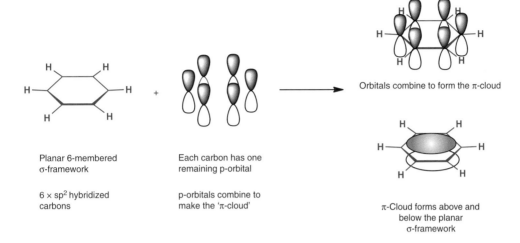

Planar 6-membered
σ-framework

6 × sp² hybridized
carbons

Each carbon has one
remaining p-orbital

p-orbitals combine to
make the 'π-cloud'

Orbitals combine to form the π-cloud

π-Cloud forms above and
below the planar
σ-framework

Figure 7.3   Representations of the benzene molecule

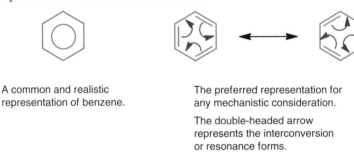

A common and realistic
representation of benzene.

The preferred representation for
any mechanistic consideration.

The double-headed arrow
represents the interconversion
or resonance forms.

Although the term 'aromatic chemistry' originally stemmed from the characteristic odour of compounds, as our understanding has increased this definition has changed and more stringent criteria are now employed. To be considered aromatic a compound must:

- be planar (or close to planar)
- have 4n+2 π-electrons. This criterion is known as Hückel's rule
- be cyclic and fully conjugated.

In Hückel's rule, n is a positive integer, meaning that aromatic compounds can have 2 π-electrons (n = 0), 6 π-electrons (n = 1 e.g. benzene); 10 π-electrons (n = 2, e.g. naphthalene); 14 π-electrons (n = 3, e.g. anthracene); 18 electrons (n = 4 e.g. [18]-annulene) and so on; see Figure 7.4.

Nuclear Magnetic Resonance (NMR) experiments have given us a new criterion for aromaticity: aromatic compounds are able to form a ring current in a magnetic field. This means that their protons produce signals in a particular region of the spectrum, about δ 7 ppm. However, aromatic compounds do not need to be completely carbon-based: pyridine is an example of a heteroaromatic compound (nitrogen is considered a heteroatom).

When the criteria for aromaticity are fulfilled (i.e. when the compound is planar, cyclic and obeys Hückel's rule) the molecule achieves a degree of extra stability. This is known as

Figure 7.4 Some simple aromatic compounds

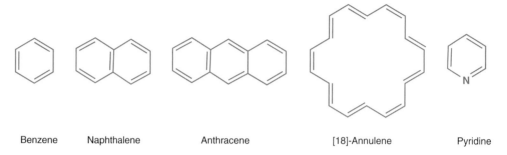

| Benzene | Naphthalene | Anthracene | [18]-Annulene | Pyridine |

'aromatic stabilization energy' and is 151 kJ mol^{-1} or 36 kcal mol^{-1} in the case of benzene. Aromatic stabilization energy has a dramatic effect on the reactivity of aromatic systems and is discussed later (Section 7.3.).

7.2 WHY IS AROMATIC CHEMISTRY IMPORTANT?

Aromatic chemistry has a long and distinguished history and was the driving force behind the rise of the chemical industry in the 1850s. Early industrial chemistry focused on dye production: dyes require extended **chromophores**, and chromophores are often aromatic. The first synthetic dye, mauveine, was prepared accidentally by William Perkin while he was trying (unsuccessfully) to synthesize the anti-malarial compound quinine. Although mauveine was initially only produced in small quantities, Perkin was able to refine the process and improve the yield. He was also astute enough to patent the invention, and in 1857 to set up a factory to manufacture the dye. Industrial chemistry began here, and, despite many changes, continues to be important today.

> More information on chromophores can be found in Chapter 1, 'The importance of pharmaceutical chemistry'.

Protosil and the sulfa drugs

Mauveine was the by-product of an attempt to produce a drug, but some of the earliest successful drugs were actually failed dyes! Prontosil, shown in Figure 7.5A, is a red azo-dye (azo refers to the characteristic nitrogen–nitrogen double bond in these dyes). Scientists at the Bayer company in Germany had shown that prontosil could kill streptococcal bacteria in mice, and, in a leap of faith, Gerhard Domagk (Bayer's Director of Pathology and Bacteriology) saved his daughter from serious complications associated with a bacterial infection by treating her with it. Domagk was awarded the Nobel Prize in Physiology or Medicine in 1939 'for the discovery of the antibacterial effects of prontosil', but, because of orders from the Nazi regime, he was not able to accept it until 1947. The compound went on to become the first commercially available antibiotic.

The active agent in prontosil is actually a metabolite, sulfanilamide; this led to the development of the so-called 'sulfa' anti-bacterial drugs. The sulfa drugs have been almost completely superseded by the pencillins, which have better activity and fewer side-effects, although sulfamethoxazole is still used in the treatment of certain types of pneumonia.

Many other familiar drugs contain aromatic structures. These include OTC (over-the-counter) analgesics, aspirin, paracetamol and ibuprofen, which ease pain by interfering with

Figure 7.5 (A) The production of sulfanilamide in the body from the azo-dye prontosil. (B) The structure of sulfamethoxazole, a sulfa drug still in use today

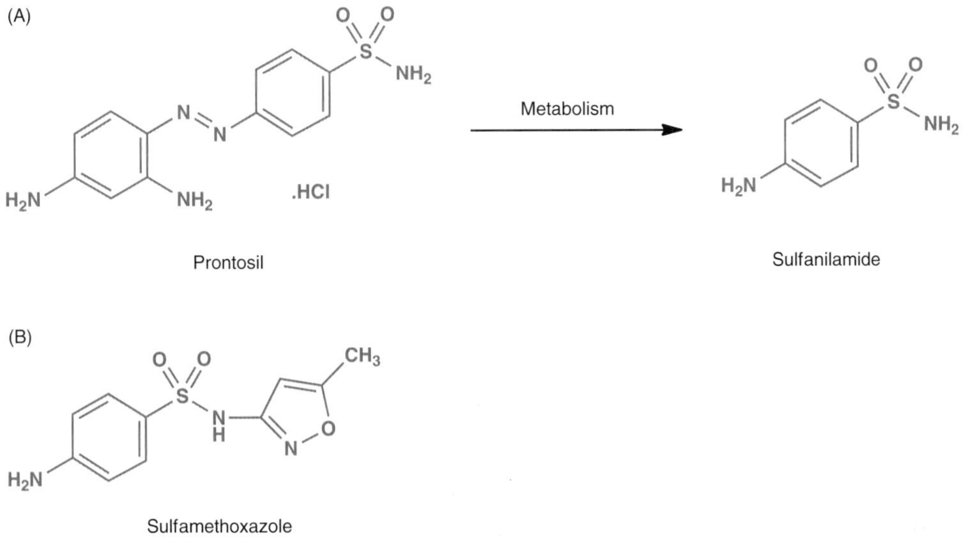

(A)

Prontosil

Metabolism

Sulfanilamide

(B)

Sulfamethoxazole

Figure 7.6 The familiar over-the-counter analgesics aspirin, paracetamol and ibuprofen

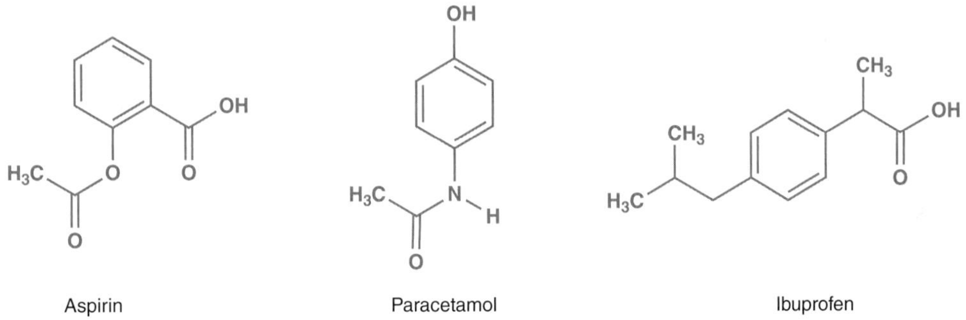

Aspirin

Paracetamol

Ibuprofen

the pain response within the body. Their structures are shown in Figure 7.6; notice how they all feature an aromatic ring.

Aspirin

The story of aspirin is an interesting one. Willow bark has been known to treat mild pain and fever for hundreds of years, and Hippocrates of Kos advocated its use for fever, pain and child-birth around 2,400 years ago. In 1763, Edward Stone published the first recorded clinical trial *via* The Royal Society of London in which he administered dried willow bark extracts in tea, water or beer to fifty patients who had fever, and then observed the effects. In 1828, Johan Andreas Buchner in Munich purified willow bark extracts and obtained a yellow powder that he called salicin (see Figure 7.7). We now know that salicin is converted to salicylic acid in the body; it is salicylic acid that causes the beneficial effects associated with willow bark extract.

Generally, trees are not a sustainable source of drugs; they take many years to grow. Further, the concentration of drug in a material like willow bark is hard to predict (this is often a problem with plant preparations.). In more recent times it became more straightforward to replace willow

Figure 7.7   The path from willow bark to aspirin

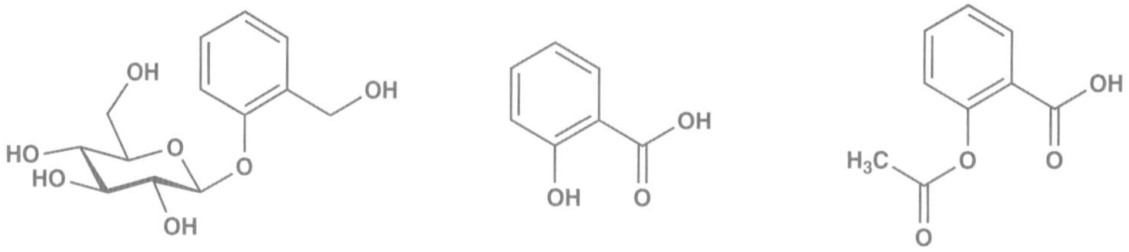

Salicin   Salicylic acid   Aspirin

bark with pure salicylic acid but, unfortunately, the pure acid causes severe irritation to the mouth, throat and stomach. The side-effects of salicylic acid were vastly reduced when the hydroxyl group was acetylated to form aspirin. This process was mastered in 1897 by Felix Hoffmann at Bayer, who was able to produce aspirin with suitable purity for therapeutic use. Incidentally, the acetylation of morphine to give diamorphine (heroin) was also first performed around the same time.

❯ For more information on these drugs, see Chapter 13, 'Origins of drug molecules'.

Fluoxetine

Aromatic compounds have even altered the way certain diseases are perceived by society, as illustrated by the drugs shown in Figure 7.8. Prior to the development of fluoxetine and other selective serotonin reuptake inhibitor (SSRI) anti-depressants, depression was rarely discussed in public. Sufferers and their families were often reluctant to admit they had a problem. The SSRIs made depression a much more easily treatable disease, benefiting both sufferers and the economy. This in turn led to much more widespread discussion of the disease.

Sildenafil

Similarly, sildenafil changed the way society views erectile dysfunction. Before the release of the drug, the topic was rarely discussed. Erectile dysfunction is now treatable in many cases and is much more easily discussed and can even form the basis of jokes. Sildenafil was initially

Figure 7.8   Fluoxetine and Sildenafil: aromatic molecules that have reduced the stigma of depression and erectile dysfunction

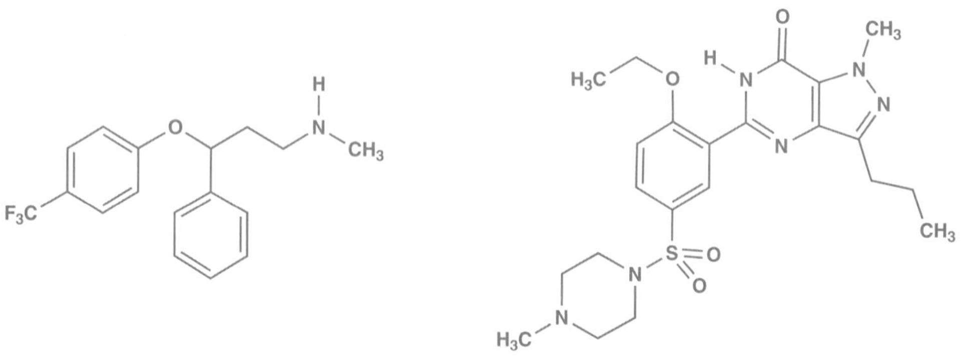

Fluoxetine   Sildenafil

developed by Pfizer as a treatment for angina. It was unsuccessful in this context but, during clinical trials in humans, a number of men were honest enough to report the side-effects that led to its release as a treatment for erectile dysfunction.

Fluoxetine and sildenafil are particularly well-known aromatic drugs, but, in fact, all the top five drugs (in terms of prescriptions issued) in 2016 contained substituted benzene rings. The drugs in question were lisinopril, atorvastatin, levothyroxine, hydrocodone/paracetamol and amlodipine (see Figure 7.9). Two of the top five drugs by sales in 2016—Harvoni® (antiviral drug used against hepatitis C) and lenalidomide (anticancer drug)—contained aromatic rings; the remaining three places were taken by biologics. Figures for sales are perhaps a little misleading. because the relatively high cost of biologics and the specific small molecule treatments distorts how widespread their use is.

Self-check 7.1

What do you think the top five most prescribed drugs are used to treat? How about those with the largest sales? Are you surprised?

Figure 7.9 The top five branded drugs

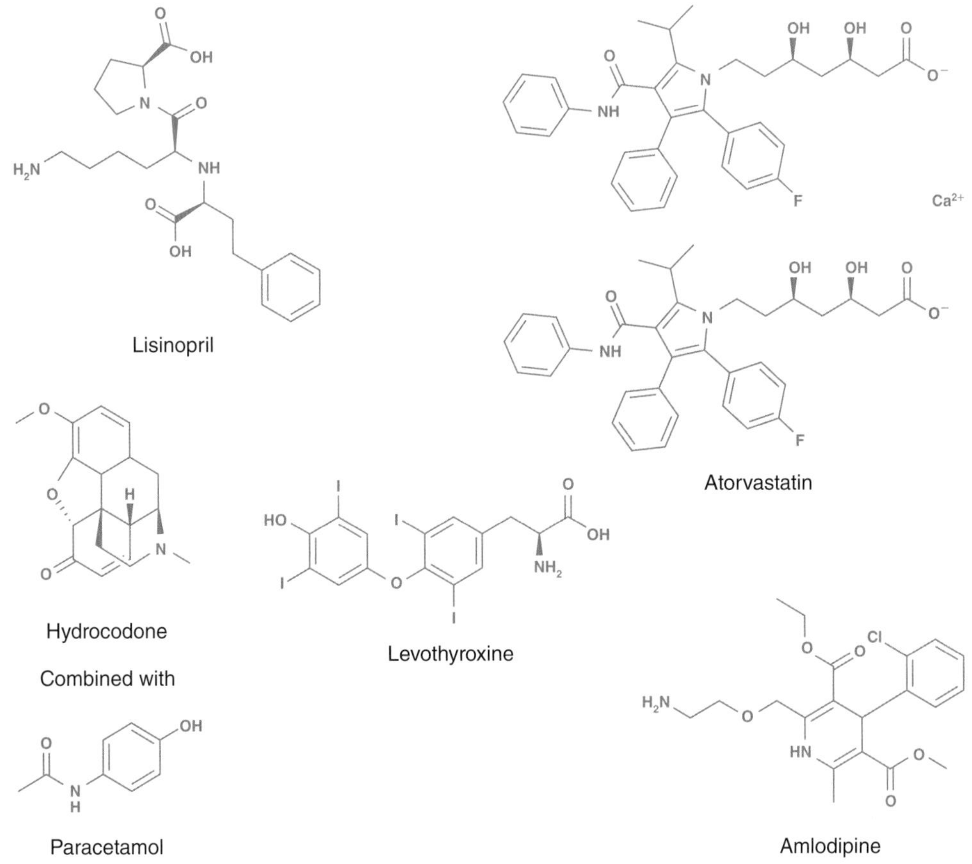

The appearance of aromatic rings in the top five prescribed drugs is not coincidence: aromatic structures feature strongly in a large percentage of successful drugs, indicating the importance of aromatic chemistry to global health.

Ecstasy and cannabis

Aromatic compounds also feature in illegal substances such as MDMA (ecstasy) and Δ^9-tetrahydrocannabinol (THC, one of the active ingredients of cannabis), shown in Figure 7.10. There is longstanding anecdotal evidence that a number of illegal compounds have therapeutic benefits, and these anecdotes have led to proper scientific trials being conducted.

Sativex® is a cannabis extract (containing THC and cannabidiol) that is now available (in the UK and Spain) as an oromucosal spray to treat the spasticity associated with multiple sclerosis. In Canada it is also used for the treatment of neuropathic pain. Small-scale clinical trials have also indicated that MDMA may be of benefit in the treatment of post-traumatic stress disorder.

Aromatic compounds are not only found in both legal and illegal drugs; read Box 7.1 to discover how they also give a spicy kick to the food we eat.

It is clear that many biologically active compounds are aromatic. If we want to be able to maximize the impact of the beneficial effects of this class of compound we must be able to construct such molecules in a predictable and controlled manner. This will allow us to discover new chemical entities with beneficial therapeutic effects and to optimize the therapeutic aspects and minimize the side-effects of current or potential new drugs. In order to do this successfully we need to understand the chemistry of benzene and related aromatic compounds.

Figure 7.10   Illegal drugs: (A) The cannabis plant and one of its active ingredients, Δ^9-tetrahydrocannabinol (Δ^9-THC). (B) The synthetic drug MDMA *Source*: https://commons.wikimedia.org/wiki/File:Cannabis_01_bgiu.jpg
Wikimedia Commons/Public Domain

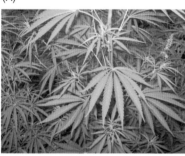

(A)

Δ^9-Tetrahydrocannabinol

(B)

MDMA 'ecstasy'

Box 7.1 Feeling the heat of chilli peppers

There is no doubting the popularity of chilli peppers as an addition to food. They have found fans across the globe since their export from South America. Chilli peppers are thought to have been cultivated in South America for a few thousand years, and it is likely that Christopher Columbus first introduced chillis to Europeans after encountering them in the Caribbean.

The main compound responsible for the 'heat' of chillis is the benzene derivative capsaicin (see Figure 7.11). The heat of chillis is measured on the Scoville scale, which gives a measure of how many times a standard extract of a particular chilli has to be diluted with dilute syrup until its heat becomes undetectable by taste. Clearly this is a little subjective, so high-performance liquid chromatography (HPLC) is now employed to provide a more accurate measurement. The common Jalapeño generally has a heat of around 3,500 Scoville Heat Units (SHU), the Scotch Bonnet ranges from 100,000 to 350,000 SHU, and the 2017 Guinness Book of Records states that world's hottest chilli, the Corolina Reaper, was measured at an eye-watering average of 1,641,183 SHU.

Figure 7.11   Red chillis and the aromatic compound capsaicin—the main compound that gives chillis their 'heat' *Source*: https://commons.wikimedia.org/wiki/File:Capsicum_-_red_chili_chilli_-_piment_rouge_-_roter_Chili_02.jpg

Norbert Nagel, Mörfelden-Walldorf / Wikimedia Commons / CC BY-SA 3.0

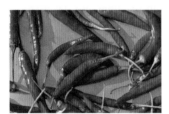

Capsaicin

7.3 THE CHEMISTRY OF BENZENE

The most important chemistry of aromatic compounds can be divided into two main reaction types:

- Electrophilic aromatic substitution (EAS or S_EAr—Substitution Electrophilic Aromatic) in which the aromatic compound reacts with an electrophile.

- Nucleophillic aromatic substitution (NAS or S_NAR) in which the aromatic species reacts with a nucleophile.

Note that in the following reactions we will show hydrogen atoms on the aromatic rings where it helps to explain the mechanistic details being discussed.

Electrophilic aromatic substitution

Firstly, let us consider the general reactivity of benzene. We can represent it as a six-membered ring containing three double bonds—but does it react like that? The answer is 'no': the reactivity of benzene is very different from that of simple alkenes. This can be illustrated by the reactivity of benzene with bromine compared with that of a simple alkene. Bromine reacts with alkenes extremely rapidly, with the red/brown colour of bromine disappearing almost instantaneously (until all the alkene is consumed). The resulting product is a dibromide formed by an **addition reaction**. However, if benzene is treated with bromine no reaction takes place and the colour of bromine persists. Benzene can be forced to react with bromine by employing a catalyst that makes the bromine more reactive (more electrophilic in this case). However, rather than undergoing an addition reaction and forming the dibromide, a **substitution reaction** occurs to form bromobenzene.

The difference in reactivity between alkenes and aromatic compounds arises from the aromatic stabilization energy (mentioned in section 7.1). Remember that this is a result of the six carbon atoms of the benzene ring sharing their six p-electrons in a cyclic delocalized system or π-cloud. For benzene to react, this delocalization has to be interrupted, which requires a relatively large amount of energy in order to compensate for the loss of aromaticity and its associated aromatic stabilization energy.

Benzene reacts with bromine only when the bromine is activated by a catalyst; when the reaction does occur it does so by forming another aromatic product, which is energetically favourable. The intermediate cationic species does not react with a bromide ion (as is the case in the bromination of alkenes) but instead loses a proton so that the molecule can re-establish its aromatic character and regain the associated stabilization energy. In effect, a hydrogen atom is substituted by a bromine atom.

In short, bromine reacts with an alkene by an **addition reaction**, but activated bromine reacts with benzene by a **substitution reaction** as shown in Figure 7.12.

> The bromination of alkenes and also addition and substitution reactions are discussed in more detail in Chapter 4, 'Properties of aliphatic hydrocarbons'.

Figure 7.12 (A) The addition of bromine to prop-2-ene; (B) bromine does not react with benzene; (C) electrophilic aromatic substitution reaction of bromine and benzene

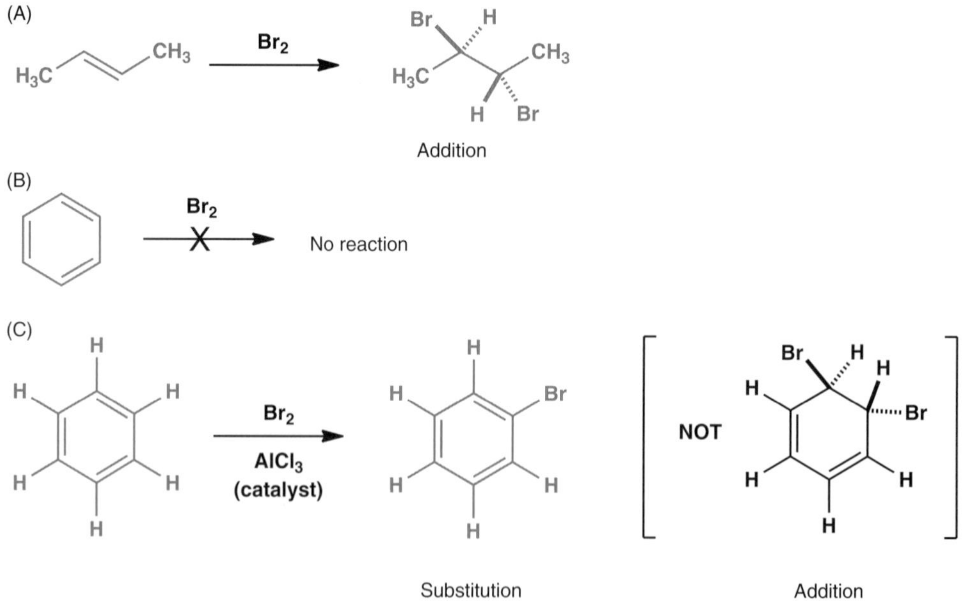

Mechanism of electrophilic aromatic substitution

In the bromination of benzene illustrated in Figure 7.13, bromine first combines with aluminium trichloride to form the active electrophile. The π-system of benzene then acts as a nucleophile and attacks the bromine complex to form the high-energy, positively charged, non-aromatic sigma-complex (σ-complex), also known as the Wheland Intermediate. Loss of a proton neutralizes the intermediate to restore aromaticity, forming HBr as a by-product and regenerating the catalyst. The addition of an electrophile, formation of the σ-complex and restoration of aromaticity is common to all EAS reactions; it is only the nature of the electrophile that changes.

It is extremely important to understand the mechanism of EAS, because if we understand one example then we understand them all. Let us therefore look at the mechanism in more detail, focusing on the aromatic ring. We will use a generic electrophile E^+ and examine the fate of the double bonds of the benzene ring.

Look at Figure 7.14, which illustrates the reaction of benzene with a generic electrophile. As benzene attacks the electrophile, one carbon of the double bond (C2) becomes positively charged whereas the other (C1) forms a bond to the electrophile. For C1 little has changed; it has four bonds in the starting material and four in the intermediate (although one bond in the π-system has been replaced by the new σ-bond). Consequently, C1 still has a full octet of electrons. However, C2 is now electron-deficient, with the electron it donated to the π-bond now used to form the new σ-bond from C1 to E. C2 has only six valence electrons (three bonding pairs) and therefore has a positive charge.

There is a large driving force for rearomatization (because of the aromatic stabilization energy), and any basic species in the reaction mixture (even a weak base) can remove the proton so that aromaticity is restored (see Figure 7.14).

Figure 7.13   Electrophilic aromatic substitution—the bromination of benzene

Active electrophile

Non aromatic sigma-complex (σ-complex) sometimes called the Wheland Intermediate

+ HBr

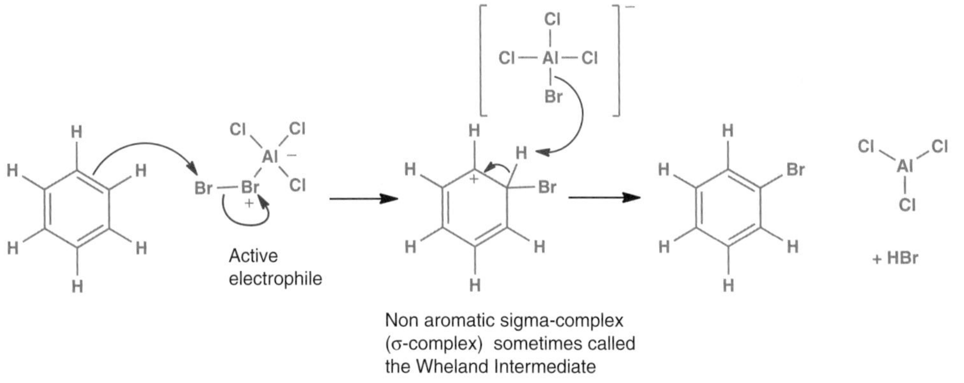

Figure 7.14   Electrophilic aromatic substitution—reaction of benzene with a generic electrophile

σ-complex 1

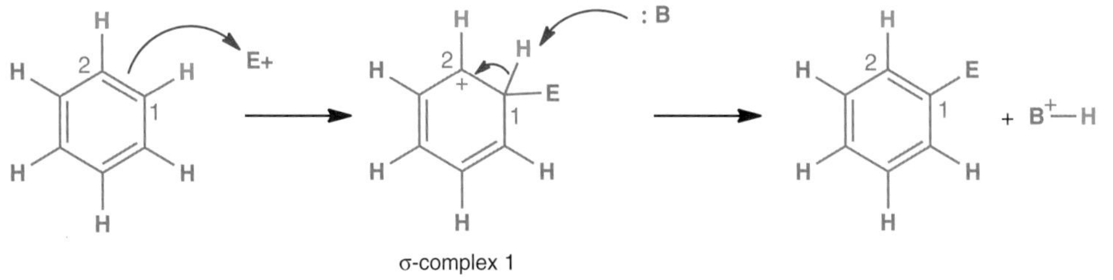

Another aspect of the reaction that needs consideration is the delocalization of electrons in the σ-complex, as illustrated in Figure 7.15. Remember that the electrons in the π-system of benzene are delocalized; we used curly arrows to represent the movement of electrons around the ring to interconvert the two resonance forms. We can also use curly arrows to represent the delocalization within the σ-complex; in this instance the positive charge moves around the ring.

The σ-complex is not aromatic: it consists of a cyclic, planar carbon framework but it no longer obeys Hückel's 4n+2 π-electrons rule. However, the delocalization of the remaining electrons stabilizes the high energy intermediate by spreading the positive charge across a number of atoms.

Consider σ-complex 1. There is a double bond (C3-C4) adjacent to a positively charged carbon, C2. Using a curly arrow, we can show that the electrons of the C3-C4 double bond move towards the positively charged carbon to form a new carbon–carbon double bond (C2-C3) leaving a positive charge on C4. We have now formed σ-complex 2. If you have trouble convincing yourself of this, count the valence electrons on each of the carbons discussed (C2-C4). Now σ-complex 2 once again has a double bond (C5-C6) adjacent to a positively charged carbon (C4). Using another curly arrow we can represent further delocalization of the electrons and move the double bond from C5-C6 to C4-C5, leaving carbon C6 with a positive charge. A proton can then be lost from σ-complex 3 to restore aromaticity.

In total, the three resonance forms shown in Figure 7.15 can be drawn to illustrate the delocalization of the electrons.

For the remainder of this section only one resonance form will normally be shown, but you should remember that another two can be drawn.

If you are having trouble understanding the advantages of delocalization then consider a potato that has finished baking and needs to be removed from the oven, in the absence of oven gloves or similar equipment. The hot potato represents the high-energy cationic species and your hands represent positions of delocalization. If you attempt to remove the potato with one hand then it is highly likely that a severe burn will ensue and that the potato will end up on the floor. However, if you make use of two hands to juggle the potato and delocalize the heat/energy then you have a much greater chance of getting the potato onto a plate safely.

Self-check 7.2

We have seen how a proton can be lost from σ-complex 1 and σ-complex 3 to restore aromaticity. Can you see how a proton can be lost from σ-complex 2 to restore aromaticity?

Figure 7.15 Interconversion of σ-complexes during electrophilic aromatic substitution

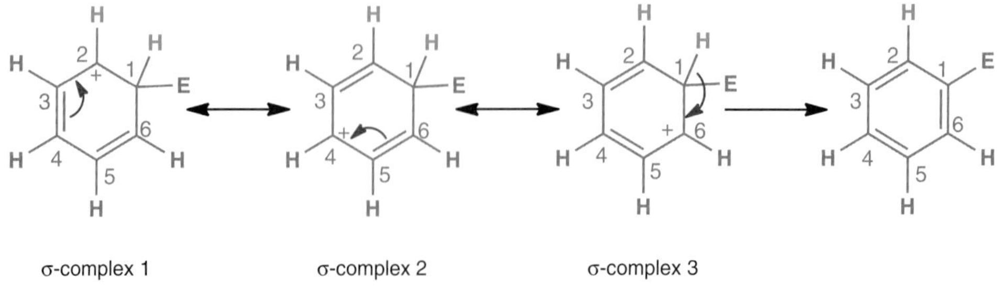

σ-complex 1   σ-complex 2   σ-complex 3

Self-check 7.3

Use the alternative initial resonance form of benzene shown in Figure 7.14 to verify that the overall mechanism and associated resonance forms (Figure 7.15) can still be employed to form a substituted benzene.

Specific reactions which employ EAS

Now it is time to apply EAS to real reactions. Note that, as far as the benzene ring is concerned, the mechanism is always the same. Bromination has already been discussed, and we will now consider four more important EAS reactions. Arguably the most important reaction in aromatic chemistry is nitration, because of the versatility of the nitro group (considered in more detail later). Mixing nitric and sulfuric acid together forms the active electrophile $[NO_2]^+$, and this reacts with benzene by the EAS reaction mechanism to form nitrobenzene (see Figure 7.16).

A similar reaction employing benzene and concentrated sulfuric acid or oleum (SO_3 dissolved in sulfuric acid) gives benzene sulfonic acid as the product, as illustrated in Figure 7.17. In this case, protonated SO_3 $[SO_3H]^+$ is the active electrophile. Sulfonic acids are very strong acids (similar in strength to sulfuric acid) and are useful for organic synthesis because they are very soluble in organic solvents (unlike inorganic acids). They also serve as precursors to the sulfa antibiotics.

Figure 7.16   Descriptor of nitrobenzene

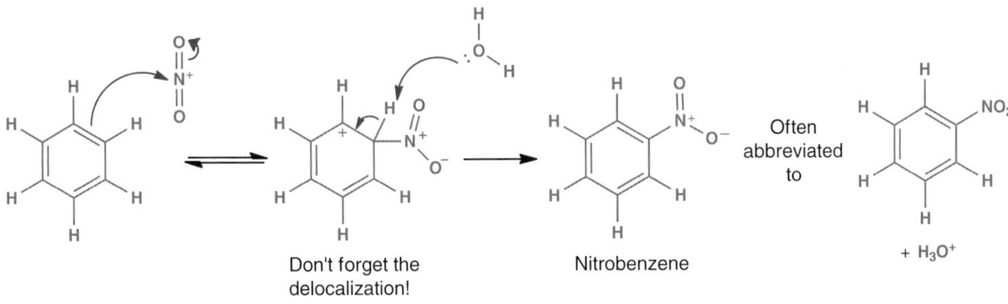

Don't forget the delocalization!

Nitrobenzene

Often abbreviated to

$+ H_3O^+$

Figure 7.17   Sulfonation of benzene

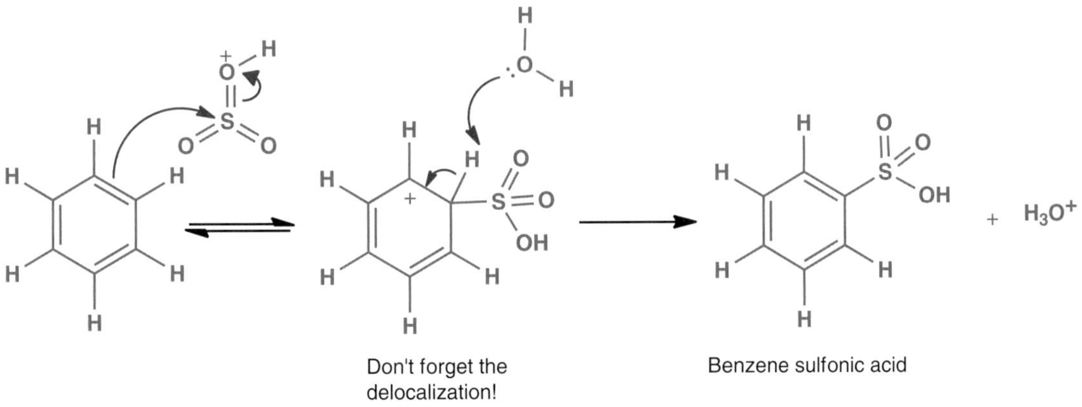

Don't forget the delocalization!

Benzene sulfonic acid

$+ H_3O^+$

Self-check 7.4

Draw all the resonance forms of the intermediate shown in Figure 7.17.

Friedel–Crafts reactions—the formation of carbon–carbon bonds

The formation of carbon–carbon bonds is of paramount importance when constructing organic molecules. Towards the end of the 1800s, Charles Friedel and James Crafts developed useful methods to couple acyl and alkyl chlorides with benzene and other aromatic species. The fact that these methods are still widely employed today illustrates their versatility, utility and importance. In both cases, aluminium trichloride (or a related compound such as tin tetrachloride) is employed to generate the active electrophile.

The Friedel–Crafts **acylation** is shown in Figure 7.18. The active electrophile is the oxonium ion (the odd-looking species with the positive charge on oxygen), which is formed by combining an acyl chloride (sometimes called an acid chloride) with aluminium trichloride. The EAS reaction proceeds in the usual manner to form an aromatic ketone. The reaction is very general, and many R groups can be employed.

The Friedel–Crafts alkylation also employs aluminium trichloride to form a cationic species which is the active electrophile as shown in Figure 7.19.

Figure 7.18 Friedel–Crafts acylation of benzene

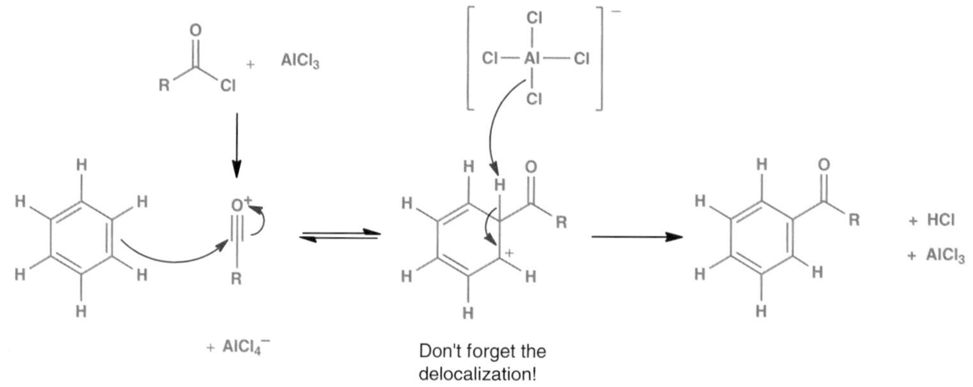

Figure 7.19 Friedel–Crafts alkylation of benzene

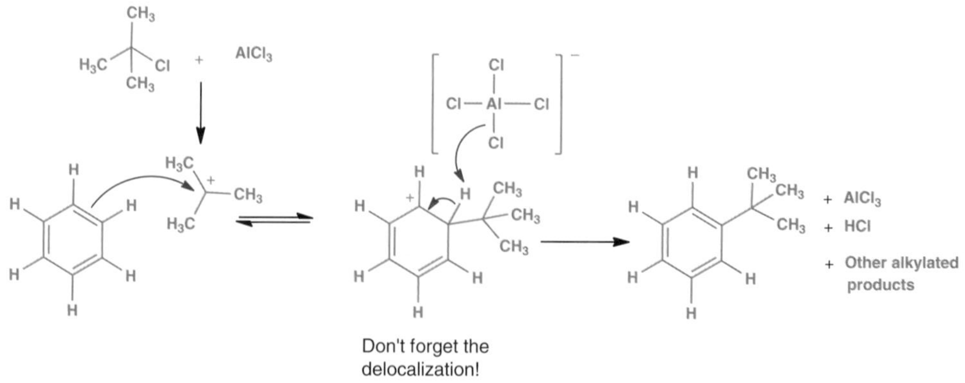

The Friedel−Crafts alkylation is a less useful reaction than the Friedel−Crafts acylation because it can give a mixture of products. The introduction of an alkyl group activates the benzene ring towards further alkylation, so that products with extra alkyl groups may be formed. Additionally, the active electrophile (a carbocation) may rearrange before it can react with benzene. The stability of carbon-based cations follows a trend: tertiary carbocations are more stable than secondary carbocations which are considerably more stable than primary carbocations, as depicted in Figure 7.20.

> Stabilities of carbocations are discussed in more detail in Chapter 4.

In practice, if the electrophile required for a Friedel−Crafts **alkylation** is a primary carbocation, it is likely to undergo rearrangement to the more stable secondary cation before reacting with benzene; this results in a mixture of products. For example, if 1-chloropropane were employed in a Friedel−Crafts **alkylation** then the major product from the reaction would be isopropylbenzene (2-phenylpropane), which would result from the rearrangement of the primary carbocation as shown in Figure 7.21.

   Fortunately there is a simple solution to this problem, although an extra reaction is required. The Friedel−Crafts **acylation** can be employed, and the ketone produced then reduced to the alkane. This sort of reduction can be carried out using various methods: for example, Figure 7.22 shows the Clemmensen reduction which employs zinc, mercury and concentrated hydrochloric acid. As an alternative, the Wolf−Kishner reduction could be employed which uses hydrazine and potassium hydroxide.

Figure 7.20   Stability of carbocations

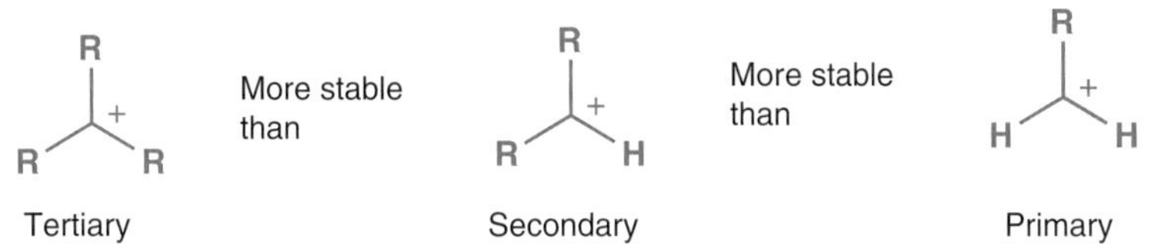

Tertiary   More stable than   Secondary   More stable than   Primary

Figure 7.21   Friedel−Crafts alkylation of 1-chloropropane with benzene

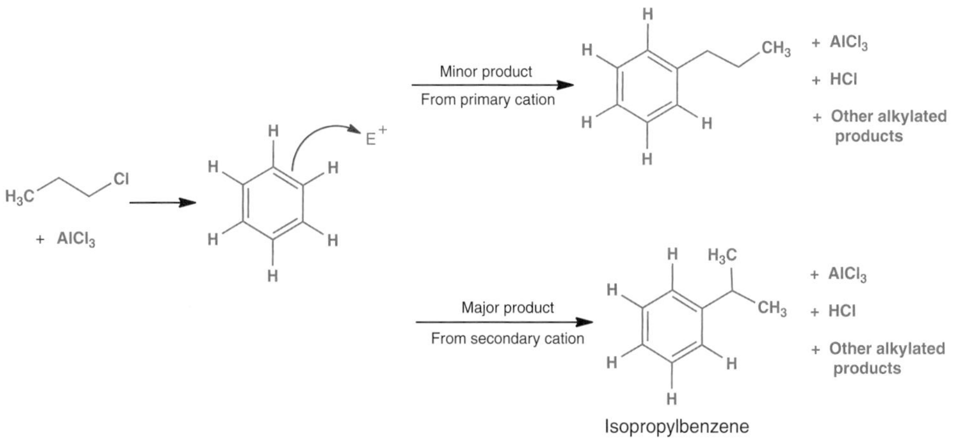

Minor product
From primary cation

+ AlCl₃
+ HCl
+ Other alkylated products

Major product
From secondary cation

+ AlCl₃
+ HCl
+ Other alkylated products

Isopropylbenzene

Figure 7.22 Preparation of 1-phenylpropane using a Friedel–Crafts acylation and a Clemmensen reduction

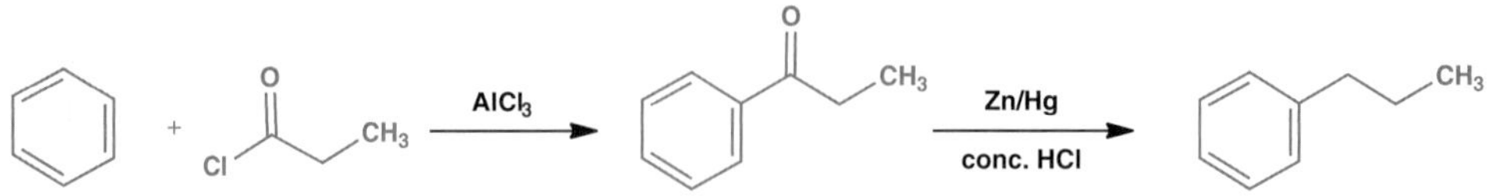

Electrophilic aromatic substitution of substituted benzenes—directing effects

The five EAS reactions that we have seen so far are not only used on benzene but are also useful for further functionalizing substituted benzenes, i.e. benzene that already has at least one substituent on the ring. However, the substituent on the ring has a strong influence on the outcome of the EAS reaction; this is known as the **directing effect**. There are three distinct classes of directing effect; in order to understand them we must first consider the nomenclature used to describe substituted benzenes, as illustrated in Figure 7.23.

Ortho, *meta* and *para* are relatively old Greek-derived terms. They are so far removed from their original meanings that English words such as orthodox, metamorphosis and parachute are unlikely to help you to remember them! The more modern way to describe aromatic substitution is numerical, and descriptors such as 1,2-, 1,3- and 1,4- to denote the relationship between the two substituents on a benzene ring are perhaps more coherent. However, the language of aromatic chemistry is dominated by *ortho*, *meta* and *para*, so we will use them where appropriate. In more complex trisubstituted systems it is usually easier to use the numerical terminology.

In Figure 7.23, note that there is a plane of symmetry down the middle of monosubstituted benzene derivatives (such as toluene (methylbenzene) or chlorobenzene), meaning that there are two equivalent *ortho*-positions, two equivalent *meta*-positions but only one *para*-position (see Box 7.2).

Figure 7.23 Directing effects in aromatic substitution

Substitution at the *ipso*-position does not yield a disubstituted benzene

Ortho-disubstituted benzene
1,2-disubstituted benzene

Meta-disubstituted benzene
1,3-disubstituted benzene

Para-disubstituted benzene
1,4-disubstituted benzene

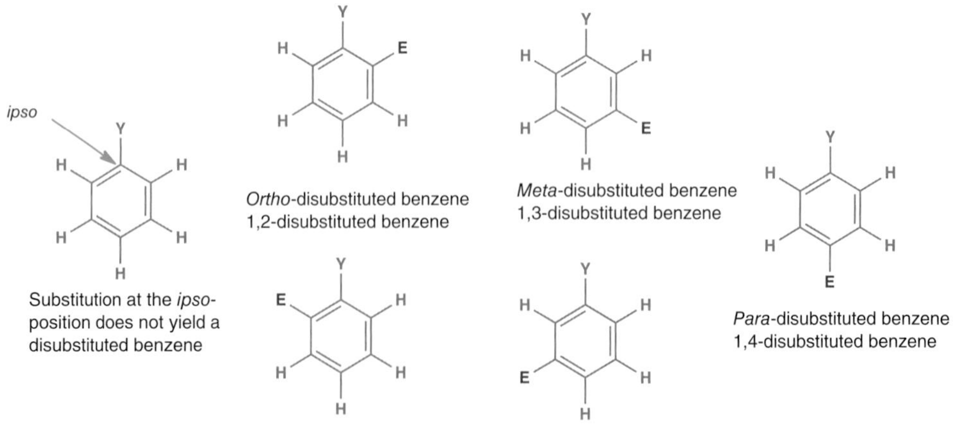

As explained in Chapter 1, when old-fashioned nomenclature is retained there is usually a good reason. The *ortho, meta, para* nomenclature tells you where substituents are relative to one another, which is useful for talking about mechanism. To use numbers you have to decide where number 1 is, which is useful for describing a final molecule. It is a bit like left and right *vs* north and south. A map shows you that Manchester is almost due east of Liverpool, but a SatNav gives directions in terms of right and left.

The directing effects of electron-donating groups

Consider the substitution reaction to install a second group onto a mono-substituted aromatic ring. The first important question is whether any particular isomer is favoured during the re-action, or whether a more even distribution of different isomers is obtained. To address this point we need to consider the intermediates in the reaction. Figure 7.24 shows the reaction of mono-substituted Y-benzene with a generic electrophile E^+ at the *ortho-, meta-* and *para-* positions. The three possible resonance forms associated with the reactions at each position are shown, and consideration of these will help us determine the directing effects of different groups.

Notice that the patterns of delocalization are the same when substitution is *ortho-* and *para-* to Y: the same three carbons relative to Y carry the positive charge. In each case, one of the resonance

223

Figure 7.24   The resonance patterns of Y-benzene reacting with a generic electrophile at the *ortho-, meta-* and *para*-positions

Ortho

Meta

Para

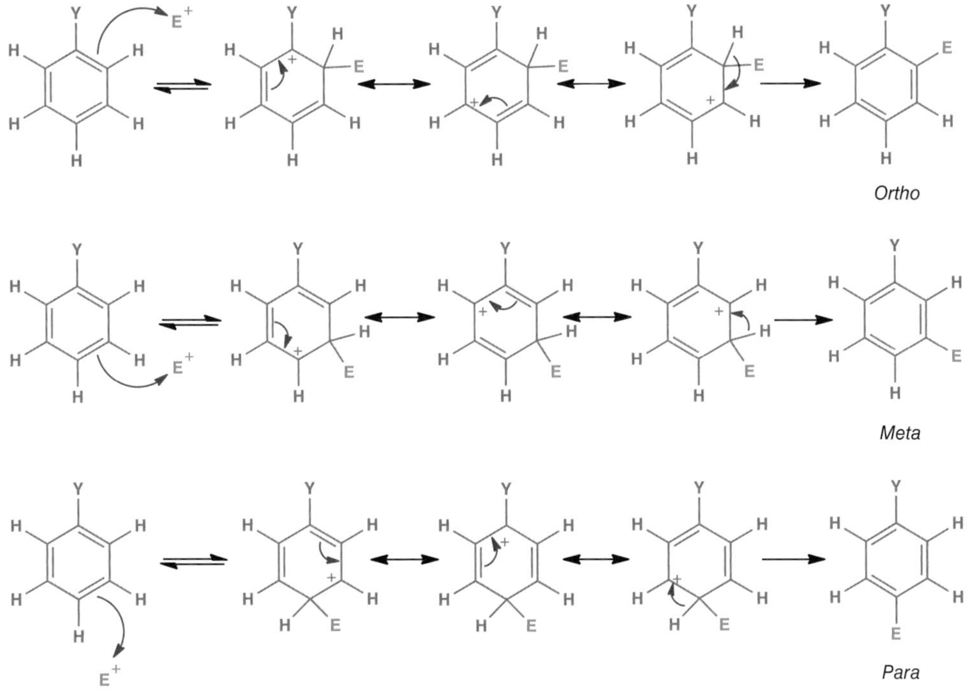

Self-check 7.5

Close the page and draw the intermediates formed by bromobenzene reacting with a generic electrophile E^+.

---

forms has the cation on the carbon bearing the group Y (the *ipso* carbon). Reaction at the *meta*-position, conversely, generates a delocalization pattern in which the other three carbons (relative to Y) carry the positive charge. You might expect therefore that Y could have an effect on the product of the reaction. We could postulate that if Y has characteristics that stabilize an adjacent positive charge then the *ortho*- and *para*-isomers will be favoured. However, if Y destabilizes an adjacent positive charge then the *meta*-isomer is likely to be favoured because reaction at this position gives a delocalization pattern without the positive charge on the carbon bearing Y.

We have already seen a group that stabilizes an adjacent positive charge—the alkyl group. Recall the order of carbocation stability: the more alkyl groups attached to a carbocation the more stable the cation. This is because electron density in one of the C–H sigma bonds of an attached alkyl group (methyl groups in the example shown) can interact with the positive charge (empty p-orbital) and help stabilize it—a phenomenon called σ-conjugation (**sigma conjugation**). The situation with EAS is remarkably similar, and one of the C–H bonds of the methyl group can align itself with the π-system and help stabilize the positive charge (see Figure 7.25).

> Sigma conjugation is also covered in Chapter 4.

So, we can hypothesize that electrophilic aromatic substitution of toluene will be predominantly *ortho*- and *para*-. But does this hypothesis bear any resemblance to reality? Yes, it does! EAS reactions of toluene (methylbenzene) have a typical distribution pattern of approximately 60% *ortho*, 5% *meta* and 35% *para*, as depicted in Figure 7.26. Bear in mind that there are two *ortho*-positions, two *meta*-positions but only one *para*-position, so, statistically, twice as much incorporation at the *ortho*- and *meta*- vs the *para*- position would be expected.

Self-check 7.6

Can you explain why the addition of an alkyl group to a benzene ring will facilitate the formation of 'other alkylated products'? What do you expect they might be?

Figure 7.25   The stabilization of carbocations by σ-conjugation

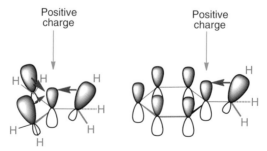

Figure 7.26 Representative distribution pattern for the reaction of toluene with an electrophile

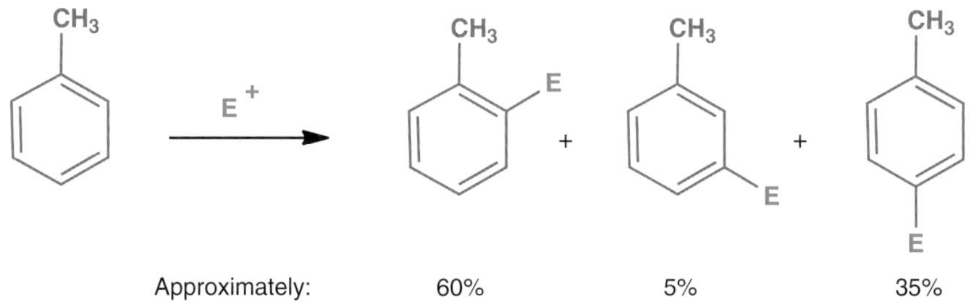

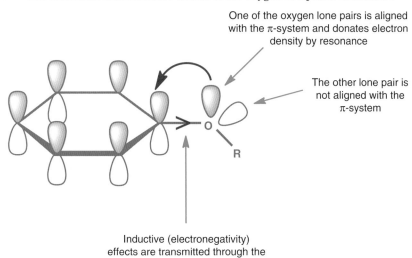

Approximately: 60%   5%   35%

Alkyl groups are described as mildly *ortho/para*-**directing** and as **activating groups**. This explains that formation of other alkylated products in the Friedel−Crafts alkylation reactions.

The stabilization of the cation by the electron density of the C–H bond (σ-conjugation) is not fantastic but it is certainly better than no stabilization at all. However, there are other (better) ways to provide stabilization—for example, by conjugation with the lone pair of an oxygen atom. The orbital containing the lone pair can align itself parallel with the π-system, and interact with it (See Figure 7.27). This means that an oxygen-based functionality such as a hydroxyl group or an ether can effectively donate electrons and stabilize an adjacent positive charge by conjugation.

But how can an element as electronegative as oxygen be electron-donating? This can seem confusing, but it is important to understand that there are two separate effects at work. The electronegative oxygen exerts an electron-withdrawing **inductive effect** on the σ-framework of the molecule. However, the oxygen lone-pair can also donate electron density into the aromatic π-system. Since the EAS reaction occurs through the π-system the inductive effect is much less significant and consequently alcohol and ether groups are overall strongly electron-donating in aromatic systems, as depicted in Figure 7.27.

Figure 7.27 The resonance and inductive effects of the oxygen of a phenol derivative

One of the oxygen lone pairs is aligned with the π-system and donates electron density by resonance

The other lone pair is not aligned with the π-system

R

Inductive (electronegativity) effects are transmitted through the σ-framework (short range)

The delocalization patterns of methoxybenzene (anisole) reacting with the generic electrophile E^+ are shown in Figure 7.28. Note how the lone pairs of the oxygen can help stabilize the adjacent positive charge when the electrophile reacts at either the *ortho*- or *para*-position. The appropriate resonance forms are shown shown in the lower structures, and note that these resonance forms are not available after meta-substitution. Additionally, there is an energetic advantage to having extra resonance forms in the non-aromatic intermediate (the hot potato analogy), and this has implications for aromatic compounds containing such groups. These functionalities are strongly ***ortho/para*-directing,** and are also **activating**: the aromatic compounds containing them are significantly more reactive in EAS reactions than benzene.

Oxygen can also act as an electron-donating group in non-aromatic systems. Examples include the chemistry of acetal formation and hydrolysis.

❯ Acetals and hemiacetals are covered in detail in Chapter 6.

Figure 7.28 Distribution and stabilization of the carbocations formed when anisole reacts with an electrophile

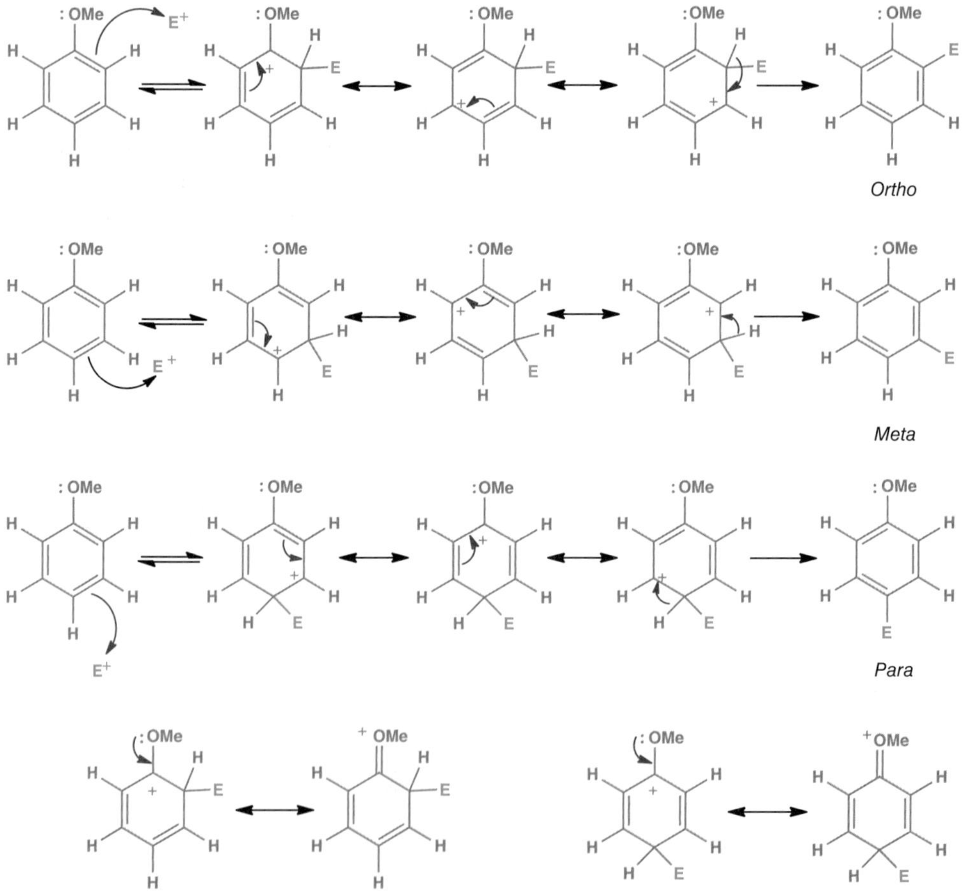

Stabilization of the cations adjacent to the methoxy group

Alternatively, the resonance forms associated with benzene derivatives substituted with electron-donating groups, for example, anisole (methoxybenzene), can be considered. In the case of anisole, Scheme 7.1 shows how the lone pair on the oxygen can interact with the π-system in such a way that the *ortho*- and *para*-positions, but not the *meta*-position, can carry a negative charge. Electrophilic aromatic substitution requires that the aromatic species acts as a nucleophile (i.e. providing electron density) so it is clear to see why the *ortho*- and *para*-positions should react in preference to the *meta*-position. Activation of the *ortho/para*-positions or stabilization of the cationic intermediate are essentially two methods of describing the same thing.

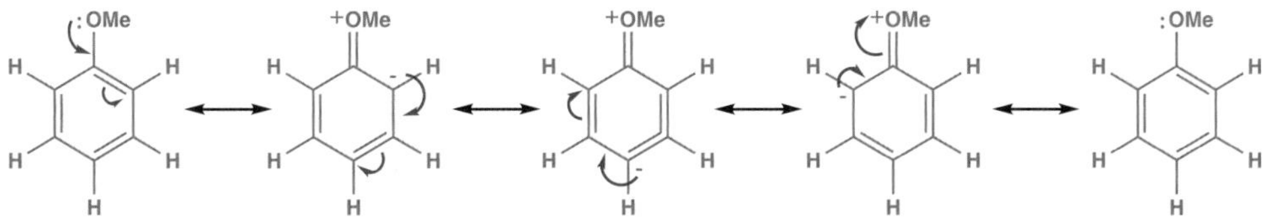

The effect of adding a powerful electron-donating group is considerable. For example, the bromination of phenol (hydroxybenzene) does not require a catalyst (unlike the bromination of benzene or toluene) and it is difficult to control the reaction—the tribromide is readily formed at room temperature. Note that only the *ortho*- and *para*-positions (with respect to the hydroxyl group) are brominated, as shown in Figure 7.29.

Replacing the hydroxyl group with the nitrogen-based amine group generates anilines (aminobenzenes) that are even more reactive than their phenol analogues. Again the lone pair is involved in the enhanced reactivity, but the lower electronegativity of the nitrogen make it better equipped to carry the positive charge. Anilines are often too reactive, and making simple disubstituted aromatics (by the addition of a single electrophile) is even more difficult than in the case of phenol. Fortunately, it is possible to reduce their reactivity by converting the amine to an amide or the alcohol to an ester.

Scheme 7.1   Activation of the *ortho*- and *para*-positions by resonance

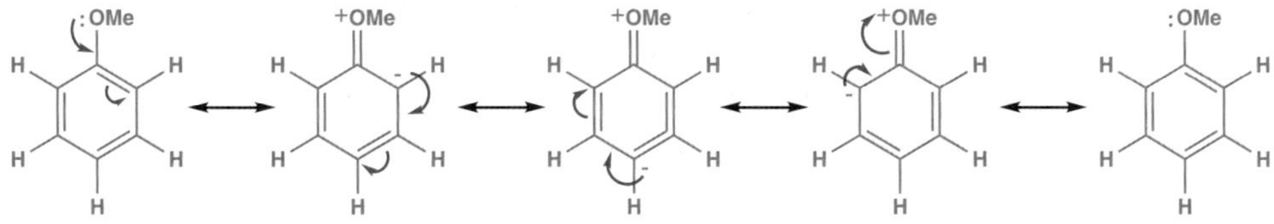

Figure 7.29   The bromination of phenol

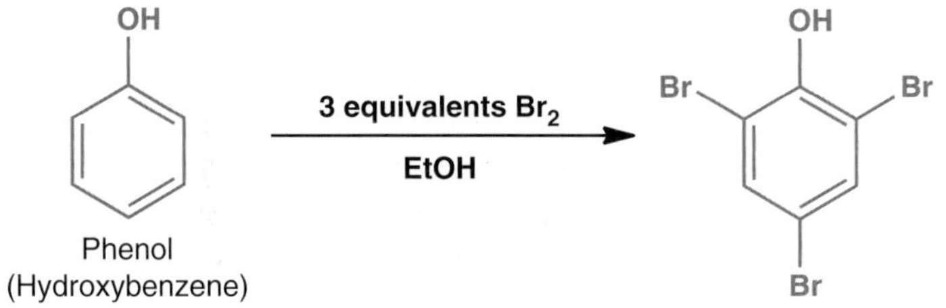

Controlling the reactivity of activated aromatics

If we were unable to use anilines or phenols in the synthesis of potential drugs we would be excluding a vast range of useful and important compounds. Chemists in the past realized this and so developed methods to circumvent the problem. In the case of aniline, one method is to derivatize the amine to make an amide. If derivatization is carried out using acetic anhydride (ethanoic anhydride), the product is acetanilide (also known as N-phenylacetamide).

The electron-withdrawing nature of the carbonyl (see Figure 7.30) creates competition for the nitrogen's lone pair, making it less available to interact with the π-system of the σ-complex. The carbonyl calms the overall reactivity of the aniline such that a single alkylation (mono-alkylation) is possible. Notice that the amide still has an activating effect and no catalyst is required to activate the bromine.

Of course, this approach would be useless if it were not possible to convert the amide back to the amine (which is achieved by treatment with acid). Do not forget that amines are basic, so they will be protonated in acidic medium to form the ammonium salt; the acid conditions will then need to be neutralized if the free amine is required. A similar approach can be used in the case of phenols by making an ester rather than an amide.

> The basicity of amines is discussed in Chapter 5.

> Protecting groups are discussed in more detail in Chapter 6.

You may be wondering why the *para*-isomer is favoured over the *ortho*-isomer when acetanilide is brominated (or indeed substituted with other electrophiles). This is because of steric hindrance: the amide group blocks reaction at the *ortho*-positions. Do not forget that molecules are not fixed, rigid structures. Rotation around the benzene–nitrogen bond is possible, and so both *ortho*-positions are hindered, making reaction at that position more difficult.

Figure 7.30   The use of an electron-withdrawing group to control the reactivity of aniline

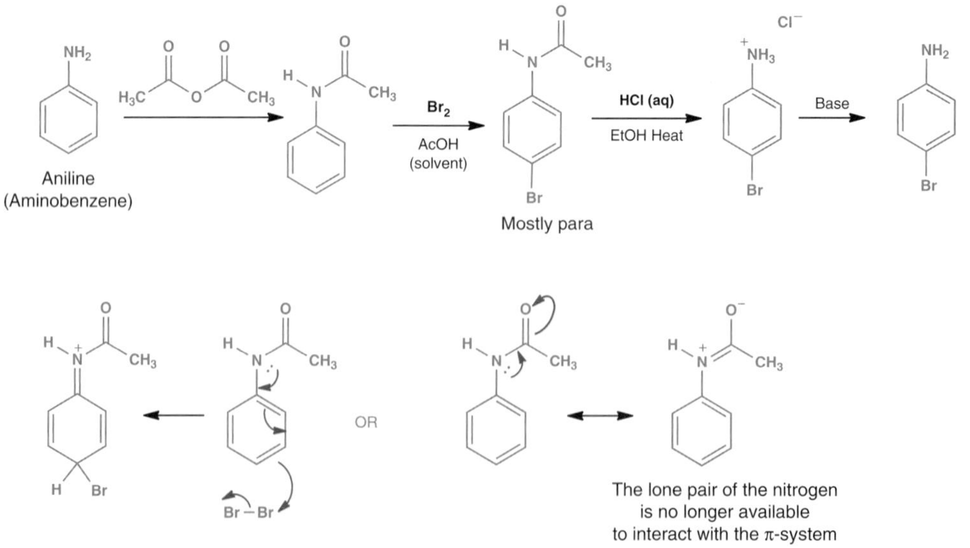

The directing effects of electron-withdrawing groups

We have seen that having a cation adjacent to an electron-donating group is energetically favourable. Naturally, it is also important to be able to describe the directing effects of an electron-*withdrawing* group, such as the extremely versatile nitro (NO_2) group. Since an electron-donating group stabilizes a positive charge, it is not really surprising that an electron-withdrawing group does the opposite: it acts to make the charge more positive—an unfavourable situation. This means that it is advantageous if the cation does not fall on the carbon bearing the substituent, i.e. if the substitution occurs at the *meta*-position. If necessary, use Figure 7.24 (with Y = NO_2) to remind yourself of the resonance patterns.

Furthermore, if you look at the resonance forms of nitrobenzene shown in Figure 7.31, you can see that the carbons in the *ortho*- and *para*-positions carry the cationic charge. If a carbon is to act as a nucleophile, as in electrophilic aromatic substitution, then it must be a provider of electrons. This is much more difficult if it is carrying a positive charge. Therefore, when an electron-withdrawing group is present on the aromatic ring, electrophilic aromatic substitution occurs at the *meta*-position, which does not carry the cationic charge in the resonance forms.

We would expect benzene substituted with an electron-withdrawing substituent to react more slowly with electrophiles than benzene itself. This is observed experimentally. Electron-withdrawing groups are both **meta-directing** and **deactivating**, as shown in Figure 7.32.

The directing effects of halogens

There is a final class of directing group that needs to be considered: namely, the halogens. They have their own unique directing effect: *ortho/para*-directing but deactivating. The inductive effect of the electronegative halogen is deactivating, but the activating effect of conjugation by the lone pair is of similar size. Overall, there is a small deactivating effect, but the

Figure 7.31   The withdrawing effect of the nitro group (by conjugation)

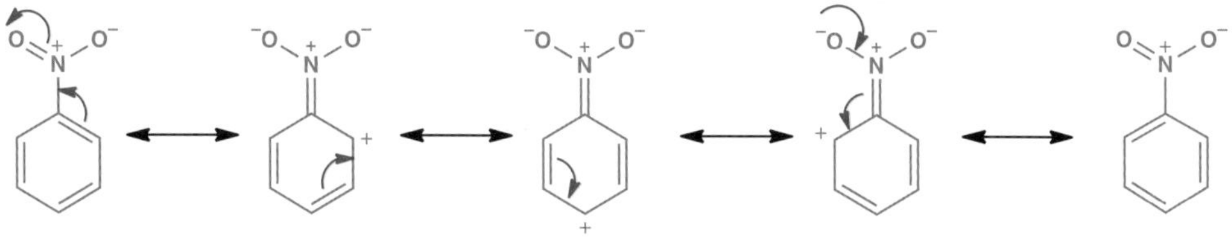

Figure 7.32   Representative distribution pattern for the reaction of nitrobenzene with an electrophile

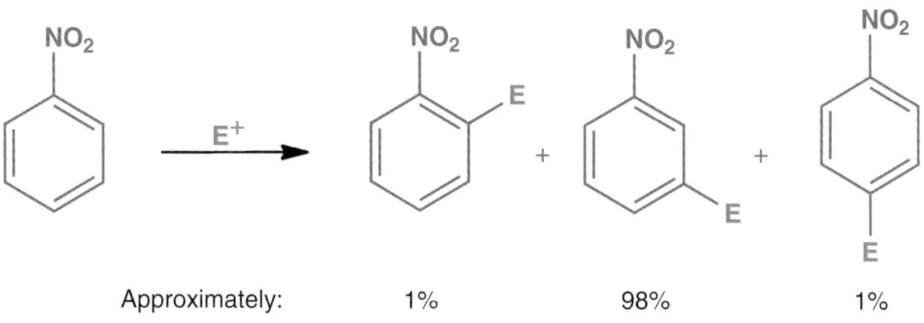

| Approximately: | 1% | 98% | 1% |

meta-position does not benefit from activation by conjugation so it is deactivated more than the *ortho-* or *para-* position.

You may also notice, in Table 7.1, that the preference for *ortho-* vs *para*-substitution is different to the electron-donating groups (activating *ortho/para*-directors) we saw previously. In the case of halogens, the preference for *para*-substitution results from two complementary effects—electronegativity and atomic radius. The inductive (deactivating) effect works through the σ-bonds and is therefore much more pronounced at the *ortho*-position than at the *para*-position. This is most important for the more electronegative halogens, especially fluorine. The halogens lower down the periodic table are less electronegative but they have much larger atomic radii, which also reduces reactivity at the *ortho*-position. So, as the electronegativity decreases down the group the atomic radii increase to maintain the preference for *para*-substitution. Halogens might be described as *para/ortho*-directing, rather than *ortho/para*-directing!

Note that in cases where conflicting directing effects exist, strong directors such as hydroxyl and amino will dominate weaker directors such as halogens. This is illustrated in the bromination of phenol in Figure 7.29.

To give you an idea of the effects of different substituents on the rates of EAS reactions, the relative rates of reaction of some substituted benzenes with a generic electrophile in an EAS reaction are shown below:

Electron-donating groups are described as ***ortho/para*-directing and activating** (i.e. they react more readily with electrophiles than benzene). It is unfortunate that most commonly mixtures of the *ortho-* and *para*-isomers are produced and these must be separated. There are some tricks to get around this problem, as we shall see later. Common electron-donating groups include alkyl, hydroxyl, ethers, amines, amides, **thiols and thioethers**.

Electron-withdrawing groups are described as ***meta*-directing** and **deactivating**. Common electron-withdrawing groups include nitro, aldehydes, ketones, esters, carboxylic acids, nitriles and sulfonic acids.

Halogens are described as ***ortho/para*-directing** and **deactivating**. They have a preference for reaction at the *para*-position, and this can be exploited.

Table 7.1 shows the distribution and relative rates of nitration of halobenzenes, with respect to benzene

X	Ortho	Meta	Para	Rate
H	-	-	-	1.00
F	12.4	0.00	87.6	0.15
Cl	29.6	0.90	69.5	0.03
Br	36.5	1.20	62.4	0.03
I	38.3	1.8	59.7	0.18

Self-check 7.7

Consider Figure 7.29—the tribromination of phenol

(a) Draw the mechanism of monobromination and indicate the major products.

(b) Explain why the second bromination leads to a mixture of 2,4-dibromophenol and 2,6-dibromophenol

(c) Arrange these reactions in order of rate: bromination of phenol, bromination of 4-bromophenol, bromination of 2,4-dibromophenol

R=	NO_2	H	Me	OMe	NMe_2
Rate	1×10^{-7}	1	4×10^3	1×10^9	1×10^{14}

Electrophilic aromatic substitution is the most important mechanism for preparing aromatic compounds because it allows an increase in molecular complexity as H is substituted with a functional group. There are other mechanisms for introducing substituents into an aromatic ring (e.g. nucleophilic aromatic substitution) but these are beyond the scope of this chapter.

Post-substitution functional group interconversion and metal-based reactions

Having prepared the desired aromatic skeleton by aromatic substitution reactions it is possible that further reactions are required. Many reactions are possible—for example, the reduction of nitro groups to amines, or ketones to alcohols or alkyl groups. Another option that is particularly versatile and widely used is organo-metallic chemistry. Aromatic bromides in particular are useful reagents in this regard. Of particular note are Grignard (organo-magnesium) reactions and palladium-based sp^2-sp^2 couplings.

You may not have realized that aromatic bromides can be converted into Grignard reagents (which we discuss in Chapter 6) and can therefore be used to make new carbon–carbon bonds. The advantage of these reactions is that they can be used to generate a series of compounds that have the same basic framework but in which functionality at a specific position is varied. This allows medicinal chemists to probe the significance of a specific portion of a potential drug molecule and to fine-tune its biological activity; this is the basis of a Structure Activity Relationship (SAR) study.

> More information on Grignard reagents can be found in Chapter 6.

Self-check 7.8

Use your knowledge of aromatic chemistry (this chapter) and your knowledge of carbonyl chemistry (Chapter 6) to design a synthesis of 1-phenylethanol, starting from benzene and acetaldehyde.

Figure 7.33 Reaction of phenyldiazonium chloride with selected nucleophiles

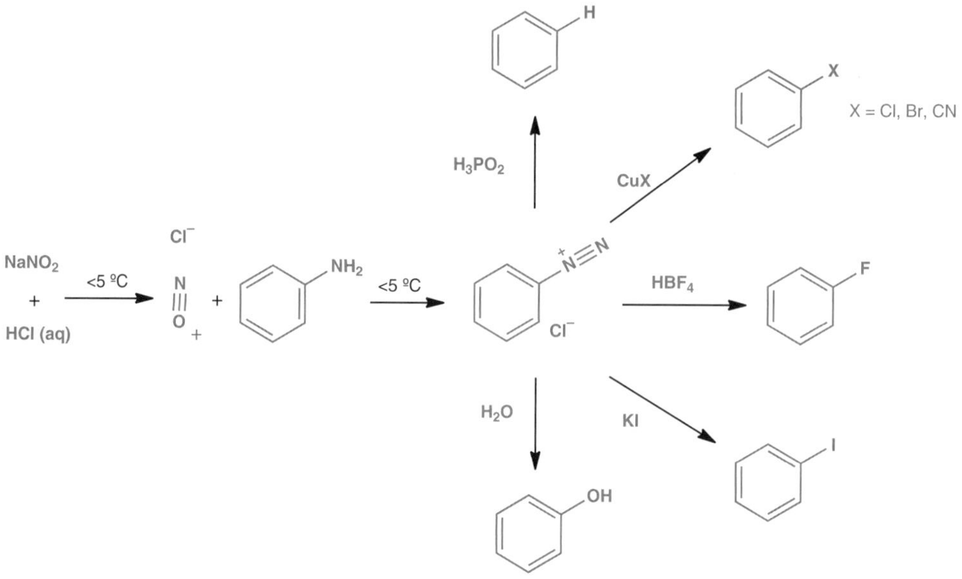

The versatility of the nitro group

We are now in a position to consider the versatility of the nitro group. The nitro group is easily installed by nitration whereupon it has a *meta*-directing effect for the installation of further electrophiles by EAS. It is easily reduced to the corresponding amine by hydrogenation with hydrogen and a catalyst of palladium on charcoal or by a mixture of tin and hydrochloric acid. The *ortho/para*-directing effects of the amino group can be exploited at this point to install another electrophile.

Substituted amino benzenes may be the desired products but they can also serve as intermediates for a range of other nucleophiles *via* the diazonium salt, see Figure 7.33.

Now we have seen some reactions of aromatic systems, it is time to see these reactions exploited in the synthesis of drugs.

7.4 THE SYNTHESIS OF DRUGS

As mentioned previously, a number of important drugs are aromatic. We can now consider some of their syntheses, starting with paracetamol, a derivative of acetanilide. Acetanilide was itself employed as an analgesic in the past but was withdrawn because of concerns about its toxicity. The preparation of paracetamol provided a medicine that is an effective analgesic with few side-effects at therapeutic doses (see Box 7.3).

Box 7.3 Paracetamol

Although paracetamol has few side-effects at therapeutic doses, it is extremely dangerous in overdose, and one of its metabolites is a major cause of liver damage (see Case study 7.1). Interestingly it has also been shown that acetanilide is metabolized to paracetamol.

Paracetamol synthesis

The first step in the synthesis of paracetamol is the nitration of phenol by electrophilic aromatic substitution, as illustrated in Figure 7.34. The high reactivity of phenol means that even the low concentration of $[NO_2]^+$ produced in dilute nitric acid is sufficient for the EAS reaction to proceed in a reasonable time. Note that the powerful deactivating effect of the nitro group means that it is possible to obtain workable yields of the mono-nitrated material.

As expected, a mixture of *ortho-* and *para*-isomers is produced, which need to be separated. In this case, the *ortho* isomer (2-nitrophenol) has a much lower boiling point than the desired 4-nitrophenol, and can be readily removed by distillation (Box 7.4). If you have noticed that the yields of the *ortho* and *para*-products do not add up to 100% you may be wondering what has happened to the remainder. It is rare that chemical reactions proceed with 100% yield because there are often side-reactions that can occur (in this case over-nitration is the main issue) and there can be problems with isolating the pure product. One of the skills required for synthetic chemistry to be able to minimize the formation of side-products and maximize the isolation of the desired compound.

❯ Intra- and intermolecular hydrogen bonds are discussed in greater detail in Chapter 2.

Box 7.4 The separation of the *ortho-* and *para*-isomers

The separation of the *ortho-* and *para*-isomers of nitrophenol is easier than normal because there is an intramolecular hydrogen bond between the hydroxyl and nitro group in the *ortho*-isomer that cannot form in the *para*-isomer. Consequently, the intermolecular attractive interactions are reduced in the *ortho*-isomer such that its melting and boiling points are considerably lower than the *para*-isomer. This difference makes separation by distillation relatively easy.

Figure 7.34 The synthesis of paracetamol

Approximately 35% – removed by distillation

Approximately 25%

Intramolecular Hydrogen bonding

Acetanilide

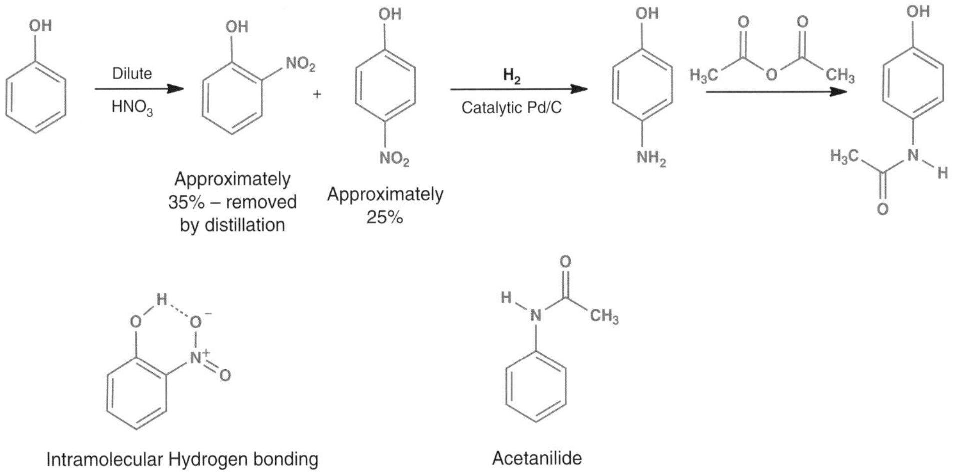

Self-check 7.9

Why is a mixture of *ortho*- and *para*- isomers formed in the nitration of phenol?
Why is mononitration of phenol simple while monobromination of phenol is not?

The next task is to reduce the versatile nitro group (NO_2) to an amino group (NH_2). A number of reagents can be used; tin and hydrochloric acid or catalytic hydrogenation (used in this case) are common. The final step in the synthesis is the acetylation of the amine with acetic anhydride (or acetyl chloride). Note that reaction occurs at the more nucleophilic amino group rather than at the hydroxyl group.

Aspirin synthesis

The synthesis of aspirin is illustrated in Figure 7.35. This synthesis also involves the electrophilic aromatic substitution of phenol; the electrophile is carbon dioxide and the desired product is *ortho*-substituted. Sodium hydroxide is used to deprotonate phenol forming the expected sodium phenoxide (an extremely active participant in EAS reactions), which reacts with electrophilic carbon dioxide. The clever aspect of this reaction is that the sodium cation associated with the negatively charged oxygen of phenoxide can coordinate to the carbon dioxide and hold it in close proximity to the *ortho*-position. This behaviour ensures a high ratio of the desired *ortho*-product. This is known as the Kolbe Reaction.

Notice the keto-enol tautomerism in the mechanism. In this case the aromatic stabilization energy means that the enol form is completely dominant. (Compare this with the keto-enol ratio of acetone.) Reaction of salicylic acid with acetic anhydride forms aspirin.

More information can be found on keto-enol tautomerism in Chapter 6.

Figure 7.35 The synthesis of aspirin

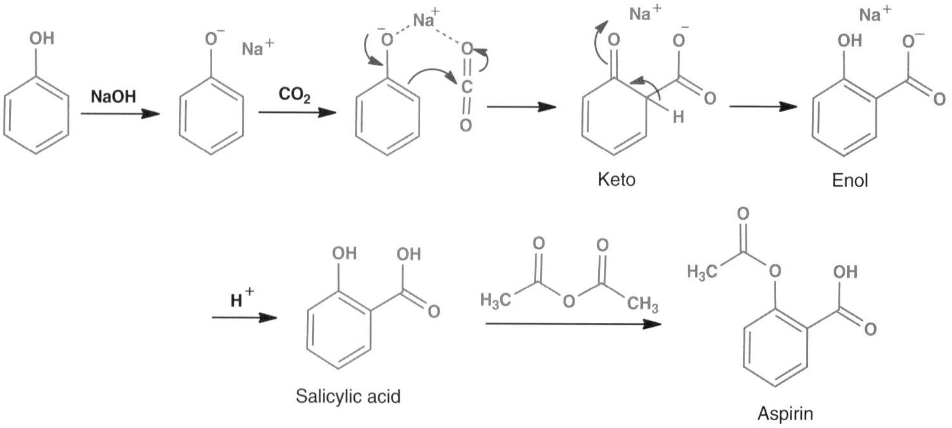

7.5 AROMATIC CHEMISTRY IN THE BODY

The body requires many aromatic compounds. Some of these are synthesized from preformed aromatic compounds such as the amino acids phenylalanine and tyrosine, which are usually obtained from the diet. However, aromatic compounds can also be synthesized from non-aromatic substrates using the shikimate pathway. Specialized aromatase enzymes can also generate aromatic steroids from non-aromatic precursors, as shown in Figure 7.38. Although these reactions are mediated by enzymes they are still examples of aromatic chemistry.

Aromatic amino acids, neurotransmitters, hormones and drugs

Aromatic compounds feature in the important catechol neurotransmitter/hormone family, which includes adrenaline, noradrenaline and dopamine. The importance of these compounds in the body cannot be overstated, and numerous drugs interact with the biochemical systems associated with them. The biosynthesis of adrenaline (*via* noradrenaline and dopamine) starts with aromatic amino acid tyrosine and is shown in Figure 7.36.

Figure 7.37 shows how aromatic rings feature strongly in drugs that interact with the biochemical systems that make these compounds and the receptors on which these compounds act. Aromatic drugs can interfere by binding in the binding site intended for the hormone or neurotransmitter. Drugs that interact with the catechol system include:

Figure 7.36   The biosynthesis and deactivation of adrenaline

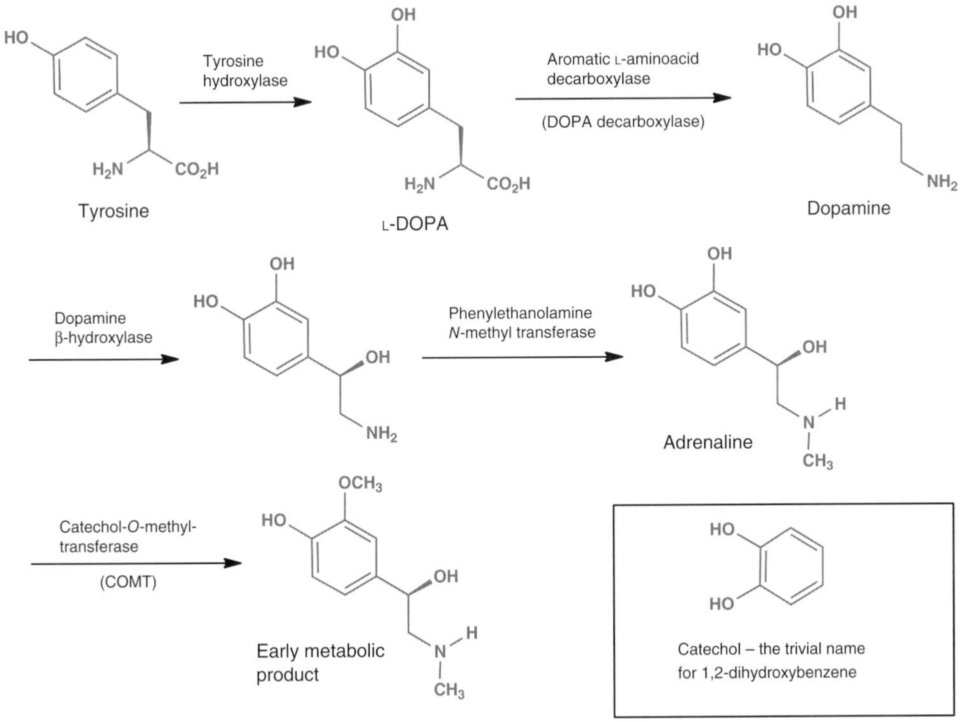

Figure 7.37 The structures of some drugs that interfere with the synthesis or action of aromatic compounds in the body

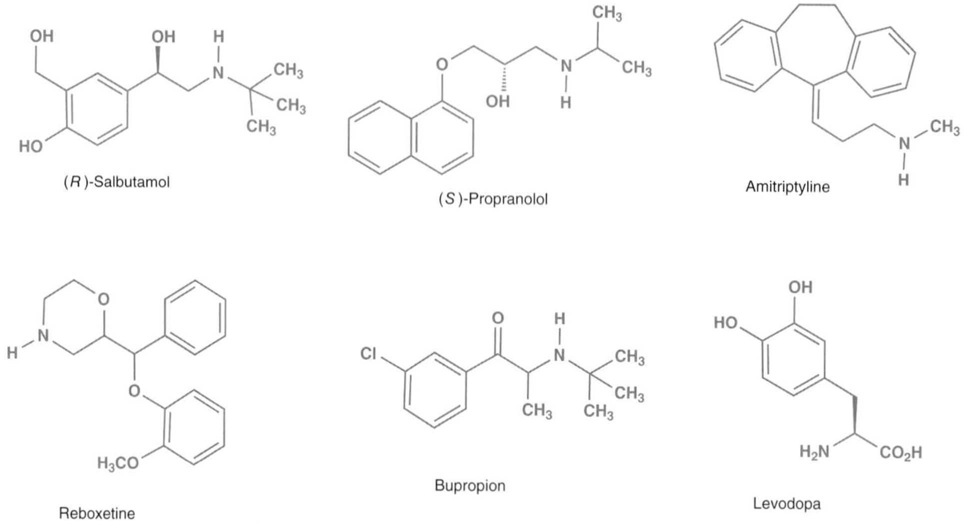

(R)-Salbutamol

(S)-Propranolol

Amitriptyline

Reboxetine

Bupropion

Levodopa

- Asthma treatments salbutamol and salmeterol (β_2-adrenoreceptor agonist).

- High blood pressure medication β-blocker antihypertensives, e.g. propranolol (β_1-adreno-receptor antagonist).

- Several classes of antidepressant, including tricyclics such as amitriptyline, and the nor-adrenaline reuptake inhibitor reboxetine.

- The smoking cessation aid bupropion, which is also an antidepressant.

- The Parkinson's Disease treatment levodopa (a dopamine precursor).

Oestrogens and aromatase enzymes

Oestrogen hormones (oestone, oestradiol and oestriol) play an important role in a class of breast cancers known as hormone-dependent cancers. If a tumour is dependent on these hormones for proliferation, then compounds that either block the action of hormones (antagonists) or prevent their biosynthesis may offer treatments. The biosynthesis of the oestrogen hormones involves the action of the enzyme aromatase on andostradione and testosterone to form oestrone and oestradiol respectively, as shown in Figure 7.38.

Tamoxifen and fulvestrant are antioestrogens (oestrogen antagonists), which block the action of the oestrogens directly. Anastrozole and letrozole (see Figure 7.39) are reversible aromatase inhibitors, and 4-hydroxyandrostenedione is a **suicide substrate** that reacts with the aromatase enzyme and renders it permanently deactivated. Anti-oestrogens and aromatase inhibitors are extremely effective treatments for hormone sensitive breast cancer, and the lives of huge numbers of breast cancer sufferers have been saved since the introduction of Tamoxifen around thirty years ago.

Figure 7.38 The action of the enzyme aromatase on steroids to form two of the oestrogen hormones

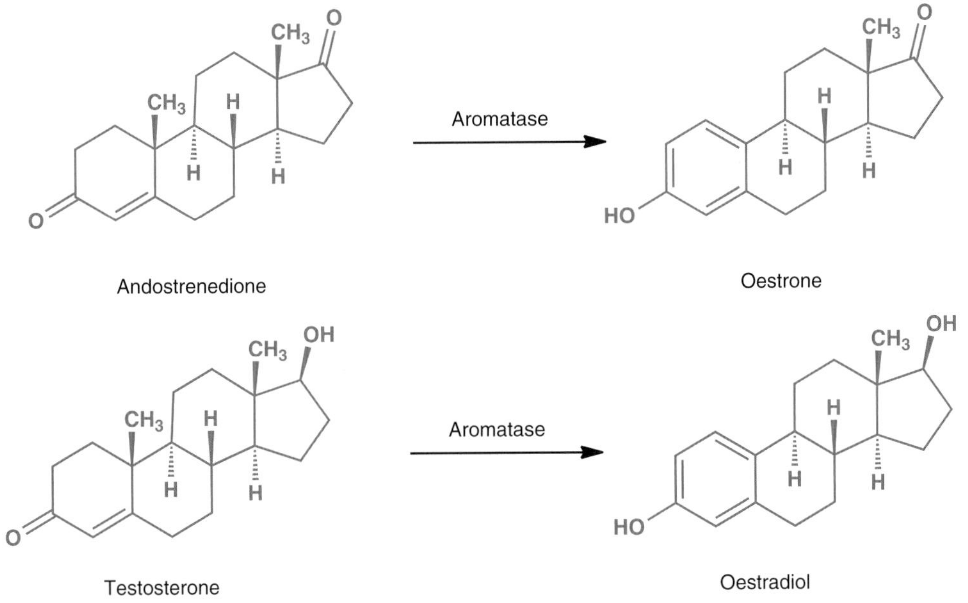

Andostrenedione → Aromatase → Oestrone

Testosterone → Aromatase → Oestradiol

Figure 7.39 Two anti-oestrogen drugs and three aromatase inhibitors

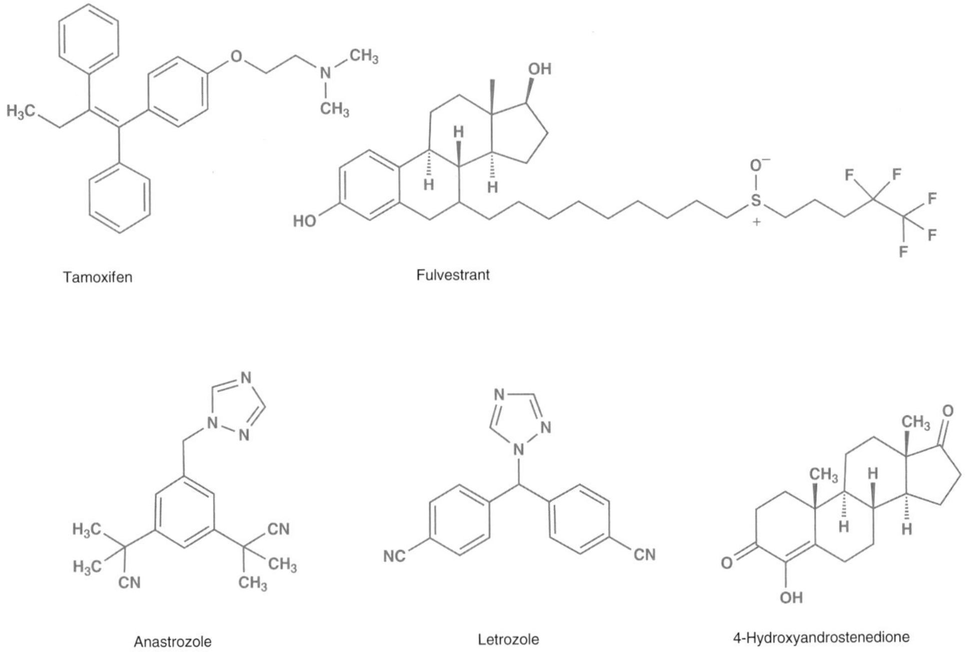

Tamoxifen

Fulvestrant

Anastrozole

Letrozole

4-Hydroxyandrostenedione

> The stereochemistry of tamoxifen is discussed in detail in Chapter 3, 'Stereochemistry and drug action'.

Metabolism of aromatic compounds

The metabolism of aromatic compounds generally involves oxidation, usually mediated by one of the **cytochrome P450 enzymes**; the initial product is often an epoxide (a three-membered ring containing two carbons and an oxygen).

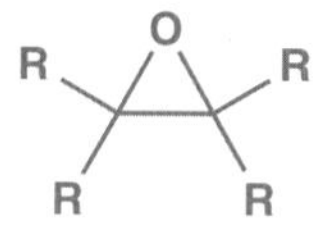

Subsequent reactions and rearrangements can take place, and the metabolic pathway often involves the installation of a hydroxyl group *via* rearrangement of the initial epoxide. Hydroxylation often takes place at the *para*-position in singly substituted aromatic rings, but the situation is more complicated in polysubstituted systems.

In some cases, metabolism of aromatic compounds can lead to an active metabolite (for example, paracetamol from acetanilide, as illustrated in Figure 7.40) but such situations are rare and a compound is more likely to be deactivated directly or conjugated and eliminated. The body has evolved mechanisms to rid itself of foreign compounds; for example, the formation of oxygenated compounds generally increases their water solubility and renders them more easily removed from the body—a process known as 'phase one metabolism'. Phase two metabolism involves the formation of conjugates between the oxygenated molecules and various polar derivatives to further enhance their water solubility and further aid their removal from the body.

> Cytochrome P450 enzymes and metabolism are also discussed in Chapter 14, 'Absorption, distribution, metabolism and excretion'.

> Epoxides are discussed in more detail in Chapter 5, 'Alcohols, phenols, ethers, organic halogen compounds, and amines'.

Figure 7.40   Metabolism of acetanilide to form the analgesic paracetamol

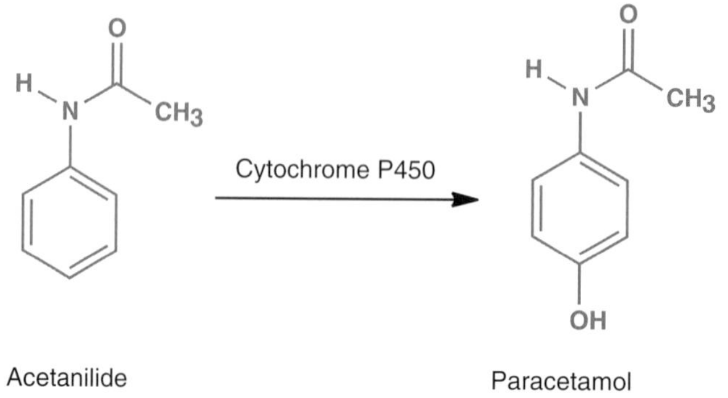

When designing new drugs, it is important to consider the possible metabolism of the new compound. As a consequence, promising drug candidates are now regularly screened against a range of P_{450} enzymes. If troublesome metabolism is detected or expected, additional functional groups can be installed to prevent or slow those metabolic processes. One method of reducing the problem of unwanted *para*-hydroxylation is to place a fluorine atom on the aromatic ring, usually in the *para*-position. Since fluorine is the most electronegative element, its presence alters the electronic nature of the aromatic ring, making it less prone to oxidation. The fluorine atom is not much larger than hydrogen (atomic radius 1.47 Å *vs* 1.2 Å), so that a single substitution of hydrogen for fluorine will not have a significant steric effect. The use of fluorine as a metabolic blocker has been employed in the drug ezetimibe (see Figure 7.41), used to treat patients with high levels of cholesterol.

Metabolism and toxicity

The toxicity data for benzene makes worrying reading: it 'may cause cancer' and 'may cause heritable genetic damage'. As such, the use of benzene is now restricted to professional chemists and similarly qualified personnel. However, we should not assume that all aromatic compounds have the same safety profile. Indeed, the fact that so many drugs contain aromatic rings is indicative of the fact that the toxicity of benzene is not commonly carried over into its derivatives.

Metabolism of benzene begins with the formation of an epoxide, mediated by P450 enzymes, as shown in Figure 7.42. The epoxide can then react further to form a variety of metabolites, which can interact with biomolecules, including DNA. It is these metabolites that have significant toxicity, rather than benzene itself. Exposure to benzene is inadvisable, but it is actually the body's attempts to metabolize and eliminate benzene that make it problematic. It is important to note that the epoxidation of benzene is a very difficult reaction to perform by simple chemical means, but it occurs in the body by the action of the P450 enzymes.

Doll and Hill famously published the statistical link between smoking and lung cancer in 1950. The exact cause (and therefore proof) of the connection was published twenty-four years

Figure 7.41 The use of fluorine as a metabolic blocker to prevent oxidation at the positions bearing the fluorine

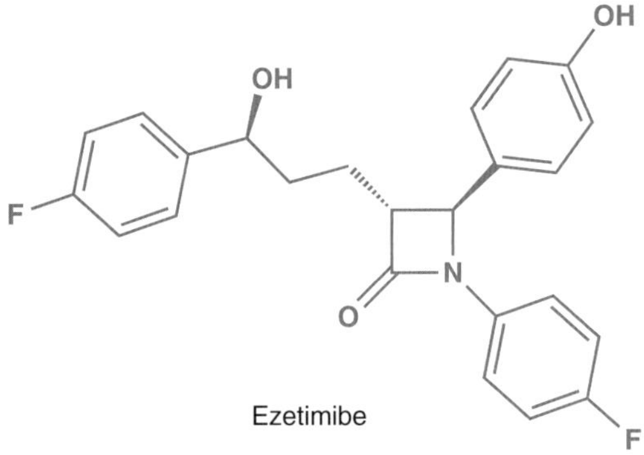

Ezetimibe

Figure 7.42 The metabolism of benzene

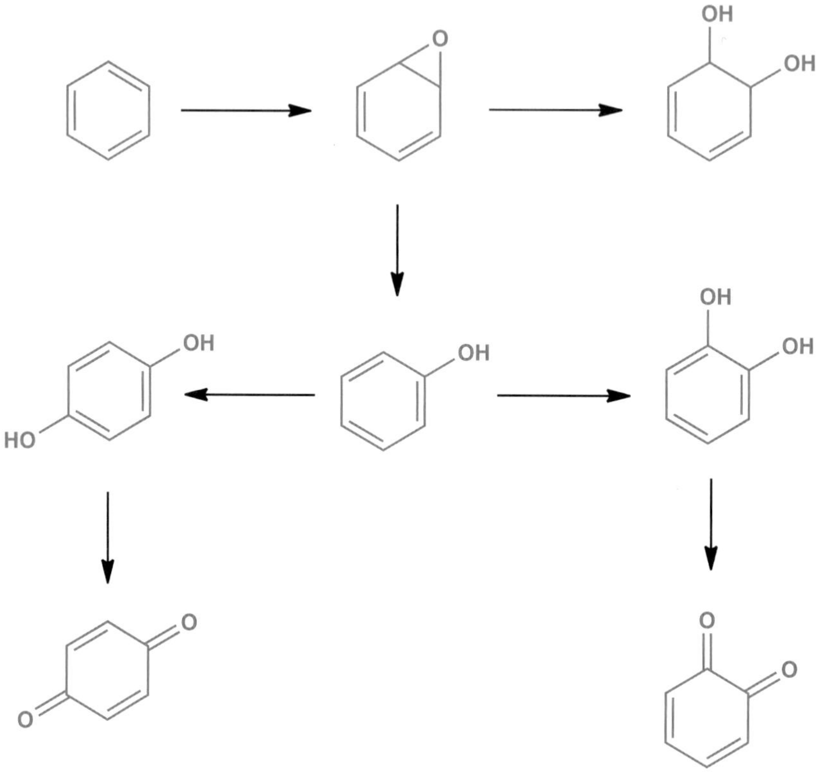

Figure 7.43 Metabolism of a constituent of cigarette smoke and the reaction of the metabolite with DNA

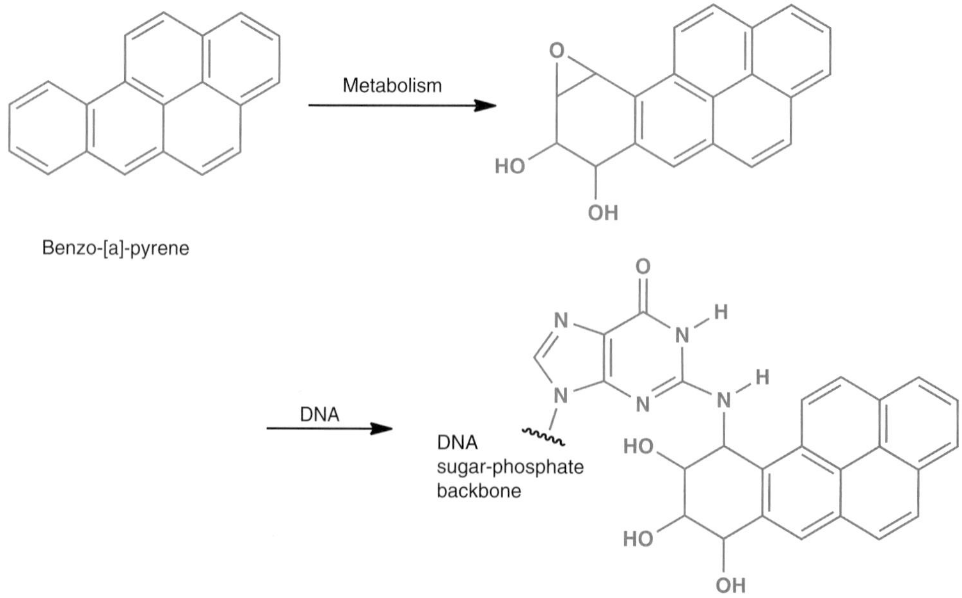

Benzo-[a]-pyrene

Case study 7.1

A customer in Tu's pharmacy wants to purchase 100 paracetamol tablets to save her from coming to the pharmacy as often. Tu has to explain to the customer that she is not allowed, legally, to purchase that number of paracetamol tablets.

Reflection questions

1. Why is the customer not allowed to buy 100 paracetamol tablets?

2. What is the mechanism of paracetamol toxicity?

For answers, visit the online resources which accompany this textbook.

later. A compound called benzo–[a]–pyrene (a member of the polyaromatic hydrocarbon family) is the villain. More specifically, it is its metabolic product that contains an epoxide and a diol that is most responsible for the carcinogenic properties, as illustrated in Figure 7.43. Reaction of the epoxydiol with DNA *via* guanine is responsible for DNA damage that can result in tumourogenesis.

- To be classed as aromatic, a compound needs to be planar, have 4n+2 π electrons and be cyclic and fully conjugated.

- Many currently used drugs contain an aromatic structure.

- The chemistry of aromatic compounds is dominated by electrophilic aromatic substitution reactions.

- Electrophilic aromatic substitution occurs rather than addition reactions because this allows the retaining of the aromatic stabilization energy.

- All electrophilic aromatic substitution reactions utilize the same reaction mechanism.

- Substituents already present on the aromatic ring can significantly influence the product(s) formed during the substitution reaction.

- Electron-donating groups are ortho/para-directing and activating and include alkyl, hydroxyl and amine groups.

- Electron-withdrawing groups are meta-directing and deactivating and include nitro, carbonyl and sulfonic acid groups.

- Halogens are ortho/para-directing and deactivating.

- Metabolism of aromatic compounds generally involves oxidation, often yielding an epoxide as the initial product, followed by conversion to an hydroxyl group.

- A knowledge of aromatic chemistry allows the design and preparation of new chemical entities in the search for new drugs.

FURTHER READING

Further information on post-substitution functional group interconversion and metal-based reactions can be found in these books:

Clayden, J., Greeves, N. and Warren, S., *Organic Chemistry*, 2nd edn. Oxford University Press, 2012.

McMurry, J., *Fundamentals of Organic Chemistry*, 7th edn. Cengage Learning, 2011. ISBN 9781439049730.
A student-friendly organic chemistry textbook.

Morrison, R. T. and Boyd, R. N. *Organic Chemistry*, 6th edn. Pearson, 1996. ISBN 978-0136436690.
A popular introduction to organic chemistry with an emphasis on chemical behaviour as determined by molecular structure.

Self-check

For the answers to the Self-Check questions in Chapter 7, visit the online resources which accompany this textbook.

INORGANIC CHEMISTRY IN PHARMACY

Geoff Hall

The elements you will be most familiar with are those that are frequently encountered in the organic molecules found in biological systems: carbon, hydrogen, oxygen and nitrogen. However, lots of inorganic chemistry occurs in the body as well, and a number of drugs are inorganic, containing no carbon. In this chapter we shall study the chemistry of these inorganic elements. The roles of some of the elements may be familiar to you whilst others may surprise you. The chapter is organized so that after a revision of atomic structure, the periodic table and types of bonding, we will study individual inorganic elements. For this chapter they are organized into the alkali and alkaline earth metals, transition metals, zinc and iron, and the precious metals, silver, gold and platinum and, briefly, the lanthanide metals. The non-metals studied will be phosphorus and sulfur. Many other elements are also important to drug development, drug action and delivery. It is not possible to go into detail about each element, but by understanding the chemical properties of an element, it should be possible to understand its biological function.

Learning objectives

Having read this chapter you are expected to be able to:

- understand concepts in inorganic chemistry namely:
  - types of bonding
  - electron distribution in orbitals
- recognize the importance of alkali and alkaline earth metals for normal cell function
- carry out calculations associated with concentrations of ions
- identify how the biological role of iron and zinc can be related to their chemistry and how some drug actions and side-effects can be explained by their interaction with these metal ions
- recognize that seemingly inert metals such as the precious metals can have biological activity

- understand the importance of phosphorus and sulfur in biological systems, and how this can be explained in terms of their chemical properties.

- identify various phosphorus and sulfur-containing functional groups in drug molecules, and be able to explain the role of these functional groups for either the formulation of the drug into a medicine or the biological action of the drug.

8.1 CONCEPTS IN INORGANIC CHEMISTRY

To introduce the chapter, try to complete Table 8.1 by listing two transition metal ions that are found in biological systems and two precious metals that are found in drugs. Give a short description of the function of each element.

The periodic table

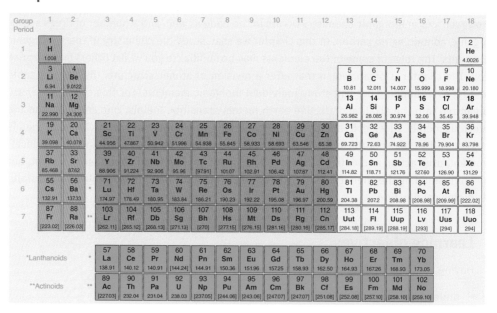

As you may remember from your previous chemistry studies, an element's position in the periodic table is based on its atomic number and on the distribution of its electrons. The vertical columns are called groups, and elements within the group have similar chemical behaviours. Traditionally, the main groups are designated by Roman numerals (I–VIII), with some more

Table 8.1   Metals in pharmacy

Metal	Action/Use
e.g. Cobalt	Found in vitamin B_{12}, used to treat pernicious anaemia

complicated arrangements for elements such as the transition metals. In the IUPAC system the groups are designated 1–18. Groups 1 and 2 are the same as groups I and II in the traditional format, with groups 13–18 being the same as groups III–VIII. The IUPAC system is used in this chapter. Therefore, lithium is in group 1 and carbon is in group 14.

The horizontal rows of the table are known as periods. Across a period there tends to be a gradual and regular change in physical properties, but the elements possess quite different chemical properties. We see an exception to this with the transition metals where adjacent elements tend to have similar chemical properties as the arrangement of electrons in the outer shell can be similar.

Chemical bonds

In addition to covalent bonds, elements studied in this chapter take part in other forms of bonding. Both ionic and **covalent dative bonding** are important in the biological action of various elements—for example, in the interactions of ligands with biological macromolecules.

> Further information on covalent bonds can be found in Chapter 2, 'Organic structure and bonding'.

An ionic bond is formed between positively and negatively charged ions. When an ionic bond is formed. both electrons come from one of the ions and there is usually a large difference in electronegativity between the elements whose ions form the bond. (Consider common salt, for example, which consists of sodium and chloride ions. Na has an electronegativity of 0.93, Cl 3.16).

Dative covalent bonds were introduced in Chapter 5. Nitrogen in quaternary ammonium salts donates a pair of electrons to form a positively charged group, as shown in this tetramethylammonium ion.

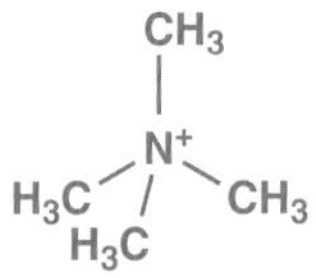

Dative covalent bonding can also occur between complex **ligands** and metal cations. Ligands can be considered to be **Lewis bases** in that they donate electrons to the metal ions; the metal ions, in turn, act as **Lewis acids** by accepting the electrons.

Dative covalent bonding can result in the formation of complexes; if the ligand can donate more than one pair of electrons to the metal then it is called a **chelating agent**. Chelating agents may be used to treat poisoning with metal ions; for example, Figure 8.1 shows the structure of desferrioxamine, which is used to treat iron poisoning.

Ligands require lone pairs of electrons, and the lone pair usually comes from oxygen or nitrogen. Ligands are often based on amino acids such as histidine, or the pyrrole ring of porphyrin. The structure

Figure 8.1 The structure of desferrioxamine

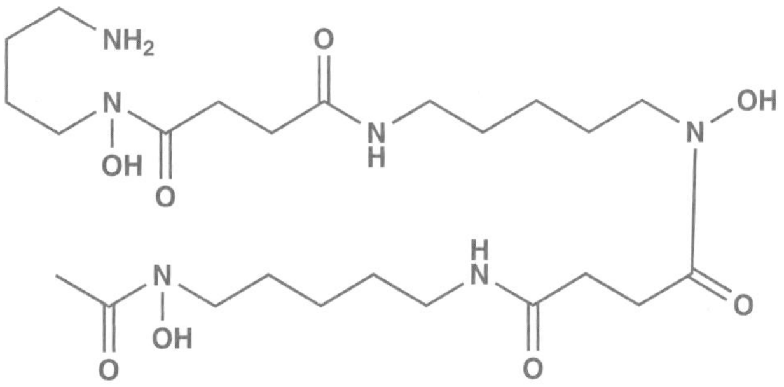

Figure 8.2   The structure of pyrrole; draw the structure of histidine alongside

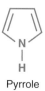

Pyrrole

Self-check 8.1

The structure of pyrrole is shown in Figure 8.2. Draw the structure of the amino acid histidine alongside it and highlight the atoms which may act as Lewis bases when histidine is one of the amino acids of a protein.

of pyrrole is shown in Figure 8.2; it is an example of an aromatic heterocyclic compound. The lone pair of electrons on the nitrogen is available for donation to a metal ion in biological complexes.

Oxidation and oxidation states (numbers)

Oxidation is the loss of electrons. Metals are oxidized to metal ions M^{n+} when they lose electrons to a more electronegative element. Metal ions in group 1, such as sodium and potassium, lose the outer s electron very easily and tend to exist as ions, e.g. Na^+ and K^+. Similarly, group 2 metals, such as calcium and magnesium, lose both electrons from the outer s shells, easily giving the divalent ions Ca^{2+} and Mg^{2+}.

The situation with transition metals is more complicated as they can have multiple oxidation states. Iron(II) results from the loss of the two $4s^2$ electrons, whilst iron(III) results from the loss of two $4s^2$ electrons and one 3d electron. As the energy difference between the 4s shell and the 3d shell is small, the transition between Fe^{2+} and Fe^{3+} can occur easily in biological situations.

The oxidation state (oxidation number) of an element refers to the number of electrons an element has lost or gained. Positive oxidation numbers mean that the element has lost electrons while a negative oxidation number means that the element has gained electrons. As discussed previously, iron commonly exists in two oxidation states, +2 as in iron(II) (Fe^{2+}), or +3 as in iron(III) (Fe^{3+}). Iron(II) is still commonly referred to as 'ferrous' (as in ferrous sulfate tablets), whilst iron(III) is 'ferric' (as in ferric chloride, which may be used in tests for phenols).

8.2 METALS: INTRODUCTION

The normal activity of cells depends on the correct concentrations of certain metal ions, both inside and outside the cell (see Box 8.1). Metal ions are also found in medicines. For instance, sodium and potassium ions are frequently used in salts of carboxylic acids. Benzylpenicillin sodium is used as a treatment for bacterial meningitis, and iron(II) salts are used for the treatment of anaemia.

Self-check 8.2

Complete Table 8.2 by calculating the missing values. Remember: number of moles = (number of grams)/(molar mass).

Table 8.2 Amounts of metals in the body and concentration of ions in serum or plasma

Metal	Average amount in the adult body (g)	Average amount in the adult body (mol)	Ion serum/plasma concentration reference range
Sodium		4	137–145 mM
Potassium	140		3.6–5.0 mM
Calcium		30	2.1–2.6 mM
Iron	4		male 11–28 μM female 7–26 μM
Zinc	2		10–24 μM

Box 8.1 Ion serum/plasma concentration reference range

Whilst watching a TV medical drama you may have heard a doctor order 'Us' and 'Es' for a patient. The 'Es' refer to electrolyte tests, which is the determination of the concentration of specific ions in the blood. These tests are very useful for the diagnosis of a patient's disease or condition. The resulting ion concentrations can be compared with a set of values known as the ion serum concentration range (see Table 8.2). The detection of an abnormal electrolyte value may facilitate diagnosis and subsequent treatment. A range of values is quoted as a reference because normal values can vary according to age and gender.

8.3 GROUP 1 METALS

The group 1 metals, known as the alkali metals, include lithium, sodium and potassium. All the group 1 metals react with water to release hydrogen, forming hydroxides. The reaction can be represented as:

$$2M + 2H_2O \rightarrow 2M^+ + 2OH^- + H_2$$

The effect of placing small pieces of these metals into water is quite spectacular. (There are a number of videos available on the internet, if you have not seen this before.) The reaction becomes more vigorous as you descend the group.

The relative molecular mass (RMM) and the electronic configuration of some group 1 and 2 metals are shown in Table 8.3.

Sodium and potassium ions are the most important of the group 1 metal ions for normal cell function, whilst lithium ions can be used in the prophylaxis and treatment of mania and other disorders.

Table 8.3 Properties of some group 1 and group 2 metals

Element	Symbol	Atomic number	RMM	Electronic configuration
Sodium	Na	11	22.99	$1s^2 2s^2 2p^6 3s^1$
Potassium	K	19	39.10	$1s^2 2s^2 2p^6 3s^2 3p^6 4s^1$
Magnesium	Mg	12	24.31	$1s^2 2s^2 2p^6 3s^2$
Calcium	Ca	20	40.08	$1s^2 2s^2 2p^6 3s^2 3p^6 4s^2$

Sodium

The normal adult body contains about 4 moles of sodium, of which approximately half is found in the extracellular fluid. Sodium levels can affect the volume of extracellular fluid, and excess sodium ions in the blood can lead to a number of conditions, including hypertension. Sodium ions are absorbed very easily from the gastrointestinal tract, and many of us ingest more than we need.

The recommended dietary intake for sodium in the UK is 1.6 g daily for adults, equivalent to 4 g of sodium chloride (salt). The target maximum daily intake is 6 g of salt, yet the average intake is approximately 9 g. Figure 8.3 shows these amounts of salt relative to a teaspoon, dessertspoon and tablespoon. The salt taste that most of us enjoy is due to sodium ions, which are able to enter ion channels in receptors on the tongue. Salt substitutes contain potassium ions, which are small enough to enter these same ion channels.

Intravenous sodium chloride solution is prescribed when there are low levels of sodium in the body. Sodium Chloride Infusion is isotonic with the physiological concentration of sodium and has a concentration of 0.9% w/v.

The levels of sodium in the body can be affected by the administration of medicines, including penicillin antibiotics. These compounds contain a carboxylic acid functional group and are formulated as sodium salts to give water solubility. The BNF specifically warns that high doses of injectable penicillins, or even normal doses given to patients with renal failure, can lead to the build up of an excess of sodium ions. Neonates can also be adversely affected by medicines with high sodium levels. The sodium intake is further increased if the medicine is reconstituted or infused with a sodium chloride solution (saline).

Figure 8.3   Amounts of sodium chloride (salt) in our diet

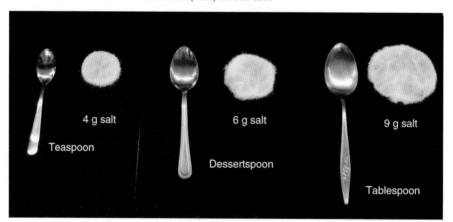

4 g salt

6 g salt

9 g salt

Teaspoon

Dessertspoon

Tablespoon

Self-check 8.3

Calculate the concentration of Na$^+$ ions in 0.9% w/v sodium chloride solution in g L^{-1} and in mM. How does the latter value compare with the value in Table 8.2?

Self-check 8.4

Draw the structure of benzylpenicillin sodium, look up its relative molecular mass, and calculate the number of moles of sodium ions in a vial containing 600 mg of benzylpenicillin sodium. Use the BNF to check your answer.

Potassium

Low levels of potassium can be caused by fluid loss and can cause muscle weakness. Fruit and vegetables are good sources of potassium. Many sportsmen and women try to combat muscle fatigue by eating bananas, which are especially rich in potassium. A medium banana contains about 420 mg potassium, equivalent to about 800 mg of potassium chloride. Figure 8.4 shows this amount of KCl relative to a banana and a two-pence piece.

Digoxin, which is used to treat some cardiac problems, normally competes with K^+ ions for the same binding site on the Na^+/K^+ ATPase pump, an enzyme essential for maintaining correct intracellular Na^+/K^+ ratios. Some patients are therefore treated with oral potassium supplements to try to minimize the unwanted side-effects of digoxin treatment. In the oral supplements, the potassium is usually formulated as the chloride salt. Severe hypokalaemia is treated with intravenous potassium chloride injections; as potassium overdose can be fatal, there are very clear guidelines for the use, labelling and storage of ampoules of potassium chloride.

Membrane potentials

Potassium ions inside cells work with extracellular sodium ions to maintain electrical potentials across cell membranes. The concentrations of Na^+ and K^+ ions inside cells are approximately 10 mM and 150 mM, respectively. If you compare these values with the values in Table 8.2, which refers to extracellular plasma concentrations, you will see that ratios of Na^+ to K^+ are reversed. In total, however, the concentrations of group 1 cations are high, both inside and outside cells.

Figure 8.4 The amount of potassium in a banana

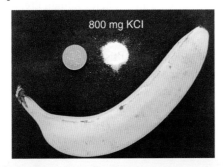

Self-check 8.5

The normal dosage for oral potassium supplements is 2–4 g KCl per day, in divided doses. Calculate the weight (in g) and number of millimoles of potassium that a patient would receive in a day if they were prescribed 10 mL, three times daily, of a solution containing 7.5% w/v potassium chloride. Compare this with the amount of potassium contained in a banana.

Box 8.2 Calculation of membrane potentials

Electrical potentials across cell membranes are generated by the difference in concentrations of ions across the cell membrane. For individual ions the potential can be calculated from the Nernst equation:

$$E = \frac{RT}{zF} \ln \frac{[ion]_{in}}{[ion]_{out}}$$

where R is the gas constant, T is the temperature in Kelvin, z is the net charge on the ion, [ion] is the concentration of the ion and F is the Faraday constant. For K^+ at body temperature this would give a value of –91 mV.

For resting membranes, the main contributor to the membrane potential is K^+, but there are small contributions from Na^+ and Cl^-. The overall potential can be calculated from the Goldman equation, which is beyond the scope of this book.

Organic anions inside the cell balance the positively charged metal ions, whilst chloride ions provide the anions outside the cell. The concentration of positive ions outside the cell is slightly higher than that inside the cell, generating a small electrical potential across the cell membrane; the membrane potential for a resting neuron is about –70 mV. For information on calculating membrane potentials, see Box 8.2.

The correct balance between sodium and potassium ion concentrations both inside and outside cells is essential to maintain electrical potentials in nerves and muscles, and for these to work efficiently. Signals are transmitted along nerve fibres by the influx of sodium ions into the cell and a corresponding movement of potassium ions out of the cell. After the signal has passed, the cell returns to its normal state due to the action of the Na^+/K^+ pump, which transports ions across the membrane against concentration gradients.

Lithium

Although lithium does not appear to be essential for human life, it is used to treat mania and recurrent depression. Despite being used since the 1950s, the exact mechanism of action is still unknown. There have been suggestions that it interferes with membrane transport of metal cations (including sodium ions), but this has not been proven. It has also been suggested that lithium blocks an enzyme pathway that uses magnesium ions, and it has been observed that lithium ions (Li^+) and magnesium ions (Mg^{2+}) are of a similar size.

Lithium is usually formulated as the carbonate salt in tablets (Li_2CO_3) or as the citrate salt in liquids $Li_3C_6H_5O_7$. Lithium toxicity is closely related to serum–lithium levels; the BNF target

Self-check 8.6

Lithium carbonate tablets contain 200 mg of lithium carbonate. Calculate the weight of lithium citrate ($Li_3C_6H_5O_7.4H_2O$) required in a 5-mL spoonful of lithium citrate oral solution to produce the same number of mmoles of lithium as are present in a 200 mg tablet of lithium carbonate, Check your answer against the figures quoted for lithium preparations in the BNF.

range is 0.4–1.0 mmol/l and should not exceed 1.5 mmol/l. Facilities for accurate monitoring of serum-lithium levels are required when initiating treatment or when changing preparations, as these can have varying bioavailablity.

8.4 GROUP 2 METALS

Group 2 metals (magnesium, calcium, strontium, barium and radium) are referred to as the alkaline earth metals. They are less reactive than the alkali metals, and their salts are not always soluble in water. Group 2 metal salts with polyvalent anions—for example, carbonate, phosphate and sulfate—tend not to be soluble. The limit test for sulfates, which can be found in the British Pharmacopoeia, is based on the formation of insoluble barium sulfate under controlled conditions.

Insoluble calcium salts can give rise to medical problems and can decrease the absorption of drugs. For instance, kidney stones, which can cause severe pain, usually consist of calcium oxalate or calcium phosphate salts.

Biologically, the most important group 2 metals are calcium and magnesium. Magnesium ions tend to be concentrated inside the cells, whilst calcium ions are mainly outside the cells.

Calcium

Over 95% of the calcium in the body is found in bone and teeth, where it exists mainly as calcium phosphate salts (hydroxyapatite, $Ca(OH)_2 \cdot 3Ca_3(PO_4)_2$). The concentration of calcium in plasma is about 2.5 mM, and, of this, 40–50% is bound to plasma proteins, particularly serum albumin. Only free calcium ions are biologically active, and so adjustments to the serum values determined need to be made if it is known that the patient has abnormally high or low levels of serum albumin.

❭ More information on phosphates can be found in Section 8.7.

Calcium ions are involved in blood-clotting, transmission of nerve signals and muscle contraction. When muscle cells are stimulated there is a rapid influx of sodium ions, which produces an action potential. There follows an influx of calcium ions, which maintains the action potential and leads to contraction of muscle. Calcium channel blockers such as verapamil and nifedipine prevent the entry of calcium ions into cells, preventing contraction of vascular smooth muscle and conduction of signals in myocardial cells. Both these drugs are used to treat several conditions; for example, verapamil is used to treat hypertension and nifedipine to treat angina.

Adults require a daily intake of approximately 700 mg calcium for maintenance of bone and plasma levels. This is increased for children, nursing mothers and in pregnancy. Dairy products are a good source of calcium, which is absorbed from the gastrointestinal tract. However, although calcium ions themselves are well absorbed they can interfere with the absorption of drugs. For example, they can form chelates with tetracycline and quinolone antibiotics, which cannot be absorbed. As a consequence, patients are advised to take tetracycline antibiotics one hour before food or two hours after meals to prevent the interaction, which can reduce absorption of the antibiotic by up to 80%.

The chelation reaction between tetracycline and calcium can have other serious effects. Tetracyclines should not be prescribed in the first trimester of pregnancy as they can affect bone

Figure 8.5 Ethylenediamine tetraacetic acid (EDTA)

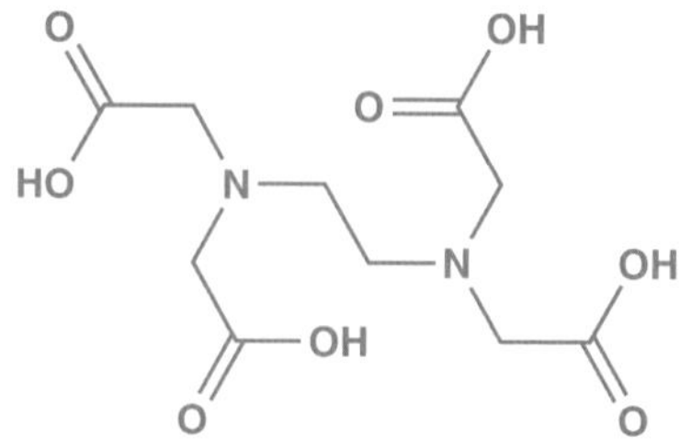

Self-check 8.7

Draw the structure of the quinolone antibiotic ciprofloxacin and identify a part of the structure that could be responsible for the interaction with Ca^{2+} ions. Are there any functional groups common to EDTA and ciprofloxacin?

development in the foetus. If possible, they should also be avoided later in pregnancy and in childhood, as they can cause serious discolouration of teeth.

Although chelation reactions may cause problems with drug interactions they are useful in pharmaceutical analysis. For instance, the British Pharmacopoeia uses a titration with ethylenediamine tetraacetic acid (EDTA), shown in Figure 8.5, to assay calcium gluconate tablets, which are used to treat calcium deficiency. The reaction is a 1:1 reaction and the titration is carried out at a high pH, as the complexes are unstable at low pH.

Magnesium

There are approximately 25 g of magnesium in the average adult. Half of this is found in bone, with most of the remainder being inside cells. Magnesium ions are important cofactors for enzymes and are therefore required for normal body function. There are about 500 kinases in the human body, which catalyse the transfer of a phosphate group from adenosine triphosphate (ATP) to an acceptor. Kinases typically contain magnesium ions, which complex with the ATP.

Magnesium levels within the body are carefully controlled, and absorption from the gut is slow. The fact that magnesium salts are not well absorbed from the gastrointestinal tract has meant that compounds such as magnesium sulfate, commonly called Epsom salts, have been widely used as osmotic laxatives.

Box 8.3 Antacids

Many of us suffer from dyspepsia (indigestion and heartburn), creating a large market for antacid preparations to relieve symptoms. Most of these medicines contain salts of aluminium or magnesium, which react to neutralize excess acid in the stomach. In general, magnesium-containing antacids tend to have a laxative effect, whilst those containing aluminium may be constipating. Not surprisingly, therefore, preparations such as Co-magaldrox, which contain both magnesium and aluminium ions, are available.

Self-check 8.8

Write equations for the reactions of aluminium hydroxide and magnesium hydroxide with hydrochloric acid. Use equations to explain why antacids that contain magnesium carbonate may make patients belch.

Group 1 and group 2 metal ions play a vital part in maintaining normal cell functions. Imbalances in concentrations of these ions usually need to be corrected as soon as possible. Concentrations of ions in body fluids and medicines are expressed in a variety of units, and you need to be very competent in working between weight per litre, percentage solutions and molarity.

8.5 **PERIOD 4 METALS**

In this section we study the metals zinc and iron in more detail. These metals are frequently known as transition metals, and some of their electrons are contained in d-orbitals. Look at Table 8.4 and notice how zinc actually has a complete set of d-electrons, and its chemistry is much simpler (and less colourful) than that of iron, copper or vanadium; for this reason inorganic chemists do not usually consider it to be a transition metal. Nevertheless, zinc, like iron, has important functions in biological systems, and it is the ability to use the d-orbitals that explains many of the biological activities of these metals. Some basic information about three of the period 4 elements is shown in Table 8.4.

Period 4 chemistry is greatly influenced by d-orbitals. There are five d-orbitals, each able to hold two electrons. Four of these have dumbbell-type shapes, each with four lobes all of which lie in a plane. The fifth orbital, the so-called d_{z^2} orbital, is different in that it has a dumbbell-shaped orbital running along the y-axis and a doughnut-shaped Taurus round the middle. Figure 8.6 shows a p orbital, the typical arrangement of the first four d orbitals and the shape of the d_{z^2} orbital.

> See Chapter 2, 'Organic structure and bonding', to remind yourself about s and p orbitals and hybridization of orbitals. There are also associated materials on the online resources which accompany this textbook.

Figure 8.6 Shapes of p and d orbitals

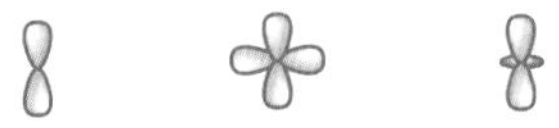

p orbital   d orbital d_{z^2} orbital

Table 8.4 Properties of some period 4 elements

Element	Symbol	Atomic number	RMM	Electron distribution
Iron	Fe	26	55.85	$1s^22s^22p^63s^23p^63d^64s^2$
Copper	Cu	29	63.55	$1s^22s^22p^63s^23p^63d^{10}4s^1$
Zinc	Zn	30	65.39	$1s^22s^22p^63s^23p^63d^{10}4s^2$

Iron

Our bodies contain about 4 g of iron, which is essential for life. It is probably best known as a carrier of oxygen in haemoglobin, but it is also found in cytochrome enzymes and in electron chain reactions. As iron is such an important component of the body, iron deficiency must be corrected by its administration (see Case study 8.1).

Biological activity associated with redox reactions

About 70% of the iron found in the body is found as haemoglobin (see Figure 8.7), where it acts to bind oxygen molecules, allowing blood to transport oxygen round the body. Haemoglobin comprises four peptide chains (globins), each of which has a haem group (a porphyrin) bound. This arrangement relies on the iron (Fe^{2+}) ion being able to form six dative covalent bonds. Four of the bonds are to nitrogen atoms in pyrrole rings in porphyrin, the fifth bond is to a nitrogen in a histidine ring in the globin, and the sixth dative covalent bond is to either oxygen (O_2) or to a water molecule. The bond between oxygen and iron is weak, allowing haemoglobin to give up its oxygen easily when required—hence making haemoglobin an efficient biological transporter of oxygen.

Figure 8.8 shows the structure of haem, illustrating the bonds between the pyrrole rings and Fe^{2+}. Also shown are simplified diagrams showing the overall arrangement of iron in haemoglobin and cytochrome c.

The bright red colour of blood is due to formation of a **complex** between the Fe^{2+} ion and the porphyrin ring. Oxidation of Fe^{2+} to Fe^{3+} in haemoglobin occurs when blood is exposed to air, resulting in a colour change from red to brown. Although iron is absorbed and largely used in its iron(II) oxidation state, it is stored in ferritin as the iron(III) state.

Iron is also an essential component of cytochrome enzymes, which are involved in respiration and drug metabolism. **Cytochromes** have a similar structure to haemoglobin, with the iron ion being bonded to four nitrogen atoms from porphyrin. The fifth bond is to a nitrogen atom from an associated protein. The difference between cytochromes and haemoglobin is that the sixth bond can be to other proteins or to a sulfur atom, as in cytochrome c (see Figure 8.8).

Case study 8.1

Iron deficiency

A patient with iron deficiency is prescribed iron(II) salts (usually as ferrous sulfate), which is the recommended salt in the BNF. Other salts may be used depending on side-effects and costs. In the BNF, it states that the oral dose of iron to treat iron deficient anaemia should be 100 to 200 mg of elemental iron daily.

Reflection questions

1. If a patient is initially prescribed ferrous sulfate tablets (200 mg), one tablet three times a day, how much elemental iron would she receive in one day?

2. The patient complains that the tablets do not suit her and so she is changed to ferrous gluconate tablets, two tablets three times a day. Can you explain to the patient why she now has to take six tablets a day instead of three?

For answers, visit the online resources which accompany this textbook.

Figure 8.7 Haemoglobin

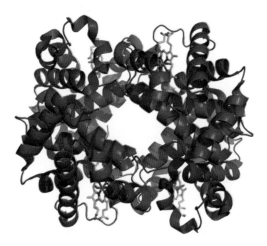

Figure 8.8 The structure of haem and cytochrome and the interaction of the iron ion with the pyrrole rings of porphyrin, globin, water molecules and sulfur

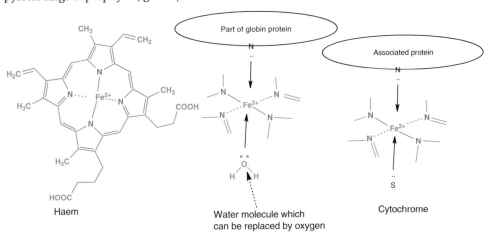

The cytochromes involved in respiration belong to three groups, a, b and c. Each cytochrome has a slightly different reduction potential (i.e. a slightly different tendency to acquire electrons and be reduced), because the haem units are associated with different polypeptides. In the respiration cycle, these are arranged in the order b, c_1, c, a, a_3 so that the energy obtained from the oxidation of glucose is released gradually and in a controlled manner. A simplified description of the electron transfer chain follows and is shown in Figure 8.9.

Initially, electrons are passed from reduced complex Q to cytochrome b, reducing Fe^{3+} to Fe^{2+}. In the next stage of the chain the Fe^{2+} in cytochrome b is oxidized back to Fe^{3+}, reducing the Fe^{3+} of cytochrome c_1 to Fe^{2+}. These cycles are repeated through cytochrome c, cytochrome a and cytochrome a_3. The final stage of the process sees the oxidation of Fe^{2+} in cytochrome a_3 back to Fe^{3+}, with the electrons released being used in the reduction of oxygen to water. The energy released by this process can be stored by the body as ATP; see Section 8.7.

Figure 8.9 Electron transport chain for cytochromes

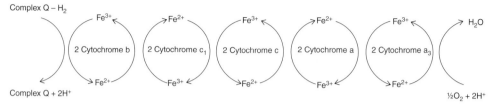

> The electron transport chain is also discussed in Chapter 11, 'Carbohydrates and carbohydrate metabolism'.

Biological activity associated with ligand binding

The cytochrome P450s (CYP450) are a family of enzymes that play an important role in the metabolism of drugs. The name P450 is based on the fact that their complexes with carbon monoxide (CO) absorb light at approximately 450 nm. Cytochrome P450s are found in many tissues in the body, but the liver, kidney and intestinal enzymes are especially important. They all have a similar structure, with the iron, Fe^{2+}, coordinated to four nitrogens of haem and the thiol group of a cysteine residue, which can act as an electron donor (see Figure 8.8). The sixth coordination position is occupied by water or other ligands which can be easily exchanged.

The role of CYP450 is usually described as activation of O_2 to allow oxidation of xenobiotics. Oxidation renders these molecules more water soluble, so that they are more easily eliminated from the body. Inhibition of CYP450s is a major cause of drug interactions, because CYP450s are not very specific and many drugs are processed on the same enzyme. For example, the anti-ulcer H_2 antagonist cimetidine binds reversibly to the iron in a number of CYP450s, including CYP450 2C9, which metabolizes warfarin. This interaction can prevent the metabolism of warfarin, leading to high levels of warfarin accumulating, which can result in excessive bleeding. Similar interactions can also occur with herbal medicines and some fruit juices; for instance, grapefruit juice can increase plasma concentrations of many drugs.

> CYP450s are also dealt with in Chapter 14, 'Absorption, distribution, metabolism and excretion'. There is more about warfarin metabolism in Chapter 3, 'Stereochemistry and drug action'.

Self-check 8.9

The structure of cimetidine is shown in Figure 8.10. Which parts of the cimetidine molecule do you think could be responsible for cimetidine binding to iron?

The activity of iron in the body depends on the fact that it can:

- act as a Lewis acid accepting electrons from electron rich ligands
- take part in redox reactions.

Zinc

The human body contains about 2 g of zinc; many enzymes have Zn^{2+} ions in their active sites. The role of zinc in biochemical processes continues to be a subject of investigation, and research has suggested that Zn^{2+} ions may be involved in modulation of insulin secretion, while a decrease in Zn^{2+} levels has been associated with type 2 diabetes. Medicines containing Zn^{2+} ions have been used for many years. They are said to promote healing, and there are frequent media reports that they can help cure the common cold.

We will consider the angiotensin-converting-enzyme (ACE) to illustrate how the chemistry of zinc relates to its biological role. ACE is a metalloprotease enzyme (i.e. it contains a metal ion) and is responsible for the hydrolysis of peptide (amide) links. **ACE inhibitors** are frequently used to treat hypertension and heart failure.

In biological systems, zinc exists as the Zn^{2+} ion, having lost its two $4s^2$ electrons. It is able to form complexes with four ligands in a tetrahedral shape. In ACE, the zinc ion is coordinated to the nitrogens of two histidine residues (see Figure 8.11) and the carboxylate group from an acidic amino acid. The fourth ligand is an activated water molecule. ACE is responsible for the hydrolysis of a peptide bond in angiotensin I, resulting in the removal of a dipeptide to give angiotensin II. The zinc ion activates the bound water molecule so that it attacks the carbonyl group of the peptide link more readily; it is this activation that acts to catalyse the hydrolysis.

All ACE inhibitors contain a functional group that is capable of interacting with the zinc ion. The thiol group (S−H) is found in captopril, the carboxylate group is found in enalaprilat, and a phosphinyl group (P=O) is found in fosinoprilat.

The interaction between the inhibitors and the zinc ion involves ligand bonding between the lone pairs of electrons on the relevant functional group and the Zn^{2+} ion.

Figure 8.10   The structure of cimetidine

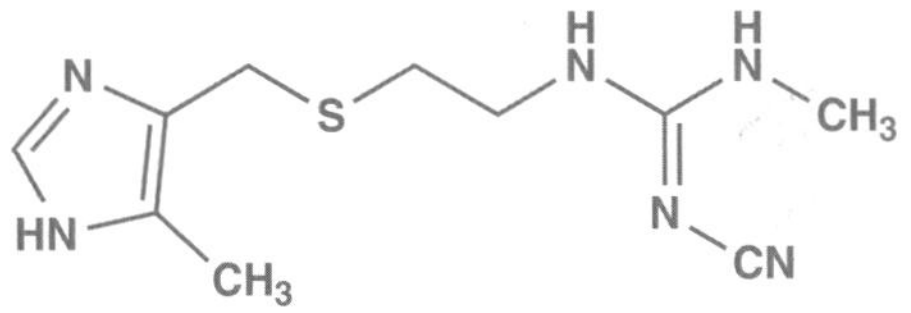

Figure 8.11   Diagram showing how Zn^{2+} ions are held in place in ACE

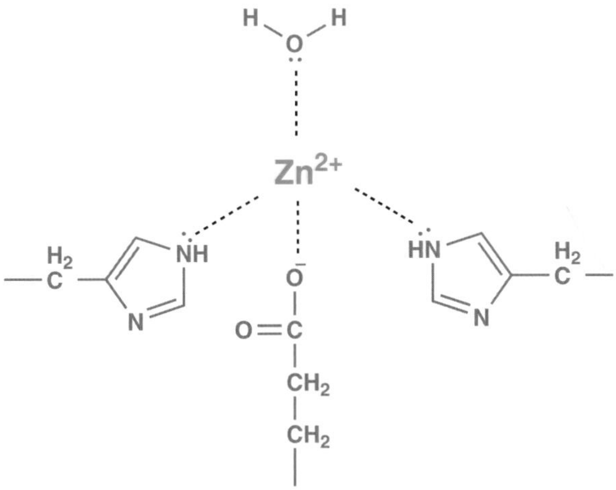

Self-check 8.10

Draw the structures of captopril, enalaprilat and fosinoprilat and highlight relevant groups that interact with the zinc ion of ACE.

The biological role of zinc in the body depends on the fact that zinc ions can interact with groups which have an excess of electrons.

8.6 PRECIOUS METALS

You might be surprised to find that precious metals such as silver, gold and platinum have a role in medicine. They are traditionally thought of as being non-reactive, and indeed, their use in jewellery relies on their low reactivity; however, their lack of reactivity does not preclude them having a role in biological systems.

Silver

Silver nitrate sticks have been used for many years to treat warts, but silver ions (Ag^{+}) also possess antibacterial activity. Silver salts such as silver sulfadiazine are therefore used in dressing wounds that might be infected. The exact mechanism of action of silver ions is not yet known, but may be related to their ability to interact with thiol groups in bacterial protein or disrupt disulfide bonds (see Section 8.8).

Gold

Gold in the form of sodium aurothiomalate, whose structure is shown in Figure 8.12, is used to treat active progressive rheumatoid arthritis. Once again the exact mechanism of action has not yet been fully established. It would appear that the compounds are most effective when the gold is in the monovalent form (Au^{+}, aurous) which is attached to a sulfur ligand.

Platinum

The last precious metal to consider is platinum, which is used in drugs such as cisplatin, a cancer therapeutic. In contrast to the silver and gold compounds, the mechanism of action of platinum compounds is well understood. Cisplatin is a complex formed between oxidized platinum, chlorine and ammonia. In this form, two chlorine atoms and two ammonia molecules are bonded to the platinum in a square planar complex as shown in Figure 8.13. This arrangement leads to the possibility of geometrical isomerism; the two chlorine atoms can either be next to each other, a *cis* arrangement, or opposite each other, a *trans* arrangement. Only the *cis* arrangement (cisplatin) makes an active anticancer drug used to treat a variety of cancers such as

Figure 8.12 Sodium aurothiomalate

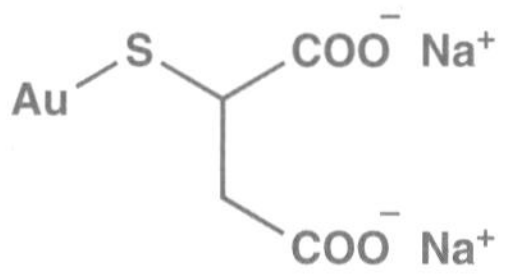

Figure 8.13 The mechanism of action of cisplatin

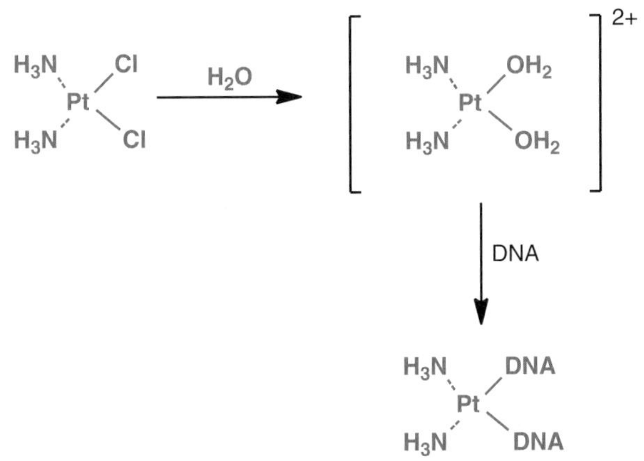

testicular cancer, ovarian cancer, bladder cancer and head and neck cancers, and examination of the mechanism of action explains why.

Inside the cell the chloro groups of cisplatin are replaced by water molecules. As the water molecules are neutral, and the leaving chloride ions take both electrons from each Pt–Cl bond, the complex now carries a positive charge. This positive charge makes the complex very reactive, facilitating its binding to nitrogen and oxygen atoms in guanine residues within DNA. Cisplatin acts to form links both within and between DNA strands, with the intrastrand links predominating. Other organoplatinum compounds with the same mode of action, such as carboplatin, have also been developed. It is thought that the *trans* arrangement of the chlorine atoms makes transplatin more reactive and so it is deactivated before it can interact with the DNA. Carboplatin is also used to treat a variety of cancers and has a bidentate dicaroxylate ligand instead of the two chlorine ligands. It is thought to act by the same mechanism as cisplatin, although it exhibits lower reactivity and slower binding to DNA. However, it has a lower excretion rate and so has a longer half-life in the body (30 hours compared to ~3 hours for cisplatin).

> Information on *cis* and *trans* alkenes can be found in Chapter 4, 'Properties of aliphatic hydrocarbons'.

Many other metals, including vanadium and copper, are important to health and can have biological activity, but here there is not space to discuss all of them. You should consider whether their reactions depend on redox-type reactions or complex formation. The metals may function as ions or as the element itself. For instance, intrauterine contraceptive devices (IUDs) appear to have their effect through the action of copper on sperm, although, once again, the exact mechanism of action is not yet known.

Self-check 8.11

Draw a structure for the *trans* isomer of cisplatin and explain why it would be likely to be deactivated.

It is worth making a mention of the medical uses of the lanthanides—a term which covers all the metallic elements from lanthanum to lutetium in the periodic table (also called the rare earth elements). Those of particular interest are cerium (atomic number 58) and lanthanum (atomic number 57), as these are potential anticancer agents. Cerium is thought to inhibit cell proliferation and promote cytotoxicity when used as a cerium-protein complex. It may replace iron in transferrin which transports iron into the cells and is needed for cell growth and replication.

The mechanism of action of lanthanum is unclear but is thought to interfere with microRNA. Lanthanum is also used in medical imaging as a 'fluorescent torch' which can aid the visualization of cell processes.

8.7 PHOSPHORUS

Phosphorus, like nitrogen, is a group 15 element in the IUPAC system, but while nitrogen is a stable gas, phosphorus can exist in several solid forms. The most common of these, white phosphorus, is far from stable and reacts vigorously with oxygen. Consequently, white phosphorus is stored under water to prevent reaction with oxygen.

In the body, phosphates are part of DNA, ATP, the buffering system for blood, and in bone in the form of calcium hydroxide phosphate, hydroxyapatite ($Ca_{10}(PO_4)_6(OH)_2$). Phosphorus in the form of phosphates is found widely in pharmacy. Phosphate esters can be produced to give solubility, phosphorus insecticides can be used to treat head lice, and phosphonates are used in the treatment of osteoporosis.

The electronic configuration of phosphorus is $1s^2 2s^2 2p^6 3s^2 3p^3$, and it can exist in two oxidation states: the III and the V state. In the III oxidation state only the 3p electrons are involved in bonding, and phosphorus is trivalent. By contrast, in the V state both the 3s and the 3p electrons are involved in bonding and the phosphorus is pentavalent. In order to have five valencies we need a situation in which there are five single electrons. This is achieved by using a 3d orbital as well as the 3s and 3p orbitals. This results in the production of five sp^3d hybrid orbitals, each with one electron and each with the same energy. These orbitals can be used to form covalent bonds; for example, in phosphorus pentachloride (PCl_5).

> Chapter 2, 'Organic structure and bonding', deals with the formation of hybrid orbitals.

In pharmacy and related disciplines, we normally encounter phosphorus in derivatives of orthophosphoric acid, more widely known as phosphoric acid (H_3PO_4). This molecule consists of phosphorus that forms single bonds to three OH groups and a double bond to the remaining oxygen. The phosphoric acid molecule is tetrahedral. as shown in Figure 8.14. The hydrogens attached to the oxygens are acidic such that each of the OH groups of phosphoric acid can act as an acid. Each has a separate pK_a; these values are shown in Table 8.5. Phosphoric acid is similar to a carboxylic acid in that it can produce esters, anhydrides and amides.

Figure 8.14   Phosphoric acid

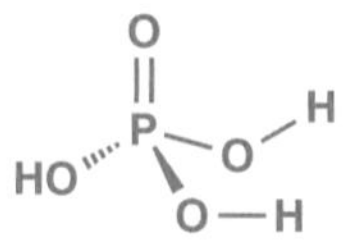

Table 8.5 Ionization reactions and pK_a values for the separate ionizations of acid.

Ionization	pK_a
$H_3PO_4 \rightleftharpoons H^+ + H_2PO_4^-$	2.14
$H_2PO_4^- \rightleftharpoons H^+ + HPO_4^{2-}$	7.20
$HPO_4^{2-} \rightleftharpoons H^+ + PO_4^{3-}$	12.37

At physiological pH (pH 7.4) the most important ionization is the second ionization, which sets up an equilibrium between dihydrogen phosphate ($H_2PO_4^-$) and hydrogen phosphate (HPO_4^{2-}). This equilibrium enables phosphate to buffer solutions at or close to pH 7.4.

When phosphoric acid is neutralized, it forms phosphate salts that can be used in medicines. Some basic drugs are formulated as water-soluble phosphate salts—for example, the analgesic, codeine phosphate (see Figure 8.15).

Phosphoesters

Phosphoric acid, like carboxylic acids, can form esters with alcohols. Each OH group can react independently to form phosphomonoesters, phosphodiesters and phosphotriesters. These, collectively, are also known as phosphate esters or organophosphates. In a phosphomonoester, one OH of the phosphate is replaced by OR (from an alcohol). The glycolysis intermediate glucose-6-phosphate is an ester formed between phosphoric acid and the OH in the 6-position of glucose. (Glucose is the alcohol.) The phosphoester group is shown in blue in Figure 8.16.

> Glycolysis is also discussed in Chapter 11, 'Carbohydrates and carbohydrate metabolism'.

In phosphomonoesters, the remaining OH groups are still capable of ionization. This property can be put to good use in the production of ionized derivatives, which are water soluble. For example, the steroid dexamethasone, which can be used to treat cerebral oedema associated with malignancy, is formulated for injection as the sodium phosphate derivative. A structure of dexamethasone is shown in Figure 8.16; again the phosphoester group is shown in blue.

When phosphoric acid reacts with two alcohol groups, a diester is formed. A good example of a phosphodiester is present in the structure of DNA, as shown in Figure 8.17, where the deoxyribonucleic acid units are connected through a phosphate group. The diester part is shown in blue.

Phosphoric acids can form anhydrides as well as esters. (You might anticipate this, because of their similarity to carboxylic acids.) These derivatives are diphosphoric acid (two molecules

Figure 8.15 Codeine phosphate

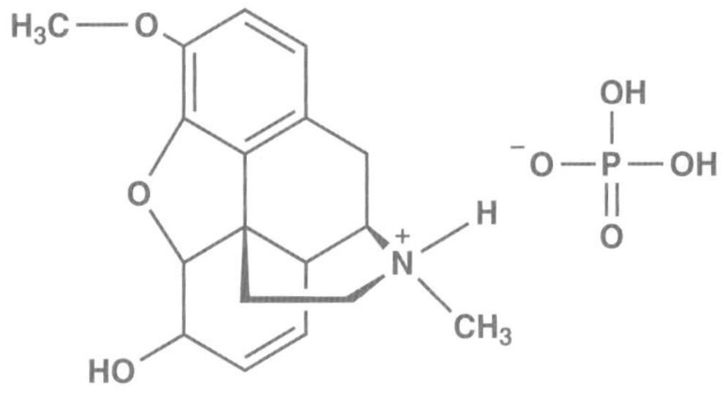

Figure 8.16   Glucose-6-phosphate and dexamethasone sodium phosphate

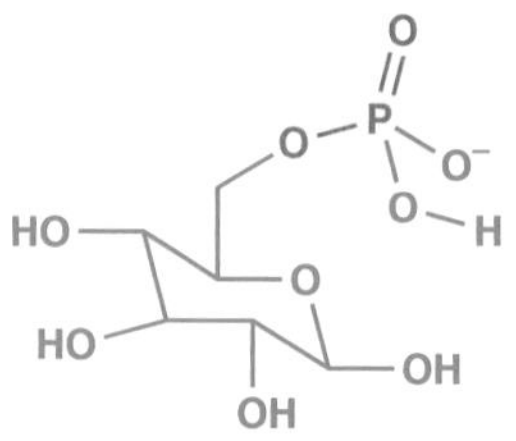

Glucose-6-phosphate

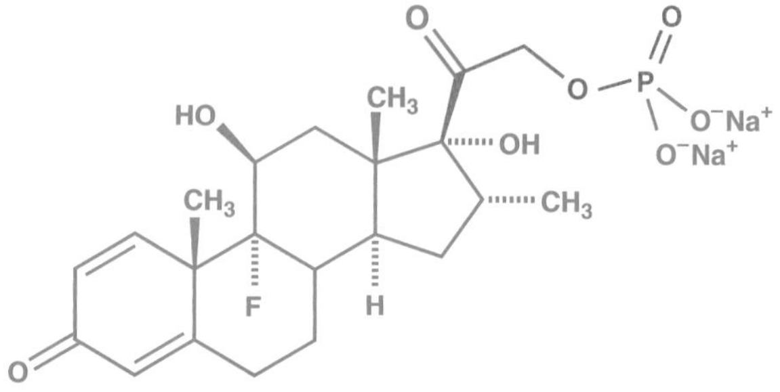

Dexamethasone sodium phosphate

Figure 8.17   DNA showing how a phosphodiester links two nucleosides together

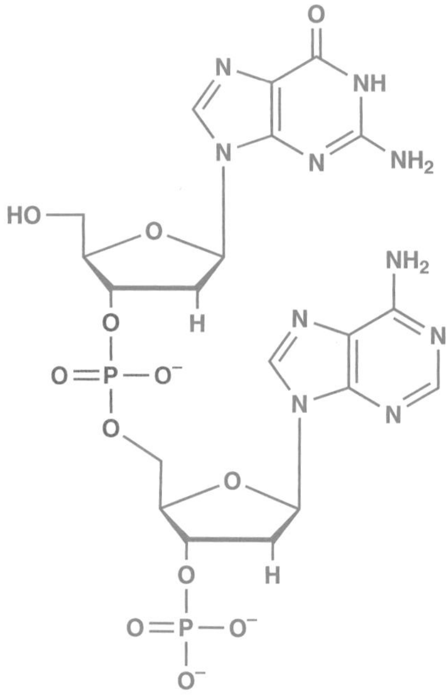

joined together), and triphosphoric acid (three molecules joined together). These condensed phosphates are formed by the loss of water, which is why they can be considered to be anhydrides. Look at Figure 8.18 to see the structures of di- and triphosphoric acid; the anhydride part is highlighted in blue.

> More details on carboxylic acid anhydrides can be found in Chapter 6, 'The carbonyl group and its chemistry'.

Examples of di- and triphosphates are seen in adenosine diphosphate (ADP) and ATP. These anhydrides (like carboxylic acid anhydrides) are easily hydrolysed, leading to the release of considerable amounts of energy: 34 kJ mol^{-1} for the conversion of ATP to ADP and the same again for ADP to AMP. The body stores energy in the form of ATP and ADP and releases it when required.

Figure 8.18   Diphosphoric and triphosphoric acid

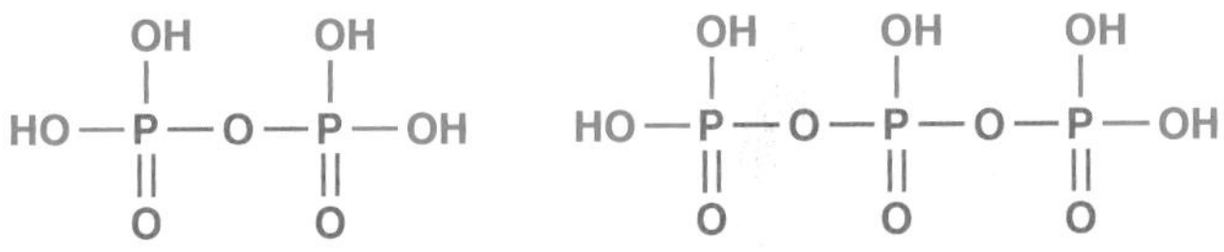

Diphosphoric acid   Triphosphoric acid

Figure 8.19   The structure of ATP

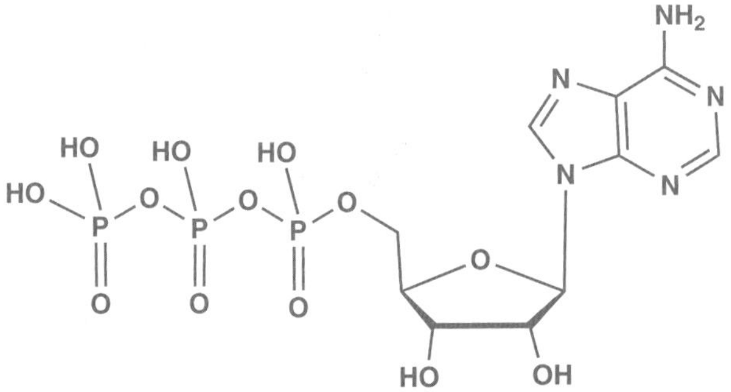

Self-check 8.12

Identify the anhydride parts of the ATP in Figure 8.19. What is the normal function of ATP in the body?

> The mechanism of the hydrolysis of ATP is illustrated in Chapter 1, 'The importance of pharmaceutical chemistry'.

ATP and ADP are part of the normal biochemistry of the body, but derivatives of phosphoric acid are used in medicines. One example is malathion, a phosphorus insecticide used to treat head lice. Malathion inhibits insect acetylcholinesterase by reacting with a serine residue at the active site of the enzyme. The reaction depends on the fact that phosphorus–oxygen double bonds (P=O) are polarized because the oxygen is more electronegative than phosphorus. There is a lower electron density on the phosphorus, making it susceptible to attack by nucleophiles. A covalent bond is formed between the oxygen of the enzyme and the phosphorus of the insecticide, which inactivates the enzyme.

At first glance, malathion may appear to be inactive because it contains a phosphorus–sulfur double bond rather than a phosphorus–oxygen double bond. Sulfur is less electronegative than oxygen, so a P=S bond is less polarized than a P=O bond (and therefore less susceptible to attack by a nucleophile). Insects, however, metabolize malathion by replacing the sulfur with oxygen, whereas mammals hydrolyse the carboxylic ester to produce inactive compounds, which are excreted. The **selective toxicity** of malathion to insects, and not humans, is achieved through the different metabolic pathways in insects and mammals. The reactions showing the different metabolic routes and the reactions resulting in inhibition are shown in Figure 8.20. Nerve gases, such as sarin, attack **acetylcholinesterase** through a similar reaction, but in this case there is no selective toxicity.

Figure 8.20   Metabolism and actions of malathion

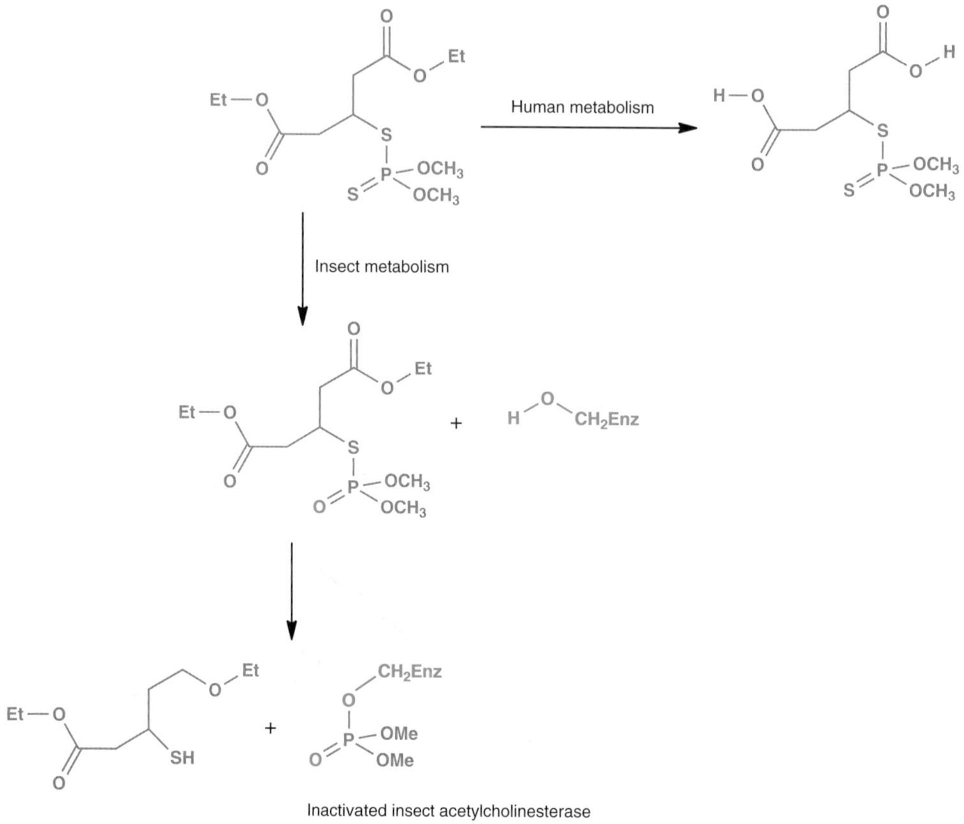

Self-check 8.13

Using the reaction between malathion and acetylcholinesterase shown in Figure 8.20 as an example, draw the mechanism for the interaction between the hydroxyl group of the enzyme and the phosphorus–oxygen double bond leading to inactivation of the enzyme.

Phospholipids are a major component of cell membranes; they are derivatives of glycerol in which one of the hydroxyl groups forms a phosphate ester. The other hydroxyl groups in glycerol form esters with fatty acids. The phosphate group usually exists as a diester with one of the other OH groups being esterified with a hydrophilic alcohol (for example, choline) to give lecithins, or ethanolamine to give cephalins. The other OH from the phosphate is ionized at physiological pH.

The ionized phosphate group of a phospholipid forms a polar, hydrophilic 'head', which is found on the outside of membranes (exposed to the aqueous surroundings). By contrast, the hydrocarbon chains from the fatty acids give phospholipids their hydrophobic lipid tails, which are directed towards the inside of the membrane.

A structure of a typical lecithin is shown in Figure 8.21, along with a diagram of a membrane showing the phospholipid bilayer, Figure 8.22.

Figure 8.21 A lecithin

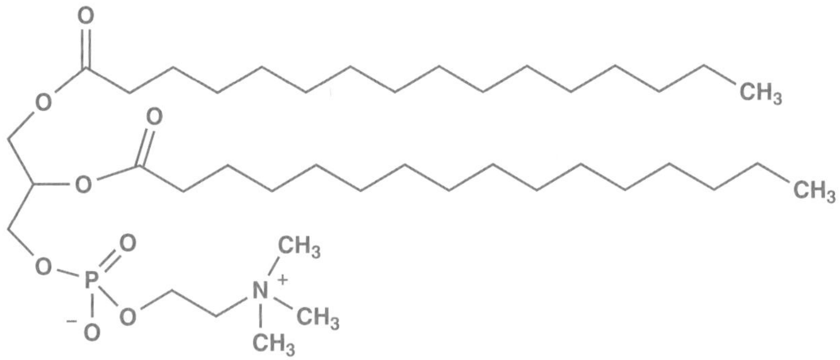

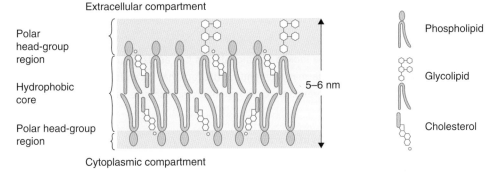

Figure 8.22 Phospholipid bilayer

Adapted from *Human Physiology: The Basis of Medicine*, 3rd edn, by Gillian Pocock and Christopher D. Richards (2006), by permission of Oxford University Press.

265

Bisphosphonates

In the phosphorus compounds that we have studied so far, the phosphorus has been directly bonded to oxygen or sulfur. However, the bisphosphonates are a class of compound in which phosphorus bonds to carbon. In bisphosphonates, a carbon atom bonds to two phosphorus atoms. (Take care not to confuse bisphosphonates with biphosphates, which are phosphoesters.) Alendronic acid is a bisphosphonate, which can be used to treat osteoporosis by mimicking pyrophosphoric acid in the body; both structures are shown in Figure 8.23.

Pyrophosphoric acid is another name for diphosphoric acid and is part of the hydroxyapatite component of bone. Bisphosphonates are adsorbed onto hydroxyapatite where they cannot be easily hydrolysed (because they are not esters). This leads to a decrease in the rate of bone turnover, allowing well-mineralized bone to be formed. Alendronic acid is usually formulated as the sodium salt, sodium alendronate, and is taken by patients once a week.

Self-check 8.14

Sodium alendronate is reported to be poorly absorbed from the gastrointestinal tract, and patients are advised to take these tablets at least 30 minutes before breakfast. Looking at the structure, shown in Figure 8.23, why do you think this is?

Figure 8.23   Alendronic acid and pyrophosphoric acid

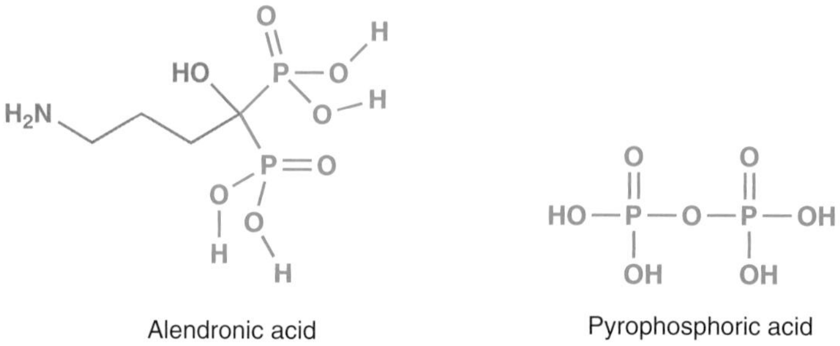

Alendronic acid

Pyrophosphoric acid

Self-check 8.15

Many of the phosphorus-containing substances have very similar names or structures. Complete Table 8.6 by identifying whether the compounds listed are salts, phosphoesters, phosphorus anhydrides or bisphosphonates.

In all the examples that we have looked at, phosphorus has an oxidation number of 5. Its biological activity and use in pharmacy depend on the fact that it can form a double bond with oxygen and still have O-H groups that can lose hydrogens to give salts or esters.

Table 8.6   Phosphorus compounds in pharmacy

Compound	Designation	Biological function or therapeutic use
e.g. ADP	phosphorus anhydride	mammalian energy store
chloroquine phosphate		
hydrocortisone sodium phosphate		
risedronate		
cyclophosphamide		

8.8 SULFUR

Sulfur and oxygen are both group 16 elements, so it should be of little surprise that some of sulfur's chemistry is similar to that of oxygen. However, there are important differences: an atom of sulfur is larger, less electronegative, and has empty 3d orbitals available. Like phosphorus, sulfur is widely distributed in nature, including the human body, and is a constituent of drug molecules.

The electronic configuration of sulfur is $1s^2 2s^2 2p^6 3s^2 3p^4$, and it can exist in oxidation states ranging from -2 to +6. Table 8.7 shows the oxidation states of sulfur and gives pharmaceutical examples of these oxidation states. Sulfur's ability to exist in so many oxidation states stems from the way it can use d orbitals to share electrons from oxygen. In the rest of this chapter we shall include examples from earlier in the chapter and try to relate the biological activity to the chemistry.

Table 8.7   Oxidation states of sulfur and pharmaceutical examples

Oxidation state	Group	General structure	Biological/Pharmaceutical example
-2	thiol	R–S–H	captopril
0	sulfoxide	R–SO–R	sulindac
+2	sulfone	$R–SO_2–R$	dapsone
+4	sulfonate ester	$R–SO_2O–R'$	busulfan
+6	sulfate esters	$RO–SO_2–OR$	sodium dodecyl sulfate

Thiols

In thiols, sulfur is in the -2 oxidation state and, like oxygen in alcohols, it has accepted electrons from other atoms. Much of the chemistry of thiols and thiophenols is similar to that of alcohols and phenols, although they are stronger acids because the larger sulfur atom is better able to spread the negative charge of the conjugate base, making it easier for a proton to be extracted. Like alcohols, thiols can react with alkyl halides to form thioethers and with acid chlorides to form thioesters, as shown in Figure 8.24.

The S–H group is sometimes called a sulfhydryl group as well as a 'thiol'. The old name for thiols was mercaptans, and this is still found in the name of pharmaceutical compounds such as the anticancer drug mercaptopurine. (Strictly, this drug is a thiophenol, since the S–H group is attached directly to the aromatic ring).

Low-molecular-weight thiols are foul-smelling—none more so than hydrogen sulfide, H_2S, which gives the characteristic smell to rotten eggs. For this reason, thiols are added to the domestic gas supply to allow us to detect leaks. Drugs containing sulfhydryl groups have an unpleasant taste.

To illustrate how the chemistry of the S–H group can explain the action of drugs and some of their side-effects, we shall again consider the ACE inhibitor captopril. In Section 8.5 we

Figure 8.24   Formation of thioethers and thioesters

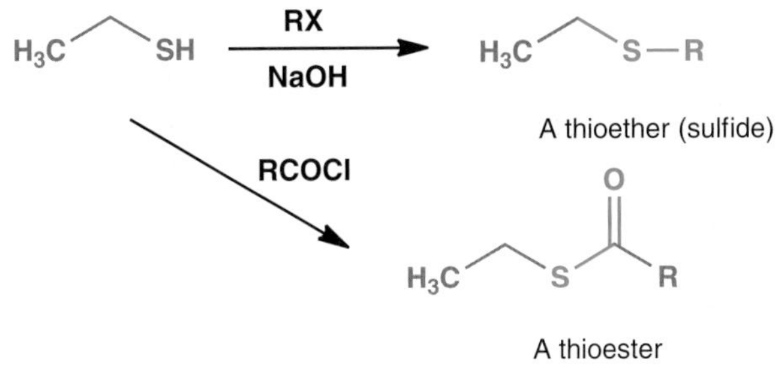

A thioether (sulfide)

A thioester

Figure 8.25   Succinyl derivative of proline and captopril

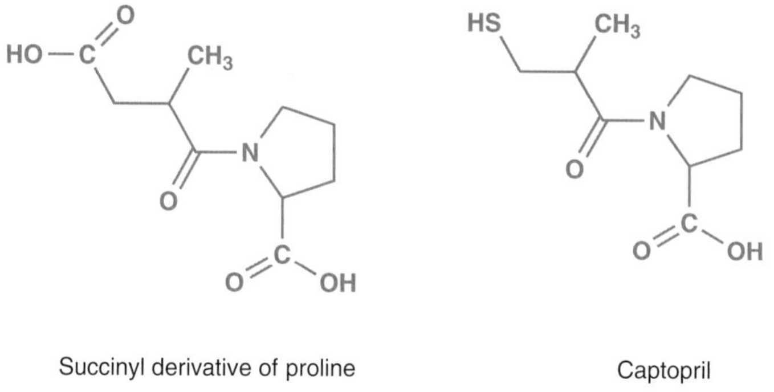

Succinyl derivative of proline   Captopril

saw that ACE contains a zinc ion at the active site. Thiols react readily with metal ions to form complexes, and captopril was developed by replacing a carboxylate group in a succinylproline derivative (the first inhibitor of ACE to be synthesized) with a thiol group, which has greater affinity for the Zn^{2+} ion. The structure of this derivative is shown in Figure 8.25.

Interestingly, patients who are given captopril may complain of a metallic taste in their mouth, and this is attributed to the presence of a thiol group.

> See Chapter 6, 'The carbonyl group and its chemistry', for more details on the development of captopril.

Thiols are able to form disulfides ($R-S-S-R'$), which are more stable than the analogous per-oxides $R-O-O-R'$. Disulfides may be formed in the laboratory from mild oxidation of thiols, but disulfides are also widely found in protein molecules. The tertiary structure of protein mol-ecules is partly determined by the presence of disulfide links between the sulfur-containing amino acid residues of peptide chains. In the example shown in Figure 8.26 the amino acid res-idues are cysteine, which contains sulfur as a thiol. Disulfide bonds are relatively weak and can be broken and reformed relatively easily.

Thioethers (sulfides)

Thioethers are more reactive than the corresponding oxygen ethers and they act as nucleo-philes: one of the lone pairs of electrons on the sulfur attacks an electrophilic centre (where there is lower electron density). In the body, the sulfur of methionine can react with ATP, as shown in Figure 8.27. This reaction results in the formation of S-adenosylmethionine (SAM), which is a very good biological methylating agent and is used by the body to add methyl groups to metabolites and to xenobiotics. For example, the enzyme catechol-O-methyltransferase transfers a methyl group onto one of the phenolic hydroxyl groups of catecholamines, such as the neurotransmitter noradrenaline. This inactivates noradrenaline, preventing it from interacting with β_2-adrenoceptors in the lungs. Airways are dilated when these receptors are occupied.

The formation of SAM is shown in Figure 8.27, and its subsequent use to transfer a methyl group to the hydroxyl group of noradrenaline is shown in Figure 8.28. Bronchodila-tors such as salbutamol and terbutaline are not catechols and therefore are not metabolized by this route.

Figure 8.26 (A) The structure of cysteine with the thiol group in green; (B) the structure of insulin showing the amino sequences of its composite chains, with the cross-linking of the chains via cysteine residues; (C) a diagram showing the links at a more detailed level. The disulfide bond is shown in green, the cysteine residues in pink

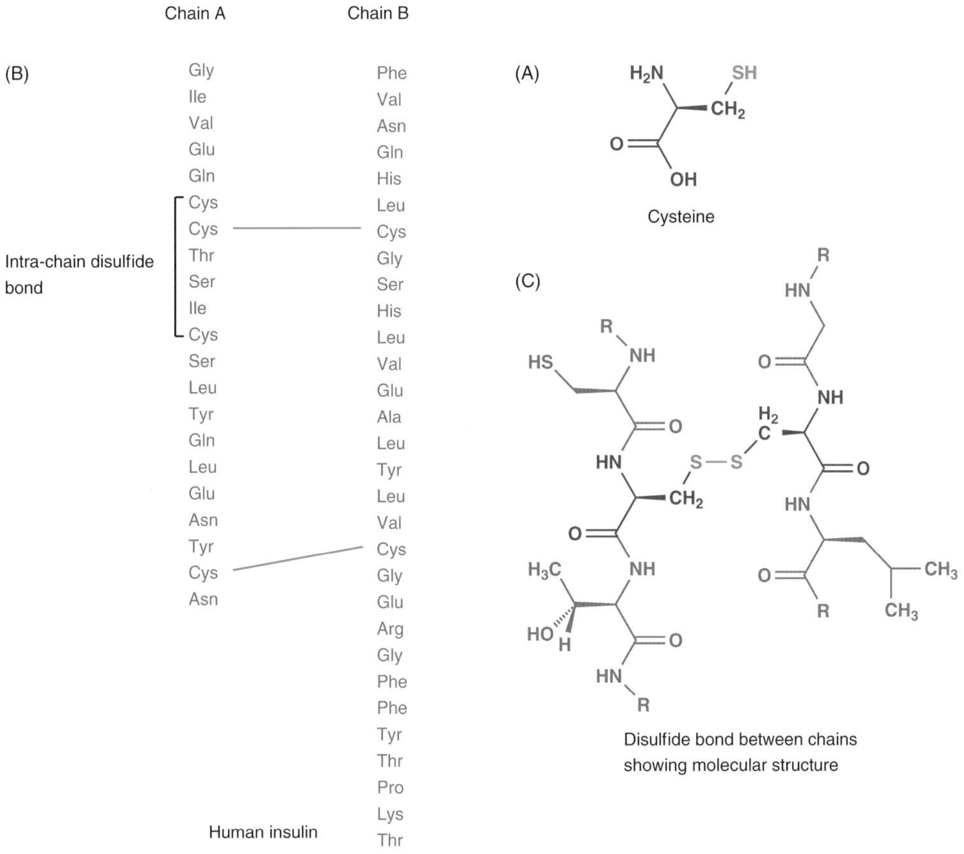

Sulfoxides, sulfones and sulfonates

Stepwise oxidation of thioethers produces sulfoxides (S=O) and then sulfones ($S(=O)_2$), as shown in Figure 8.29. In sulfoxides, sulfur has an oxidation number of 0, and in sulfones it is +2.

Sulfoxides are often represented as having an S=O double bond, but this representation requires overlap of a $2p$ orbital of oxygen with a much larger $3p$ orbital from sulfur. Such overlap is not very effective, and the SO group is so polarized that it is often represented as S^+-O^-, with the greater electron density on the oxygen. This increased polarization makes sulfoxides more water-soluble than sulfides and therefore easier for the body to excrete. The body can metabolize sulfides by oxidation to produce sulfoxides.

Usually the body oxidizes xenobiotics (such as drugs), but occasionally reductions do occur. For example, sulindac, which is used to treat pain and inflammation in rheumatic disease, is a sulfoxide. Sulindac is actually a pro-drug, which is reduced in the body to a lipophilic sulfide, as shown in Figure 8.30. The structural requirements for non-steroidal anti-inflammatory drugs require that they should be lipophilic, so in this case the body reduces the hydrophilic sulfoxide group to the sulfide which is the active species.

Figure 8.27 The formation of S-adenosylmethionine (SAM)

Methionine

ATP

S-Adenosylmethionine (SAM)

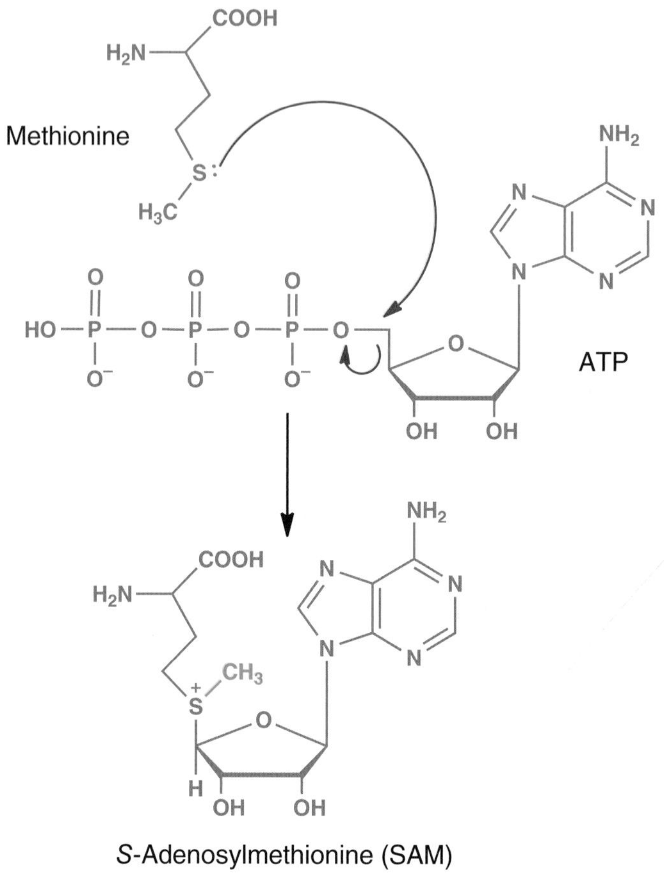

Sulfoxides are non-planar, and sulfoxides with two different substituents are chiral. The pharmaceutical significance of this is demonstrated with the proton pump inhibitor omeprazole, which is used to reduce gastric acid secretion in gastro-oesophageal reflux disease (GORD). Omeprazole, whose structure is shown in Figure 8.31, exists as both R and S isomers and is usually administered as the racemate because both isomers are active. The S isomer is, however, marketed as esomeprazole, which is claimed to lead to higher plasma levels of omeprazole. This is attributed to the S isomer being less susceptible to metabolism than the R isomer, such that it is removed from the body more slowly.

> R and S isomers are discussed in more detail in Chapter 3, 'Stereochemistry and drug action'.

Dapsone, which has been used to treat leprosy and tuberculosis, is an example of a sulfone. Sulfones are produced by the oxidation of sulfoxides, after which sulfur has an oxidation number of +2, with double bonds to two oxygen atoms. Dapsone, like sulphonamide antibacterials, blocks the synthesis of folic acid.

Sulfonates where sulfur has an oxidation number of +4 are the next oxidation state from sulfones. Sulfonic acids, RSO_3H, where R=H or an aliphatic or aromatic carbon, are strong acids and are ionized at physiological pH, as depicted in Figure 8.32. They form water–soluble salts (sulfonates)

Figure 8.28 Transfer of a methyl group from SAM to noradrenaline

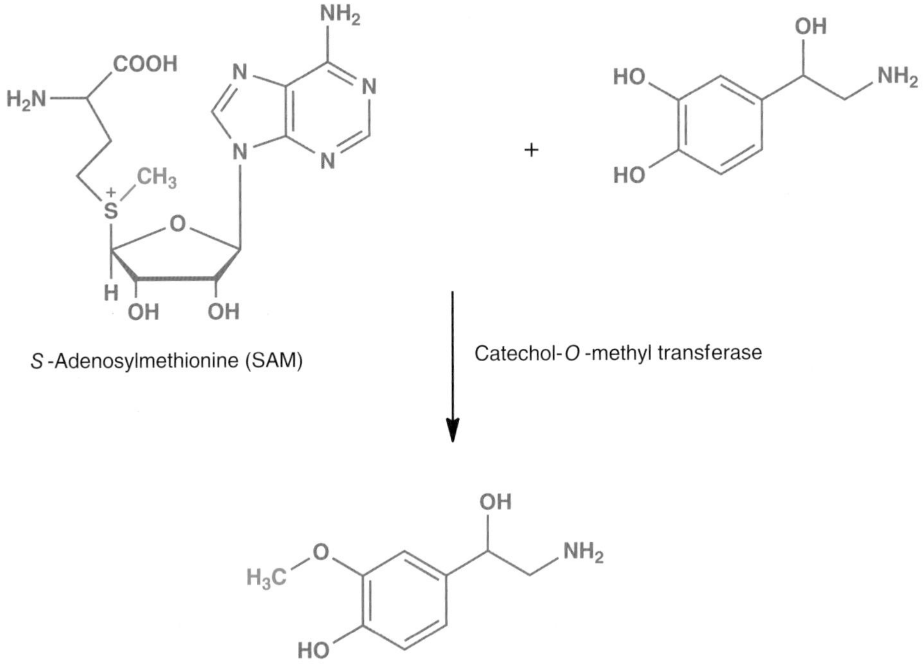

S-Adenosylmethionine (SAM)

+

Catechol-O-methyl transferase

Figure 8.29 Oxidation products from thioethers

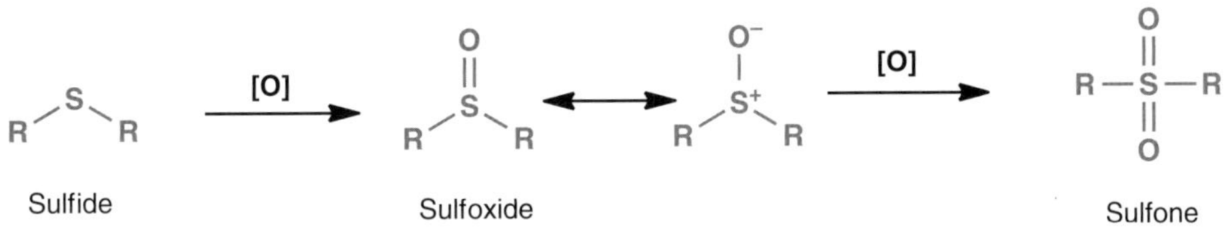

Sulfide

Sulfoxide

Sulfone

Box 8.4 Sulphur or sulfur?

It is often said that the British and the Americans are divided by a common language. The spelling of 'sulfur' has been standardized to the American. Several drug classes, discovered in Europe before standardization of spelling, retain the British English spelling; for example, cephalosporins, sulphonamides. Individual drugs (cefalexin, sulfasalazine) are often spelt in American English. It is the duty of the pharmacist (the same spelling in British and American English) to be concerned about spelling. Drug names (digitoxin and digoxin, for example) are sometimes very similar.

with organic bases and quaternary ammonium ions. For example, the neuromuscular blocking agent atracurium is formulated as its benzene sulfonate (besilate) salt, as shown in Figure 8.33.

Sulfonic acids are similar to carboxylic acids in that they can form esters and chlorides. The chlorides can be used as intermediates in the preparation of sulphonamides, as shown in Figure 8.34.

Figure 8.30   Reduction of sulindac

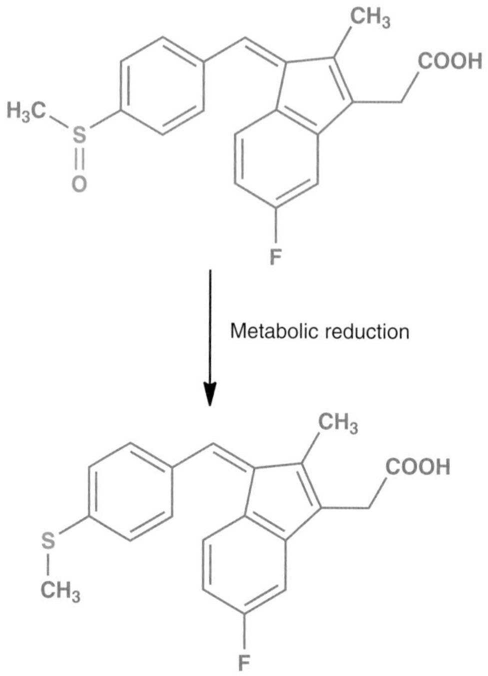

Metabolic reduction

Figure 8.31   Omeprazole

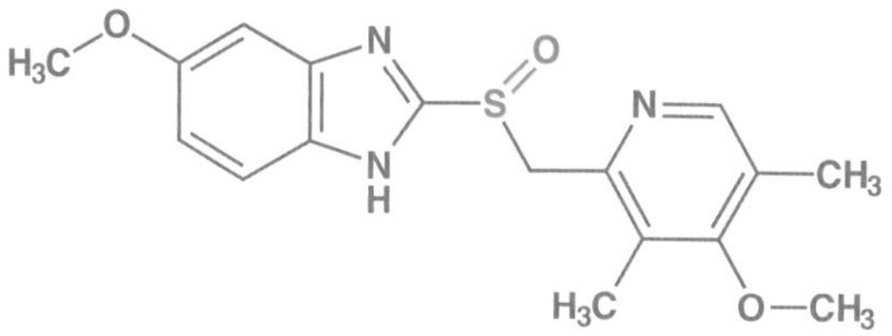

Figure 8.32   Sulfonic acid and sulfonate ion

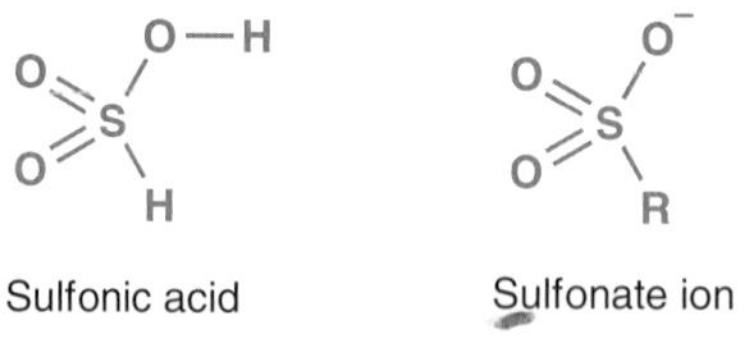

Sulfonic acid   Sulfonate ion

Figure 8.33   Atracurium besilate

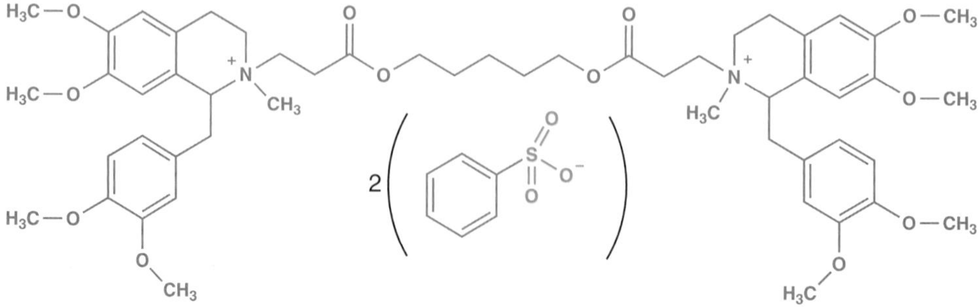

Figure 8.34 Synthesis and ionization of sulphonamides

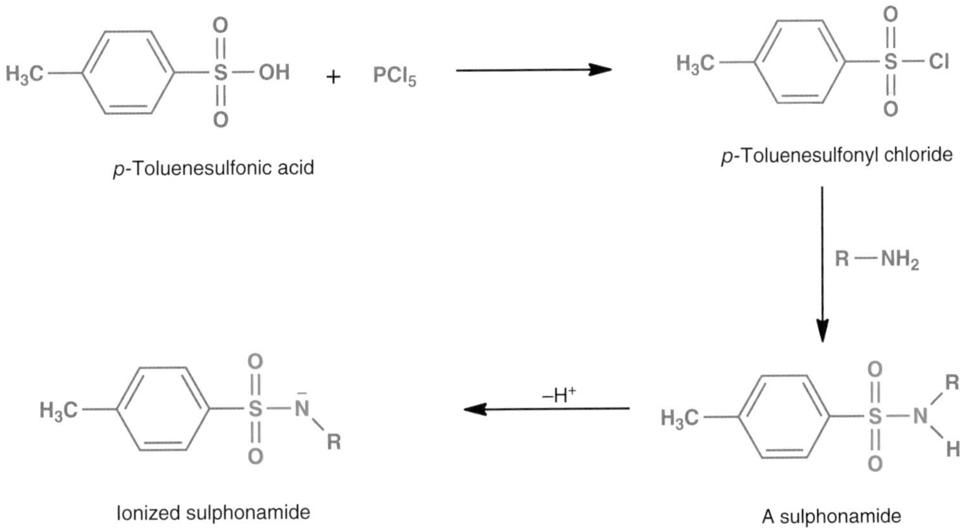

p-Toluenesulfonic acid

p-Toluenesulfonyl chloride

$R-NH_2$

$-H^+$

Ionized sulphonamide

A sulphonamide

The best known use of sulphonamides is as antibacterial agents. However, they also act as inhibitors of carbonic anhydrase, a zinc-containing enzyme that catalyses the interconversion of carbon dioxide and water to carbonic acid; the carbonic acid is subsequently converted into hydrogen carbonate (bicarbonate) ions by the loss of H^+.

$$CO_2 + H_2O \rightleftharpoons H_2CO_3 \rightleftharpoons H^+ + HCO_3^-$$

Sulphonamides have an acidic hydrogen and are ionized by the loss of a proton at physiological pH. The ionized sulphonamide interacts with the zinc ion at the active site of carbonic anhydrase. Acetazolamide, whose structure is shown in Figure 8.35, is an example of a sulphonamide carbonic anhydrase inhibitor that may be given by injection. It can be used to treat glaucoma, because the inhibition of carbonic anhydrase that it promotes reduces pressure in the eye. The BNF recommends that the injection is given intravenously, as intramuscular injections may be painful because of the alkalinity of the solution.

The sulfonyl group readily attracts electrons. Consequently, sulfonates are good leaving groups. This characteristic is exploited in sulfonate esters such as busulfan, where the C–O

Self-check 8.17

Why do you think that aqueous solutions of acetazolamide are alkaline? Hint: acetazolamide (see Figure 8.35) is formulated as the sodium salt.

Figure 8.35 Acetazolamide

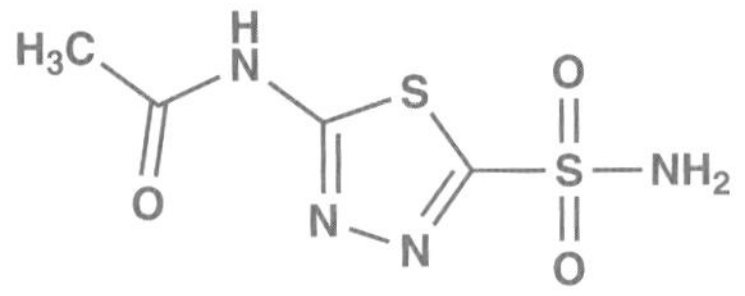

Figure 8.36 Mechanism of action of busulfan

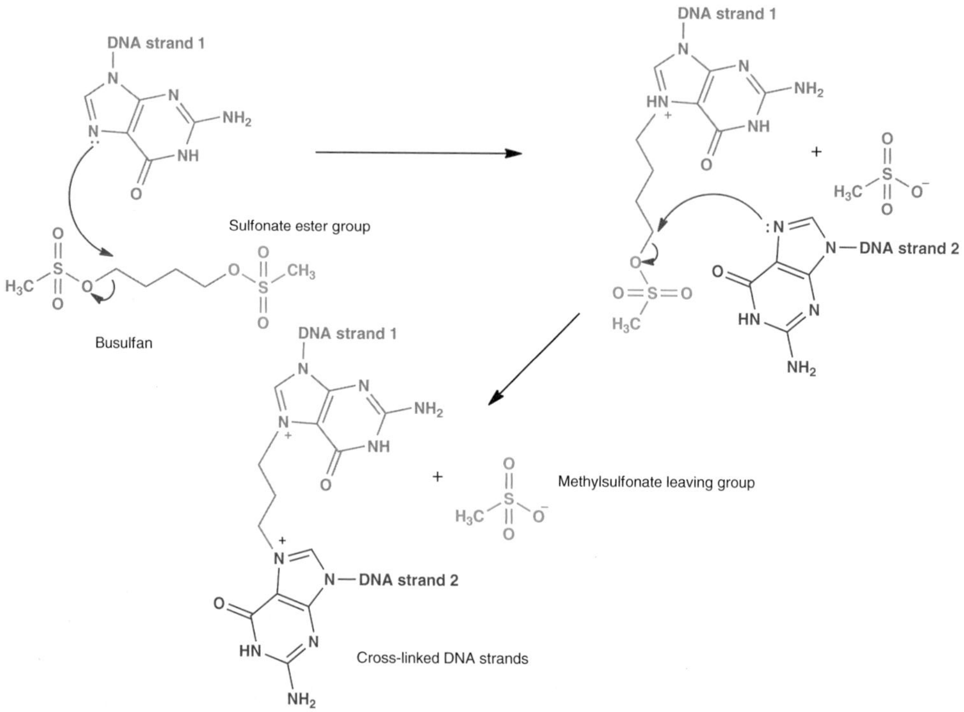

bond is readily broken. The reaction is an S_N2 type reaction and results in cross-linking DNA and the release of methyl sulfonate, as illustrated in Figure 8.36.

> S_N2 reactions are discussed in greater detail in Chapter 5, 'Alcohols, phenols, ethers, organic halogen compounds, and amines'.

Derivatives of sulfuric acid

The highest oxidation state of sulfur is +6, as seen in sulfuric acid. The sulfur in this compound forms two double bonds with oxygen atoms and two single bonds to hydroxyl groups. Sulfuric acid is a strong dibasic acid and is capable of forming hydrogen sulfate (HSO_4^-) and sulfate (SO_4^{2-}) ions. Amine drugs are formulated as sulfate salts to give water solubility; examples include morphine sulfate and quinine sulfate.

Sulfuric acid can form sulfate esters (also called sulfoesters or organosulfates) in the same way that phosphoric acid can form phosphoesters (phosphate esters).

Sodium dodecyl sulfate is a widely used detergent. It can be formed by treating dodecyl alcohol with sulfur trioxide to form dodecyl hydrogen sulfate, which, if neutralized with sodium hydroxide or sodium carbonate, gives sodium dodecyl sulfate. The structure of sodium dodecyl sulfate is shown in Figure 8.37, with the sulfate ester group shown in green.

Dodecyl alcohol may be obtained from coconut oil, and has the trivial name lauryl alcohol. Consequently, sodium dodecyl sulfate is usually known as sodium lauryl sulfate outside the laboratory. Sodium dodecyl sulfate is amphipathic: it has a polar head and a long non-polar tail, which is capable of solubilizing oils and fats and does not form insoluble salts with calcium and magnesium ions. It is therefore very often used in the laboratory to dissociate and

Figure 8.37   Sodium dodecyl sulfate

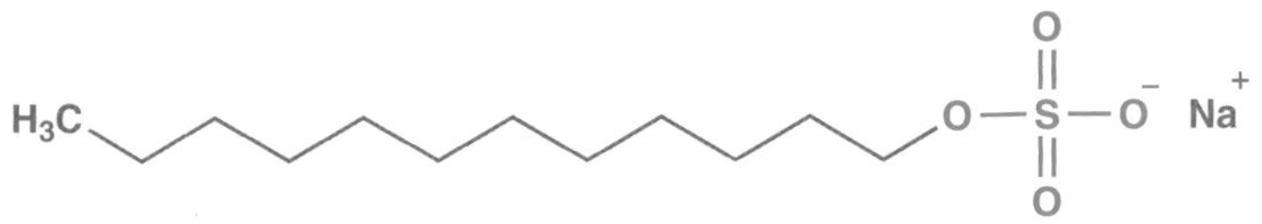

Box 8.5   Sodium lauryl sulfate in toothpaste

Not surprisingly, sodium lauryl sulfate (SLS) is an irritant, because it solubilizes proteins. Indeed, anecdotal evidence suggests that SLS in toothpastes exacerbates the pain caused by mouth ulcers. Mouth ulcers can be caused by serious disease, but they are more usually symptoms of stress or benign hormonal imbalance. Sufferers may benefit from using an SLS-free toothpaste.

---

solubilize macromolecules such as proteins. (We say that it is an 'anionic surfactant'.) It is also used in most toothpastes—which is why they foam (see Box 8.5).

> Surfactants are discussed in Chapter 5, 'Alcohols, phenols, ethers, organic halogen compounds, and amines'.

Sulfate esters are also formed in the body; sulfates conjugate to alcohol and phenol functional groups. For example, the phenolic hydroxyl in salbutamol is a site for sulfate conjugation. The reaction shown in Figure 8.38 leads to the formation of a sulfate ester which is inactive and polar, and so is easily excreted in the urine. The sulfate ester is polar because only one of the available oxygen atoms is esterified; the remaining –OH acts as a strong acid (pK_a 1–2) so it will be ionized at physiological pH. Sulfotransferase enzymes, which transfer sulfate from 3′-phosphoadenosine-5′-phosphosulfate to hydroxyl groups, are found in the liver, intestine and kidney, which are the main sites of drug metabolism in the body.

Thiocarbonyl compounds (thiones)

In the previous few sections we have been looking at the different oxidation states of sulfur. In the following examples we will consider the replacement of oxygen in carbonyl groups, by sulfur, to give thiocarbonyl compounds, which are commonly called thiones. Thiones can have significantly different properties from their parent carbonyls, though they can tautomerize in the same way that carbonyl groups undergo keto–enol tautomerism, as illustrated in Figure 8.39.

Figure 8.38   Metabolic sulfate ester formation

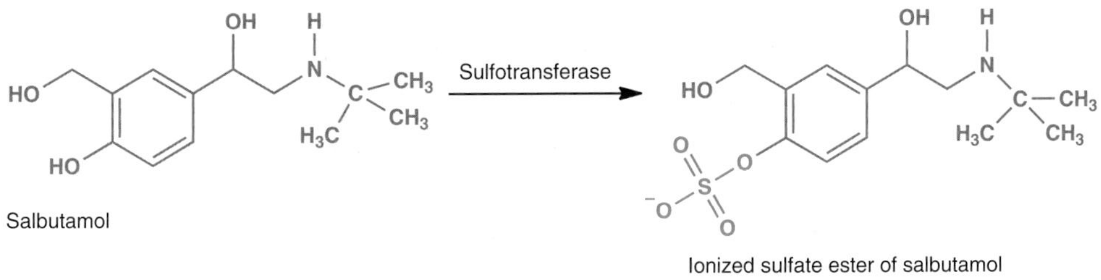

Salbutamol

Ionized sulfate ester of salbutamol

Figure 8.39 Keto–enol and thione–lactam tautomerism

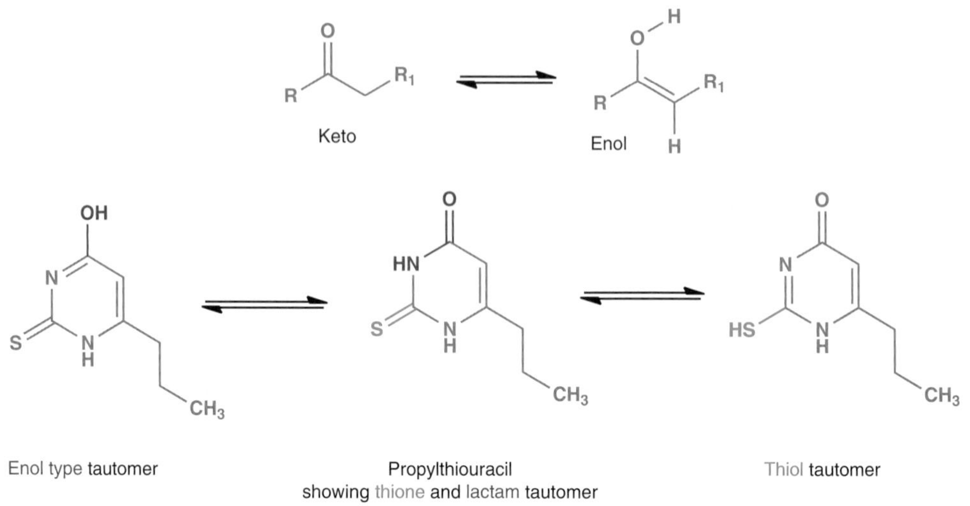

Keto

Enol

Enol type tautomer

Propylthiouracil
showing thione and lactam tautomer

Thiol tautomer

> More details on keto-enol tautomerism can be found in Chapter 6, 'The carbonyl group and its chemistry'.

The antithyroid compound propylthiouracil, whose structure is shown in Figure 8.39, illustrates how amides and the thione equivalent can tautomerize. The action of propylthiouracil may partly depend on its ability to function as a thiol.

The thione double bond is normally less polarized than the double bond of carbonyls, resulting in the compounds being less polar. The biological effect of this can be seen by considering the barbiturates, pentobarbital and thiopental. The only difference between the two compounds is that pentobarbital has three oxygen functions, whereas one of the oxygen atoms in thiopental is replaced by sulfur, as shown in Figure 8.40. The change in polarity in the compounds is reflected in the log P values—2.1 for pentobarbital and 2.9 for thiopental—with thiopental being more lipophilic. This change in log P has a significant effect on the biological properties of the drugs, which influences their therapeutic use.

Pentobarbital belongs to the barbiturate class of drugs, which were introduced as hypnotics in the early part of the twentieth century. These drugs were very popular until the 1960s

Figure 8.40 Pentobarbital and thiopental

Pentobarbital

Thiopental

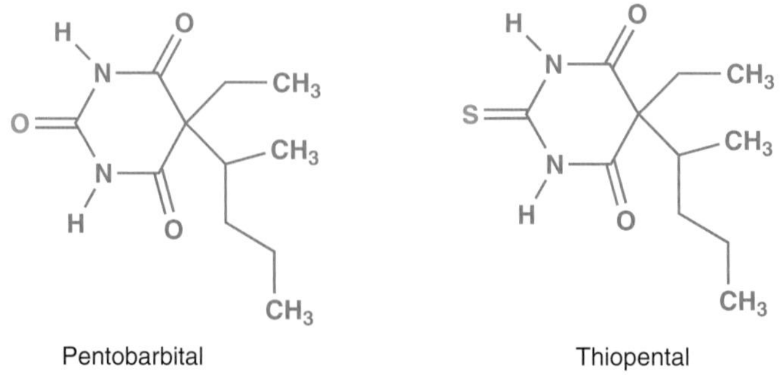

when apparently safer drugs, such as the benzodiazepines, started to replace them. In the BNF, the only barbiturates appropriate for treating insomnia are amobarbital, butobarbital and secobarbital—and even these are only on a named-patient basis. Thiopental as the sodium salt, however, is still used as a short-acting intravenous anaesthetic. Because it is very lipophilic, it quickly crosses the blood–brain barrier, producing very rapid anaesthesia; it can take effect before the patient can count to 10.

The action of thiopental ends when it is redistributed into the fat deposits of the body. The resulting equilibration lowers the concentration of thiopental in the brain, and the anaesthetic effect wears off. The uptake of pentobarbital into the brain is slower, so that the patient takes longer to go to sleep; the redistribution of pentobarbital into other tissues is also slower, so it takes much longer for the blood level in the brain to fall and the patient to wake up.

- Sulfur can exist in oxidation states from −2 to +6, and all states are found in pharmaceutical and biological molecules. The wide range of oxidation states results from its ability to use d-orbitals to accept electrons.
- The sulfur atom is bigger than the oxygen atom and is less electronegative.
- Thiols and thiophenols have similar chemistry to alcohols and phenols.
- Thiols can form complexes with metal ions.
- Oxidation of thioethers can produce sulfoxides and sulfones.
- Sulfonic acid and sulfuric acid derivatives are strong acids and can be used to produce water-soluble derivatives.

Self-check 8.18

To test your understanding of the role of sulfur-containing compounds in pharmacy, look up the structures of the compounds listed in Table 8.8. For each compound, identify the functional group that contains sulfur, predict the oxidation state of the sulfur and indicate the therapeutic use of the compound or its role in metabolism.

Table 8.8 Sulfur-containing compounds in pharmacy

Compound	Functional group	Oxidation state of sulfur	Therapeutic use or biological function of compound
e.g. gentamicin sulfate	sulfate	+6	antibiotic
thioridazine			
bretylium tosilate			
sulfamethoxazole			
dimercaprol			
carbimazole			
glutathione			

Our bodies need elements other than carbon, hydrogen, nitrogen and oxygen to allow us to function; imbalances in these elements can have serious effects on our health. Many drugs and medicines rely on the presence of both metallic and non-metallic elements to produce their biological effect and for their formulation.

For metals:

- Most metals usually function as the cation.

- Metal ions can usually interact by ionic bonding or complex formation.

- Iron has activity both through complex formation and through redox reactions.

- Ligands are molecules that contain groups capable of acting as Lewis bases by donating electrons.

Phosphorus is found in both the normal biochemistry of the body and in drugs.

- Phosphorus is usually pentavalent in pharmaceutical and biological molecules because it can make use of d orbitals.

- Phosphoric acid is tribasic and the 2nd ionization is important for regulating body pH.

- Phosphoric acid can form esters and anhydrides in the same way as carboxylic acids.

- Phosphate esters are important for biological molecules and can be used to produce water-soluble derivatives of drugs.

Sulfur can have an oxidation number from –2 to +6, and all states are found in pharmaceutically relevant molecules. It has so many oxidation states because it can use the d orbitals to share electrons from oxygen atoms.

- Some of the uses of sulfur in drugs depend on the fact that it is a bigger atom than oxygen.

- Thiols have a similar chemistry to alcohols.

- Although thiones can undergo tautomerism in the same way that ketones can, they tend to be less polar because of the larger size of the sulfur atom.

- Sulfonate and sulfate esters are polar and can increase water-solubility of drugs.

Although most drug action can be explained in terms of the chemistry of the elements, there are still a number of drugs for which the exact mechanism of action has not been determined.

More in-depth coverage of inorganic chemistry may be found in books such as:

Overton, T., Rourke, J. and Weller, M. *Inorganic Chemistry*, 7th edn. Oxford University Press, 2018. ISBN 9780198768128.

Dewick, P. M., *Essentials of Organic Chemistry, for Students of Pharmacy, Medicinal Chemistry and Biological Chemistry*. Wiley, 2006.

This provides good detail on hydrolysis of ATP and ADP and release of energy.

Patrick, G. *Introduction to Medicinal Chemistry*, 6th edn. Oxford University Press, 2017.

This provides mechanisms for the action of drugs.

Rayner-Canham, G. *Descriptive Inorganic Chemistry*, 6th edn. W. H. Freeman, 2014.

Other books you might find helpful are:

The British National Formulary (BNF).

Kean, S. *The Disappearing Spoon*. Doubleday, 2011.

> This is a slightly different book which is full of anecdotes about the elements and their discovery and effects.

Pocket clinical pharmacy reference books such as:

Wiffen, P., Mitchell, M., Snelling, M. and Stoner, N. *The Oxford Handbook of Clinical Pharmacy*, 3rd edn. Oxford University Press, 2017.

> These are good for providing normal ranges of ions in body fluids and infusion fluids.

http://www.chemguide.co.uk

> Provides good clear explanations and diagrams based on A-level syllabi, which may help you with revising some of your previous chemistry.

Online, you might like to research related news articles. For example:

- Zinc can be an 'effective treatment' for common colds: http://www.bbc.co.uk/news/health-12462910

- Zinc tablets may shorten the duration of a cold: http://www.independent.co.uk/lifestyle/health-and-families/health-news/zinc-tablets-may-shorten-the-duration-of-a-cold-7720704.html

Meyers, S and Norouzi, S, Diabetes Management Vol 6 90–91, The relationship between zinc and insulin signalling - the implications for type 2 diabetes, 2016.

Lankshear, A. J., Sheldon, T. A., Lowson, K. V., Watt, I. S. and Wright, J. 'Evaluation of the implementation of the alert issued by the UK National Patient Safety Agency on the storage and handling of potassium chloride concentrate solution', *Qual. Saf. Health Care* 2005, 14:196–201.

Self-check

For the answers to the Self-Check questions in Chapter 8, visit the online resources which accompany this textbook.

CHAPTER 9

NUCLEIC ACIDS
Alex White And Andrew Evans

In order to appreciate the varied roles of the molecules which are the subject of the next four chapters, it is necessary to describe the classes of cells which form the basis of all life. Information will be presented on the basic structure and functions of cells before considering the molecules involved in their structure and function. This chapter will then outline the chemistry of nucleic acids. These biologically important molecules are larger than most molecules we have met in the preceding chapters, and they are often referred to as macromolecules. At first glance the study of such complex molecules may seem demanding, but the principles of chemistry, presented in the preceding chapters of this book, can be applied to the study of these molecules to help us understand their functions in the cells of our body. In addition the involvement of nucleic acids in the genetic code will be explored, covering how it is stored, used, protected, repaired and passed from generation to generation. Diseases that can come about when our genetic code is damaged and not repaired will also be discussed.

Learning objectives

Having read this chapter you are expected to be able to:

- appreciate the difference between prokaryotic and eukaryotic cells
- explain the chemical nature of nucleotides and nucleic acids
- discuss the biochemistry of nucleic acids and how they function at the molecular level
- know how the genetic code works
- understand how the code is transcribed and translated into protein
- describe the basic processes of DNA replication
- explain how, as a result of damage to DNA, diseases may arise
- recognize the potential of current and future genetic therapies.

9.1 THE UNIT OF LIFE: THE CELL

We can consider the cell as a self-sustained parcel or *unit of life*. This is because cells are present in all living organisms, whether they exist as a single cell or a collection of cells. Cells also contain all the necessary information and machinery to be able to sustain and perpetuate life.

Common features of cells

Despite the vast diversity of life we have on Earth, living organisms are made from cells and all cells have some common features. These include:

- They have all inherited from their predecessors, and can also pass on to their daughter cells, the *instruction manual of life*, or the genetic code. We will look into this further in Section 9.3 'The instruction manual of life: the genetic code'.

- All cells also have a *cellular membrane,* sometimes called a *plasma membrane*. This cellular membrane is a lipid bilayer (consists of two layers of lipids) that acts as a barrier to separate the inside of the cell from the external environment. Although some molecules are able to pass though the cellular membrane, it is a selective barrier to most. Many proteins are incorporated into the cellular membrane, and these have various functions. Some of them act as transporters or channels that use energy to actively transport specific molecules such as nutrients, waste products, or ions into or out of the cell. Others form selective transporters or channels that allow passive (energy-free) movement of specific molecules, such as drugs, across this barrier. Thus, the cellular membrane regulates what enters and exits the cell.

- All cells carry out metabolism to produce energy and make new molecules

- Finally, all cells are capable of movement of some form. This can be just the movement of individual components within the cell to assist certain cellular processes, or the movement of the whole cell.

> Chapter 11, 'Carbohydrates and carbohydrate metabolism', goes into more detail about cellular metabolic pathways.

Basic cell structure of prokaryotic and eukaryotic cells

Most cells can be classified into one of the two main evolutionary branches. The first branch is the *prokaryotes*, which are the simplest forms of life and tend to exist as single-celled entities. The second branch is the *eukaryotes*; these cells are more complex and whereas some can exist in a single-celled form, others form multicellular organisms like you and me. Although there are similarities between all cells, there are also fundamental differences between these two classifications, which we will look at next.

The fundamental difference between a prokaryotic and eukaryotic cell is the fact that eukaryotes have a membrane-bound nucleus (also known as a *karyon*) that separately contains the genetic material, whereas prokaryotes do not. Prokaryotes are relatively small cells, with a total volume about a thousand times smaller than that of a typical eukaryotic cell. We have about ten times more prokaryotic cells in our gut than the eukaryotic cells that make up our whole body!

Eukaryotes are subdivided into plants, animals, fungi or protists (protozoa and algae), whereas prokaryotes have traditionally been subdivided into *bacteria* and *archaea*. You are probably familiar with bacterial genera such as *Streptococcus*, *Salmonella*, and *Escherichia* because they are associated with disease. However, the genera of archaea, for example *Haloarchaea* or *Pyrococcus*, are not that well known, probably because they are generally not thought to cause disease. Archaea are about the same size and shape as bacteria, but the cell wall and cellular membrane of archaea are made of components different from those of bacteria. Box 9.1 further explores the classification of archaea.

Archaea are often found living in some of the most extreme environments on earth, in conditions where humans would not be able to survive. These include high temperatures, often above 100 °C, such as those seen in deep-sea vents. Some of the chemical processes carried out by archaea are similar to those of bacteria, but some have also been found to be similar to those of eukaryotes. More recently, a number of genetic differences and similarities between archaea, bacteria and eukaryotes have been revealed. Because of these differences and similarities, many researchers now believe that archaea should actually be classified separately from prokaryotes and eukaryotes.

Surrounding the cell

All cells have a cellular membrane, which allows the passage of water and gases such as oxygen and carbon dioxide. Therefore, if there is a higher osmotic pressure within the cells than in the environment outside the cells, water can enter, swell and ultimately burst (*lyse*) the cells. This would result in cell death (*cytolysis*). If you look at Figure 9.1(A) you will see that prokaryotic cells, in addition to the cellular membrane, usually also have a rigid *cell wall* that is sometimes surrounded by a *capsule*. The rigid cell wall is a simple yet effective way of preventing cytolysis from occurring. It consists of *peptidoglycans*, chains of amino acids and sugars which have a strong lattice structure. The cell wall is the target of a number of classes of antibiotic drugs that we use, including the β-lactam antibiotics (such as penicillin), that work by inhibiting the production of the cell wall. The capsule in prokaryotic cells provides an additional protective layer. It is a slimy layer, full of polysaccharides and water, which acts as a shield preventing the cell from being destroyed by other cells, or being dehydrated, and it can even act as a reserve of nutrients for the cell.

Plants, fungi, and algae also have a peptidoglycan cell wall, whereas animal cells do not because they are able to control their osmotic pressure. Animal cells, however, have a *cytoskeleton*, which allows them to adapt to a variety of shapes and structures. For example, a single nerve cell in our body can be extremely thin but over 1.5 metres in length, whereas cuboidal epithelial cells are an approximately 0.02 millimetre cube! Figure 9.1(B) shows a typical eukaryotic animal cell.

You will also notice from Figure 9.1 that prokaryotes often have structures protruding from their surface whereas eukaryotes generally do not. The *pili* are hair-like additions that allow the cell to attach to other cells and facilitate the sharing of genetic material. Some prokaryotes also have tail-like features called *flagella*, which rotate to propel the cell forward, enabling the cell to swim.

Inside the cell

The interior of all cells (prokaryotic or eukaryotic) is bathed in a highly regulated aqueous solution called the *cytoplasm*. Within the cytoplasm of eukaryotes there are membrane-bound structures, collectively known as organelles, each filled with its own specific fluid. An important organelle already mentioned is the nucleus. Prokaryotes do not have this level of structure. As they have no nucleus, prokaryotes usually carry their genetic code in the form of a condensed single circular DNA molecule within the cytoplasm. This is sometimes referred to as

Figure 9.1 Basic structure of (A) prokaryotic and (B) eukaryotic cells

(A) Prokaryotic cell

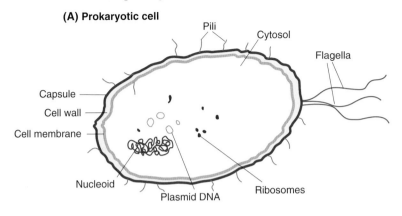

(B) Eukaryotic cell

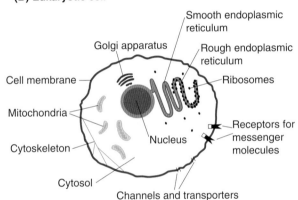

the *nucleoid*. In addition, prokaryotes can also have relatively small circular DNA molecules called *plasmids*. Plasmids can be transferred from one cell to another via their pili. This means that certain genes can be shared. For example, if a bacterium develops genetic resistance to an antibiotic it can quickly share this with the whole population, making it resistant to that antibiotic.

The organelles present in eukaryotic cells carry out specialized functions within the cell, similar to the way our organs carry out specialized functions in our bodies. Different eukaryotes have defined differences in their organelles, some of which are described below:

- *Chloroplasts* are only present in plants and protists. These organelles can generate energy from sunlight.

- *Mitochondria* are present in virtually all eukaryotic cells. They are often described as the power stations of the cell because they produce most of the cell's energy in the form of adenosine-5′-triphosphate (ATP). Mitochondria are about the size of a typical prokaryotic cell, and eukaryotic cells may contain in excess of 2,000 of them. They have their own DNA, the origins of which are discussed in Box 9.2.

- *Ribosomes* are where proteins are assembled from amino acids.

> **Box 9.2 Endosymbiotic theory**
>
> The endosymbiotic theory was first proposed in 1905 (*endo* means 'within' and *symbiotic* means 'cooperative'). Owing to some striking similarities between free-living prokaryotes called cyanobacteria and the chloroplasts found in plant cells, it was proposed that chloroplasts were once also free-living cyanobacteria-like prokaryotes. However, it was not until the 1960s, with the use of more advanced techniques in cell and molecular biology, that this theory was taken seriously. Many scientists now believe that chloroplasts and mitochondria are actually direct descendants of prokaryotic cells—cells that were engulfed by ancestral eukaryotes and existed and evolved within them! These organelles have their own DNA, which has similarities to prokaryotic DNA, and they replicate independently of the cell.

- The *endoplasmic reticulum* is a network of membrane-bound folds that surrounds the nucleus. The rough endoplasmic reticulum appears rough because it is covered with ribosomes, which carry out the processing and folding of new proteins. Lipids are produced by the smooth endoplasmic reticulum, which does not contain ribosomes.

- The *Golgi apparatus* further modifies and packages the proteins and lipids produced by the endoplasmic reticulum.

> There is more detail about the role of ATP in cellular energy production in Chapter 11, 'Carbohydrates and carbohydrate metabolism'.

From single cells to multicellular organisms

Eukaryotic cells often exist within multicellular organisms, like the human body, and communication between cells is essential for the survival of the whole organism. Cells communicate with each other by releasing or receiving messenger molecules. These messages are received by receptors found within cells or on the cellular membranes of responding cells.

In addition to communicating with each other, cells within multicellular organisms must become *specialized* to fulfil specific needs required by the organism as a whole. These specialized cells make up tissues, organs and body systems. Specialization of cells occurs during development, by a process called **differentiation**. As cells divide during development, the daughter cells receive all the genetic information from the parental cell. However, the genes expressed by the daughter cell may be different compared with those of the parental cell, making the daughter cell functionally different. This concept is further explained in Box 9.3 later in this chapter. Clearly, the expression of genes has to be a highly controlled process, with only the appropriate genes being used at the appropriate time in the appropriate cells. In cancer, cells often lose this control and express a number of genes inappropriately, which can lead to the progression of the cancer. Before we explore gene expression, however, we must first draw our attention to the molecules that make up the genetic information.

All our cells contain identical genetic information; however, the cells differentiate to make up the various types of tissues, organs and body systems of which we are made.

Self-check 9.1

What are the two major physical differences between prokaryotes and eukaryotes?

9.2 NUCLEIC ACIDS AND NUCLEOSIDES

Two nucleic acids, DNA (DeoxyriboNucleic Acid) and RNA (RiboNucleic Acid), are of fundamental importance to biochemistry and all life on Earth. DNA is the carrier of genetic information, and is divided into specific sequences called genes. Genes are typically packaged into separate chromosomes, the distinctive structures found in nearly every cell, in every multicellular organism.

Most genes are sequences of DNA that carry instructions for making proteins. RNA, a molecule whose chemical composition is very similar to DNA, is mostly concerned with the processing of the information contained within DNA as part of the process of 'reading' the information stored in the DNA to make proteins.

Understanding the chemistry of nucleic acids is essential for many aspects of pharmaceutical science. Many important anticancer, antiviral and antibacterial drugs target nucleic acids. An understanding of nucleic acid chemistry shows us how nucleic acids work, and how drugs interact with them.

Nucleic acid structure: the backbone

DNA (see Figure 9.2A) and RNA are relatively simple biopolymers, each composed of just four monomers, known as nucleotides. Each nucleotide has three components, a phosphate group, a ribose sugar and a heterocyclic organic base. A nucleotide unit is highlighted in purple in Figure 9.2B. As nucleotides are joined together, alternating phosphate and sugar groups form the nucleic acid backbone. In DNA, the sugar component of the nucleotide is 2′-deoxyribose—a molecule of ribose lacking a hydroxyl (OH) group. In RNA, the sugar component is ribose itself.

Look at Figure 9.2 and notice how the phosphate groups are covalently bonded to two sugar groups, forming a functional group analogous to an ester. For this reason, this functional group is classified as a phospho*diester*. The acidic nature of DNA and RNA arises from the presence of this group. The P–OH group acts as an acid at physiological pH (that is, it donates its proton), making the phosphodiester negatively charged. The stability of the negatively charged oxygen group is the driving force for the loss of the proton. DNA and RNA are usually drawn with negatively charged phosphodiester groups since proton donation is always assumed to occur.

> The chemistry of phosphodiesters is dealt with in Chapter 8, 'Inorganic chemistry in pharmacy'.

Nucleic acid structure: bases

The varying nature of the base distinguishes individual nucleotides and influences the composition of the nucleic acid. DNA contains four heterocyclic bases: adenine (A), guanine (G), cytosine (C) and thymine (T). RNA differs from DNA in that uracil (U) replaces thymine. The structure of each base is shown in Figure 9.2. The single-letter abbreviations (in brackets) are usually used to denote the nucleic acid bases and have widespread acceptance. They will be used

Figure 9.2 Nucleic acid structure. (A) A model of a short sequence of DNA (12 base pairs). The nucleic acid backbone is highlighted by a grey ribbon. The bases are shown in the ball and stick format (carbon—grey; nitrogen—blue; oxygen—red. Hydrogen is omitted for clarity). (PDB code: 423d.) (B) The structure of two single base pairs. A nucleic acid nucleotide unit is highlighted in purple. Hydrogen bonds are indicated by dashed lines

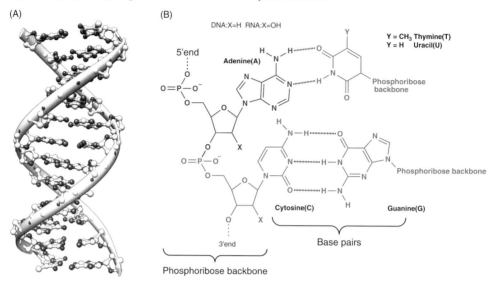

(A)　　　　　　　　　(B)

DNA:X=H　RNA:X=OH

Y = CH₃ Thymine(T)
Y = H　Uracil(U)

5'end
Adenine(A)
Phosphoribose backbone

Cytosine(C)　　Guanine(G)

3'end
Base pairs

Phosphoribose backbone

DNA and RNA are made up of nucleotides that are joined together by phosphodiester groups.

Self-check 9.2

Be sure you can identify the base pairs in Figure 9.2A. These are the *rungs* of the DNA *ladder*. Make sure you understand how these base pairs are related to the base pair structures shown in Figure 9.2B.

---

in this chapter and you will encounter these abbreviations throughout scientific literature. It is very useful to learn and remember them. Each base is bonded to the nucleic acid backbone via the sugar group.

Base pairing in nucleic acids

The interaction between bases is the key to understanding nucleic acid function. The bases are examples of heterocycles, organic ring systems that contain an element other than carbon as part of that ring. The bases come in two varieties, purines and pyrimidines. A pyrimidine contains a single six-membered ring, whereas a purine has a bicyclic structure with a six-membered ring fused to a five-membered ring. Both purines and pyrimidines are nitrogen-containing heterocycles. The presence of electron rich heteroatoms and other functional groups such as amino (NH2) and carbonyl (C=O) groups allow for the formation of hydrogen bonds between base pairs. As we see in Chapter 2, individual hydrogen bonds are rather weak, typically 1–5%

of the strength of a covalent bond. Despite their weakness, networks of *many hydrogen bonds* within a molecule are much stronger and convey great stability to macromolecules.

The pairing between bases is very specific. In DNA, *A always pairs with T and G always pairs with C*. RNA does not contain T so A pairs with U instead. Note that two hydrogen bonds are formed in the A−T and A−U base pairs, whereas three hydrogen bonds stabilize the G−C base pair. Each base pair contains a purine and pyrimidine. These pairings result from the structure of each base; look at the base pairs in Figure 9.2 and notice how the functional groups complement each other perfectly. This is essential for the formation of the hydrogen bond network.

The DNA double helix

The properties outlined above give rise to the well-known and very distinctive DNA double helix. Looking at the model of DNA in Figure 9.2, we see two separate DNA backbones wrapping around each other about a central axis. The structure is held together by the network of hydrogen bonds formed between the inward facing bases. It is hard to detect or visualize hydrogen bonds by common physical techniques (e.g. NMR), but their existence is strongly suggested by the orientation of the bases towards each other within the double helix.

As a consequence of this structure, the base sequence is complementary between the two strands. Recall that A always pairs with T and C always pairs with G. Therefore, if you know the sequence of one strand, you can deduce the sequence of the other. The strands run in opposite (or antiparallel) directions to each other. The direction of each strand is defined by the unbonded groups at its extreme ends: a ribose 5′-OH is located at one end (the 5′ end), with the strand running towards an unbonded ribose 3′-OH at the other (3′) end. By convention, bases are always listed in the 5′ to 3′ direction. Therefore, a particular sequence of DNA could be communicated in the following way:

5′-AAGCGATAGCTC-3′

This is much easier than drawing the full chemical structure! This shorthand method is used to communicate information about nucleic acids, and it ignores the common, repetitive parts of the structure. But you should always remember the more complex structure behind the shorthand notation!

Ribonucleic acid (RNA)

RNA differs from DNA: it usually exists as a single strand and folds into a greater variety of three-dimensional shapes than DNA. The structure of each folded strand is stabilized by the strand interacting *with itself* by base pairing. There are three main types of RNA: messenger

> The structure of DNA is a double helix of two antiparallel polynucleotide strands. The two strands are joined together by a network of hydrogen bonds between purine and pyrimidine bases on the inside of the helix.

Self-check 9.3

If 5'-AAGCGATAGCTC-3' is the sequence of one strand of a short section of DNA, what is the sequence of the other strand? Remember that a DNA sequence is always listed in the 5'→3' direction.

> RNA molecules, which contain copies of the genetic code, are produced by transcription from DNA.

RNA (mRNA), transfer RNA (tRNA) and ribosomal RNA (rRNA). The functions of these molecules are covered in more depth elsewhere in this chapter, but to summarize: single stranded mRNA is transcribed from a complementary strand of DNA and travels to the ribosome, a structure that is composed of rRNA and protein. The ribosome translates the mRNA sequence into proteins, using the amino acids attached to tRNAs.

> Genetic code, genes, transcription and translation are discussed in more detail in Section 9.3.

9.3 THE INSTRUCTION MANUAL OF LIFE: THE GENETIC CODE

The *instruction manual of life*, the genetic code, containing all the information that is required to make, sustain and proliferate life, is stored in DNA molecules packaged into chromosomes. When our cells require specific proteins, the corresponding sections of the genetic code that contain the relevant information, the *genes*, are expressed, as described in Box 9.3. Expression of genes means that the coded instructions within the specific genes are copied into RNA molecules (this process is called *transcription*) in the first instance, followed by decoding and protein assembly (this process is known as *translation*).

Transcription

For gene expression to occur, the information held within the genetic code must move from the nucleus, where it is stored, to the ribosomes in the cytoplasm, where proteins are made. The entire DNA within the nucleus is too big to be effectively moved and it would be too risky to expose the original copy of the genetic code to degradation by certain **enzymes** present in the cytoplasm. Therefore, the genetic code is first copied and this copy, in the form of an RNA molecule, then carries the information to the ribosomes. This process is called *transcription*.

> Transcription results in the production of complementary RNA molecules that contain copies of sections of the genetic code which then relocate to the cytoplasm.

Box 9.3   One size fits all!

Everything we are at the molecular and microscopic level is determined by our individual genetic code. This genetic code is held in each of our cells, yet our cells are not all the same. This is because different genes are expressed in different cells. Of course, many genes are expressed or 'switched on' in all cells and these give rise to common proteins that all cells require. The differences between cells arise because they express a different selection of genes and so contain a different array of proteins. A different array of proteins within cells gives rise to different cell structures and different cell functions. However, your cells each still contain all the instructions that would be needed to create a whole new you.

Transcribed RNA molecules have exactly the same sequence of bases as the **coding strand** of the DNA gene sequence, except that thymine (T) is substituted by uracil (U). It is worth noting that not all of the transcribed RNA molecules are destined to be translated into proteins. The cell uses some RNA for other purposes. There are several different types of RNA molecules in cells, including:

- Ribosomal RNA (rRNA) is used to form part of the ribosome.
- Transfer RNA (tRNA) is used to transfer amino acids to the ribosome, where they are attached to the newly forming protein.
- Messenger RNA (mRNA) contains the copy of the gene code that is used to make proteins.
- Micro RNA (miRNA) is small RNA molecules that bind complementary nucleotide sequences found in target mRNA molecules to form double-stranded RNA. Double-stranded RNA is destroyed by cellular enzymes and therefore miRNAs can regulate the translation of mRNA into protein.
- Small nuclear RNA (snRNA) has a functional role within the nucleus.

Genes that code for proteins are, however, copied into *messenger RNA (mRNA)* molecules. Enzymes found in the cytoplasm eventually degrade the transcribed RNA molecules. The original genetic code, however, remains intact as DNA within the nucleus, and can be copied into more RNA when next required.

Key features of transcription

Transcription is a complex process that involves a large number of different molecules within the nucleus. We will only outline the key features of the process here. Figure 9.3 shows how all the molecules involved interact during the process of transcription.

Figure 9.3 The RNA Pol II transcription initiation complex and the arrangement of regulatory sequences. RNA Poll II, RNA polymerase II; URE, upstream regulatory elements; Inr, initiator

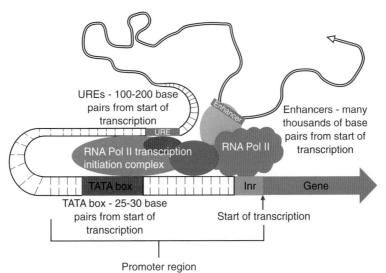

- *RNA polymerases* are enzyme complexes that are responsible for producing the comple-mentary RNA transcripts from genes. Humans and all other eukaryotes have three different versions of this enzyme complex: RNA polymerase I, II, and III, each responsible for tran-scribing different RNA molecules. We will specifically look at the role of RNA polymerase II (RNA Pol II), as this enzyme complex, consisting of 12 subunits, is involved in the transcrip-tion of the protein-coding genes into mRNA.

- *Promoters* are regulatory sequences of nucleotides within the DNA and act as signals to the nuclear proteins. As they are found upstream of the genes they promote transcription. These signals are diverse in nature and may contain a number of different sections, including:

  - *Initiator (Inr)* sequences, where transcription of a gene starts.

  - *TATA boxes*, which have a sequence of 5'-TATA(A or T)A(A or T)-3' and are located about 25 to 30 bases upstream from the start point of transcription.

  - *Upstream regulatory elements* (*UREs*), which regulate the level of gene expression. Genes that have UREs are more actively expressed than genes without them. These URE se-quences are located 100 to 200 bases upstream of the start point of transcription. Pro-moters may have one or many UREs and may also have more than one copy of the same URE. *Regulatory proteins* bind to UREs and stimulate the RNA Pol II initiation complex to start transcription.

- *Enhancers* are nucleotide sequences outside of the promoter region. *Activator proteins* bind to enhancer sequences and very strongly stimulate expression of their associated genes. These sequences can be about 200 bases in length and can be found many thousands of bases up-stream or downstream from the start point of transcription, though they are usually spa-tially very close to the promoter due to the highly packaged nature of DNA in our nuclei.

- *Transcription factors* are a series of nuclear proteins, including regulatory and activator pro-teins, which bind to the enhancer and/or promoter sequences of a gene. These transcription factors can then interact with the RNA Pol II enzyme complex to form the RNA Pol II initia-tion complex to promote the initiation of transcription.

- *Polyadenylation signals* are sequences of nucleotides found at the end of a gene-coding region of DNA. This sequence signals the end of transcription of a gene into mRNA by the RNA Pol II enzyme complex. The corresponding sequence on the mRNA transcript (5'-AAUAAA-3') triggers cleavage of the transcript and the addition of a couple of hundred adenine (A) nu-cleotides (*polyadenylation*) by specific proteins at the 3' end, forming what is known as the *poly(A) tail*.

Key stages of transcription

Transcription proceeds through three stages:

- *Initiation* involves the formation the *RNA Pol II transcription initiation complex*, consisting of many proteins or transcription factors that associate in a sequential fashion upon the TATA box within the promoter of a gene. Some of these proteins have a role in locally unravel-ling the packaged DNA, so allowing other proteins to access the promoter. One of the last proteins to join this growing complex is RNA Pol II, which is positioned at the site of the start of transcription. The RNA Pol II transcription initiation complex is shown in Figure 9.3. In highly active genes the regulatory proteins bind to UREs, and activator proteins bind to the enhancer sequences. These regulatory and activator proteins interact directly with and stimulate the RNA Pol II transcription initiation complex to initiate the start of transcription.

- *Elongation* occurs once transcription has been triggered. RNA Pol II separates from the RNA Pol II initiation complex and moves along the template strand of DNA in the 3′ → 5′ direction, unwinding the DNA double helix as it forms the mRNA transcript. Complementary nucleotides are added to the growing mRNA transcript in the 5′ → 3′ direction. The double-stranded DNA reassociates behind the progressing RNA Pol II. The mRNA molecule will have exactly the same base sequence as the coding strand gene sequence of the DNA, except that thymine (T) will be replaced by uracil (U). This mRNA molecule is known as *pre-mRNA* and requires further processing to produce a mature mRNA molecule. This processing includes the addition of a 'chemical cap' (7-methylguanosine) to the 5′ end of the growing pre-mRNA transcript, which protects the molecule from being quickly degraded by other enzymes found in the cell.

- *Termination* occurs when RNA Pol II releases the mRNA transcript. This takes place about 1,000 to 2,000 base pairs downstream of the polyadenylation signal (5′-AATAAA-3′) found at the end of a gene. The mechanism of terminating transcription in eukaryotes is not fully understood. The corresponding polyadenylation signal (5′-AAUAAA-3′) that is copied within the mRNA transcript acts as a signal for further modification by polyadenylation, which is the addition of a couple of hundred adenine (A) nucleotides at the 3′ end to form the poly(A) tail. One of the roles of the poly(A) tail is to inhibit rapid degradation of the mRNA by enzymes in the cytoplasm, thereby allowing time for the translation of the mRNA into protein to take place. Some genes contain sequences called *introns*, which do not code for protein. The protein-coding sequences of these genes are known as *exons*. Any intron sequences copied within the mRNA are removed, and the coding sequences are joined up together. This step, known as *splicing*, results in the production of a mature mRNA molecule. The mature mRNA is then transported to the cytoplasm to be translated into protein.

Translation

Translation is the process that generally follows transcription of mRNA. In translation, the nucleotide sequence, initially transcribed from the genes into an mRNA molecule, is translated into a polypeptide sequence. Before we discuss the process of translation we must first consider how the genetic code is read.

We previously likened the genetic code to a language, and the nucleotides to the letters of that language. The words of the genetic code language, however, are only ever written in a sequence of three letters or base sequence triplets called *codons*. There are 64 possible words or codons in the language of our genetic code, as shown in Table 9.1. These codons code either for a single amino acid or for the process of translation to start or stop.

From Table 9.1 you can see that the codon AUG codes for methionine, but it also acts as a 'start' signal for translation. Therefore, methionine is the first amino acid added during translation. Codons UAG, UGA, and UAA, however, all act as 'stop' translation signals and do not code for any amino acid.

Transcription is a complex three-phase process whereby genes are copied into RNA molecules.

Table 9.1 The genetic code

First letter		Second letter: U		Second letter: C		Second letter: A		Second letter: G		Third letter
		U		C		A		G		
U	UUU	Phenylalanine	UCU	Serine	UAU	Tyrosine	UGU	Cysteine	U
U	UUC		UCC		UAC		UGU		C
U	UUA	Leucine	UCA		UAA	Stop condon	UGA	Stop codon	A
U	UUG		UCG		UAG	Stop condon	UGG	Tryptophan	G
C	CUU	Leucine	CCU	Proline	CAU	Histidine	CGU	Arginine	U
C	CUC		CCC		CAC		CGC		C
C	CUA		CCA		CAA	Glutamine	CGA		A
C	CUG		CCG		CAG		CGG		G
A	AUU	Isoleucine	ACU	Threonine	AAU	Asparagine	AGU	Serine	U
A	AUC		ACC		AAC		AGC		C
A	AUA		ACA		AAA	Lysine	AGA	Arginine	A
A	AUG	Methionine; Start condon	ACG		AAG		AGG		G
G	GUU	Valine	GCU	Alanine	GAU	Aspartic Acid	GGU	Glycine	U
G	GUC		GCC		GAC		GGC		C
G	GUA		GCA		GAA	Glutamic acid	GGA		A
G	GUG		GCG		GAG		GGG		G

The start codon is extremely important because it signals the exact start of the translation process, and so ensures that the codons are read in the correct *reading frame*. Consider a simple mRNA sequence such as 5′-CAUGGCUCUAGUUA-3′. Scanning along the sequence you can see a AUG codon, so using the genetic code, the sequence will be read as 5′-C(AUG)(GCU) (CUA) (GUU)A-3′ and translated as start/methionine-alanine-leucine-valine. If there were not a definitive start signal in this genetic language, the sequence could be read in a number of different reading frames and so interpreted as completely different codons. For example, the codons in our simple sequence could be wrongly read, as 5′-(CAU)(GGC)(UCU)(AGU)UA-3′, translating it into a *mis-sense* polypeptide sequence of histidine-glycine-serine-serine, or it could be read as 5′-CA(UGG)(CUC)(UAG)(UUA)-3′, translating into tryptophan-leucine-stop, producing a *truncated* and incorrect polypeptide.

Key features of translation

Translation occurs when the code within the mRNA molecule is translated into a polypeptide by the ribosomes. Some of the key proteins and molecules involved are outlined here. Figure 9.4 shows the sequence of events in translation.

Figure 9.4 mRNA translation. (A) Initiation factors modify the mRNA's 5′ chemical cap and bind the mRNA to the 40s ribosomal sub-unit. (B) The 40s sub-unit scans the mRNA for the AUG start codon and then joins the 60s ribosomal sub-unit. (C) Initiation: the initiator tRNA delivers methionine (Met). (D) Elongation: the ribosome complex scans along the mRNA in the 5′ → 3′ direction. tRNAs bring in the amino acids which link to the growing polypeptide. (E) Termination: the ribosome complex reads a stop codon, the polypeptide is released and the complex dissociates

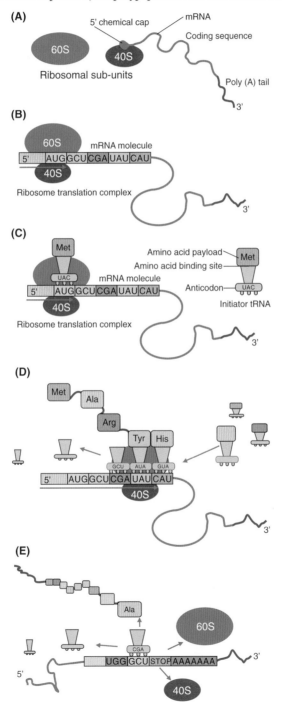

> The tRNA molecule with an anticodon sequence complementary to the codon on the mRNA will bring the correct amino acid to the ribosome.

- *tRNA molecules* have the role of transferring their amino acid cargo to a newly forming protein. There is a specific tRNA for every amino acid and each tRNA molecule has an *amino acid binding site* and an *anticodon sequence*. The anticodon is a triplicate RNA nucleotide sequence that is complementary to the codons in an mRNA molecule. The anticodon therefore specifies which amino acid the tRNA carries. The amino acid binding site on the tRNA is specific for the amino acid coded by the anticodon. The *initiator* tRNA is the first tRNA at the site of translation and always carries methionine. *Ribosomes* consist of a mixture of ribosomal RNA (rRNA) in conjunction with ribosomal proteins. The ribosomes in eukaryotic cells have two parts, a small subunit (known as 40S) and a large subunit (60S), which join together during translation.

- *Initiation factors* are proteins that have a number of roles in initiating translation. For example, they melt the 5' chemical cap on the mRNA molecule and deliver the mRNA to the ribosomes. Other roles include delivering the initiator tRNA. Initiation factors are also involved with the formation of a complex between the ribosome subunit, the initiator tRNA, and the mRNA molecule.

Key stages of translation

Translation, like transcription, proceeds through three phases:

- *Initiation* begins when the initiator tRNA binds to the small 40S ribosome subunit with the help of initiation factors. The 5' chemical cap on the mRNA molecule is used by other initiation factors to also bind the mRNA molecule to the 40S subunit. The mRNA sequence is then scanned for the first AUG start codon and this triggers the 60S subunit to join the 40S subunit and form the active ribosome. The ribosome starts translation with methionine from the initiator tRNA at the AUG start codon.

- *Elongation* is the process by which the ribosome scans along the mRNA, codon to codon, in the 5'→3' direction. Each subsequent codon is matched with the complementary anticodon on the specific tRNA molecules that carry the appropriate amino acid. These amino acids are linked together in a chain by peptide bonds to form a polypeptide. After each amino acid is added to the growing polypeptide, the empty tRNA molecule is released from the ribosome.

- Termination occurs when the ribosome reaches a stop codon in the mRNA sequence and the newly synthesized polypeptide is released.

The sequence of events in translation is summarized in Figure 9.4. The synthesized polypeptide has to undergo *post-translational modifications* before it becomes a fully functioning protein and is transported to its site of action. Post-translational modifications are alterations to the polypeptide and may include, but are not limited to, hydroxylation, glycosylation, alkylation, and the addition of disulfide bridges or hydrophobic groups. Proteins have diverse functions, from being receptors and enzymes to having structural or signalling roles.

Nonetheless, they are all produced in a similar way.

> The structure and functions of proteins is covered in detail in Chapter 10, 'Proteins and enzymes'.

The sequence of the amino acids in a protein polypeptide is dictated by the codon sequence of the mRNA, which, of course, is dictated by our genes.

9.4 HOW IS OUR GENETIC CODE PROTECTED AND PASSED ON?

So far we have looked at our genetic code in terms of how it is used by our cells to produce different RNA molecules and, of course, proteins. Humans are known as diploid organisms, i.e. they contain two complete sets of chromosomes in their somatic cells. Thus these cells contain 46 chromosomes, one set of 23 chromosomes from each parent. However, the genetic code also has to be passed on from parent to daughter cells during cell division. This process starts at the very beginning of our early development in the womb and continues until our death. As we grow, our cells divide and differentiate to produce the different tissues, organs and body systems. Even as adults, many of our cells still have to divide when a tissue needs to be repaired or when old cells need to be replaced. Our genetic code is passed down through many generations of cells. Before we consider how a cell facilitates this transfer of genetic information we must first understand the process of cell division.

The cell cycle

The cell cycle could, perhaps, be better described as the cell 'division' cycle, as this is the sequence of events that occurs when a cell is triggered to divide. It is termed a 'cycle' because these events are repeated every time cells divide.

The series of events in the cell cycle are shown in Figure 9.5, and fall into four broad phases:

1. *Gap 1 (G1)*: The cell prepares itself to make a new copy of its DNA. Genes that encode proteins and enzymes involved in the synthesis of new DNA are switched on.

2. DNA *Synthesis (S)*: The cell synthesizes a copy of its entire genetic code, resulting in duplication of every pair of chromosomes. This process is called *DNA replication* and we will look at this under the next section of this chapter.

It is imperative that our cells are able to accurately duplicate their genetic code to pass on to their daughter cells, so that each cell contains an identical copy of the full genetic code.

Figure 9.5 The cell cycle

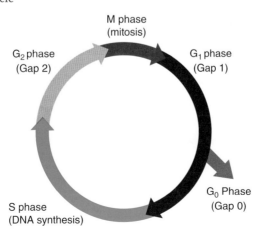

M phase
(mitosis)

G_2 phase
(Gap 2)

G_1 phase
(Gap 1)

G_0 Phase
(Gap 0)

S phase
(DNA synthesis)

> Most of our cells divide numerous times during our life; however, some cell types, such as nerve and heart cells, once mature, do not divide, and are with us for life.

3. *Gap* 2 (*G2*): The cell prepares for cell division. Genes coding for **microtubules** are switched on. Microtubules are needed during the act of cell division and are also required by the daughter cells for cell structure.

4. *Mitosis* (*M*): The cell divides into two duplicate daughter cells. These daughter cells, when the time is right, will begin the cycle again from the G1 phase.

Some cells temporarily or permanently drop out of the cell cycle during the G1 phase. These cells are called *quiescent* cells and are in what is known as the G0 phase. Cells can drop out of the cell cycle to preserve energy or if the cell has sustained damage to its DNA.

DNA replication

The process of DNA replication takes place during the S phase of the cell cycle and is a highly regulated event. Each of our chromosomes has a double helix DNA molecule that may be hundreds of millions of base pairs in length, which needs to be replicated with minimal error. The general process of eukaryotic replication is illustrated in Figure 9.6.

Replication of each chromosomal DNA molecule begins at sites within the DNA sequence known as *origins of replication*, and proceeds in both directions away from these origins. In eukaryotes, a single chromosome may contain several thousand origins of replication. To initiate replication, a protein complex called the *origin recognition complex* (ORC) must bind to each of the origin of replication sites. The ORC then recruits a series of other proteins, including *helicases* and *topoisomerases*. Helicases are enzymes that function to unwind the double helix, locally opening up the DNA to allow replication to occur. However, this results in increased coiling ahead

Figure 9.6   Eukaryotic replication

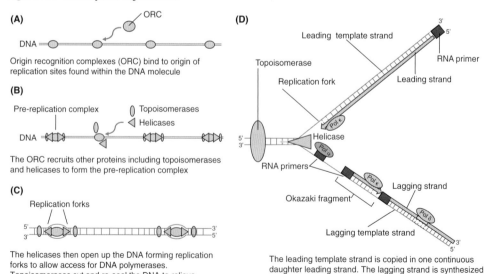

(A)

ORC

DNA

Origin recognition complexes (ORC) bind to origin of replication sites found within the DNA molecule

(B)

Pre-replication complex   Topoisomerases
                                 Helicases

DNA

The ORC recruits other proteins including topoisomerases and helicases to form the pre-replication complex

(C)

Replication forks

5'
3'   3'
                                                      5'

The helicases then open up the DNA forming replication forks to allow access for DNA polymerases. Topoisomerases cut and re-seal the DNA to relieve the tension formed in the DNA

(D)

Leading template strand

Topoisomerase

Replication fork

RNA primer

Leading strand

Pol ε

5'
3'

Helicase

Pol α

RNA primers

Pol ε

Okazaki fragment

Lagging strand

Pol δ

Lagging template strand

3'
5'

The leading template strand is copied in one continuous daughter leading strand. The lagging strand is synthesized in a discontinuous fashion via the production of Okazaki fragments. The primers are replaced with the appropriate DNA nucleotides and ligases seal any gaps with phosphodiester bonds

O DNA polymerase can only synthesize a new DNA strand in the 5'→3' direction.

Self-check 9.4

Why are Okazaki fragments formed during eukaryotic cell DNA replication?

of the replication fork. Topoisomerases therefore work ahead of the replication fork by cutting, uncoiling and resealing the DNA strand. The complex consisting of the ORC, helicases and some other proteins is known as the *pre-replication complex*. This complex needs to be triggered by a protein known as the *licensing factor* in order for replication to be initiated. The licensing factor ensures that replication occurs at precisely the right time, and only once during the cell cycle.

When the helicases in the pre-replication complex locally unwind the double helix, both strands of DNA become accessible and they both act as templates. The point where the strands separate is known as the *replication fork*. This leaves the nucleotide bases of each strand temporarily exposed so that they can base pair with 'new' complementary nucleotide bases as replication proceeds. A family of enzymes called *DNA polymerases* (Pol) carry out this process. In eukaryotes this family consists of Pol α, Pol ε, and Pol δ, each with distinct roles. At the replication fork, due to the antiparallel nature of DNA, one of the template strands runs in the $5' \rightarrow 3'$ direction, while the other runs in the $3' \rightarrow 5'$ direction. However, DNA polymerase is only capable of synthesizing a new strand of DNA in the $5' \rightarrow 3'$ direction, and therein lies a problem. The *leading template strand* runs in the $3' \rightarrow 5'$ direction and so its new complementary strand has a $5' \rightarrow 3'$ direction and can be synthesized in one continuous run, following the replication fork as it progresses and opens up the DNA. However, the *lagging template strand* runs in the $5' \rightarrow 3'$ direction, so its new complementary strand has to be synthesized in the opposite direction to the progression of the replication fork. To circumvent this problem, the DNA polymerase that is copying the lagging strand synthesizes small DNA fragments known as *Okazaki fragments*.

Replication starts by the addition of *RNA primers*—short strands of RNA that are complementary to a short DNA sequence in the template strand. These primers are made and added to the template DNA strands by Pol α. The leading strand requires only one primer, but Pol α continually adds primers to the lagging strand as the replication fork opens up. Pol ε uses the RNA primer as an anchor to start adding complementary nucleotides to the leading strand in a continuous run. Pol δ fills in the gaps between the primers with complementary nucleotides and replaces the primer RNA with DNA. Adjacent Okazaki fragments are finally joined with phosphodiester bonds by the enzyme *DNA ligase*, creating the new DNA strand that is complementary to the lagging template strand. There may be several thousand active replication forks within a single chromosome, all simultaneously copying the whole DNA molecule. When all the replication forks meet, the result is two identical complete copies of the chromosome's linear, double-stranded DNA molecule.

9.5 WHAT CAN HAPPEN WHEN THINGS GO WRONG?

During replication, DNA polymerase occasionally adds or removes nucleotides from a sequence, or adds the wrong nucleotide. This is thought to occur at a rate of about 1 in 100,000 nucleotides, which may seem pretty rare, but results in more than 100,000 mistakes being made every

Box 9.4   Not all mutations are bad

Some good or advantageous mutations can exist in our genetic code and are passed on for generations. Sickle cell anaemia (SCA), an inherited disease affecting the red blood cells, is an example of when certain mutations can be advantageous.

Malaria can be lethal and before modern medicine and procedures for mosquito control it was widespread in West Africa. When the British Empire first colonized West Africa, thousands of the British died from malaria. West Africa was nicknamed 'the white man's grave'. Yet the West Africans themselves did not die in such numbers. This was because SCA was prevalent in West Africans. Those that had two copies of the chromosome with the sickle cell mutation, one from each parent, had the disease and were often ill and died young. Those, however, that had one normal and one mutated chromosome were carriers of SCA. In genetic terms, carriers are those people who carry a copy of the mutated gene but do not show or have only mild symptoms of the disease. Therefore, these SCA carriers did not have the disorder themselves. However, these individuals were found to be resistant to malaria. These carriers were more likely to survive to adulthood and pass on the advantageous SCA gene to their children. Those that inherited normal chromosomes were susceptible to malaria and were less likely to survive to adulthood and have children. This is how an advantageous mutation can be passed on from our ancestors and can persist in our genetic code.

time a cell divides. This level of error would be unsustainable, as it would result in too significant a number of changes in the genetic code. Our cells have therefore developed mechanisms to repair damaged DNA, and most, but not all, of these mistakes are mended. During replication, DNA polymerases, in addition to duplicating the DNA molecule, carry out *proofreading* functions and thus correct the majority of faults. In addition, after replication, *mismatch repair enzymes* examine the newly formed double-stranded DNA for mismatched nucleotide base pairs and replace the wrong nucleotide with the correct one.

In addition to errors caused during replication, the cells of our bodies are also constantly exposed to environmental factors that damage our DNA, some of which we will consider in 'Causes of mutations' within this section. If the damage or mistakes in our DNA are not repaired, then changes in the DNA sequence of our genetic code become permanent and could be passed on to daughter cells. These permanent changes are known as *mutations*. If the mutations occur in germ cells they can be passed on from ancestors through generations and generations, leading to *inherited genetic mutations*. Some of these inherited genetic mutations result in diseases, others may be harmless, and some may even be advantageous, as is explained in Box 9.4.

Causes of mutations

The environmental causes of DNA damage that can lead to mutations mostly fall into one of three broad groups:

- *Physical causes* include ultraviolet (UV) light, which is part of the sunshine we all enjoy, and ionizing radiation. UV light has a higher energy than visible light, and can penetrate our skin cells and damage DNA. UV light can cause new chemical bonds or cross-links to form between adjacent cytosine and thymine bases, forming *pyrimidine dimers,* or create free radicals that can damage DNA. It is the damage to our DNA from UV light that gives rise to sunburn. If this DNA damage is too severe to be fixed, our cells self-destruct in a process called *apoptosis*. This results in our skin peeling off and being replaced by new skin. Apoptosis therefore can help to protect us against mutations. Ionizing radiation, such as X-rays, gamma rays, and cosmic radiation from space, has enough energy to penetrate our entire bodies and cause damage to the DNA in all of our cells. This damage can include single- or double-strand breaks in the chromosomal DNA molecule, and destruction of bases or sugars in nucleotides.

- *Chemical causes* can come from the environment we live in, such as from cigarette smoke or pollution. People who work in certain industries may be exposed to DNA-damaging chemicals, such as the arylamines found in some dyes used in textile production, and the polycyclic aromatic hydrocarbons used in the petroleum industry. The food we eat may also contain DNA-damaging agents: well-cooked meat and sodium nitrate, used as a food preservative, have been associated with DNA damage. Many of these agents that we are exposed to do not directly damage DNA, but are broken down by the liver to produce DNA-damaging by-products. For example, spices, cereals, beans, nuts and other crops, if stored incorrectly, may become contaminated with aflatoxin, produced by the fungus *Aspergillus*. Aflatoxin is metabolized by the liver to produce a powerful mutagen and carcinogen. Chemical damage to DNA includes single- or double-strand breaks, bond formation between adjacent bases or between DNA strands, the addition of chemical groups to bases, and the removal of bases.

- *Biological causes* primarily involve cellular parasites such as viruses. The majority of viruses cause little or no permanent harm to us, but a few are associated with serious diseases and cancers. During infection, viruses take command of the host's replication machinery to replicate their own genes. Their DNA is inserted into our own, often causing mutations to our genes, which may destroy the genes or alter the activity of the gene products. DNA mutated by the insertion of viral DNA might not directly result in problems for the cell, but the proteins expressed from the viral DNA can. Viruses also commandeer other cellular proteins to assemble or package more viruses in order to infect other cells.

DNA damage can also occur without the presence of environmental causative factors. It can be caused in error by normal cellular enzymes and proteins during cell division and, if left unrepaired, can lead to spontaneous mutations.

Our cells can respond to and repair DNA damage, thus minimizing the effect it may cause. In addition to the mismatch repair enzymes mentioned before, during any part of the cell cycle, *excision repair enzymes* inspect our DNA for damage. When damage is discovered, these enzymes remove the damaged DNA and DNA polymerase replaces the missing nucleotides.

Probably the most important protein that is activated by DNA damage is called *tumour protein 53* or just *P53*. P53 is known as the 'guardian of the genome' for its role in protecting the integrity of our genetic code. P53 halts the cell cycle in the G1 phase just before the DNA synthesis (S) phase (at the G1/S checkpoint). If DNA damage is detected, P53 activates the excision repair enzymes to repair the damage. If the damage is successfully repaired, the cell is allowed to continue through the cell cycle; if not, P53 triggers the cell to destroy itself by undergoing apoptosis. In this way, P53 prevents mutations being passed on to daughter cells. However, despite the mechanisms our cells have to protect the fidelity of our genetic code, mutations are inevitable.

Types of mutations

Unrepaired DNA damage can give rise to a number of different types of mutations as detailed below:

- *Substitution* or *point* mutations are caused if a single nucleotide base is changed in the DNA sequence. There are two types of substitution mutation: *transition* and *transversion* mutations. In a transition mutation, a purine base is changed for another purine base (A to G or G to A) or a pyrimidine base is altered to another pyrimidine base (C to T or T to C). In a transversion mutation, a pyrimidine is substituted by a purine or vice versa.

- *Frameshift* mutations are caused when the reading frame of the gene is altered. This is the consequence of nucleotides being added to or removed from the DNA. Mutations that occur when a nucleotide or a number of nucleotides are added to a DNA sequence are called *insertion* mutations, and mutations where they are removed from the sequence are called *deletion* mutations.

- *Chromosomal translocations* occur when a fragment from one chromosome is incorrectly added to another chromosome.

Consequences of mutations

So far we have looked at how mutations might arise in cells, but what are the consequences of getting mutations in the genetic code? The consequences are largely dependent on which and how many genes are affected, in addition to the location of the mutation within the gene. In the case of a substitution mutation there might not be any consequences. For example, if the codon GCU were mutated to GCC, there would be no change in the amino acid sequence of the protein as they both code for the same amino acid (alanine). On the other hand, substitution mutations can result in considerable consequences if the change produces a stop codon in the middle of a protein-coding sequence, or codes for an incorrect amino acid to be inserted into a significant part of the polypeptide chain. For example, a substitution mutation of the 6th codon in the sequence of the β-**globin** gene results in glutamic acid being changed to valine. This change in the amino acid in the β-globin protein gives rise to *sickle cell anaemia* (see Box 9.4). Another substitution mutation within the β-globin gene at the 39th codon forms a stop codon (CAG is mutated to UAG), resulting in a useless short protein chain that does not function as a β-globin protein. This gives rise to the clinical symptoms of β-thalassaemia.

Single gene disorders

Inherited genetic diseases affecting single genes fall into two categories: *recessive* and *dominant*. Recessive diseases require the mutation to be present in both inherited copies of a chromosome to generate the most severe disease state, whereas dominant mutations need the mutation in only one inherited chromosome for there to be clinical symptoms. Based on the chromosome type that bears the mutation, there may be autosomal or sex chromosome-linked (both X and Y) disorders. Many genetic diseases exist that result in a diverse range of clinical symptoms. Some examples of genetic diseases resulting from mutations are given in Table 9.2.

An example of an **autosomal** recessive single gene disorder is cystic fibrosis (CF). CF is particularly prevalent in Caucasians. A mutation within the cystic fibrosis transmembrane regulator (CFTR) gene in both copies of chromosome 7 affects the secreting glands in the body, particularly in the lungs. If a child inherits a mutated copy of the CFTR gene from one parent

Table 9.2 Genetic diseases that result from inherited mutations

Inheritance trait	Disease	Mutation type
Autosomal recessive	Cystic fibrosis	Frameshift (deletion)
	Sickle cell anaemia	Substitution (transversion)
	Tay-Sachs disease	Numerous types of mutation give rise to disease
	β-Thalassaemia	Substitution (transition)
Autosomal dominant	Lynch syndrome (hereditary non-polyposis colorectal cancer)	Can result from mutation in a number of different DNA mismatch repair enzyme genes
	Huntington's disease	Frameshift (insertion of multiple nucleotides)
	Hypercholesterolaemia, type B	Numerous types of mutation give rise to disease
X-linked recessive	Duchenne muscular dystrophy	Frameshift (deletion)
	Haemophilia	Numerous types of mutation give rise to disease
X-linked dominant	Hypophosphataemic rickets	Frameshift (deletion)

and a normal copy from the other parent they will be symptom free; however, they will also be a CF *carrier*, meaning they may pass on the genetic disorder to their offspring. About 1 in 25 people in the UK are estimated to be CF carriers. Children born to parents who are both CF carriers might inherit the mutated chromosome 7 from each parent and have CF (there is a 25% chance of this occurring). They could, however, inherit the normal chromosome 7 from both parents and neither have CF nor carry the defective gene to pass on to the next generation (also a 25% chance). Case study 9.1 further explores the inheritance pattern of CF. Sickle cell anaemia, described earlier in Box 9.4, is also a recessive single gene disease.

Some inherited single gene disorders are sex chromosome-linked. For example, a mutation in the dystrophin gene found on the X chromosome results in the muscle-wasting disease Duchenne muscular dystrophy. The disease is carried by females and is considered to be recessive. However, as males have only one copy of the X chromosome the disease is prevalent in males; females have two X chromosomes and therefore can have a normal copy of the dystrophin gene to compensate for the faulty one. If a carrier has a child, the child has 50:50 chance of receiving the mutated X chromosome from the mother. Therefore, if the child is female she will be a carrier, if male he will have the disease.

Although many genetic diseases are caused by inherited mutations, some are also caused by spontaneous mutations. Duchenne muscular dystrophy may also occur due to spontaneous mutations in the dystrophin gene. Often, no familial genetic link is evident and the disease is considered to have arisen by spontaneous mutation during prenatal development. Of course, this means that it is also possible that, during prenatal development, spontaneous mutations could occur in the normal copy of a gene in recessive disorders such as CF, giving rise to disease.

DNA as a drug target

When a cell divides, its DNA unwinds before being copied and distributed to new daughter cells. Cancer is a disease that is characterized by excessive cell division. Many anticancer drugs work by inhibiting cell division; some drugs achieve this by directly targeting DNA. For example, doxorubicin is an intercalating drug in common use for the treatment of cancer. It contains a planar aromatic ring system that targets DNA by sliding between two adjacent base pairs in the DNA ladder (see Figure 9.7). The binding of the drug is stabilized by hydrophobic interactions between the aromatic rings of the drug and the base pairs. This stable complex helps to prevent the unwinding of DNA and so blocks cell division; the binding of the drug to DNA ultimately leads to the death of the cancer cell.

9.6 NUCLEOSIDE DERIVATIVES AS DRUGS

Nucleoside derivative drugs are often not naturally occurring nucleosides, but have very closely related structures. Nucleoside analogues are an important class of drugs, being mainly used as anti-viral and anti-cancer drugs. The nucleoside analogues acting as anti-viral drugs can be exemplified by zidovudine and aciclovir, although there are many other examples of this class of drug. Examples of nucleoside analogues as anti-cancer agents are cytarabine and mercaptopurine.

Zidovudine (also known as AZT or azidothymidine) is a nucleoside used to treat HIV infection. It contains an unusual azido (N_3) functional group at the $3'$-position. Zidovudine is added to a growing strand of viral DNA, whereupon the azide group blocks the addition of further nucleotides, and therefore the virus cannot replicate further (see Figure 9.8).

Aciclovir is often encountered as an effective treatment for cold sores (a viral infection of the lips). It has a nucleoside-like structure that is missing part of the sugar group, including the $3'$-OH required for elongation of the nucleic acid chain. Once added to the chain, aciclovir halts nucleic acid synthesis by blocking its elongation; this deactivates the virus.

Figure 9.7 A model of the cancer drug doxorubicin binding to DNA. This model shows doxorubicin (carbon atoms highlighted in green) inserting between two DNA base pairs (PDB code: 1D12)

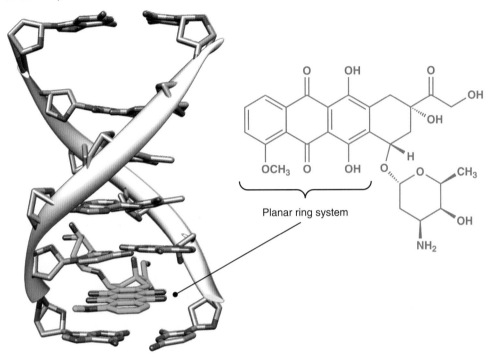

Planar ring system

Figure 9.8 Two nucleoside derivative drugs, including an illustration of the mechanism of action of zidovudine

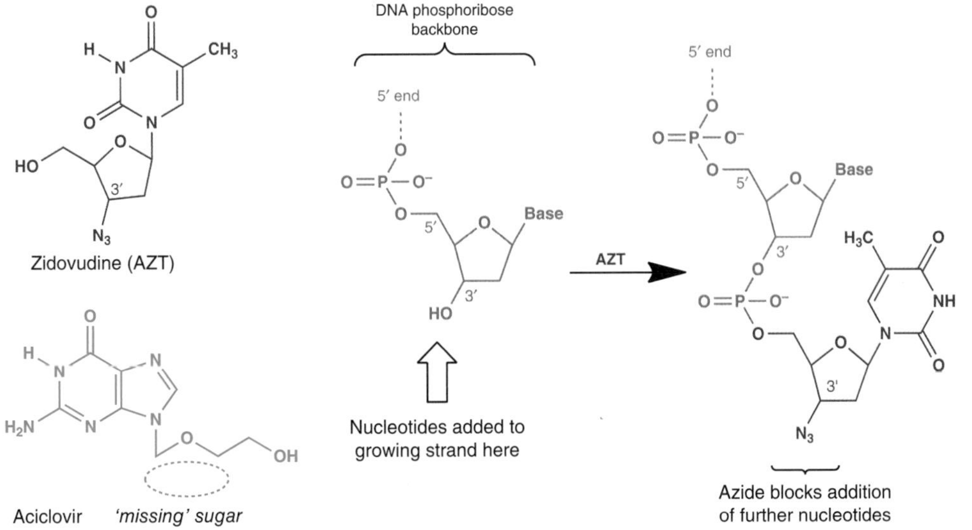

Figure 9.9 Examples of nucleoside anti-cancer agents

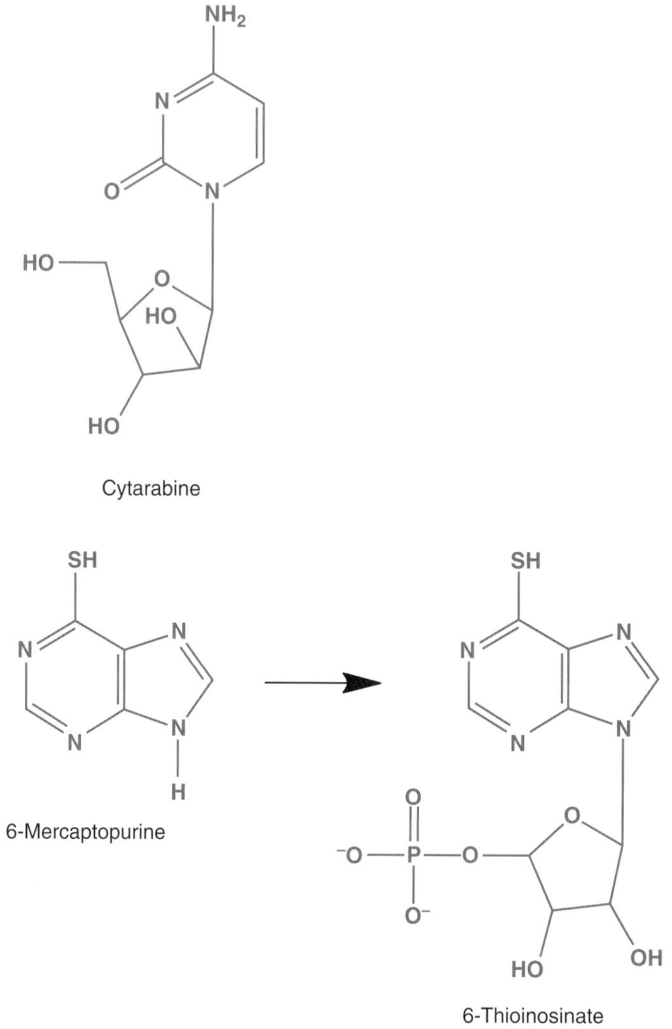

Cytarabine

6-Mercaptopurine

6-Thioinosinate

Cytarabine is an anti-cancer agent used to treat a number of leukaemias and non-Hodgkin's lymphoma. Structurally it combines the base cytosine with an arabinose sugar and acts as an antimetabolite (see Figure 9.9). It is incorporated into human DNA where it interferes with the synthesis of new DNA during replication.

Mercaptopurine (see Figure 9.9) is also used to treat a number of leukaemias as well as some autoimmune diseases such as Crohn's disease and ulcerative colitis. Like cytarabine it is an antimetabolite which interferes with nucleic acid biosynthesis. However, mercaptopurine is not, in itself, a nucleoside but needs to be converted *in vivo* to a 6-thioinosinate. which is a nucleoside.

Many anticancer and antiviral drugs interfere with replication and synthesis of nucleic acids.

9.7 CURRENT AND FUTURE GENETIC THERAPIES

We have seen how disease can arise because of changes or mutations made to our genetic code. Current treatments for some of these disorders only address the symptoms and not the underlying cause. Scientists have now, through the work of the Human Genome Project, decoded the entire 3 billion or so base pairs that make up our genetic code. So is it possible that scientists can use this knowledge to create medicines to cure genetic diseases? The answer is maybe, and research to this end is currently ongoing.

One approach currently being explored is the silencing of genes that are over-expressed in diseases. To silence or suppress an overactive gene, the expressed mRNA is targeted for destruction and so less mRNA is translated into protein. Short interfering RNA (siRNA) molecules are designed to bind to the complementary nucleotide sequence found in the target mRNA and, in a similar way to that of endogenous miRNA molecules, label the mRNA for destruction by cellular enzymes. This general approach is known as RNA interference (RNAi), and research using RNAi is now being carried out in the search for possible treatments for diseases such as cancer.

'Fixing' a mutation is the central goal of *gene therapy*. Gene therapy involves administering *therapeutic DNA* which, when expressed by the cell, acts as a substitute for the mutations present in the patient. It was used successfully for the first time in 1990 to treat a 4-year-old girl who had **severe combined immunodeficiency disease (SCID)**. People with this very rare disease have a very poor or non-existent immune system owing to a mutation in the gene for an enzyme called adenosine deaminase (ADA). Scientists inserted a normal copy of the ADA gene into the girl's white blood cells. The 'fixed' cells were propagated to increase their numbers and then administered to the child. When these fixed cells then divided, their daughter cells carried the new gene. The girl regained an immune response and the gene therapy was considered a success. Since then, a number of patients with SCID have been successfully treated with gene therapy.

The initial success in gene therapy triggered researchers to search for other applications and methods in the treatment of genetic diseases. The main problem, however, is how to get a correct copy of a gene into the DNA of enough cells to relieve the symptoms or cure the disease. A number of approaches to this problem have been investigated. One such idea was to add a therapeutic gene into a virus. Logically, viruses should make excellent carriers for therapeutic DNA because that is what they do—invade cells and add their DNA into the host cell's DNA. This approach is extremely efficient in the laboratory, but has proved problematic in humans because our **immune system** can mount an immune response to the viral carrier. In the USA in 1999, a healthy teenage boy died after taking part in a **clinical trial** for a gene therapy treatment when he had a severe reaction to the viral therapeutic gene carrier used in the trial. Subsequently, it was found that the research practices of those involved in the trial were questionable and unethical, and this has influenced the revision of the guidelines and documentation involving clinical trials. This outcome was of course very sad for the boy's family, but was also a massive setback for gene therapy research.

Scientists are also trying other, non-viral, means of delivering therapeutic DNA that are less likely to illicit immune responses in recipients. These include the use of **liposomes** and **polymers** as vehicles. Future research will undoubtedly result in permanent cures for some of the genetic disorders that conventional medicines today can only treat symptomatically.

Gene therapy has the potential to actually cure a genetic disease whereas most current therapies can only treat the symptoms.

- Cells can be divided into prokaryotes and eukaryotes.

- Eukaryotic multicellular organisms like humans exist because cells differentiate into specialist cells that make up the tissues and organs that contribute to the whole organism.

- The basic units of DNA and RNA molecules are the nucleotides.

- The 'letters' of the genetic code come from the bases guanine(G), cytosine(C), adenine(A) and thymine(T). In RNA, uracil(U) replaces thymine(T).

- The 'words' of the genetic code are written in base sequence triplets called codons.

- DNA has to be highly packaged into chromosomes to fit into the nucleus.

- Coding genes have base sequences that promote transcription.

- Enzymes called RNA polymerases carry out transcription of DNA to make RNA.

- Translation of mRNA into protein occurs in the ribosomes.

- The cell cycle has four phases, known as G_1 (Gap 1), S (synthesis), G_2 (Gap 2) and M (mitosis) phases.

- DNA replication occurs during the S phase.

- DNA damage can occur because of mistakes during DNA replication, or from physical, chemical or biological damage.

- Mutations occur when unrepaired DNA damage is passed on to daughter cells and can be advantageous, harmless or cause disease.

- Mutations in germ cells can be passed down through generations

- Chromosomal problems can result in disease.

- Some anticancer drugs interfere with replication and synthesis of nucleic acids.

- Some antiviral drugs have closely related structures to nucleosides but prevent replication by blocking viral nucleic synthesis.

- The treatment of some inherited disorders may lie within gene therapy.

Papachristodolou, D., Snape, A., Elliott, W. H. and Elliott, D. C. *Biochemistry and Molecular Biology*, 6th edn. Oxford University Press, 2018, ISBN 978-0-19-8768111.
This is a well-written textbook that covers molecular biology in depth.

King, R. I. B. and Robins, M. W. *Cancer Biology*, 3rd edn. Pearson Prentice Hall, 2006. ISBN 978-0-13-129454-7.
This textbook will give you a detailed understanding of how mutations can lead to cancer.

Patrick, G. L., *An Introduction to Medicinal Chemistry*, 6th edn. Oxford University Press, 2017. ISBN 978-0-19-8749691.
A very accessible textbook that expands upon the chemistry of drugs and their mechanisms of action against target macromolecules

Self-check

For the answers to the Self-Check questions in Chapter 9, visit the online resources which accompany this textbook.

PROTEINS AND ENZYMES
Alex White And Helen Burrell

Proteins make up a highly important class of macromolecules in biochemistry. Proteins are biopolymers constructed from amino acid monomers. Compared with nucleic acids (see Chapter 9), proteins have varied and complex three-dimensional structures, due in part to the greater variety of monomers used to construct them. As a result, each protein has a unique three-dimensional structure which is directly related to the function it performs, and this chapter describes the detail of the structures.

Proteins have a myriad of functions in cells and organelles. To pick some examples: antibodies (part of the immune system), collagen (involved in physical structures), membrane-bound receptors and enzymes. Enzymes and receptors are of particular importance to pharmacy as many drugs interact with them to bring about their therapeutic activity. This chapter discusses the kinetics of enzyme activity and the pathways by which they are inhibited or activated.

Learning objectives

After reading this chapter you should be able to:

- define the three different types of protein and give examples of where they can be found in the body
- differentiate between the primary, secondary, tertiary and quaternary structure of a protein and identify the forces or bonds that help to stabilize each structure
- describe what an active site is within an enzyme and how it is structurally formed
- give examples of the four types of reversible enzyme inhibitor and describe how they affect K_m and V_{max}
- describe how the types of irreversible inhibitor affect enzymes
- recognize the types of protein that can act as drug targets.

10.1 STRUCTURE AND FUNCTION OF PROTEINS

Proteins can generally be classified into three groups according to their shape and solubility:

1. *Globular proteins* are almost spherical and are highly soluble in aqueous solutions. Their solubility is due to the positions of **hydrophobic** and **hydrophilic** amino acids within the protein.

The hydrophilic amino acids are on the outside, where they interact with the aqueous environment, whereas the hydrophobic amino acids are protected on the inside of the molecule. Globular proteins have many roles; they include enzymes with catalytic activity, for example acetylcholinesterase, transportation devices to aid the passage of molecules through membranes, for example potassium channels, messenger signals such as hormones, for example insulin, or they can be regulatory molecules, for example histone or transcriptional factors. These proteins are easily denatured.

2. *Fibrous proteins* are linear proteins that are insoluble in aqueous solutions. They form aggregates owing to the hydrophobic side chains on the outside of the molecule. They are involved in cell structure to provide protection and support, and as a consequence they are components of connective tissue, tendons, muscle fibres and the bone matrix. Examples of fibrous proteins include keratin, collagen and elastin. In general, fibrous proteins are not denatured as easily as globular proteins.

3. *Membrane proteins* are integral, peripheral or lipid-anchored proteins associated with cell membranes, and each has different functions. Many are receptors for endogenous and therapeutic molecules. They have hydrophobic amino acids pointing outwards from the protein molecule, which enable interaction with the non-polar phase of the membrane, and have fewer hydrophilic amino acids than globular proteins. They are generally insoluble in aqueous solutions unless a detergent is present.

Although there are different classifications of proteins, all protein structures have similarities. There are four levels of protein structure; the *primary, secondary, tertiary* and *quaternary* levels.

Amino acids

All proteins are built from twenty naturally occurring amino acid monomers, which share the same general structure. An acidic carboxylic acid group and a basic amino group are both bonded to a central carbon, which is referred to as the α-carbon. The α-carbon is also bonded to a hydrogen atom and a variable side-chain group, unique for each amino acid. The amino acids are classified, as shown in Figure 10.1, by the chemical properties of the side chain. Take note of the abbreviations used for each amino acid. These are used throughout the scientific literature, so it is well worth spending some time learning both the three-letter and single-letter abbreviations (as well as the structures of the twenty side chains).

Amino acid stereochemistry

With the exception of glycine, all the amino acids in Figure 10.1 have four different groups bonded to the α-carbon atom. This means that nineteen of the twenty amino acids contain a chiral centre and can exist as pairs of enantiomers. In practice, all naturally occurring amino acids are single enantiomers and rotate plane-polarized light. The amino acids in proteins have the L-configuration. The L/D notation is an 'old fashioned' system but its use is widespread in protein chemistry. All L-amino acids have the same orientation of groups around their α-carbon as the reference compound L-glyceraldehyde (which, rather confusingly, is

Self-check 10.1

What are the differences between the main types of protein?

Figure 10.1 The twenty naturally occurring amino acids that form the building blocks of proteins, grouped by sidechain properties

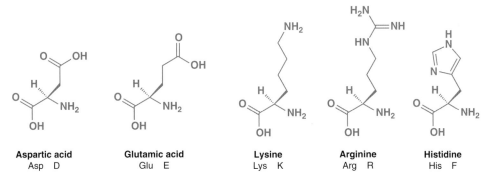

General formula for an L-amino acid

* = α-carbon
R = sidechain

| Glycine | Alanine | Valine | Leucine | Isoleucine | Proline |
| Gly   G | Ala   A | Val   V | Leu   L | Ile   I | Pro   P |

Amino acids with aliphatic (non-polar) sidechains

| Phenylalanine | Tyrosine | Tryptophan | Serine | Threonine |
| Phe   F | Tyr   Y | Trp   W | Ser   S | Thr   T |

Amino acids with aromatic (generally non-polar) sidechains

Amino acids with alcohol (polar) sidechains

| Aspartic acid | Glutamic acid | Lysine | Arginine | Histidine |
| Asp   D | Glu   E | Lys   K | Arg   R | His   F |

Amino acids with acidic (very polar) sidechains

Amino acids with basic (very polar) sidechains

| Asparagine | Glutamine | Cysteine | Methionine |
| Asn   N | Gln   Q | Cys   C | Met   M |

Amino acids with amide (polar) sidechains

Amino acids with sulfur containing sidechains

a simple sugar). The opposite enantiomers, D–amino acids, do exist in nature but they are very rare and are not coded for by DNA. (They are synthesized by microorganisms, often by isomerization from a naturally occurring L–isomer.)

> More details on stereochemistry can be found in Chapter 3, 'Stereochemistry and drug action'.

Amino acids: acid-base chemistry

Amino acids are more acidic than you might expect. Although acidity varies somewhat between the twenty amino acids, the carboxylic acid (CO_2H) group has a pKa of approximately 2. Compare this with acetic acid (CH_3CO_2H), an organic compound we normally consider to be quite acidic, which has a pKa = 4.7. Since pKa is a logarithmic expression of acidity, a change of one unit equals a ten-fold difference in that property. Therefore amino acids are over 100 times more acidic than acetic acid. The pKa of the protonated amino (NH_2) group in amino acids is approximately 9. Therefore, under physiological conditions (in other words, an aqueous solution with neutral pH), the carboxylic acid protonates the amino group, resulting in a neutral ion that contains two opposite charges. We refer to this type of species as a zwitterion (see Figure 10.2). Zwitterions are quite stable, which accounts for the high acidity, high polarity and generally good water solubility of amino acids.

Protein structure: primary sequence

Amino acids are linked together by amide bonds, which are also known in protein biochemistry as peptide bonds. They are formed by a condensation reaction between a carboxylic acid and an amine. This forms a continuous peptide backbone, highlighted in Figure 10.3 by the continuous bold line. Note that there is an amino group not involved in a peptide bond at one end of the protein, and similarly an unbonded carboxylic acid group at the opposite end. Consequently, the ends of a peptide are called the N-terminus (where the free—NH_2 is found) and the C-terminus (where the free CO_2H is located).

Figure 10.2 An amino acid zwitterion

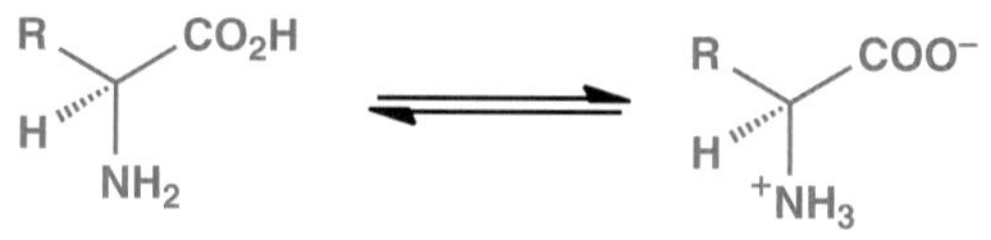

Figure 10.3 Protein primary sequence. Amino acid monomers, linked by peptide bonds, form an extended chain. The peptide backbone, highlighted by bold bonds, runs unbroken from the N-terminus to the C-terminus of the protein. The sidechains, abbreviated as R_1, R_2 etc., point outwards from the backbone

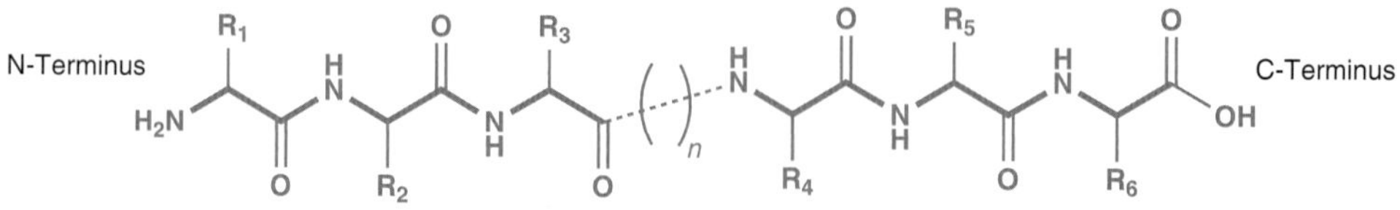

Figure 10.4 Three different methods to illustrate the same small protein. A structural formula; the three-letter amino acid abbreviations; and the single-letter amino acid abbreviations are all shown. In each case, the amino acids are always drawn/listed from the *N*- to the *C*-terminus

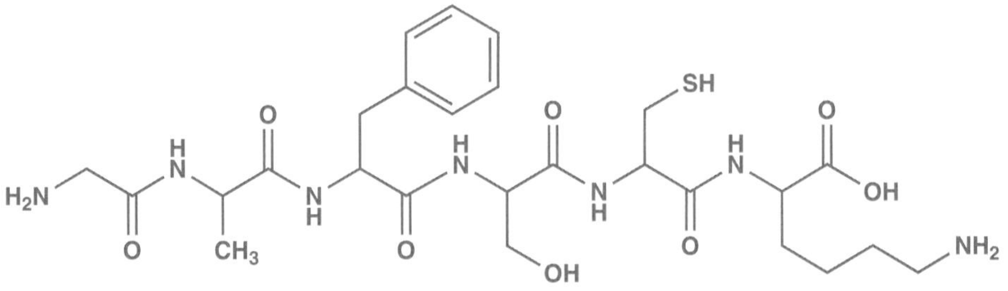

Gly-Ala-Phe-Ser-Cys-Lys

GAFSCK

Self-check 10.2

Test your knowledge of amino acid and protein structure. Pick a word made up from just the letters used as single-letter abbreviations for amino acids (only J, O, U and X are not used). Draw the structure of the protein resulting from that sequence of letters. Try PHARMACY for starters!

Proteins are made from the twenty naturally occurring L-amino acids, joined together in linear chains by peptide bonds. The order of amino acid residues in a protein is its primary structure.

By convention, the primary sequence (or primary structure) of a protein is described by listing the amino acids in the correct sequence, starting from the N-terminal amino acid and finishing at the C-terminus. Either three-letter or single-letter abbreviations can be used for individual amino acids.

Figure 10.4 shows three different ways of representing the same short protein. The full structural formula is given on top, and below are two abbreviated methods. It is common, and far easier, to describe proteins in an abbreviated form, but do not forget the chemical structure that underlies this shorthand.

Peptides

Small proteins with less than fifty amino acids are usually classified as peptides. Peptides comprising just two amino acids are dipeptides; those with three amino acids are tripeptides and so on. Therefore, Figure 10.4 illustrates a hexapeptide.

Protein folding

In practice, proteins do not exist as linear peptide chains. Immediately after synthesis, proteins fold into more complex structures. (Large proteins even start to fold up before their synthesis is complete.) There are several factors that influence the folding of a protein:

- The peptide bond. The peptide bond has approximately 40% double bond character due to resonance. This can be explained by the curly arrows in Figure 10.5. Recall that double

Figure 10.5 Factors affecting protein folding

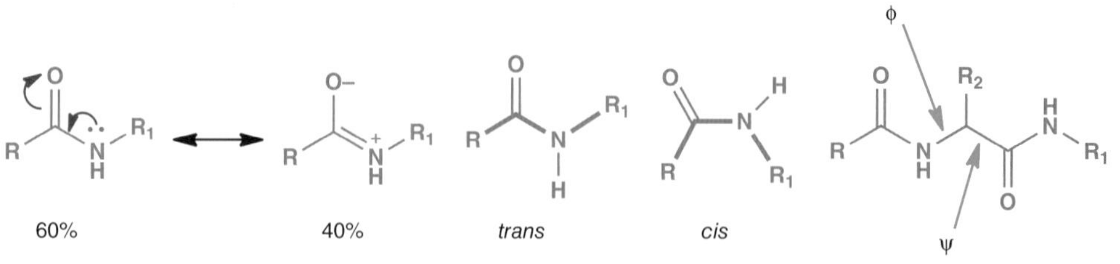

60%   40%   trans   cis

bonds are rigid and cannot rotate. This restricts the movement of the peptide backbone. Furthermore, almost all peptide bonds in proteins exist as *trans*-amides to avoid the unfavourable steric interactions that arise from *cis*-peptide bonds (e.g. between R and R1 in Figure 10.5).

- Rotation of single bonds. Since the peptide bond is generally rigid, a protein folds by movement of the remaining single bonds in the peptide backbone. As shown in Figure 10.5, these are known as the Φ and Ψ bonds.

- Interactions. **Bonding interactions** occur between different parts of a protein chain. These might be hydrogen bonds, ionic bonds, van der Waals (hydrophobic) interactions or covalent bonds. These are intramolecular interactions (i.e. within the same molecule) and are vital for maintaining a protein's shape.

> For more details on stereochemistry, see Chapter 3, 'Stereochemistry and drug action'; *cis* and *trans*-isomers are discussed in greater detail in Chapter 4, 'Properties of aliphatic hydrocarbons'.

Protein structure: secondary structure

Secondary protein structure can be described as the repetitive three-dimensional arrangement of parts of the primary structure. There are two main types of secondary structure, the α-helix and the β-sheet.

- The α-helix results from the folding of a single backbone strand of the peptide backbone into a coil around a central axis to form a **single helix**. This must not be confused with the double helix of DNA which contains two backbones—a common mistake! The coil is tight: just 3.6 amino acids are required for each complete turn. The structure is stabilized by a network of hydrogen bonds between the amide carbonyl (C=O) and NH groups along the length of the helix.

- The β-sheet forms when two or more adjacent segments of a peptide backbone interact with each other. Usually several sections of the backbone, called β-strands, interact with each other to form a relatively flat, sheet-like structure. Hydrogen bonding between strands is the most common stabilizing interaction, although hydrophobic interactions can occur between adjacent non-polar amino acid side chains.

The β-sheet exists in two varieties: parallel and antiparallel. The antiparallel sheet is more common and arises when β-strands run in opposite directions to each other. The opposite is seen in the parallel sheet, where β-strands run in the same direction.

Figure 10.6 Secondary protein structure. (A) Two representations of the α-helix showing a partial structure highlighting the backbone (bold) and a cartoon single helix; (B) antiparallel β-sheet; (C) parallel β-sheet. For clarity, all amino acids sidechains are abbreviated as R

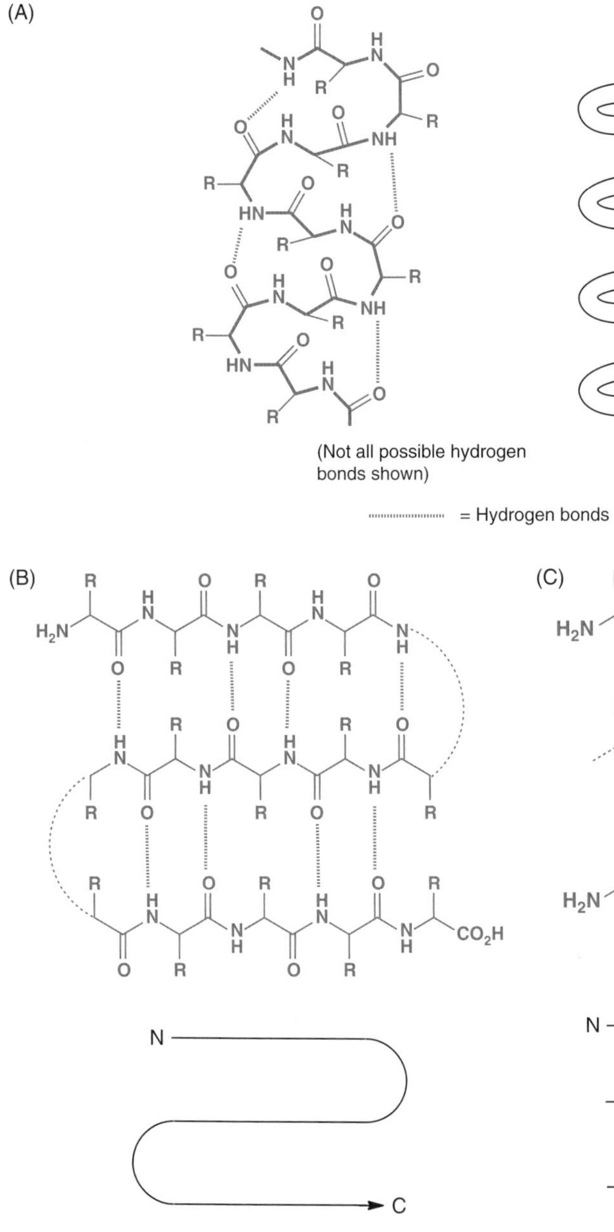

(A)

(Not all possible hydrogen bonds shown)

•••••••••••••• = Hydrogen bonds

(B)

(C)

Even though Figure 10.6 shows diagrammatic representations of the β-sheet structure, study the arrangement of the stabilizing hydrogen bond interactions. Throughout chemistry, bonding is more efficient when the groups involved are favourably aligned. You can see the hydrogen bonds are regularly aligned in the antiparallel β-sheet. This forms a more stable structure than the parallel β-sheet. This observation is confirmed in nature; antiparallel β-sheets are far more common, and exist in sheets of 2–15 strands (although the average number of strands is six).

Hydrogen bonds stabilize polypeptide chains to form different secondary protein structures.

Parallel β-sheets are far less common; the largest discovered contains just five strands. This is an excellent illustration of the stabilizing ability of a network of relatively weak hydrogen bonds.

Protein structure: tertiary structure

Proteins with more than about fifty amino acids adopt complex three-dimensional shapes, which we call tertiary structures. Each protein folds into a very specific shape, known as the native conformation, which is usually the biologically active form of the protein. Protein tertiary structures usually contain two or more elements of secondary structure. The following examples, enzymes and collagen, show how the structure of a protein relates to its biological activity (see Figure 10.7).

Enzymes are excellent examples of proteins with tertiary structure. The structures of many enzymes contain both α-helices and β-sheets. The three-dimensional arrangement of these structures creates an overall shape that is unique for every protein. Most enzymes have a roughly spherical native conformation and contain a cleft in their surface known as the active site. The active site is the location within the enzyme at which the reaction it catalyses occurs. (For more details on enzymes, see section 10.2).

Collagen is one of the most abundant proteins in nature. It has a very simple tertiary structure (in fact some texts may classify collagen as just having secondary structure). It consists of three independent peptide backbones wound together in a triple-coil. This forms a very rigid fibre-like structure that provides mechanical support in tissues such as skin, tendons and bones. α-Keratin is a related protein with a similar structure. It has a double coil of α-helices and is a principal component of hair.

Protein structure: quaternary structure

The final level of protein structure is the quaternary structure, which describes the formation of proteins containing multiple interacting polypeptide chains called subunits. A protein with two or more subunits is called a multimer. If its subunits are identical the protein is a

Figure 10.7 The structure of a typical enzyme, carbonic anhydrase (A) and collagen (B). Note the regular elongated structure of collagen (each of the three peptide chains is coloured separately), and the compact, spherical, but irregular structure of the enzyme (PDB code: 1CA2)

(A)   (B)

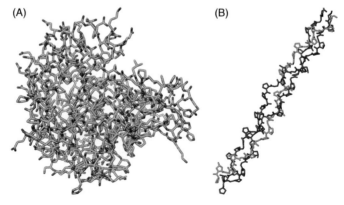

Not all proteins have the quaternary level of structure, as some can exist in a monomeric state (tertiary level).

homomultimer, and if its subunits are different it is a heteromultimer. It is more economical for an organism's proteins to contain multiple identical subunits, as less DNA is required to code for it and simultaneous translation using multiple ribosomes on the same piece of DNA can occur. The simplest form of quaternary structure is a dimer, with two subunits. This configuration is found in some DNA binding proteins. A protein with three subunits is a trimer and one with four subunits is a tetramer. Haemoglobin, the protein that transports oxygen in the blood, is composed of four distinct tertiary protein subunits. There are two identical α-subunits and two identical β-subunits.

10.2 ENZYMES AND ENZYME INHIBITION

Nearly all known enzymes are proteins (there are a few RNA-based enzymes, particularly in the ribosomes). Enzymes therefore also have a primary, secondary and tertiary structure, and some even a quaternary structure. They are generally globular in structure, and range in size from tens to over two thousand amino acids.

The enzyme molecule, when folded, forms a three-dimensional cleft or crevice, called the active site, which excludes water and other non-substrate molecules. This is where the substrate binds and is where catalytic activity occurs.

The amino acids forming the active site are few in number and may be several residues apart. Residues that are adjacent to each other are more likely to be sterically prevented from interacting with each other. Residues that are further apart, however, can interact more strongly with a substrate. The predominantly non-polar environment enhances substrate binding and catalysis via the formation of multiple relatively weak interactions, including hydrogen bonds, ionic bonds and van der Waals interactions, which would otherwise be disrupted in a polar environment. The rest of the molecule forms a protective scaffold to support the active site, and forms regulatory sites or channels to bring the substrates to the active site.

Enzymes are named according to the types of reaction that they catalyze. There are six main types of enzyme, which are classified by the Enzyme Commission (EC) as shown in Table 10.1.

Enzymes control vital biological pathways by catalyzing the chemical reactions, either enhancing or reducing the speed at which they occur. The activity of enzymes is not permanent as most can be denatured—the process by which heat or chemicals cause the protein chains to unfold, destroying the configuration of amino acids in the active site. Denaturation can be reversible or irreversible, depending on the enzyme.

The term *catalytic power* is defined as the ratio of the enzyme-catalyzed speed to the uncatalyzed speed of a reaction. The term *specificity* refers to the ability of the enzyme to selectively interact with its substrates. Specificity is achieved by bringing together substrates in an optimal configuration using multiple weak attractions mediated by hydrogen bonds and electrostatic and van der Waals interactions. The interaction of the enzyme with its substrate subsequently provides the level of specificity. In particular, the directional nature of hydrogen bonds helps to

Enzymes are proteins that have catalytic functions.

Table 10.1 Enzyme nomenclature according to the Enzyme Commission (EC)

EC number	Systematic Name	Type of reaction catalysed
1	Oxidoreductases	Oxidation–reduction reactions
2	Transferases	Transfer of functional groups from donor to acceptor
3	Hydrolases	Hydrolysis reactions of C–O, C–N, C–C, and some other bonds, including phosphoric anhydride bonds
4	Lyases	Cleavage of C–C, C–O, C–N, and other bonds by elimination, or the addition of double bonds
5	Isomerases	Geometric or structural changes within one molecule—called isomerization reactions
6	Ligases	Joining of two molecules, coupled with the hydrolysis of a diphosphate bond inadenosine-5'-triphosphate or a similar triphosphate

enforce a high level of specificity between an enzyme and its substrate (see Box 10.1 for further information on enzyme specificity).

Many enzymes have a quaternary structure. Each monomer or protein chain may contain part of an active site, and so function is only achieved when multiple polypeptides interact to form the complete active site. Enzymes with multiple subunits may also have multiple active sites. These are called **allosteric** enzymes. The catalytic activity of enzymes with quaternary structure is regulated by *cooperativity*. Multimers can contain multiple active sites for a specific substrate. If one active site is occupied, there can be a subsequent change in affinity for the substrate at the other active sites. If increases in affinity occur there is *positive cooperativity*, whereas if there is a decrease in affinity there is *negative cooperativity*. As such, the quaternary structure provides a mechanism by which the enzyme subunits can communicate to alter their function.

Box 10.1 Enzyme specificity

There are two hypotheses for how an enzyme achieves specificity. The first is called the 'lock and key' model, proposed by Emil Fischer in the 1890s. In this model, in the same way that a key fits the shape of a specific lock in order to be able to make the mechanism open, the enzyme substrate is a complementary shape to the active site of the enzyme. However, enzymes also stabilize an intermediate part of a biological reaction called the transition state, making it more likely to occur. Although the lock-and-key model explains how specificity occurs, it cannot explain how stabilization occurs, and so is now thought to be incorrect. The second model is the 'induced fit' model proposed by Daniel Koshland Jr in 1958. This model not only explains how specificity occurs but also how the transition state is stabilized. In this model, the enzyme is flexible and is constantly reshaped by interactions with the substrate. The active site can therefore bend into shape to enable a substance to bind, and is only a complementary shape once full binding occurs.

The most important features of enzymes are that they have catalytic power, specificity and are highly regulated.

Enzyme cooperativity is a phenomenon whereby the affinity for the substrate at an active site changes in accordance to the binding of the substrate at another active site within the quaternary enzyme.

For full activity, many enzymes also need to bind to other small molecules called *cofactors*. These can be substrates or products of the reaction being catalyzed or molecules further down the pathway. Binding by a cofactor causes either an increase or decrease in the enzyme activity. An enzyme in the absence of its cofactor is called an *apoenzyme* and when the cofactor binds to enable full catalytic activity the enzyme is called a *holoenzyme*. Cofactors can be divided into two main groups: metals and small organic molecules called **coenzymes**. Coenzymes are often derived from vitamins, such as vitamin B1 (thiamine), B2 (riboflavin), B3 (niacin), B6 (pyridoxine), B9 (folic acid), B12 (the cobalamins) and vitamin C, and can be bound tightly (called *prosthetic groups*) or loosely (called *cosubstrates*) to the enzyme. Enzymes using the same coenzyme will often catalyze a reaction using a similar mechanism. Examples of cofactors and the enzymes they regulate are shown in Table 10.2.

Table 10.2 Cofactors and the enzymes they regulate

Cofactor	Enzyme(s) regulated
Metal (ion)	
Copper (Cu^{2+})	Cytochrome oxidase
Iron (Fe^{2+} or Fe^{3+})	Cytochrome oxidase
	Catalase
	Peroxidase
Potassium (K^+)	Pyruvate kinase
	Propionyl-CoA carboxylase
Magnesium (Mg^{2+})	Hexokinase
	DNA polymerase
	Glucose-6-phosphatase
Manganese (Mn^{2+})	Arginase
	Superoxide dismutase
Molybdenum (Mo^{6+})	Nitrate reductase
Nickel (Ni^{2+})	Urease
Selenium	Glutathione peroxidase
Coenzyme	
Biotin	Propionyl-CoA carboxylase
	Pyruvate carboxylase
Coenzyme A	Acetyl-CoA carboxylase
5′-Deoxyadenosylcobalamin (vitamin B_{12})	Methylmalonyl-CoA mutase
Flavin adenine dinucleotide (FAD) (vitamin B_2)	Succinate dehydrogenase
	Monoamine oxidase
Nictotinamide adenine dinucleotide (NAD^+) (vitamin B_3)	Alcohol dehydrogenase
	Lactate dehydrogenase

Continued

Table 10.2 Continued

Cofactor	Enzyme(s) regulated
Pyridoxal phosphate (vitamin B$_6$)	Aspartate aminotransferase Glycogen phosphorylase
Tetrahydrofolate (folic acid)	Thymidylate synthase
Thiamine pyrophosphate (vitamin B$_1$)	Pyruvate dehydrogenase

Self-check 10.3

What is an enzyme active site and how is it produced?

Enzyme kinetics

Although biological reactions will take place without an enzyme present, they may occur too slowly for the demands of our bodies. Enzymes increase the speed of reactions so that essential products are formed quickly enough to keep us alive. Enzyme kinetics describes the rate at which enzymes catalyze biological reactions. The maximum rate of a reaction and the binding affinities for substrates and potential inhibitors are vital for the understanding of cellular metabolism, where each reaction is catalyzed by a different enzyme. As drug molecules are often specific inhibitors targeted to particular enzymes, the pharmaceutical industry requires this information to design and create new therapeutic agents.

It is important to appreciate that the amount of product formed stays the same, no matter whether the enzyme is present or absent. The only difference is the speed at which this amount is reached. Enzymes decrease the activation energy required for the reaction to take place, thus the reaction can proceed at an accelerated rate. Figure 10.8 shows the rate of product formation with time when in the presence and absence of an enzyme.

Enzymes are catalysts and can only alter the rate of reaction, not the position of the equilibrium of a reaction, since the latter would be against the laws of thermodynamics.

Figure 10.8 Enzymes accelerate the rate of a reaction but not the position of equilibrium. The same equilibrium point is reached by reactions in the presence or absence of an enzyme

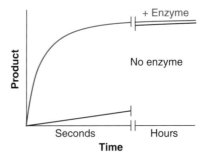

An enzyme reaction will reach a saturation point at which the concentration of substrate saturates the enzyme and V no longer increases.

When a graph of concentration of product (on the y-axis) is plotted against time (on the x-axis), the steepness of the line shows us how quickly it is being formed. A steep line means that the product is formed more quickly than when the slope of the line is more gradual. The rate of production is measured by calculating the slope (also called the gradient) of the line at any desired time point. Figure 10.8 shows that the rate of product formation decreases over time as the gradient of the line becomes less steep as time increases. This is owing to a *steady-state equilibrium* being attained. meaning the amount of substrate being converted into product in the forward reaction is equal to the amount of product being converted back into substrate in the reverse reaction. For each reaction there is a corresponding rate constant (k). Each rate constant is dependent on the concentration of substrate and has the unit of time^{-1}, normally quoted in sec^{-1}.

As mentioned previously, enzymes aid the formation of a transition state. This transition state is an unstable structure that is neither the product nor the substrate. Because it is highly unstable, the transition state molecule only exists for a short amount of time. By comparison, the substrate or product molecules are relatively stable and so exist for much longer periods of time. After the reaction has taken place, the enzyme is unchanged and so it can be used repeatedly when required.

Equations to define enzyme kinetics

When a substrate binds to an enzyme, the speed or rate at which the product is formed is given the letter V for *velocity*. The rate of catalysis at the start of the reaction, V_0, is the number of moles of product formed per second. However, if the concentration of substrate is increased, the rate of catalysis begins to level off and approaches a limit called the *maximum rate* (V_{max}).

In 1913, Leonor Michaelis and Maud Leonora Menten proposed a model to explain the concept of enzyme kinetics. Their model stated that when an enzyme E is in the presence of a substrate S, it first binds to the substrate forming an enzyme–substrate (ES) complex. The ES complex then has two fates: to dissociate back to enzyme and substrate, or for the substrate to be broken down to give a product P and release the enzyme. The reaction is reversible at each stage, and the mechanism can therefore be given the equation:

$$E + S \underset{K_{-1}}{\overset{K_1}{\rightleftharpoons}} ES \underset{K_{-2}}{\overset{K_2}{\rightleftharpoons}} E + S$$

Each reaction has its own rate constant (k_1 and k_2 for the forward reactions and k_{-1}, and k_{-2} for the reverse reactions). At equilibrium, the enzyme is still actively converting substrate into product, but the product is converted back to substrate at the same rate. At the start of the reaction, as close to zero as possible, there is negligible formation of product and likewise no reverse reaction. The substrate concentration ($[S]$) that gives a speed of half of V_{max} ($V_{max/2}$) is known as the *Michaelis constant* (K_m) and is expressed in units of concentration, usually molar (M). If a graph of V_0 is plotted against $[S]$, a saturation curve is produced as shown in Figure 10.9.

The *Michaelis–Menten equation* shown below relates the rate of reaction with the concentration of substrate, which explains the data given in Figure 10.9.

$$V_0 = V_{max} \frac{[S]}{K_m + [S]}$$

Figure 10.9 A typical saturation curve showing how the initial reaction rate increases with substrate concentration until saturation. At saturation, the speed is maximal and is correspondingly called V_{max}

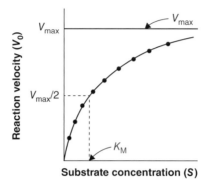

The Michaelis–Menten equation assumes that a steady state has been reached, in which the rate of formation of ES will equal the rate of breakdown of the ES complex. There are a number of other assumptions made when using this equation:

- K_m and V_{max} only define the rate of an enzyme-catalyzed reaction when there is only one substrate; if there are multiple substrates then the concentration of only one can vary while the others stay constant.

- All other variables that can alter kinetics, such as temperature, pH and ionic strength, must be constant.

- K_m and V_{max} are only valid when observing the initial rate of reaction when the product has not yet had time to be made, meaning that the concentration of product is essentially zero.

- The initial concentration of substrate must be greater than the total concentration of enzyme, which stays constant.

Once all these assumptions are agreed, the K_m and V_{max} can then be determined. However, as V_{max} is the rate of reaction at equilibrium, to measure it experimentally is impossible. Likewise, as K_m is a function of V_{max}, this too is impossible to measure. Although we now have curve- fitting software to elucidate these equations, this was not possible before computers were available. Therefore, the curved data were transformed into a straight line with the equation $y = mx + c$. There are a number of ways of doing this. If the reciprocal of both sides of the Michaelis–Menten equation is taken, this gives us the *Lineweaver–Burk* or *double reciprocal equation*:

$$\frac{1}{V_0} = \frac{K_m + [S]}{V_{max}[S]}$$

When plotted graphically with $1/V_0$ on the *y*-axis and $1/[S]$ on the *x*-axis, the line is linear and the gradient is equal to K_m/V_{max}, as shown in Figure 10.10.

   This method has the inherent problem that the double reciprocal means that the errors from measurement are consequently increased. To find the intercept on the *x*-axis also involves a large amount of extrapolation, which is inaccurate. To combat this, other linear plots have been developed as described in Box 10.2.

   K_m and V_{max} are important as they are a measure of the effectiveness of a particular enzyme. K_m for enzymes varies greatly, from 10^{-7} M to 10^{-1} M, and indicates how much substrate is needed

Figure 10.10   A Lineweaver–Burk plot. This is a double reciprocal plot generated by plotting $1/V_0$ on the y-axis against $1/[S]$. The intercept on the x-axis is $-1/K_m$, and the intercept on the y-axis is $1/V_{max}$. The gradient of the line is K_m/V_{max}

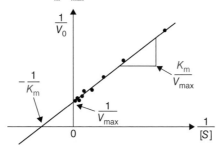

10.2   Enzymes and enzyme inhibition

Box 10.2   Alternative enzyme kinetics plots

The Eadie–Hofstee plot, with V on the y-axis and $V/[S]$ on the x-axis, gives a straight line with the intercept of the y-axis equal to V_{max} and the gradient equal to $-K_m$. However, neither axis uses independent variables as both are dependent on V. This means that any errors in measurement will be present on both axes. In addition, the Hanes–Woolf plot with $[S]/V$ on the y-axis and $[S]$ on the x-axis gives a straight line with the intercept on the x-axis equal to $-K_m$ and the intercept on the y-axis equal to K_m/V_{max}. In this case the gradient of the line is equal to $1/V_{max}$. Again, neither axis involves independent variables as both rely on $[S]$. None of the ways of plotting the data or the enzyme kinetics are perfect, but we use them accepting their inaccuracies and assumptions.

for significant catalysis to occur. A high K_m indicates weak binding of substrate with the enzyme, whereas a low K_m indicates strong binding of substrate with the enzyme. It therefore indicates the *affinity* of the ES complex. By contrast, V_{max} provides information on the turnover of the enzyme and gives a measure of the number of substrate molecules converted into product in a unit of time, when the enzyme is fully saturated with substrate.

Allosteric enzymes, with their multiple subunits and multiple active sites, do not obey the rules of Michaelis–Menten kinetics. Here, the binding of a substrate at one active site induces changes to the molecular structure that can change the binding at other active sites. This cooperativity causes the plot of V_0 against $[S]$ to be an 'S' shape. Allosteric enzymes may also be altered by molecules that can be reversibly bound to regions other than the active sites. Their catalytic nature can therefore be adjusted to meet the needs of the cell, and for this reason these enzymes are key regulators of metabolic pathways.

Enzyme inhibition

Since important biological reactions are catalyzed by enzymes, it follows that many drugs have been developed to interfere with the reaction kinetics. These therapeutic agents, called *enzyme inhibitors*, may be small molecules or ions. Enzyme inhibition can be irreversible or reversible.

Self-check 10.4

Why does an enzymatic reaction form a saturation curve when the reaction rate is plotted against the substrate concentration?

Following coronary artery bypass surgery, Lynda has been prescribed daily low dose (75 mg) aspirin. As she is collecting her prescription she asks her pharmacist, Tu, why she has been prescribed this medication and why she could not just take the aspirin tablets she has in the medicine cabinet. Tu explains to her the reason for the medication and why it is important to take the daily low dose aspirin rather than the higher dose aspirin tablets from her medicine cabinet.

Reflection questions
1. What is the rationale for prescribing the low dose of aspirin?
2. Why is the normal dose of aspirin not necessary?
3. Why would the normal dose of aspirin be inadvisable in these circumstances?

For answers, visit the online resources which accompany this textbook.

In general, the most potent inhibitors tend to be analogues of transition state molecules. A common enzyme inhibitor that is used as a drug is aspirin, which inhibits the cyclooxygenase enzymes that produce prostaglandins during inflammation. By reversibly inhibiting these enzymes, pain and inflammation are therefore suppressed (see Case study 10.1).

Irreversible inhibitors and slow-binding reversible inhibitors

Irreversible enzyme inhibitors covalently modify the structure of the enzyme active site. They dissociate from the enzyme very slowly because the bonds between the enzyme and inhibitor are strong, thus preventing inhibition from being reversed. Dilution or dialysis will therefore not dislodge the inhibitor and cannot be used to reverse the effect of an irreversible inhibitor. They are normally specific for a type of enzyme. Inhibition by these molecules is not instantaneous but depends on the time spent in contact with the enzyme—the longer the inhibitor is in contact with the enzyme, the stronger the interaction between the enzyme and inhibitor.

Irreversible inhibitors bind to the enzyme as a normal substrate would, thus initiating catalysis. However, an intermediate molecule is generated that covalently modifies the active site and thus irreversibly inhibits the enzyme. Examples of irreversible inhibitors are the monoamine oxidase enzyme inhibitors selegiline and tranylcypromine, which are used to treat Parkinsonism and depression, respectively. Another example is the antibiotic penicillin, which covalently modifies the serine residues in the active site of the transpeptidase enzyme and so prevents bacterial cell wall synthesis, effectively killing the bacteria.

There are also some slow-binding reversible inhibitors that bind non-covalently but resemble irreversible inhibitors because their binding is so strong. One example is methotrexate, which inhibits the dihydrofolate reductase enzyme involved in folic acid metabolism and is used in the treatment of cancer and autoimmune disorders.

Reversible inhibitors

Reversible inhibitors interact with the enzyme using non-covalent interactions, including hydrogen bonds, hydrophobic interactions and ionic bonds. The strength of inhibition is maximized by multiple weak bonds between the enzyme active site and the inhibitor. Reversible inhibitors

Box 10.3   Competitive inhibitors

Nitisinone is a competitive inhibitor of 4-hydroxyphenylpyruvate oxidase. It is used to treat type I tyrosinaemia, which is a disease that leads to the build-up of tyrosine in the blood. Other examples of therapeutic competitive inhibitors include ibuprofen, which competitively inhibits the enzymes involved in inflammation, and statins, which competitively inhibit an enzyme in the cholesterol biosynthesis pathway to reduce blood cholesterol levels (see also Section 10.3). Even some foodstuffs can act as competitive inhibitors. One example is grapefruit juice, which contains bergamottin. Bergamottin competitively inhibits the cytochrome P450 enzyme, which is involved in the metabolic breakdown of statins and other drugs. If grapefruit juice is consumed at the same time as statins, it can lead to the accumulation of an excessively high level of statins in the body, resulting in liver damage. Similarly, consumption of grapefruit juice with some hayfever drugs, for example terfeadine, is equally dangerous for the same reason.

can often be easily removed from the enzyme by dilution or dialysis, and their activity is characterized by a rapid association/dissociation with the enzyme. Reversible inhibitors are classified under four groups according to the method of inhibition:

1. *Competitive inhibition* is where the substrate and the inhibitor try to bind at the same active site and compete for the same space. Examples of clinically relevant competitive inhibitors are given in Box 10.3. This type of inhibition can be overcome by increasing the concentration of the substrate, as it will then out-compete the inhibitor for the active site. This can be shown graphically in terms of both reaction rate versus substrate concentration graphs and Lineweaver–Burk plots, as shown in Figure 10.11.

2. *Uncompetitive inhibition* is where the inhibitor binds to the ES complex, but not the free enzyme, and forms an enzyme–substrate–inhibitor (ESI) complex. This makes the ES complex inactive and prevents the formation of product. The uncompetitive inhibitor's binding site is only formed once the ES complex occurs. In the presence of an uncompetitive inhibitor, the ESI complex cannot form product and so V_{max} is therefore reduced by comparison with the complex in the absence of inhibitor. Figure 10.12 shows the effects of an uncompetitive inhibitor. This type of inhibition is rare. Lithium, which is used as a mood stabilizer in the treatment of bipolar disorder, has been suggested to work as an uncompetitive inhibitor, although its precise mechanism of action is unknown.

3. *Mixed inhibition* involves the inhibitor binding to both the free enzyme and the ES complex, although the affinity for each is different. This is because the inhibitor and the substrate bind to the enzyme at separate sites. However, the binding of the inhibitor affects that of the substrate, and vice versa, due to either a conformational change when one binds or by the two sites being close together, enabling interactions to occur. Increasing the substrate concentration can reduce the effects of a mixed inhibitor, but will not remove the inhibition entirely. Mixed inhibitors interfere with the substrate binding, which causes an increase in K_m, while they hinder catalysis of the ES complex, which causes a decrease in V_{max}. This type of inhibition is common and usually results from an allosteric effect. Fluoxetine, a drug that is licensed for treatment of major depression, obsessive–compulsive disorder and severe premenstrual disorder, is thought to act as a mixed inhibitor in some circumstances and a competitive inhibitor in others.

Figure 10.11 Kinetics of a competitive inhibitor. (A) The rate of reaction (*V*) against substrate concentration ([*S*]) shows that higher concentrations of substrate are required for a certain reaction rate to be achieved by out-competing for the active site. (B) Lineweaver–Burk plot showing that K_m is increased by V_{max} is unaffected

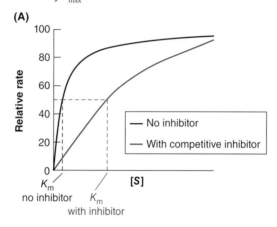

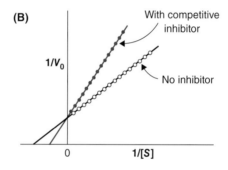

4. *Non-competitive inhibition* can be described as one form of mixed inhibition; however, the inhibitors have identical affinities for both the free enzyme and the ES complex. The binding of the inhibitor to the enzyme again causes a reduction in the enzyme activity but without altering the ability of the substrate to bind. The extent of the inhibition therefore relies only on the concentration of the inhibitor. One example of a non-competitive inhibitor is donepezil, which is a **cholinesterase** inhibitor used in the treatment of Alzheimer's disease. People with this disease have a low level of acetylcholine and so the enzyme that breaks down the acetylcholine in the brain must be inhibited to help maintain a functional level of acetylcholine. A further example is the antiretroviral drug nevirapine, which is a non-nucleoside reverse transcriptase inhibitor used in the treatment of human immunodeficiency virus and acquired immunodeficiency syndrome. Figure 10.13 shows the effect of a non-competitive inhibitor.

Self-check 10.5

Irreversible inhibitors can be used to map enzyme active sites, but how?

Figure 10.12 Kinetics of an uncompetitive inhibitor. (A) The rate of reaction (V) against substrate concentration ($[S]$) shows that V_{max} is not reached, even at high concentrations of substrate. K_m decreases as more inhibitor is present. (B) Lineweaver–Burk plot showing that the gradients of the lines in the presence and absence of inhibitor are identical, as both V_{max} and K_m decrease by the corresponding amounts

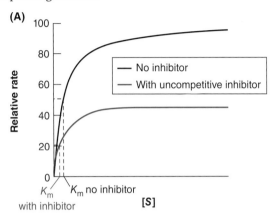

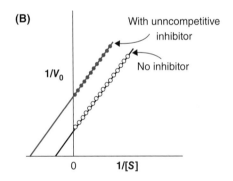

10.3 PROTEINS AS DRUG TARGETS

Proteins, especially enzymes and receptors, are important molecular targets for many drugs. Initially we will focus on the example of a drug targeting an enzyme, although receptors, particularly those which are membrane-bound, are also very important drug targets.

The unique tertiary structure of an enzyme often leads to the formation of a very specific active site. Enzymes are biological catalysts that regulate a wide range of biochemical reactions and their active sites bind specific substrates. Although other mechanisms of action are possible, a drug that targets an enzyme often binds to the active site, blocking the binding of the substrate, and hence inhibiting the function of the enzyme. This is commonly referred to as *enzyme inhibition*.

A good example of a drug that causes enzyme inhibition is the widely prescribed drug, atorvastatin, which is used to treat high cholesterol levels. It works by inhibiting HMG-CoA reductase, an enzyme involved in the production of cholesterol. As illustrated in Figure 10.14, the drug has been designed to bind perfectly in the active site, forming a number of interactions

Figure 10.13 Kinetics of a non-competitive inhibitor. (A) The rate of reaction (V) against substrate concentration ($[S]$) shows that V_{max} is not reached, as the inhibitor binds to both the free enzyme and the enzyme–substrate complex. K_m is unchanged but the reaction rate increases more slowly at low concentrations of substrate. (B) Lineweaver–Burk plot showing that K_m is unaffected but V_{max} is reduced

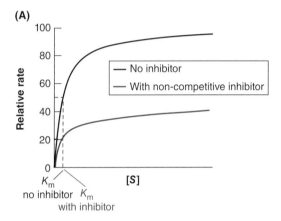

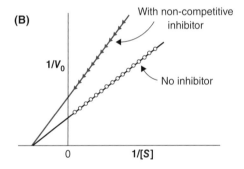

Figure 10.14 A detailed view of atorvastatin bound to the active site of HMG-CoA reductase. The various bonding interactions between the drug and protein are highlighted as black solid lines (hydrogen bonds) and black dashed lines (non-polar interactions)

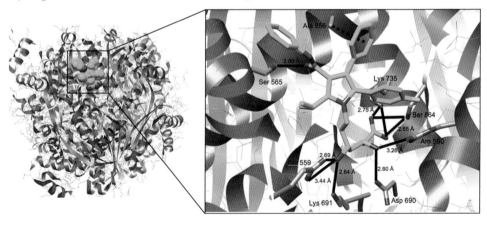

with specific amino acids. The shape of the drug complements the shape and the amino acid functional groups of the enzyme active site.

The wide variety of protein structures means that usually a drug is very specific for a certain protein target (see Chapter 1). This is in contrast to drugs targeting DNA where any planar compound could potentially intercalate with DNA. DNA targeting drugs are therefore much less specific for their target and serious side-effects are common for DNA targeted therapeutics (see Section 9.1).

Endogenous molecules and exogenous molecules such as drugs (often referred to as ligands) interact with specific recognition sites known as receptors. The interaction of such molecules with a receptor leads to a specific biological response. Receptors may be intracellular or extracellular. Extracellular receptors are usually found on cell membranes, often possessing an exofacial binding site linked to an endofacial protein molecule. Receptors are classified into four main types often known as superfamilies. These are ion channel receptors where the endogenous ligands are fast neurotransmitters; G-protein-coupled receptors (GPCRs) where the endogenous ligands are hormones and slow neurotransmitters; tyrosine kinase receptors with insulin and growth factors as endogenous ligands; and nuclear receptors with steroid hormones, thyroid hormones and certain vitamins as endogenous ligands.

GPCRs are probably the most common type of receptor to be utilized as drug targets. It is estimated that 45% of all drugs target GPCRs in some way, although this percentage is gradually falling as new targets are discovered and exploited. Activation of the receptor causes a G-protein to activate a membrane-bound enzyme, leading to the production of a second messenger.

· ·

- Proteins are grouped into three major groups called globular, fibrous and membrane proteins, each of which has different functions which result from their differing structures.

- Protein structure can be described in terms of four levels—primary, secondary, tertiary and quaternary.

- The primary structure of proteins is the sequence of amino acids.

- The secondary structure explains how a polypeptide chain is stabilized by formation of an α-helix or a β-sheet.

- The tertiary structure describes how the protein forms a more compact shape that further enhances stability.

- The quaternary structure describes how some proteins have multiple interacting subunits that come together to give function.

- Enzymes are proteins that have catalytic function by virtue of their active site. They are specific and have affinity for their substrate.

- Allosteric enzymes contain multiple active sites and multiple subunits.

- Enzymes stabilize the formation of a transition state and alter the rate of reaction but not the equilibrium.

- Enzyme inhibition can be irreversible, via modification of the structure of the active site, or reversible via non-covalent interactions that are easily broken.

- Protein molecules, particularly enzymes and receptors, are often drug targets.

Buxbaum, E. *Fundamentals of Protein Structure and Function*, 2nd edn. Springer, 2015. ISBN 9783319199191.

This book covers all the basics of protein structure and function in great detail.

Papachristodolou, D., Snape, A., Elliott, W. H. and Elliott, D. C. *Biochemistry and Molecular Biology*, 6th edn. Oxford University Press, 2018. ISBN 9780198768111.

This is a well-written textbook that covers molecular biology in depth.

Patrick, G. L. *An Introduction to Medicinal Chemistry*, 6th edn. Oxford University Press, 2017. ISBN 9780198749691.

A very accessible textbook that expands upon the chemistry of drugs and their mechanisms of action against target macromolecules.

Self-check

For the answers to the Self-Check questions in Chapter 10, visit the online resources which accompany this textbook.

CARBOHYDRATES AND CARBOHYDRATE METABOLISM

Alex White And Helen Burrell

Carbohydrates (literally meaning *carbon* and *water*) are molecules composed almost exclusively of carbon, hydrogen and oxygen. Carbohydrate monomers are called *monosaccharides* (trivially called *sugars*) and are found throughout nature. Carbohydrates are synthesized in plants during the process of photosynthesis, with their carbon atoms being obtained from atmospheric carbon dioxide. The carbohydrates are a huge class of organic molecules, so we must limit the discussion here to selected examples. Carbohydrates are the main fuel source in our bodies and are divided into two groups: simple sugars and complex carbohydrates. Simple sugars like glucose are metabolized directly via *glycolysis* and the *citric acid cycle*, whereas complex carbohydrates like starch and **glycogen** are first broken down into simple sugars. The process of glycogen breakdown is called *glycogenolysis*. If the intake of carbohydrates exceeds the amount the body needs, the excess is converted into **triacylglycerols** and glycogen for long-term storage. However, if carbohydrate intake is low, for example during fasting, fatty acid breakdown in the liver or kidney occurs. Fatty acids and triacylglycerols are the subunits of lipids, which will be considered in Chapter 12.

Learning objectives

Having read this chapter you are expected to be able to:

- describe the structural features of monosaccharides and their ability to exist as open-chain and cyclic forms
- appreciate the stereochemistry of carbohydrates
- identify the ways in which large carbohydrates are constructed from simple monosaccharides
- appreciate the metabolic pathways by which carbohydrates can provide energy for the body
- explain the process of glycolysis
- describe how the citric acid cycle provides energy in the form of ATP
- explain how glucose can be generated, when required, in the body from other substances
- appreciate the importance to human health of regulating carbohydrate metabolism.

11.1 STRUCTURE OF CARBOHYDRATES

Carbohydrates are classified into simple carbohydrates or monosaccharides, oligosaccharides and complex carbohydrates or polysaccharides.

Simple carbohydrates—monosaccharides

Monosaccharides are the simplest carbohydrates and are classified by the number of carbons they contain. Most common monosaccharides contain five carbons (classified as *pentoses*) or six carbons (known as *hexoses*). The general structure of these carbohydrates features a carbon chain functionalized with several hydroxyl groups and one or two more oxidized groups; aldehydes, ketones or carboxylic acids are all encountered.

Monosaccharides exist in two isomeric forms: open-chain and cyclic. In aqueous solution, these structures are in equilibrium. (Remember that biological systems are aqueous and that all biochemistry occurs in water.) The cyclic form is, generally, more stable and therefore the more likely structure.

Understanding carbohydrate structure is complicated by the large number of stereoisomers that are possible. This issue is addressed by the use of Fischer projections, a convenient way to represent three dimensions on the page of a book. In Figure 11.1, Fischer projections are used to show the structure of the open-chain forms of two common carbohydrates: glucose (a hexose) and ribose (a pentose).

> More details on Fischer projections can be found in Chapter 3, 'Stereochemistry and drug action'.

Figure 11.1 Monosaccharide structure. Different ways to represent the structures of: the hexose sugar, glucose; and ribose, a pentose sugar

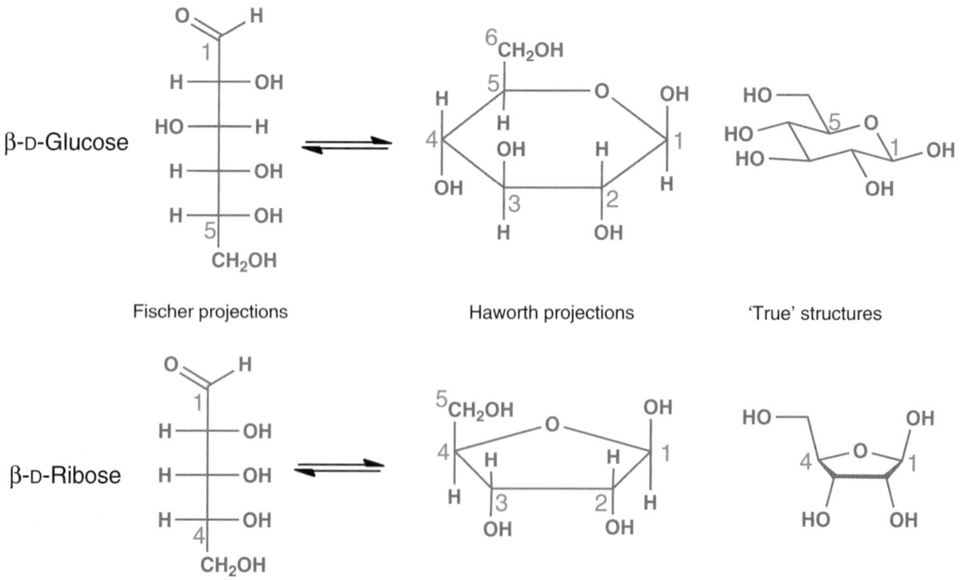

Figure 11.2 D and L glyceraldehyde

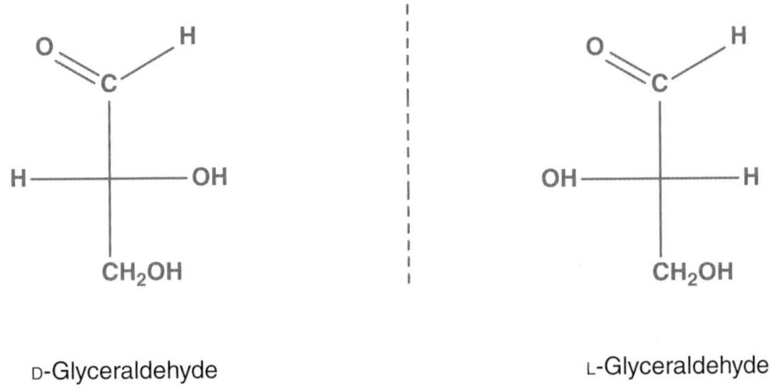

D-Glyceraldehyde

L-Glyceraldehyde

Monosaccharide stereochemistry

The D- and L-notation is used to describe carbohydrate stereochemistry, as well as amino acid stereochemistry. The three-carbon monosaccharide glyceraldehyde is the reference compound. This sugar contains a single chiral centre, resulting in two mirror image enantiomers, assigned D (*dextro*) and L (*levo*) (see Figure 11.2).

Monosaccharides matching this configuration at the highest numbered chiral carbon are named D, and those matching the configuration of L-glyceraldehyde are labelled L. It is important to note that the D/L system is independent of both the R/S system and of optical activity. For example, L-monosaccharides may rotate plane-polarized light in either direction. Although the R/S system is arguably more logical than the D/L method, most common carbohydrates are found in the D form and so the D/L system has become the accepted standard in carbohydrate chemistry.

> Stereochemistry is discussed in more detail in Chapter 3, 'Stereochemistry and drug action', and amino acid stereochemistry is discussed further in Section 10.1.2.

Hemiacetal formation

The cyclic forms of glucose and ribose arise from a nucleophilic reaction between one of their hydroxyl groups and the aldehyde functional group present in both these monosaccharides. Compare the structures in Figure 11.1 and the generalized mechanism shown (see Figure 11.3).

Figure 11.3 Hemiacetal formation

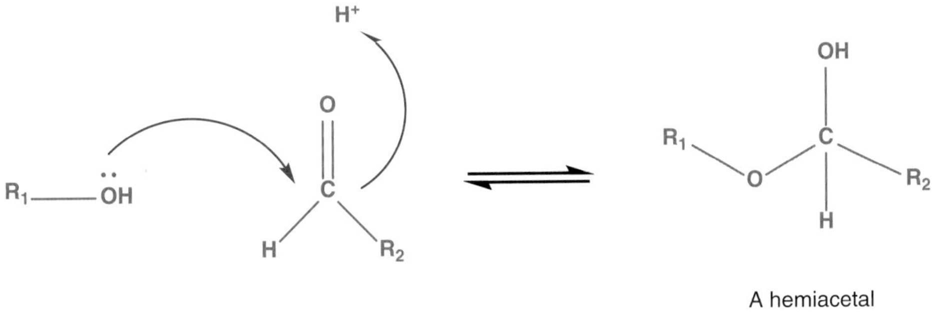

A hemiacetal

Another type of drawing can be used to represent the cyclic form of carbohydrates. Known as *Haworth projections*, they also help us see the three-dimensional shape of the molecule, especially the chiral centres; this type of projection is particularly favoured in biochemistry textbooks. This is still a diagrammatic (easy to draw) way of showing a structure. For comparison, more accurate structures are also shown in Figure 11.1. Note that hexoses such as glucose normally have stable 'chair' conformations.

Included on the Haworth projections in Figure 11.1 is the numbering system used in carbohydrates. By convention, the hemiacetal carbon (also called the anomeric carbon) is labelled C1; the remaining carbons then follow in order.

We might think that any of the hydroxyl groups within an open-chain carbohydrate could react with the highest oxidized group (carbon-1) to yield a hemiacetal. In principle this can and does happen, but at equilibrium the most stable (that is, energetically favoured) cyclic structures are more likely to form. Therefore, in Figure 11.1 the cyclic structures shown for glucose and ribose are those most commonly encountered at equilibrium.

> More information on chair and boat conformations can be found in Chapter 3, 'Stereochemistry and drug action', while hemiacetals and acetals are discussed in greater detail in Chapter 6, 'The carbonyl group and its chemistry'.

Monosaccharide isomerism: anomers

The formation of cyclic monosaccharides can result in two isomers, called the α- and β-anomers. In cyclic D-glucose and D-ribose, the hemiacetal carbon (the aldehyde carbon in the open-chain isomer) is known as the anomeric carbon. The hemiacetal functional group and the *anomeric carbons* are highlighted in Figure 11.4 as a 'C' with related bonds in bold.

The stereochemistry of the anomeric centre is assigned on the basis of stereochemical priorities. In most cases, including D-ribose and D-glucose, the α-anomer has the hydroxyl group in the axial (or down) orientation, whereas in the β-anomer the hydroxyl group is equatorial (or up). Remember that carbohydrates are in equilibrium between the open-chain and cyclic forms. Therefore, in aqueous solution, D-glucose and D-ribose exist as a mixture of the α- and β-anomers. In both these examples, the more stable β-anomers are the major form.

Oligosaccharides

As we have already observed, nucleic acids (see Section 9.2) and proteins (see Section 10.1) are complex biochemical molecules built from simple monomer building blocks. This is also the case for polysaccharides, which are large carbohydrates constructed from simple monosaccharides.

> Cyclic monosaccharides can form two isomers called anomers.

Figure 11.4   Monosaccharide isomerism: anomers

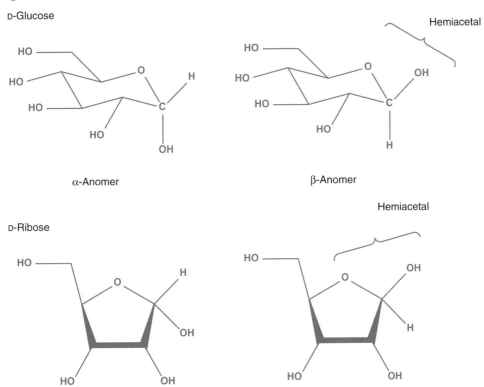

D-Glucose

Hemiacetal

α-Anomer

β-Anomer

Hemiacetal

D-Ribose

Figure 11.5   Sucrose and lactose, two disaccharides (oligosaccharides composed of *two* carbohydrate monomers). The glycosidic bonds are highlighted in bold

α-D-Glucose

β-D-Galactose

β-D-Glucose

β-D-Fructose

Sucrose

Lactose

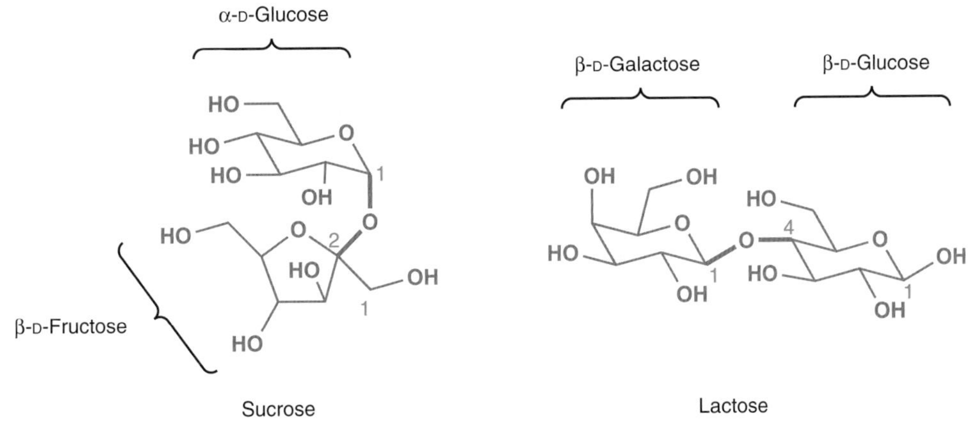

Oligosaccharides are small polysaccharides containing fewer than ten carbohydrate monomers. A good example is sucrose, a molecule familiar to us as table sugar. Sucrose is a **disaccharide** of D-glucose and D-fructose joined by a linkage known as a **glycosidic bond**. These bonds are formed, by loss of water (another condensation reaction), between two adjacent hydroxyl groups, and are highlighted in bold on the structures in Figure 11.5.

Study the structure of sucrose in Figure 11.5 carefully. The D-glucose monomer is the α-anomer (the O-group at carbon 1 is 'down'), and bonds directly to the anomeric carbon

> **Self-check 11.2**
>
> Using the structures within this chapter, draw the structure of the disaccharide D-galactose-(α1→6)-β-D-fructose.

of β-D-fructose. This is the first time we have met fructose. Note that it contains six carbon atoms, so is a hexose carbohydrate, but forms a five-membered ring, because the carbonyl group in the open-chain form was at C2, rather than C1. Therefore carbon-1 is outside the ring system and the anomeric carbon is at position 2.

Glycosidic bonds are described using a convention that describes both the number of each carbon involved in the bond and its anomeric form. In sucrose, the glycosidic bond is between two anomeric carbons and is described as D-glucose-(α1→β2)-D-fructose.

Lactose is a disaccharide of D-galactose (a hexose) and D-glucose. It is present in the milk of many mammals, including cows and humans. The glycosidic linkage between the β-anomeric (C1) hydroxyl group of galactose and the hydroxyl group of C4 in glucose (not an anomeric carbon) is described as D-galactose-(β1→4)-D-glucose. (See Boxes 11.1 and 11.2 on lactose intolerance and the use of lactulose in laxatives.)

The advantage of this system to describe glycosidic bonds is hopefully obvious—with so many variations possible this simple method helps anyone easily determine the nature of the bond between two monosaccharides.

Complex carbohydrates—polysaccharides

Large carbohydrates contain greater numbers of monosaccharide building blocks. Known as polysaccharides, they can be composed of repeats of a single monosaccharide monomer or a mixture of different sugars. A distinctive feature of these macromolecules is their ability to form *branched structures*; this is never seen in nucleic acids or proteins.

> **Box 11.1 Lactose intolerance**
>
> Lactose is an important dietary carbohydrate, especially for infant mammals who consume large quantities of milk. Young children express an intestinal enzyme, β-D-galactosidase (commonly known by the trivial name lactase) that breaks down (or digests) lactose into the two constituent monosaccharides which are readily absorbed into the bloodstream. However, most mammals do not consume large quantities of milk beyond infancy, so the production of this enzyme decreases into adulthood.
>
> Some humans, notably those living in the West, continue to express lactase into adulthood and are able to consume milk and dairy products throughout life. By contrast, most Southeast Asian adults do not express lactase and cannot digest lactose. Milk and dairy products are rarely consumed in these parts of the world.
>
> A minority of Western adults do not express lactase and are said to be lactose intolerant. Eating dairy products causes abdominal discomfort, as bacteria in the lower gut ferment the lactose. Fortunately this condition is easily treated. A variety of preparations of the enzyme lactase are available that can be added to milk, or taken during a meal, to digest lactose and help prevent symptoms occurring.

Box 11.2 Lactulose in laxatives

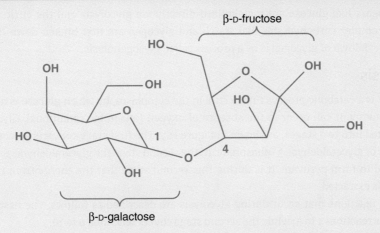

Lactulose is a disaccharide of D-galactose and D-fructose linked by a β1→4 glycosidic bond. Lactulose is used widely as a laxative for the treatment of constipation; it does not occur naturally and is manufactured synthetically. It is taken orally as a syrup and remains un-digested until it reaches the colon. There it causes water to concentrate by osmosis; this softens the accumulated stools, making them easier to pass.

Figure 11.6   The structure of glycogen. Note the branch point (only one is shown) from car-bon-6 of one of the glucose monomers

Glycogen is a common animal polysaccharide used to store glucose. When energy is required, glycogen is rapidly degraded to release glucose monomers. Glycogen is a polymer composed entirely of glucose monomers joined by (α1→4) bonds. The structure of glycogen, shown par-tially in Figure 11.6, contains many branch points. Additional (α1→6) glycosidic bonds start a new branch of the polymer.

Polysaccharides have numerous additional functions in biology. The ABO blood group system is a good example. Oligosaccharides of four or five monosaccharides attached to the surface of the cell membranes of red blood cells act as antigens that determine the blood group of any individual.

11.2 CARBOHYDRATE METABOLISM

Simple sugars like glucose are metabolized directly via glycolysis and the citric acid cycle, whereas complex carbohydrates like starch and glycogen are first broken down into simple sugars. Breakdown of glycogen is by a process called glycogenolysis.

Glycolysis

Glycolysis is a catabolic process that occurs in the cytoplasm, by which glucose is degraded to produce energy. It can occur in the absence of oxygen (anaerobic conditions). Glycolysis can be separated into two stages, as shown in Figure 11.7. The first stage converts glucose into two molecules of glyceraldehyde 3-phosphate. In the second stage the glyceraldehyde 3-phosphate is oxidized to form pyruvate. It is during this second stage that the energy from the glucose molecule is extracted.

The ten reactions that occur during glycolysis are described as follows. The first stage encompasses reactions 1 to 5, while the second stage covers reactions 6 to 10.

1. *Phosphorylation of glucose at the 6-carbon position to form glucose 6-phosphate.* To prevent glucose diffusing out of the cell it is phosphorylated. This irreversible reaction, catalyzed by hexokinase, requires energy, and so one ATP molecule is broken down to ADP. This enzyme, as per all kinases, requires Mg^{2+}, and is allosterically inhibited by the product, glucose 6-phosphate. This stage is highly regulated and inhibition is only removed by subsequent reactions consuming the glucose 6-phosphate. In liver cells this reaction is catalyzed by the enzyme, glucokinase, not hexokinase.

2. *Formation of fructose 6-phosphate.* This is a reversible isomerization step, catalyzed by glucose-6-phophate isomerase, in which an aldose, glucose 6-phosphate, is converted to a ketose, fructose 6-phosphate. The glucose 6-phosphate is initially a cyclic molecule and so the ring is first opened before the isomerization can take place. The ring then reforms to give fructose 6-phosphate.

3. *Phosphorylation of fructose to form fructose 1,6-bisphosphate.* The prefix 'bis' means that the two phosphate groups are on separate carbon atoms. This irreversible reaction again requires Mg^{2+} and utilizes another molecule of ATP. It is catalyzed by phosphofructokinase, which is an allosteric enzyme that determines the speed of glycolysis. The reaction ensures that the cell metabolizes glucose rather than allowing its conversion to another sugar for storage. It is therefore highly regulated.

4. *Cleavage of fructose 1,6-bisphosphate to form two triose phosphates.* This reaction, catalyzed by fructose-bisphosphate aldolase (often just aldolase), gives rise to two triose phosphate products: glyceraldehyde 3-phosphate and dihydroxyacetone phosphate. While glyceraldehyde 3-phosphate is on the direct pathway of glycolysis, dihydroxyacetone phosphate is not. It is, however, converted to glyceraldehyde 3-phosphate during the next step and thus re-enters glycolysis.

5. *Interconversion of glyceraldehyde 3-phosphate and dihydroxyacetone phosphate.* This rapid and reversible reaction is catalyzed by triose phosphate isomerase. At equilibrium, 96% of the triose phosphate is dihydroxyacetone phosphate; interconversion is triggered as the further stages of glycolysis reduce the amount of glyceraldehyde 3-phosphate. This reaction completes the first stage of glycolysis.

Figure 11.7 The glycolytic pathway

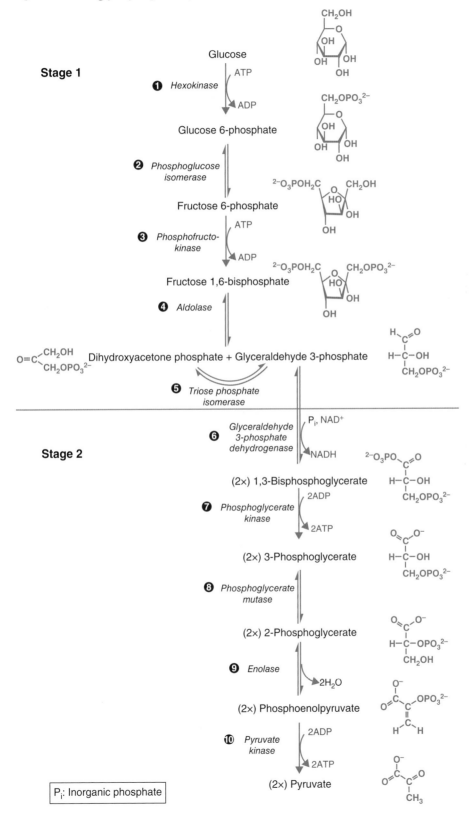

P$_i$: Inorganic phosphate

The overall net reaction of glycolysis is:

$$Glucose + 2ADP + 2P_i + 2NAD^+ \rightarrow 2Pyruvate + 2ATP + 2NADH + 2H^+ + 2H_2O$$

where P_i denotes inorganic phosphate.

6. *Conversion of glyceraldehyde 3-phosphate into 1,3-bisphosphoglycerate.* This reaction involves two steps. The aldehyde group is first oxidized to a carboxylic acid by NAD^+, and second, the carboxylic acid is then joined to an orthophosphate (PO_4^{3-}). The NAD^+ is reduced to NADH. This reaction is catalyzed by glyceraldehyde-3-phosphate dehydrogenase.

7. *Transfer of a phosphoryl group from 1,3-bisphosphoglycerate to ADP to form ATP and 3-phosphoglycerate.* This reaction, catalyzed by phosphoglycerate kinase, is known as a substrate-level phosphorylation and requires a Mg^{2+} ion. As each glucose molecule gives two molecules of glyceraldehyde 3-phosphate, there are therefore two molecules of ATP produced at this stage. With the production of ATP during this reaction, the energy debt from the first stage of glycolysis is paid off.

8. *Movement of the phosphoryl group from 3-phosphoglycerate to form 2-phosphoglycerate.* Phosphoglycerate mutase catalyzes this reaction and produces a substrate molecule that can be further transformed during the next reaction.

9. *Dehydration of 2-phosphoglycerate.* This reaction is catalyzed by enolase, and introduces a double bond to create an enol called phosphoenolpyruvate, which is an unstable molecule and is further transformed during the next reaction.

10. *The conversion of phosphoenolpyruvate to pyruvate, generating ATP.* Phosphoenolpyruvate quickly releases its phosphoryl group to a further molecule of ADP, forming ATP and a molecule of pyruvate. Pyruvate is a more stable molecule than phosphoenolpyruvate. This final reaction is catalyzed by pyruvate kinase and regulated by the concentration of ATP. Again, as there are two molecules of glyceraldehyde 3-phosphate entering stage two of glycolysis, there are two molecules of pyruvate and a further two molecules of ATP formed by the end of glycolysis.

At the end of glycolysis, the important process is to prevent a lack of NAD^+ from becoming limiting. Pyruvate is therefore further metabolized so that NAD^+ is regenerated from NADH. Under anaerobic conditions, for example in contracting muscle cells during intense activity, pyruvate can be reduced by NADH to form lactate (also known as lactic acid—the substance known to cause muscle cramps after intense exercise) and NAD^+. However, under aerobic conditions, pyruvate is further metabolized in the citric acid cycle (also known as the tricarboxylic acid cycle or Krebs cycle).

Citric acid cycle

The pyruvate generated during glycolysis is first transported from the cytoplasm into the mitochondria by a specific carrier protein. Once in the mitochondrial matrix, the pyruvate is oxidatively decarboxylated by pyruvate dehydrogenase to form acetyl coenzyme A (acetyl-CoA). This produces carbon dioxide (CO_2) and a molecule of NADH. The NADH is then reoxidized in the mitochondrial electron transport chain. Pyruvate dehydrogenase is a multienzyme complex that is a non-covalent group of three enzymes and five coenzymes. The acetyl-CoA formed is the fuel for the citric acid cycle, which is a series of eight oxidation–reduction reactions, as shown in Figure 11.8.

Figure 11.8 The citric acid cycle

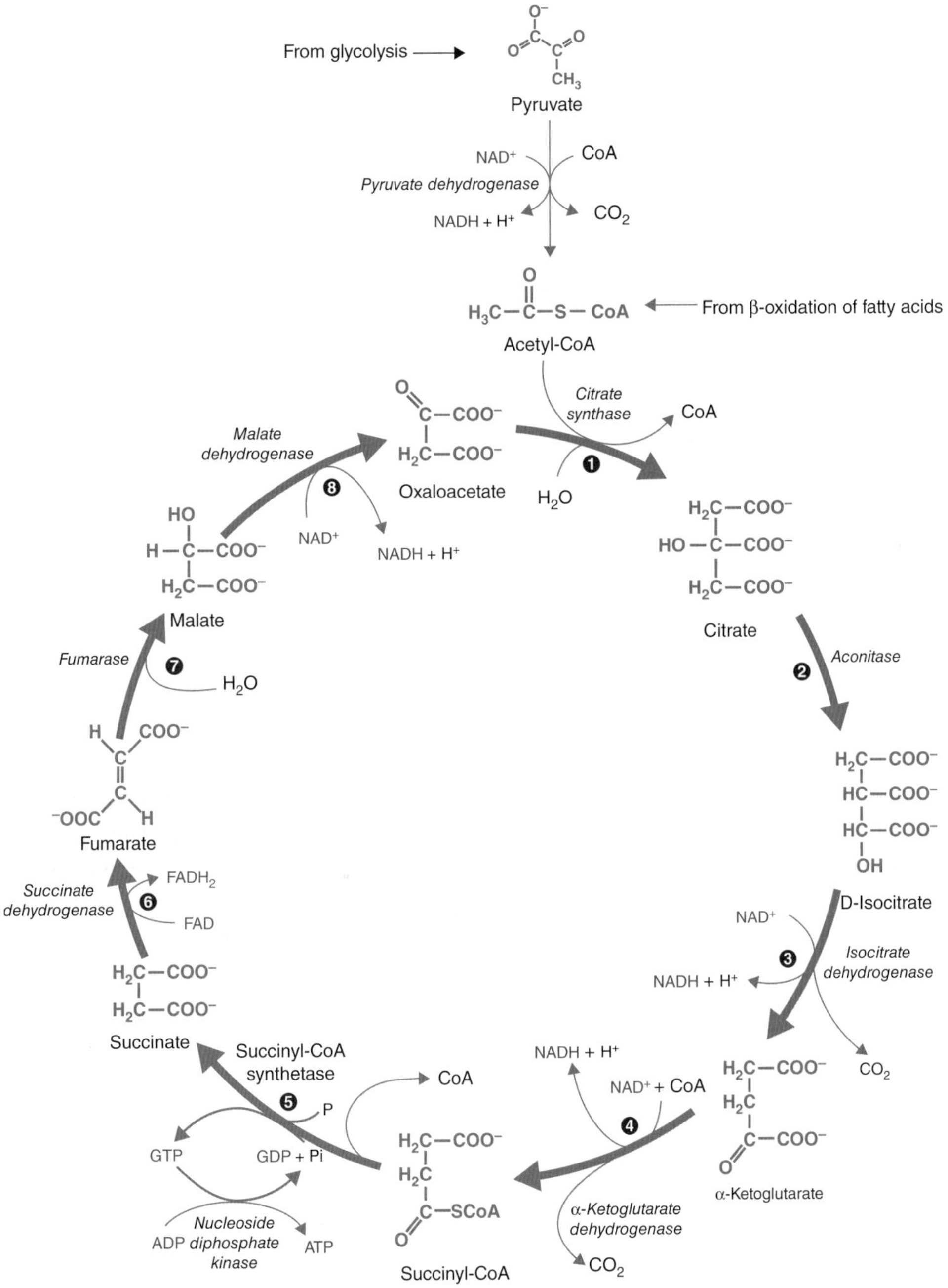

From glycolysis →

Pyruvate

NAD⁺   CoA
Pyruvate dehydrogenase
NADH + H⁺ CO_2

$H_3C-\overset{O}{\overset{\|}{C}}-S-CoA$ ← From β-oxidation of fatty acids

Acetyl-CoA

Citrate synthase   CoA
❶ H_2O

Oxaloacetate

Malate dehydrogenase
❽   NAD⁺   NADH + H⁺

Malate

Citrate

❷   *Aconitase*

Fumarase ❼ H_2O

Fumarate

D-Isocitrate

Succinate dehydrogenase ❻   FADH₂   FAD

NAD⁺
❸   *Isocitrate dehydrogenase*
NADH + H⁺

Succinate

Succinyl-CoA synthetase ❺   CoA   P

GTP   GDP + Pi

NADH + H⁺
NAD⁺ + CoA
❹

α-Ketoglutarate

α-Ketoglutarate

α-Ketoglutarate dehydrogenase
CO_2

Nucleoside diphosphate kinase   ADP   ATP

Succinyl-CoA

CO_2

The eight reactions occurring in the citric acid cycle are described as follows:

1. *Condensation of acetyl-CoA with oxaloacetate.* This produces citrate and is catalyzed by citrate synthase. This enzyme is a dimer that is conformationally changed when oxaloacetate binds to the active site. This change in shape aids the binding of acetyl-CoA and closes the active site to stop water from entering. This prevents the hydrolysis of acetyl-CoA to acetate, which

> The citric acid cycle occurs in the mitochondria and is the final pathway for the oxidation of fuel molecules.

would be detrimental to the citric acid cycle. Both succinyl-CoA, from later in the citric acid cycle, and NADH are allosteric inhibitors of citrate synthase and thus exert some control of the citric acid cycle.

2. *Citrate isomerization into isocitrate.* This reaction is catalyzed by aconitate hydratase (known as aconitase), and the isocitrate produced is the start of four oxidation–reduction reactions.

3. *Isocitrate is oxidatively decarboxylated to α-ketoglutarate, with the concomitant reduction of NAD^+ to NADH.* The rate of α-ketoglutarate formation, catalyzed by isocitrate dehydrogenase, determines the overall rate of the citric acid cycle.

4. *The α-ketoglutarate is oxidatively decarboxylated to form succinyl-CoA, with the further concomitant reduction of NAD^+ to NADH.* This reaction is catalyzed by 2-oxoglutarate dehydrogenase (α-ketoglutarate dehydrogenase), which again is a multienzyme complex with four enzymes and five coenzymes. Succinyl-CoA is a high-energy intermediate used to drive the phosphorylation of guanosine-5'-diphosphate (GDP) to guanosine-5'- triphosphate (GTP).

5. *Cleavage of the thioester bond within succinyl-CoA to form succinate.* The reaction is catalyzed by succinyl-CoA synthetase (also known as succinyl-CoA ligase) and forms a molecule of GTP. This GTP is interconverted to ATP by nucleoside diphosphokinase, whereby the terminal phosphate from the GTP is donated to ADP to form ATP in the following reaction:

$$GTP + ADP \leftrightarrow ATP + GDP$$

6. *Oxidation of succinate to fumarate.* This oxidation involves the removal of hydrogen atoms. The enzyme involved is succinate dehydrogenase, which is a membrane-bound enzyme that is part of the mitochondrial electron transport chain. This reaction is exergonic enough to reduce FAD to $FADH_2$. Succinate dehydrogenase is a dimer and the FAD covalently binds to one of the subunits.

7. *Fumarate is hydrated to form l-malate.* The hydration step, catalyzed by fumarate hydratase (fumarase), converts fumarate into an oxidizable product (malate), enabling further conversion in the cycle.

8. *Oxidation of malate to oxaloacetate.* Malate dehydrogenase catalyzes this final reaction in the citric acid cycle, which is coupled to the reduction of a final molecule of NAD^+. The concentration of oxaloacetate within the mitochondrial matrix is usually low, as the reaction involving citrate synthase (the first reaction within the citric acid cycle) is more favourable and quickly removes the final product.

The twelve reduced coenzymes (10 NADH and 2 $FADH_2$) generated from one molecule of glucose which has undergone glycolysis and the citric acid cycle then produce a further maximum of thirty-four ATP molecules in the electron transport and oxidative phosphorylation pathways, since each NADH molecule can yield three ATP molecules, and each $FADH_2$ can yield two ATP molecules. Box 11.3 emphasizes the importance of the pathways involving carbohydrates.

> The overall net equation of the citric acid cycle is:
> $$Acetyl\text{-}CoA + 3NAD^+ + FAD + ADP + P_i + 2H_2O \rightarrow CoA + 2CO_2 + 3NADH + ATP + H^+$$

Box 11.3 Diseases of carbohydrate metabolism

As changes to the key stages within the citric acid cycle would be severely detrimental, diseases involving them are rarely seen as they are more than likely lethal to the individual. However, diseases due to altered glycolysis can occur. In particular, red blood cells can be severely affected as they have no mitochondria and so cannot obtain energy through the citric acid cycle. Deficiency of one or more enzymes in the glycolysis pathway within red blood cells results in their destruction, as their energy needs are not met. This causes haemolytic anaemia, the most common cause of which is pyruvate kinase deficiency, which leads to the accumulation of 3-phosphoglycerate.

McArdle's syndrome is an autosomal recessive disorder in which a defect in the glycogen phosphorylase gene results in an inability to break down glycogen in the muscle. People with McArdle's syndrome cannot intensively or excessively exercise as they cannot break down glycogen to glucose. Instead, glucose 1-phosphate is formed and, since this molecule has a phosphate group attached, it means it cannot leave the cell via the glucose transporters. Muscle activity is then dependent on the availability of glucose circulating in the bloodstream, rather than from storage.

When glycolysis and the citric acid cycle are taken together, the net equation is:

$$\text{Glucose} + 2H_2O + 10NAD^+ + 2FAD + 4ADP + P_i \rightarrow 6CO_2 + 10NADH + 10H^+ + 2FADH_2 + 4ATP$$

341

Gluconeogenesis

Both the brain and red blood cells use glucose as their only fuel. This leads to the question of what happens if the supply of glucose runs out. The answer is that there are mechanisms in place to generate glucose from other substances. One of these processes is called gluconeogenesis, and it occurs in the liver or kidney during starvation or fasting. This pathway converts pyruvate into glucose, as shown in Figure 11.9.

In addition to pyruvate, three other fuels can also enter the gluconeogenesis pathway. These are lactate from skeletal muscle, glycerol from storage, and amino acids from the diet or from the breakdown of muscle. The breakdown of muscle occurs particularly during periods of starvation; some of the amino acids released enter the gluconeogenesis pathway via oxaloacetate or pyruvate. Lactate is converted to pyruvate using lactate dehydrogenase, and the pyruvate then enters gluconeogenesis. The hydrolysis of triacylglycerols in the adipose tissue forms glycerol and fatty acids. The glycerol then enters the gluconeogenesis pathway via dihydroxyacetone phosphate.

Gluconeogenesis is not simply the reverse of glycolysis, as some of the steps are irreversible and involve the use of different enzymes, as detailed in Figure 11.9. The first step, conversion of pyruvate to oxaloacetate, takes place inside the mitochondria but the rest of the pathway takes place in the cytoplasm. The oxaloacetate is then reduced to malate by an NADH-linked malate dehydrogenase inside the mitochondria. Malate can cross the mitochondrial membrane, and once in the cytoplasm it is reoxidized to oxaloacetate by NAD$^+$-linked malate dehydrogenase. The next stages then take place in the cytoplasm, until the final step, where glucose is formed from glucose 6-phosphate. This final step takes place inside the lumen of the endoplasmic

Figure 11.9 Gluconeogenesis and the entry points for alternative fuels

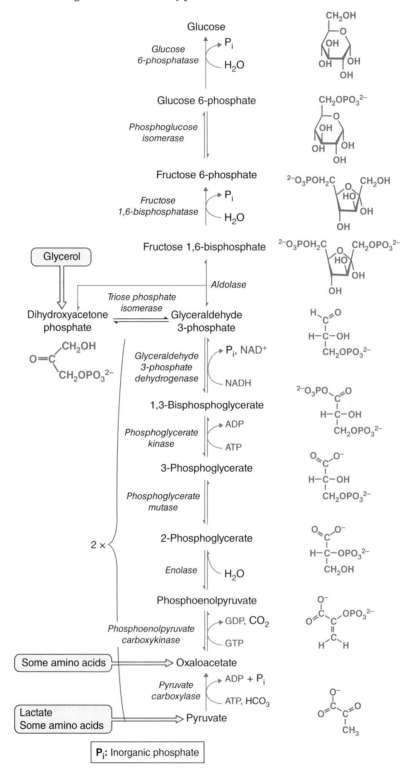

P$_i$: Inorganic phosphate

> Gluconeogenesis is the formation of glucose from pyruvate and should not be confused with glycogenesis, which is the formation of glycogen from glucose.

reticulum of liver or kidney cells only. In other tissues, gluconeogenesis finishes with glucose 6-phosphate, which cannot be transported out of the cell and so accumulates to be stored as glycogen in the process of *glycogenesis*.

11.3 **REGULATION OF CARBOHYDRATE METABOLISM**

Carbohydrate metabolism is fundamental in generating energy for biological processes under normal circumstances. Controlling the blood glucose level is important for the functioning of many organs, and it is therefore not surprising that there are numerous regulatory stages in carbohydrate metabolism.

Phosphofructokinase is the most important controlling enzyme in glycolysis and is inhibited by high levels of ATP. It has two ATP binding sites. The first is a high-affinity catalytic site, and the second is a low-affinity regulatory site. When ATP binds to the catalytic site, the enzyme's affinity for its other substrate, fructose 6-phosphate, is reduced. AMP prevents permanent inhibition of phosphofructokinase by competing with ATP for the allosteric regulatory site. As the concentration of ATP falls due to consumption, the ratio of ATP to AMP is reduced, and this stimulates glycolysis. In muscle, a decrease in pH also inhibits phosphofructokinase. The pH falls due to the formation of lactic acid during intense activity that induces anaerobic conditions (for example a sprint). Inhibition prevents muscle damage by accumulation of too high a concentration of lactic acid. By contrast, in aerobic conditions such as a long, slow run, the citric acid cycle is activated and the pyruvate is converted to CO_2 and H_2O rather than lactate. In the liver, lactate is not normally formed and so low pH is not regulatory here. Instead, phosphofructokinase is inhibited by citrate, a metabolite formed in the citric acid cycle, which enhances the inhibitory effect of ATP. A high level of cytoplasmic citrate ensures that there are sufficient metabolic precursors, meaning further glycolysis is unnecessary.

When phosphofructokinase is inactive, the level of fructose 6-phosphate is elevated and this elevates the concentration of glucose 6-phosphate as the two products are in equilibrium. The glucose 6-phosphate can then be converted to glycogen for storage.

This is not the only glycolysis step to have physiological regulation; the pathway is also regulated at the first step, whereby hexokinase is inhibited by its product, glucose 6-phosphate. In the muscle, accumulation of glucose 6-phosphate signals that glucose is no longer needed for energy, and it therefore remains in the bloodstream and is subsequently stored as glycogen (in the liver) or used to synthesize fatty acids.

While hexokinase is involved in most cells, glucokinase is used in the liver when blood glucose levels are high. Glucokinase has approximately 50-fold lower affinity for glucose than hexokinase. This lower affinity ensures that when glucose levels are low, the glucose is used up by the brain and muscles first. This is also a point at which positive feedback can occur, as outlined in Box 11.4.

The final reaction within glycolysis is also regulated. There are several isoforms of the enzyme pyruvate kinase: the muscle contains type M, whereas the liver contains type L. ATP allosterically inhibits pyruvate kinase, and when concentrations of ATP are high, the rate of glycolysis is reduced. This allosteric inhibition is also achieved by the amino acid alanine, which

Box 11.4 Positive feedback

Glucokinase is also present in the β-cells of the pancreas. The resulting formation of glucose 6-phosphate in this organ leads to the secretion of insulin, the hormone involved in stimulating the uptake of glucose by the cells. This type of positive feedback signals for glucose to be removed from the bloodstream. The glucose is then metabolized by glucokinase to form more glucose 6-phosphate, which is the precursor for glycogen formation.

Case study 11.1

Huri is a type 1 diabetic and has been on insulin all of his life. He has gone to the GP after feeling very tired and nauseous and having passed out on a number of occasions. The GP took a routine blood and urine sample and told him he has high levels of ketones in his urine. The GP explained to Huri that he has developed ketoacidosis because of his diabetes.

Reflection questions

1. What is diabetes, and what are the different types of diabetes?

2. Why do ketone bodies form in diabetic patients?

3. What are the symptoms of ketoacidosis?

For answers, visit the online resources which accompany this textbook.

can be synthesized from and broken down to pyruvate. When the level of ATP is low, fructose 1,6-bisphosphate from earlier in the pathway activates pyruvate kinase to enhance the rate of glycolysis. In the liver, there is an additional controlling feature via reversible phosphorylation. When blood glucose is low, the pancreatic hormone **glucagon** triggers a messenger cascade involving **3',5'-cyclic adenosine monophosphate (cAMP)**. This phosphorylates the pyruvate kinase type L and thus reduces its activity to prevent glucose consumption by the liver when the brain's need is greater.

- Carbohydrates are classified as monosaccharides, oligosaccharides and polysaccharides.
- Monosaccharides exist in two isomeric forms, open-chain and cyclic, which are in equilibrium in aqueous solution.
- There are a number of ways of representing the structure of carbohydrates: Fischer projections for the open-chain form and, for the cyclic form, Haworth projections and the form which more closely resembles the 3-dimensional structure—the conformational structure.
- Oligosaccharides generally contain fewer than ten monomeric units.
- The monosaccharides in oligosaccharides are joined together by a variety of glycosidic linkages.

- Polysaccharides contain larger numbers of monosaccharide units, either of a single monosaccharide or a number of different monosaccharide units.
- Carbohydrates are the main fuel for metabolic processes.
- Glycolysis is the breakdown of glucose to pyruvate. There are a number of enzymes involved, and the key stages are regulated to ensure appropriate use of energy resources.
- The citric acid cycle is an aerobic process which converts pyruvate to acetyl-CoA and energy (in the form of ATP). It occurs in a cyclical series of reactions involving different enzymes at each stage.
- Physiologically, the regulation of glycolysis and the citric acid cycle depends on the tissue, the level of physical activity and the intake of fuel in the diet. The liver and muscle are the key tissues.
- Depending on the blood glucose level, the body either metabolizes what it has taken in or demands fuels from stores.
- If too many fuel molecules are taken in, the components are sent for storage.

FURTHER READING

McKee, T. and McKee, J. R. *Biochemistry: The Molecular Basis of Life*, 6th edn. Oxford University Press, 2015. ISBN 978-0-19-029896.

A very accessible textbook which covers all aspects of carbohydrates and carbohydrate metabolism.

Papachristodolou, D., Snape, A., Elliott, W. H. and Elliott, D. C. *Biochemistry and Molecular Biology*, 6th edn. Oxford University Press, 2018. ISBN 978-0-19-88768111.

This is a well-written textbook that covers molecular biology in depth.

Patrick, G. L., *An Introduction to Medicinal Chemistry*, 6th edn. Oxford University Press, 2017. ISBN 978-0-19-8749691.

A very accessible textbook that expands upon the chemistry of drugs and their mechanisms of action against target macromolecules.

Self-check

For the answers to the Self-Check questions in Chapter 11, visit the online resources which accompany this textbook.

CHAPTER 12

LIPIDS

Alex White And Helen Burrell

In previous chapters we looked at aspects of the classes of macromolecules which are nucleic acids, proteins and carbohydrates. In this chapter we will consider the final class of macromolecules: lipids. They possess a greater variety of structural types than the previous classes of macromolecules and include fatty acids, triglycerides, phospholipids and steroids. Lipids can be broadly defined as water-insoluble molecules from biological systems that are readily soluble in non-polar organic solvents. In other words, they are hydrophobic. This property is unusual; the previous classes of macromolecules we have studied so far are hydrophilic and dissolve readily in water. The non-polar properties of lipids are vital to several important aspects of their biochemical roles. Finally, lipids differ from the other macromolecules we have considered in that they do not form large polymeric structures. They are mainly smaller and simpler molecules.

Learning objectives

After reading this chapter you should be able to:

- recognize the variety of types of molecule which are classified as lipids
- discuss the biochemistry of lipids and outline how these molecules function at the molecular level
- explain how the variety of structures of lipids is related to their biological function
- appreciate what happens to fatty acids within the body in terms of their metabolic pathways and how these pathways are regulated.

12.1 FATTY ACIDS

Fatty acids are the best-known examples of lipids, though they are usually found in biochemistry as components of larger molecules. Fatty acids have a single carboxylic acid functional group attached to an unbranched hydrocarbon chain. The length of this chain, and the degree of saturation, characterizes individual fatty acids. The chain length can be classified as short (less than six carbons), medium (six to twelve carbons) or long (greater than twelve carbons). These chains may be fully saturated (no double bonds) or unsaturated (containing one or more double bonds). Almost all naturally occurring fatty acids contain an even number of carbons.

Medium- and long-chain fatty acids are **amphiphilic**, a term used in biochemistry to describe molecules with both polar and non-polar characteristics. This property arises because the carboxylic acid is a very polar functional group, but the long hydrocarbon chain is very non-polar.

> Properties of amphiphilic molecules are discussed in Chapter 5, 'Alcohols, phenols, ethers, organic halogen compounds, and amines'

You have met acetic acid (ethanoic acid), the most important short-chain fatty acid, many times in this book. Most important fatty acids in human biochemistry are long-chained, with up to about twenty carbon atoms. Figure 12.1 illustrates three typical long-chain fatty acid structures. Each is a *free fatty acid*, meaning that the carboxylic acid functional group is not bonded to another group. Stearic acid is an 18-carbon, saturated fatty acid. Oleic acid is an unsaturated fatty acid with a Z (*cis*) double bond at carbon-9 (see also Box 12.1).

Figure 12.1   Examples of common fatty acids. Compare each drawn structure against the accompanying molecular model showing the precise three-dimensional structure

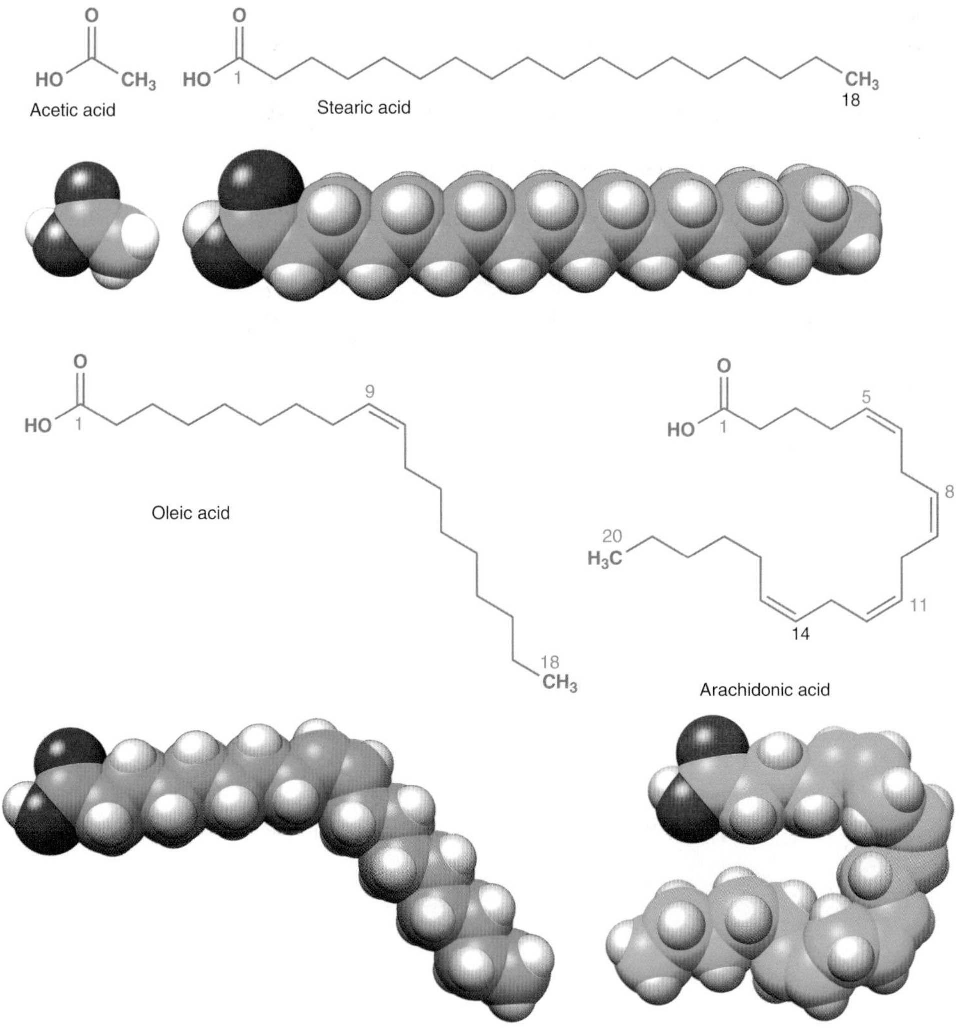

Fatty acids contain one carboxylic acid group, almost always have an even number of carbons and, if the alkyl chain is unsaturated, the double bond(s) will be *cis*.

Arachidonic acid is a *poly*unsaturated fatty acid—in other words, it contains *many* double
bonds. All four double bonds have the Z (*cis*) geometry. Arachidonic acid is notable as the precursor for the 20-carbon eicosanoids, a group including the prostaglandins, thromboxanes and
the leukotrienes, which are all important molecules in cellular signalling. Fatty acids with such
a high degree of unsaturation are otherwise unusual.

Study Figure 12.1 and note the effect that double bonds in the hydrocarbon chain of each fatty
acid have on the structure of the molecule. Stearic acid has a straight and elongated structure.
Oleic acid has a distinctive kink due the double bond. Arachidonic acid, with four double bonds,
has a very different three-dimensional shape. Since double bonds do not rotate, the geometry
of the double bonds maintains these fatty acids in distinctive and fixed shapes.

12.2 TRIGLYCERIDES

Triglycerides are a class of lipids commonly referred to as fats, and are an important part of our
diet. A triglyceride is derived from a molecule of glycerol that is bonded to three fatty acids by
ester functional groups, as illustrated in Figure 12.2. Triglycerides are even less polar than free
fatty acids. This is because the polarity of the free carboxylic acid groups has been masked by
conversion into non-polar fatty acid esters.

> Carboxylic acids and esters are discussed in Chapter 6, 'The carbonyl group and its chemistry'.

In Figure 12.2, the structure of glycerol alone is included for reference, next to a typical triglyceride. The glycerol part of this large molecule is highlighted in bold. Two saturated fatty acids, palmitic acid (sixteen carbons) and myristic acid (fourteen carbons) and one unsaturated fatty acid,
palmitoleic acid, are bonded via esters to glycerol forming a triglyceride. The three fatty acids

Figure 12.2 The structure of a typical triglyceride

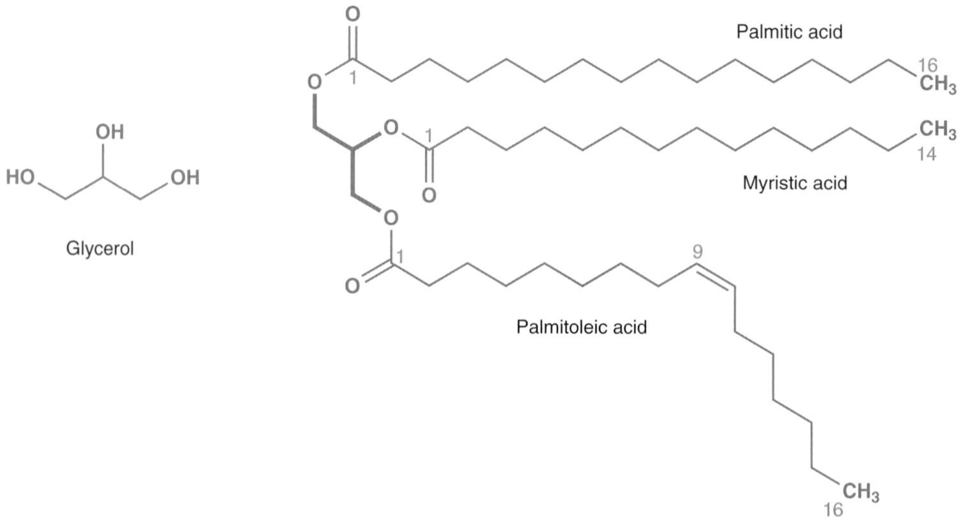

Self-check 12.1

Study the triglyceride structure and identify the ester functional group and the central glycerol molecule. Think about why esters are less polar than carboxylic acids rather than just learning this as a fact.

Self-check 12.2

You should also remind yourself about the reactivity of esters. Are esters more or less reactive to water than (a) acyl chlorides (b) amides?

Box 12.1 Fats and diet

The popular press is full of articles about fat in our diet. Newspapers often use *cis*/*trans* terminology (e.g. 'trans fats') to describe unsaturated fats instead of the scientifically correct convention of E/Z, so it is important that you are familiar with both nomenclatures.

Saturated fatty acids are generally found in animal fats, whereas unsaturated fatty acids are obtained from plants—unsaturated fatty acids tend to be liquids and, therefore, the triglycerides from plants tend to be oils. This property arises because of the distinctive 'kink' in their structure, caused by the double bond. This kink causes the hydrophobic interactions between the non-polar side-chains in adjacent lipid molecules to be less effective. Saturated fatty acids tend to be solids; their more regular structure promotes efficient non-polar interactions between adjacent molecules. In the fatty acids we have seen so far, all the unsaturated examples have contained *cis* double bonds. This is because most double bonds in naturally occurring fatty acids have this geometry.

In the food industry, liquid polyunsaturated plant oils are partially hydrogenated, by a chemical process, to manufacture solid (or more often, semi-solid) fats. This process is used in the manufacture of margarine. In processed foods of this type, some of the *cis*-fatty acids are isomerized to *trans*-fatty acids; although unsaturated, these *trans*-fatty acids have a similar shape to their saturated equivalents. *Trans*-fatty acids are linked to an increased risk of cardiovascular disease, whereas polyunsaturated (cis) fatty acids are considered to be much better for you. A minor change in the chemistry and shape of a molecule can have significant effects on its properties!

used in this example are for illustration; any combination of fatty acids can be used to form a triglyceride. In nature, mixed triglycerides (glycerol esterified with three different fatty acids) are very common. By contrast, triglycerides with three identical fatty acid side chains are rare.

12.3 PHOSPHOLIPIDS

The most significant role of lipids in biology is their function as a major component of cell membranes. Cell membranes are formed from a bilayer of a particular type of lipid known as a phospholipid. Looking at the chemistry of these lipids in more detail will help us understand

Figure 12.3 Phospholipids and the cell membrane

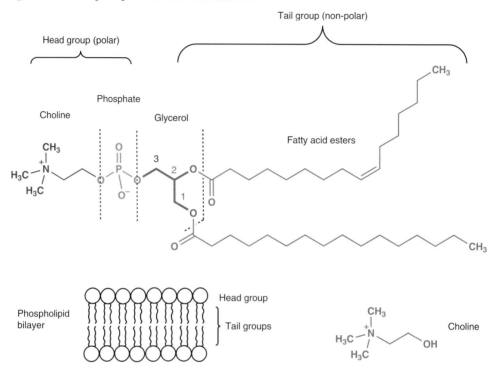

how cell membranes work. Figure 12.3 illustrates the structure of phosphatidylcholine. This is the most common phospholipid in the mammalian cell membrane, so we will focus on the chemistry of this example.

Phospholipids are related to triglycerides; the only difference is that one fatty acid is replaced by a polar *head group*. The two fatty acids constitute the non-polar *tail*. In phosphatidylcholine this consists of two fatty acids, joined by ester linkages, to carbon-1 (C1) and carbon-2 (C2) of glycerol. The fatty acid chain at C1 is usually saturated and sixteen or eighteen carbons in length. Attached to C2 of glycerol is a fatty acid that is often mono-unsaturated and is sixteen, eighteen or twenty carbons in length. A choline molecule is bonded to glycerol C3 by a phosphodiester linker. The polarity of the head group arises from the two charged functional groups, a positively charged quaternary amino group and a negatively charged phosphodiester group. By contrast, the tail of the molecule is extremely non-polar, being composed of two long-chain fatty acids.

⟩ Phosphodiesters, as part of DNA, are discussed in Chapter 8, 'Inorganic chemistry in pharmacy', and Chapter 9, 'Nucelic acids'.

This is another example of an amphiphilic molecule. The head group is soluble in polar solvents (i.e. water, the *only* available solvent in a biological system), whilst the tail has an affinity for other non-polar groups. When large numbers of amphiphilic phospholipids are packed together they form the cell membrane lipid bilayer, illustrated as a cartoon in Figure 12.3. The hydrophilic, polar head groups on both sides of the membrane (i.e. the extracellular/outside and cytoplasmic/inside) are in contact with water. In the interior of the bilayer, the hydrophobic

Phospholipids possess very polar or ionic sites in addition to long hydrocarbon chains. This makes them ideal for forming the cell membrane lipid bilayer.

fatty acid hydrocarbon chains strictly exclude water. Hydrophobic interactions between tail groups further stabilize the bilayer.

So we see how the structure of the membrane is directly related to the strongly amphiphilic properties of the phospholipid. It is important to remember that other phospholipids, with differing head and tail groups but very similar physical properties, are also found in a typical cell membrane.

The existence of a lipid bilayer is essential for forming very stable cells, but it often provides the pharmaceutical scientist with a significant challenge when a drug needs to cross a cell membrane and enter a cell to find its biological target!

12.4 STEROIDS

Steroids are an important class of lipids that share the characteristic hydrocarbon skeleton shown in Figure 12.4. They contain four fused, usually saturated, hydrocarbon rings, named, by convention, A, B, C and D. The A, B and C rings are six-membered, and the D ring is five-membered. All steroids have this basic structure.

Cholesterol, the most common steroid in animals, is a molecule that you may well have heard of, and is an important component of the cell membrane. It is a typical steroid that illustrates some common features of this class of lipids. Steroids often contain an oxygen–containing functional group at C3; in the case of cholesterol this is a hydroxyl group. The presence of this group allows further classification of this molecule as a *sterol*, the 'ol' suffix denoting an alcohol. Steroids often contain methyl groups at C10 and C13 and larger hydrocarbon groups at C17. This is further illustrated by studying the structure of ergosterol (see Figure 12.4). You can tell immediately from its structure that it is a steroid (and a sterol) and has hydrocarbon groups in the characteristic positions.

Steroid structure

You will find steroids frequently drawn as shown in Figure 12.4, because it is a convenient way to illustrate a complex structure on a flat page. However, it is important to remember that *all* molecules have three-dimensional structures. To emphasize how different three-dimensional

Figure 12.4 A general steroid structure (showing the ring naming and steroid numbering system) and two examples of typical steroids

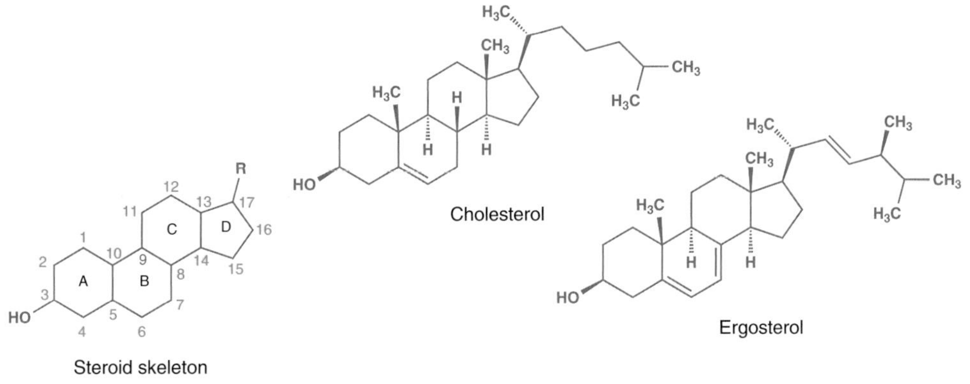

Steroid skeleton

Cholesterol

Ergosterol

Figure 12.5 A computer-generated model of the three-dimensional structure of cholesterol. Carbon atoms are shown in green, hydrogen atoms are grey, and the oxygen atom is red. The A, B, C and D rings are labelled

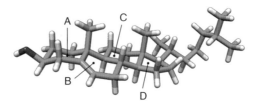

structures can be from flat representations, Figure 12.5 shows a computer-generated model of cholesterol. Note how the structure is far from flat. The model is orientated to highlight the shape of the steroid A-ring. Note how it adopts the 'chair' conformation typical of six-membered saturated rings. Ultimately, this arises from the tetrahedral conformation that most of the saturated, sp^3-hybridized, carbons in the structure adopt.

❯ Conformational isomerism is discussed in more detail in Chapter 3 'Stereochemistry and drug action'.

Steroid biochemistry

Steroids have many important roles in the body and are used widely as drugs (see Figure 12.6). For example, cholesterol is a major component of animal cell membranes. Because it is non-polar, cholesterol interacts with the tail groups of phospholipids, and together these two types of lipids determine the overall properties of a membrane.

Cholesterol is also important as the **biosynthetic precursor** for the steroid hormones, molecules vital to human physiology. For example, cholesterol is converted into the sex hormones testosterone and oestradiol, responsible for male and female sexual development and characteristics, respectively. Cortisol is a hormone synthesized in the body from cholesterol that

Figure 12.6 Some steroid hormones and drugs. Despite the similarity of these structures (they all contain the steroid ring system) they have very different biological activities

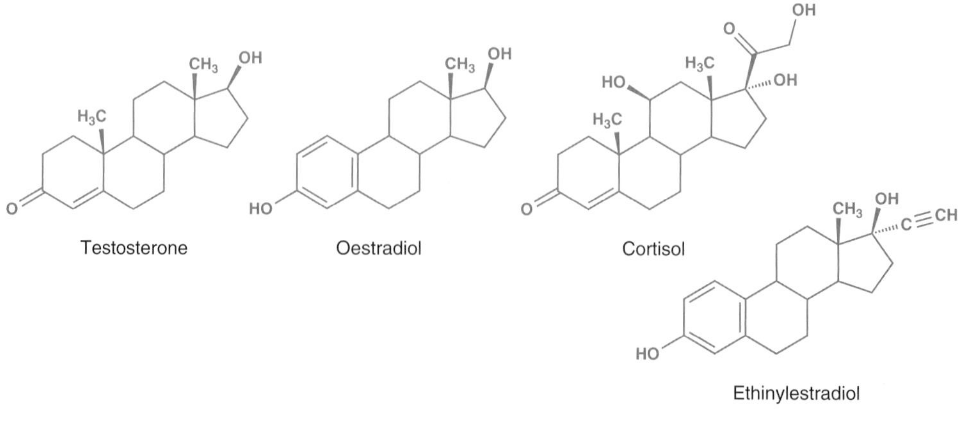

Testosterone   Oestradiol   Cortisol

Ethinylestradiol

Cholesterol is one of the most important steroid molecules. It is an important component of cell membranes and is a precursor of steroid hormones.

Case study 12.1

A teenage girl attends Tu's pharmacy requiring emergency hormonal contraception. Although worried about needing this treatment, she is also anxious about taking the drug. How does Tu do her best to reassure her?

Reflection questions

1. How does the drug work?

2. Are there any risks associated with the drug?

For answers, visit the online resources which accompany this textbook.

---

regulates the metabolism of lipids, proteins and carbohydrates. It is also used as a therapeutic drug (under the name hydrocortisone) for a variety of uses, ranging from ulcerative colitis of the bowel to skin conditions such as eczema.

However, many steroid-based therapeutics are not naturally occurring molecules. Ethinylestradiol is a synthetic derivative of oestradiol containing an unusual carbon–carbon triple bond functional group. It is widely used in many oral contraceptives ('the pill') and possibly one of the most widely prescribed drugs in the world (see also Case study 12.1).

> Ethinyloestradiol is also discussed in Chapter 4 'Properties of aliphatic hydrocarbons'.

12.5 LIPIDS AS A SOURCE OF ENERGY

Fatty acids are an important source of energy, yielding more energy than the equivalent quantity of carbohydrate. They are stored as triglycerides in specialist tissue (adipose cells), and broken down by lipase enzymes to free fatty acids and glycerol when energy is needed. Each free fatty acid molecule is then metabolized by the addition of a hydroxyl group—a process known as β-oxidation, since oxygen is added specifically to the second carbon from the carboxylic group. Since fatty acids are less oxidized than carbohydrates (which have large numbers of oxygen functional groups), they require further oxidation to be degraded and are therefore a very efficient energy store (see Figure 12.7).

The fatty acids are first linked to coenzyme A (CoA) via a thiol ester bond. This reaction is catalyzed by acyl-CoA synthetase (also called fatty acid thiokinase) in the mitochondria or at the endoplasmic reticulum surface. It requires energy, and so one molecule of ATP is broken down to AMP.

For saturated fatty acids, β-oxidation occurs in a cycle of events as shown in Figure 12.8. One cycle of these reactions results in a fatty acid that has been shortened by two carbon atoms and one molecule of acetyl-CoA. The cycle is repeated several times until two molecules of acetyl-CoA remain. For unsaturated fatty acids, an isomerase and reductase are required to first modify the double bond.

Figure 12.7   Overall reaction scheme for the cellular breakdown of fatty acids

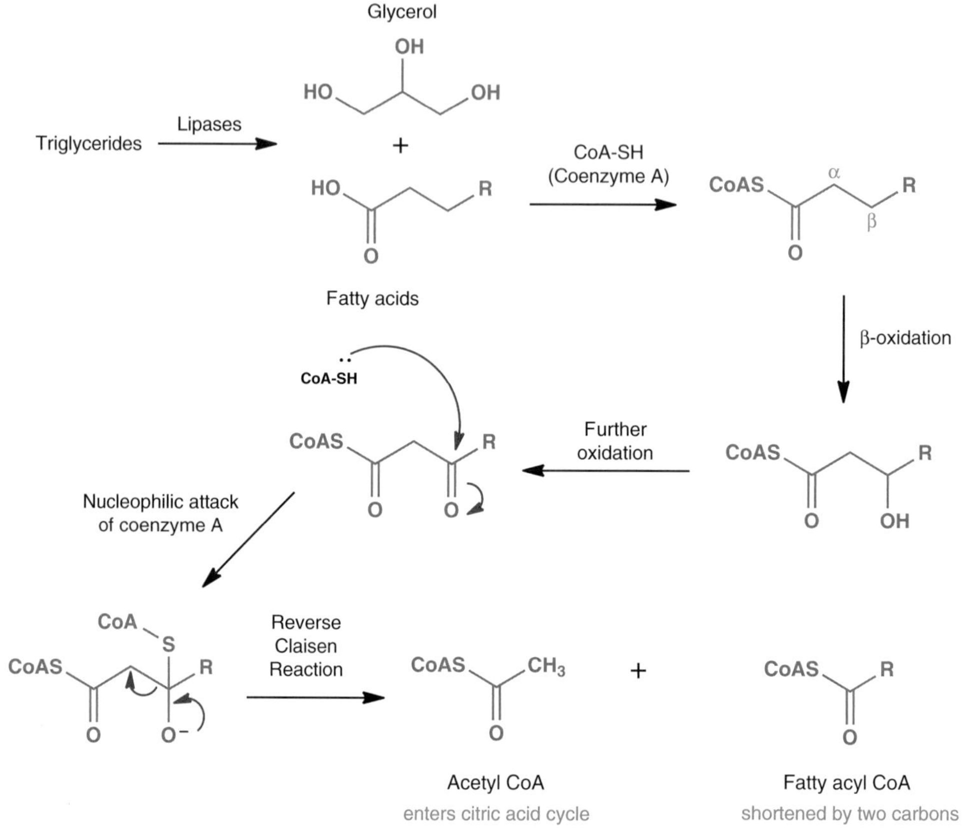

Fatty acid breakdown (β-oxidation) is a four-step cycle which is repeated until the long-chain fatty acid is broken down into numerous acetyl-CoA products.

Acetyl-CoA is released by this process and enters the citric acid (or Krebs) cycle, leading to the production of energy in the form of ATP. More acetyl-CoA is synthesized from fat than from the comparable amount of carbohydrate. Therefore, you might expect fats to be the body's preferred energy source. However, carbohydrates are preferred because they can enter the citric acid cycle more quickly than fats and thus release their energy more rapidly. Thus dietary carbohydrate is used for energy in preference to fat stores, which explains why a diet low in carbohydrate promotes fat metabolism—and why people choose low-sugar diets to reduce body fat and weight.

The acetyl-CoA from each stage enters the citric acid cycle if there is a balance between fat and carbohydrates: there must be sufficient oxaloacetate from carbohydrate catabolism to combine with the acetyl-CoA. Under fasting conditions or conditions such as diabetes, the oxaloacetate is used to produce glucose by the gluconeogenic pathway. The acetyl-CoA cannot then enter the citric acid cycle as there is no oxaloacetate and instead forms acetoacetate and D-3-hydroxybutyrate. These products are collectively known as ketone bodies. The acetoacetate is slowly decarboxylated to acetone, which can be detected in the breath and urine of a diabetic person (see Case study 11.1).

Figure 12.8 β-Oxidation of saturated fatty acids

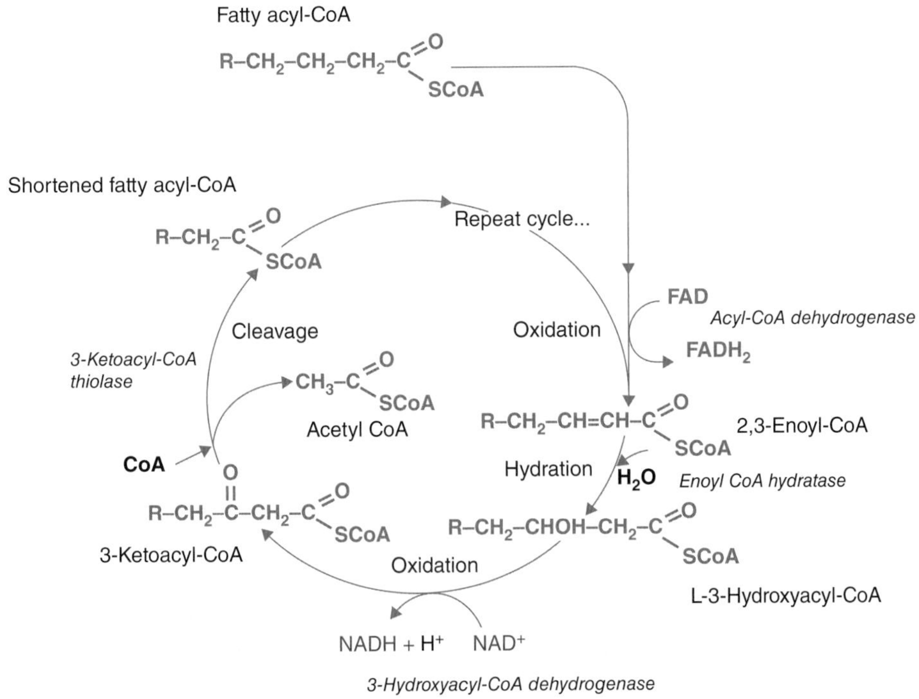

Fatty acyl-CoA

$R-CH_2-CH_2-CH_2-C$ =O SCoA

Shortened fatty acyl-CoA

$R-CH_2-C$ =O SCoA

Repeat cycle...

FAD
Acyl-CoA dehydrogenase
FADH$_2$

Cleavage

Oxidation

3-Ketoacyl-CoA thiolase

CH_3-C =O SCoA
Acetyl CoA

$R-CH_2-CH=CH-C$ =O SCoA   2,3-Enoyl-CoA

CoA

Hydration H$_2$O Enoyl CoA hydratase

$R-CH_2-C-CH_2-C$ =O SCoA
3-Ketoacyl-CoA

$R-CH_2-CHOH-CH_2-C$ =O SCoA
L-3-Hydroxyacyl-CoA

Oxidation

NADH + H$^+$ NAD$^+$

3-Hydroxyacyl-CoA dehydrogenase

If lipids are consumed in excess of usage, the surplus is stored as triglycerides within the adipose tissue. However, some can be deposited within the vessels of the cardiovascular system and can cause atherosclerosis and heart disease. Excess fat is also associated with an increased risk of some cancers, including breast and colon cancers. Conversely, if intake of lipids is low there is a risk of deficiency diseases, as some fatty acids are essential—that is, they cannot be made in the body. These include linoleic acid, linolenic acid and arachidonic acid.

CHAPTER SUMMARY

- Fatty acids can be saturated, mono-unsaturated or polyunsaturated and have an even number of carbons.
- All double bonds in unsaturated fatty acids have the *cis* orientation.
- Triglycerides are composed of the trihydric alcohol glycerol esterified with three fatty acids.
- Triglycerides may be simple (all three fatty acids are identical) or, more usually, mixed, where the three fatty acids are different.
- Phospholipids are similar to triglycerides except that one fatty acid is replaced by a polar phosphate group.
- Phospholipids are a major component of cell membranes.
- All steroids possess the same basic structure of four fused rings, labelled A, B, C and D rings. The A, B and C are six-membered whilst the D ring is five-membered.

- Cholesterol is an important steroid with a number of key biological functions including being a component of cell membranes and the biochemical precursor for steroid hormones.

- Fatty acids can be an important source of energy when required, yielding more energy, molecule for molecule, than carbohydrates.

- Fatty acids are broken down to acetyl-CoA by β-oxidation. The acetyl-CoA provides energy via the citric acid cycle.

- Excessive fatty acid breakdown can lead to the formation of ketone bodies and, if not controlled, ketoacidosis.

FURTHER READING

Patrick, G. L. *An Introduction to Medicinal Chemistry*, 6th edn. Oxford University Press, 2017. ISBN 978-0-19-8749691.

Papachristodolou, D., Snape, A., Elliott, W. H. and Elliott, D.C., *Biochemistry and Molecular Biology*, 6th edn. Oxford University Press, 2018. ISBN 978-019-8768111.

A well-written textbook that covers molecular biology in depth.

Ridgeway, N. and McLeod, R. (eds.). *Biochemistry of Lipids, Lipoproteins and Membranes*, 6th edn. Elsevier Science, 2015. ISBN 978-0-444634382.

A comprehensive textbook covering all aspects of lipid biochemistry

A very accessible textbook that expands upon the chemistry of drugs and their mechanisms of action against target macromolecules.

Self-check

For the answers to the Self-Check questions in Chapter 12, visit the online resources which accompany this textbook.

ORIGINS OF DRUG MOLECULES

Tim Snape

Our ancestors chewed tree bark and drank herbal tea to relieve their illnesses, whereas today we are more likely to visit the doctor and take prescribed medication. The medication generally appears in tablet or capsule form, and the active ingredient will have first appeared in pure form on a chemist's bench. This chapter addresses the origins of the active ingredient.

Some of today's drugs are still derived from tree bark and herbal teas, and others from more sustainable (easily replaced) biological sources, such as moulds and soil bacteria. Some drugs are synthetic (they are made wholly by chemists using chemical reactions), and some are a mixture (semi-synthetic). You will learn to recognize the structures of natural products based on their complexity and to understand that fully synthetic drugs are usually a lot simpler than natural products.

Despite the structural complexity of natural products they can be used by chemists as a source of inspiration for the development of new drugs, not only to optimize their biological activity but also to prepare novel compounds for **patent** protection. Genetic engineering is of ever-increasing importance in the production of drug molecules, enabling us to use whole proteins as drugs.

Learning objectives

Having read this chapter you are expected to be able to:

- explain the main origins of drugs, including drugs which originate from nature and those which are totally synthetic, and those with hybrid origins
- identify those drugs whose structures originated in or were inspired by nature and those that were not
- appreciate that complex drugs can be prepared using biotechnology techniques.

13.1 DRUGS, DYES AND CLEANING FLUID: SIMILARITIES AND DIFFERENCES

Most drug molecules are small and organic, made up of carbon and a small number of other elements, most of which are commonly found in living things. Drug molecules are typically based on carbon and contain hydrogen, oxygen, nitrogen, perhaps chlorine, sulfur or phosphorus.

Self-check 13.1

There is one element frequently found in drug molecules that is hardly ever found in living organisms. What is it?

These drug molecules typically have molar masses of a few hundred grams per **mole**, and can be found as clinically approved medicines (for example, aspirin, antibiotics, anti-angina drugs) or as illicit substances used to alter the mind (for example, cocaine, heroin, LSD etc.). Both types of 'drug' exert their effects by altering the biochemical processes in our bodies. From a molecular point of view, there is no difference between a legal and an illicit drug.

Figure 13.1 shows the structure of diamorphine, alongside morphine and codeine, which are closely related. Diamorphine is a strong analgesic, used clinically to treat severe, including cancer-related, pain. However, the same substance is also known as heroin, an illegal recreational drug. The distinction between diamorphine and heroin is not a molecular distinction, but a social and legal distinction.

Organic molecules are found in food, drugs, plastics, all living things, household cleaning products, fabrics, dyes and more. For the most part, they are made up of a small number of different chemical elements, arranged in a limited number of ways, yet these quite subtle variations in structure can lead to major differences in properties. For example, Figure 13.2 shows the chemical structure of the local anaesthetic lidocaine, alongside the most bitter compound yet discovered, denatonium benzoate (Bitrex®). Bitrex® was discovered by chance in 1958, by chemists trying to develop novel local anaesthetics, and was approved for use in the early 1960s as an additive to ethanol to make it undrinkable. (Ethanol for industrial use is not subject to the same taxes as alcoholic beverages, and may also contain harmful impurities.) Since then, denatonium benzoate has found many applications. For example, it is added to cleaning products and antifreeze to prevent accidental poisoning and is used in nail-biting preventions. The chemical structures of denatonium benzoate and lidocaine are almost identical (shown in blue); a small difference in molecular structure (in this case the addition of a benzyl group) may cause a hugely different biological effect.

The main difference between drugs and other small organic molecules is cost. A new drug not only requires some desirable medicinal effect, but also low toxicity and no serious unwanted side-effects—and it is far from easy to make such a drug. In fact, roughly, for every

Figure 13.1 The analgesics morphine, codeine and diamorphine that originate from poppies
Poppy: Image by Websi from Pixabay

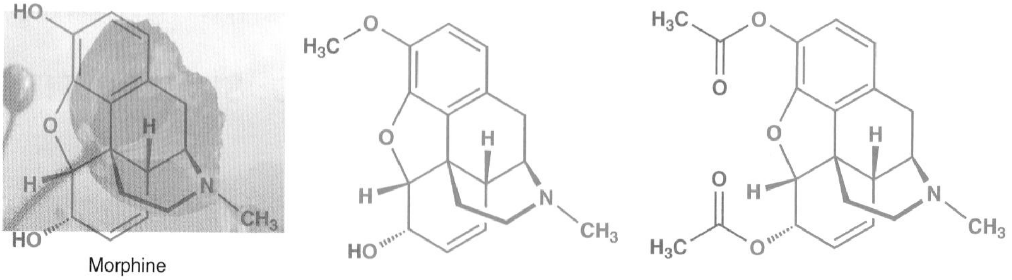

Morphine

Codeine

Diamorphine

Self-check 13.2

Four of the compounds shown below are medicinal drugs; the other is a potent poison. Can you identify it?

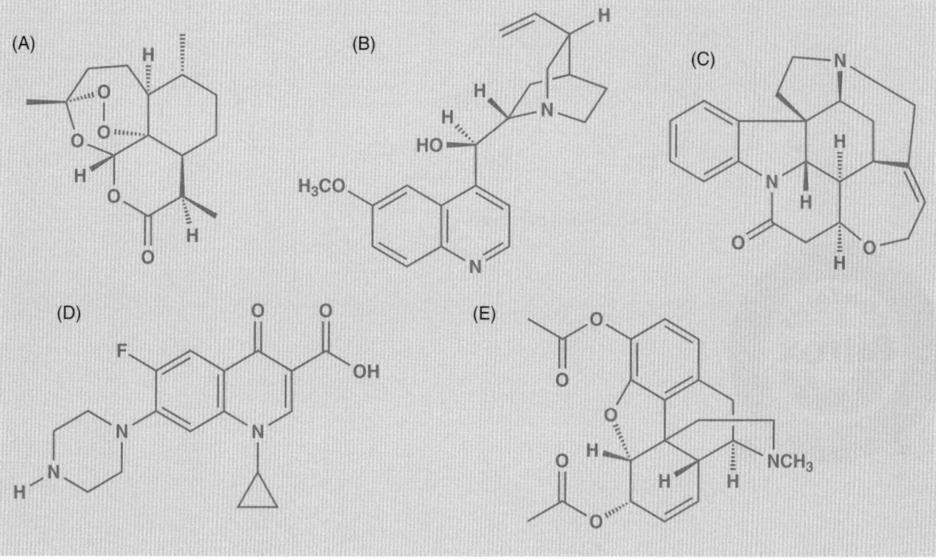

(A)

(B)

(C)

(D)

(E)

10,000 structures made or discovered, 500 will reach animal testing, ten will reach phase I clinical trials, and only one will get to market, usually at a cost of about £450 million. Before any new drug is approved for the market it must be shown to be an improvement on existing therapies. Extensive legislation requires that lengthy clinical trials are carried out, and, at the end of these, a new drug must be able to generate a profit so that the costs of its production can be recouped.

The drug discovery process raises numerous ethical questions to which there are no easy answers. Like any industry, the pharmaceutical industry must pay its employees (a very large and skilled workforce), offset its costs and reward its shareholders (such as pension funds). It is undoubtedly more profitable to invest in long-term illness of the rich nations (hypertension, cancer, diabetes) than short-term illness of the poor nations (tuberculosis, trypanosomiasis, malaria). Charities, notably the Bill and Melinda Gates Foundation, and the World Health Organisation work alongside the pharmaceutical industry to fill these gaps.

Thorough, expensive drug-testing ensures that our medicines (with some well-documented exceptions) are safe and efficacious (they work). However, the regulation of alternative therapies is very weak, as herbal teas are classed as food, not medicines. This same testing means that new drugs are so expensive that even a rich nation cannot always afford them. In the UK, the National Institute for Health and Care Excellence is charged with determining whether the country should pay for a particular therapy, or whether the money would be better spent on a different therapy. Governments decide how much money to spend on healthcare overall.

Ethics is now an important component of pharmacy courses, and although the ethics of dealing with patients is the main focus of most of this teaching and learning, you should be

Figure 13.2 The chemical structures of denatonium benzoate (Bitrex®) and the label used to denote its presence in products, and the local anaesthetic lidocaine. The structural similarity is shown in blue

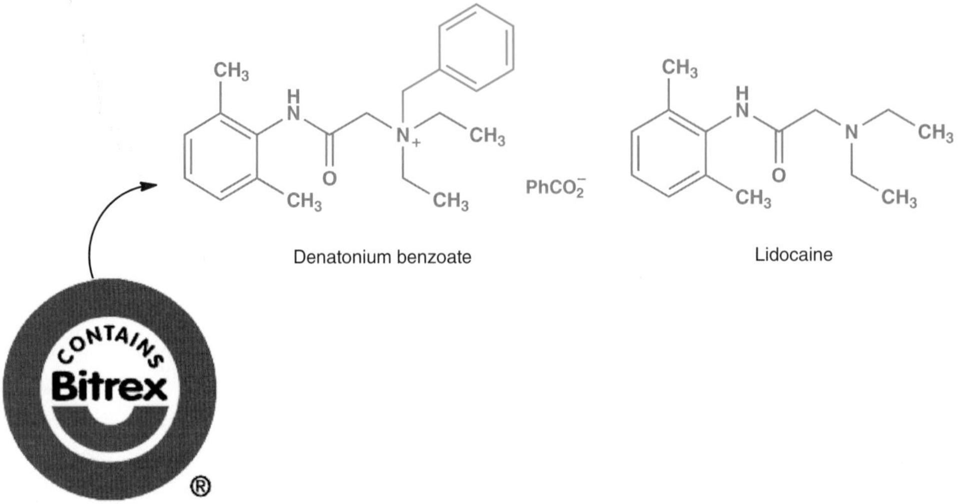

Denatonium benzoate

Lidocaine

aware that there are ethical considerations underlying all aspects of the production and use of medicines.

Let us now take a look at some of the drugs on today's market that are products from nature.

13.2 NATURAL PRODUCTS AS DRUGS AND MEDICINES

A hundred years ago almost all the medicines in the pharmacopoeia were of natural origin, and even today it is estimated that a third of the compounds we use as drugs are derived from nature. Our complex relationship with nature has developed over tens of thousands of years. It is almost inevitable that products of nature, found in animals and plants, will have some kind of medicinal effect on our bodies. Whether this effect is beneficial or not will depend on a number of factors, including the amount taken (the dose) as well as the nature of the chemicals (see Case study 13.1).

Case study 13.1

Dilip, a pharmacist, catches his mother using some dried leaves brewed in hot water to treat her aches and pains. He is worried about her and asks what they are. She says it is just herbal medicine she got from a friend, and tells Dilip not to worry because they are natural, so they must be OK.

Reflection question

1. Dilip advises his mother to stop using the dried leaves immediately. Why is this?

For answers, visit the online resources which accompany this textbook.

In the following sections we will look at several well-known medicines, where the active drug is made from, or based on, a natural product.

Aspirin

Aspirin (chemical name, acetylsalicylic acid), the well-known pain-killer, was developed from a natural source: the bark of the willow tree. You will have seen aspirin in the form of over-the-counter medicines such as Anadin®, Aspro® and Disprin®, but have you ever wondered how aspirin became a drug with a worldwide production of several thousand tonnes per year?

Aspirin itself is not a natural product. In fact it was the first drug to be prepared syntheti-cally. Its structure is, however, very similar to salicin, the active product isolated from willow tree bark. Nature was an inspiration for aspirin rather than its source—a distinction that will be made in more detail in the following sections of this chapter. Shown in Figure 13.3 are the structures of salicin, salicylic acid and aspirin. The areas of structural similarity are highlighted in blue. Aspirin, salicin and methyl salicylate are all pro-drugs and are converted to salicylic acid in the body.

> For more details about salicin, salicylic acid and aspirin, see Chapter 7 'Introduction to aromatic chemistry'.

Willow bark is still sold as an alternative therapy. The sales literature claims that it is slower to act than aspirin but that the effects last longer. As you can see from Self-Check 13.5, salicin in willow bark requires two chemical reactions to convert it into salicylic acid; the acetal function is hydrolyzed and then the drug is oxidized in the liver. The active ingredient is released more slowly than in the case of aspirin.

Self-check 13.3

Find the active ingredient of the topical pain-killer wintergreen oil and draw its structure alongside the structures in Figure 13.3. Mark the areas of structural similarity.

> If you find these questions difficult, look at the reactions of carbonyl compounds in Chapter 6.

Figure 13.3 The chemical structures of salicin, salicylic acid and aspirin. The structural similarity is shown in blue *Source*: https://pixabay.com/photos/pasture-tree-depend-59737/ Willow: Image by Hans Braxmeier from Pixabay

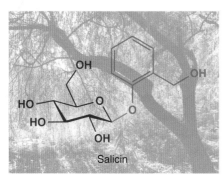

Salicin

Salicylic acid

Aspirin

Self-check 13.4

Draw the mechanisms for the conversion of aspirin to salicylic acid and the conversion of methyl salicylate to salicylic acid.

Self-check 13.5

Draw the mechanism for the conversion of salicin to 2-hydroxybenzyl alcohol. Hint: salicin is an acetal.

Opioid analgesics

Opioids are molecules which interact with the opioid receptors in the central nervous system. The body makes its own opioids, of which endorphins (produced in response to injury or exercise) are the most well known, and their effects can be mimicked by other compounds. Opioid drugs are used to relieve moderate to severe pain.

Naturally occurring opioids are extracted from opium (hence their name), which comes from the seed head of the opium poppy. Opium contains morphine (5–20%) and smaller amounts of related compounds, including codeine; it is one of the oldest herbal medicines known. So sought after were the extracts of the opium poppy that wars were fought in its name (Opium Wars, 1839–42 and 1856–60), and such were the problems associated with its use that the Opium Commission and later the League of Nations were set up to regulate its use and production. This goal was not wholly met, and illicit trade in opium continues in certain parts of the world today.

In Figure 13.1 you can see the structures of morphine and codeine, which are both natural products, together with the structure of diamorphine (heroin), which is prepared in a chemical laboratory from morphine. The structural differences between the molecules have been highlighted in blue. As you can see, these three chemical structures are extremely similar. Both codeine and diamorphine are metabolized to morphine in the body.

Opioid analgesics are some of the most effective pain-killers available to medicine; the compounds act in the brain and appear to work by elevating the pain threshold of the patient, thus decreasing the brain's awareness of pain. The side-effects of morphine are quite broad, and include nausea, constipation, drowsiness, respiratory depression, euphoria, **tolerance** and **dependence**. While side-effects are not usually desirable, euphoria can actually be helpful for treating pain in terminally ill patients. You may wish to think of the consequences of euphoria as a side-effect in those people taking drugs for recreational use! Tolerance and dependence are of course very negative side-effects of morphine, but the most dangerous side-effect is depression of breathing. The most common cause of death from a morphine overdose is suffocation.

One person's unwanted side-effect can be another person's treatment, and there are numerous examples in medicine of careful observation of side-effects being put to good use. Opioid

Self-check 13.6

Describe the differences between the structures of morphine, diamorphine and codeine. Would you expect codeine and diamorphine to be more or less hydrophobic than morphine?

The observation of side-effects with a particular drug can often lead to drugs being used to treat conditions other than the one for which they were initially used.

Self-check 13.7

Can you draw the mechanism for the conversion of diamorphine to morphine? (Think about the hydrolysis of aspirin.)

Self-check 13.8

We make diamorphine from morphine, and then diamorphine acts as a pro-drug for morphine. At first sight this looks like a waste of time and money, yet diamorphine is actually more effective than morphine. Why?

drugs, including morphine and codeine, which can have the side-effect of causing constipation, are now used for the treatment of diarrhoea and of irritable bowel syndrome. Conversely, derivatives of erythromycin (whose side-effects include diarrhoea) are used to treat constipation in intensive care patients.

Antibiotics

There is a large selection of naturally occurring antibiotics available for the treatment of bacterial infections. These include penicillins, cephalosporins, tetracyclines and macrolides. Examples of these antibacterial drugs can be seen in Figure 13.4. As you can see from their chemical structures, they are structurally very different, yet they are all antibacterial drugs. This is quite different from the opioid analgesics which all have similar chemical structures and thus have similar biological activities. It takes a little thought to appreciate that there is no contradiction here.

There is more than one way of killing a bacterium. The bacterial cell contains many different biological targets, and these are targeted by different drugs. A crude way of looking at this is to say:

Different biological target = Different chemical structure of drug

This makes sense; we would expect proteins and nucleic acids with different functions to be structurally different and to bind differently structured drugs.

> See Chapter 9, 'Nucleic acids', and Chapter 10, 'Proteins and enzymes', to refresh your memory on biologically important drug targets.

Macrolide antibiotics

Macrolides are molecules which contain a large carbon-based ring containing an ester. Cyclic esters are known as lactones.

Erythromycin (Figure 13.4) belongs to the macrolide class of antibacterial agents. It was isolated from a soil organism in the 1950s in the Philippines, and is one of the safest antibacterial agents in clinical use. Erythromycin works by binding to the 50S subunit of the bacterial ribosome, which prevents the bacteria from synthesizing essential proteins. Its specific shape and

Figure 13.4 Common antibiotics. Note the structure of erythromycin and its ball-and-stick and space-filling models which provide more realistic insights into the shape of this molecule

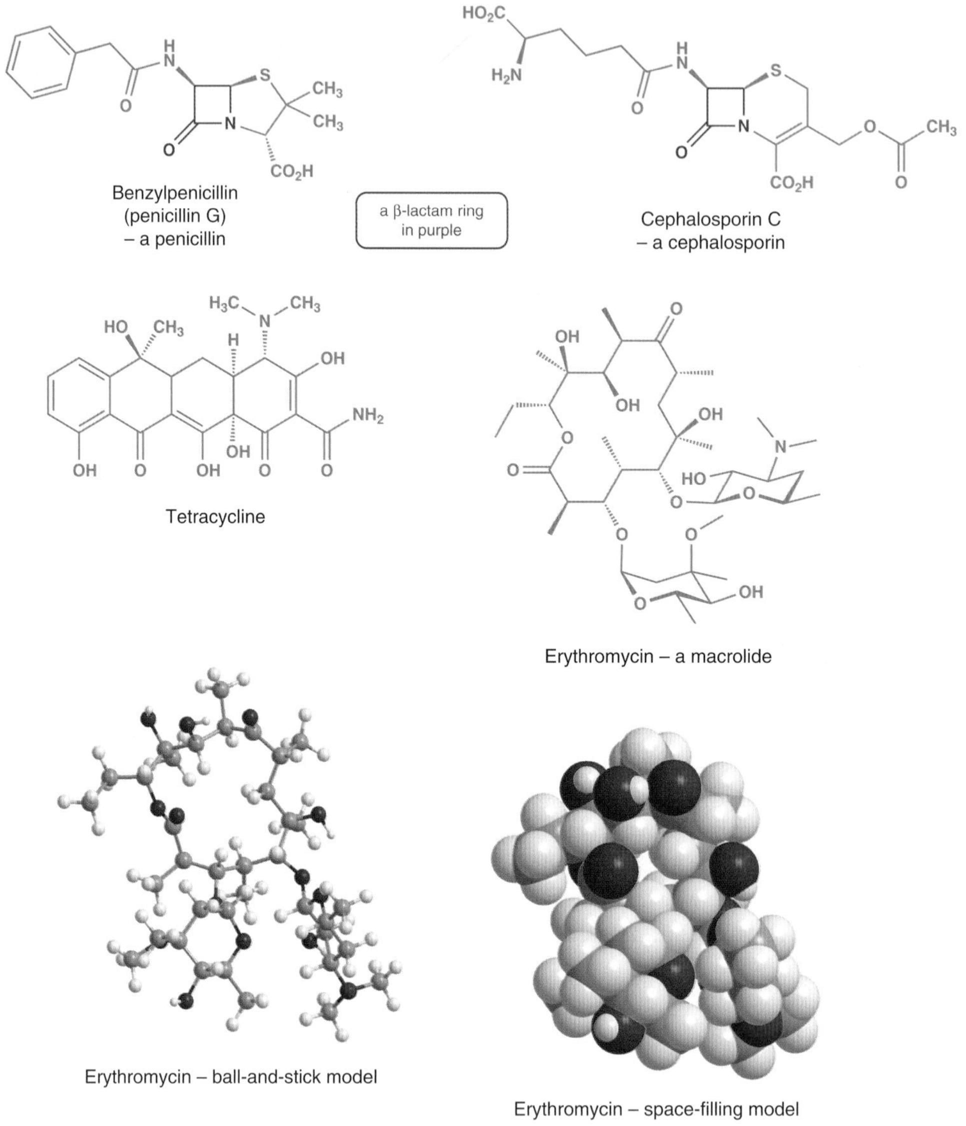

Benzylpenicillin
(penicillin G)
– a penicillin

a β-lactam ring
in purple

Cephalosporin C
– a cephalosporin

Tetracycline

Erythromycin – a macrolide

Erythromycin – ball-and-stick model

Erythromycin – space-filling model

the position of functional groups enable it, and a few derivatives, to bind to a particular binding site on the ribosome.

> See Chapter 1, 'The importance of pharmaceutical chemistry', for information on the formulation and drug delivery of erythromycin.

β-Lactam antibiotics

The β-lactam class of antibiotics include the penicillins and cephalosporins, plus a couple of other related structures (Figure 13.4). β-Lactam antibiotics work by inhibiting the enzymes responsible for bacterial cell wall synthesis. They all possess a β-lactam ring (shown in purple

Self-check 13.9

Look at the chemical structures to decide why the penicillin and cephalosporin antibiotics may trigger a similar allergic response.

in Figure 13.4), which is essential for their activity. Without this structural feature these compounds are inactive. Perhaps surprisingly, this essential β-lactam ring is partly responsible for the allergic reaction to the penicillins experienced by many patients. When the β-lactam ring is attacked by specific cellular proteins, it creates an antigen which can stimulate an immune response, resulting in hypersensitivity to the drug. This also accounts for the cross-sensitivity to cephalosporin antibiotics, which share the β-lactam ring structure. If you are allergic to the penicillin antibiotics, the similar chemical structures should also alert you to the fact that you may be allergic to the cephalosporins and other β-lactam antibiotics too. An understanding of chemical structures could save your life (see Case study 10.2)!

Penicillin G was famously discovered by Alexander Fleming as the product of a mould, *Penicillium notatum*. Moulds, like soil bacteria, can be cultured and developed to produce very high yields of drugs. Cephalosporins are also produced by fungi of the *Acremonium* species.

Glycopeptide antibiotics

Glycopeptide antibiotics work by targeting the building blocks of the bacterial cell wall, preventing cell wall synthesis and leaving the cell vulnerable. A common glycopeptide antibiotic is vancomycin (Figure 13.5). Vancomycin is important because of its ability to combat deadly

Case study 13.2

Six-year-old Maya has an upper respiratory tract infection. The doctor has prescribed her amoxicillin. Before she did so, she checked that Maya was not allergic to penicillin.

Reflection questions

1. Why did the doctor need to check Maya's allergies?

2. The original penicillin was benzylpenicillin. As you can see, the structures of amoxicillin and benzylpenicillin are very similar:

Amoxicillin   Benzylpenicillin (Penicillin G)

3. Why was benzylpenicillin not prescribed to Maya?

4. Maya quite enjoys taking her medicine. Why could this be?

For answers, visit the online resources which accompany this textbook.

Figure 13.5   Vancomycin

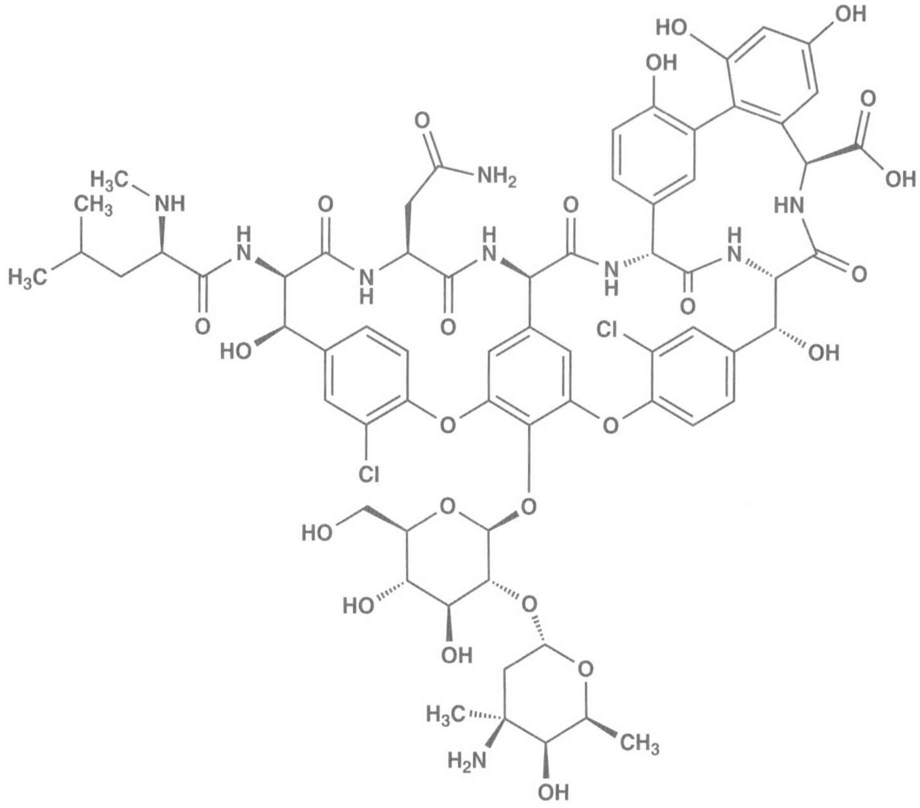

Vancomycin

meticillin-resistant strains of *Staphylococcus aureus* (MRSA). Unfortunately, we are now begin-ning to see vancomycin-resistant strains of bacteria too.

The structure of this antibiotic is hugely complex. It was first isolated in 1956 from the fer-mentation broth of the soil bacterium *Streptomyces orientalis*. Remarkably, given its complexity, it was synthesized chemically in 1998 (see Box 13.1). However, as is usually the case with com-plex molecules, the chemical synthesis is not economic, and the drug continues to be produced from the soil bacterium.

Look at the structure of vancomycin and note the number of chiral centres present: eighteen in a single molecule! Each one of these chiral centres is fixed and exists in nature as drawn. Such complexity is only ever found in natural products. Chemists making new drugs would never dream of designing such a complex molecule from scratch unless they were being inspired by a natural product.

You should be able to look at the chemical structures of the drugs that are spread through-out this chapter and identify which ones are synthetic and which ones are natural products based on their structures alone.

> **Box 13.1   Stereoisomers**
>
> For each chiral centre present in a molecule there are 2^n isomers possible (where n = the number of chiral centres). Vancomycin is a single isomer, not 2^{18} = 262,144 different molecules. Making a single compound of such complexity means making one out of 262,144 possible variations (very low odds indeed); however, chemists achieved this in 1998—a remarkable feat!

There are many different classes of antibiotics and they kill bacteria by a variety of mechanisms.

> Refer to Chapter 3 'Stereochemistry and drug action' for a refresher on stereoisomers, if you need to.

Anti-cancer agents

Cancer is the second most common cause of death in the Western world, exceeded only by heart disease. There are more than 200 different types of cancer as a result of different cellular defects, and so a treatment for one particular cancer may not be effective in controlling another type of cancer. The continuing battle we have against cancer means that we continue, as ever, to look for new drugs and treatments for the disease. Since 1980, Cancer Research UK has advanced over 100 novel anti-cancer agents through various stages of pre-clinical and early-phase clinical trials. A comparison of the BNF from September 2001 to March 2011 shows an increase in the number of cytotoxic drugs included from fifty-seven up to eighty-six. This has now increased significantly due to the inclusion of biopharmaceutical products. Some of the natural product drugs used to combat cancer are shown in Figure 13.6.

The first thing that should strike you is the sheer size and complexity of the compounds in Figure 13.6. As previously discussed, these complex compounds are natural products. For example, vincristine is found in the Madagascan periwinkle.

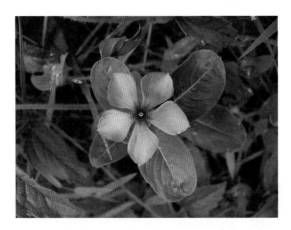

> See Chapter 2, 'Organic structure and bonding', and Chapter 3, 'Stereochemistry and drug action', for a more in-depth coverage of chiral centres and hybridization.

Figure 13.6 The chemical structures of a few anti-cancer drugs

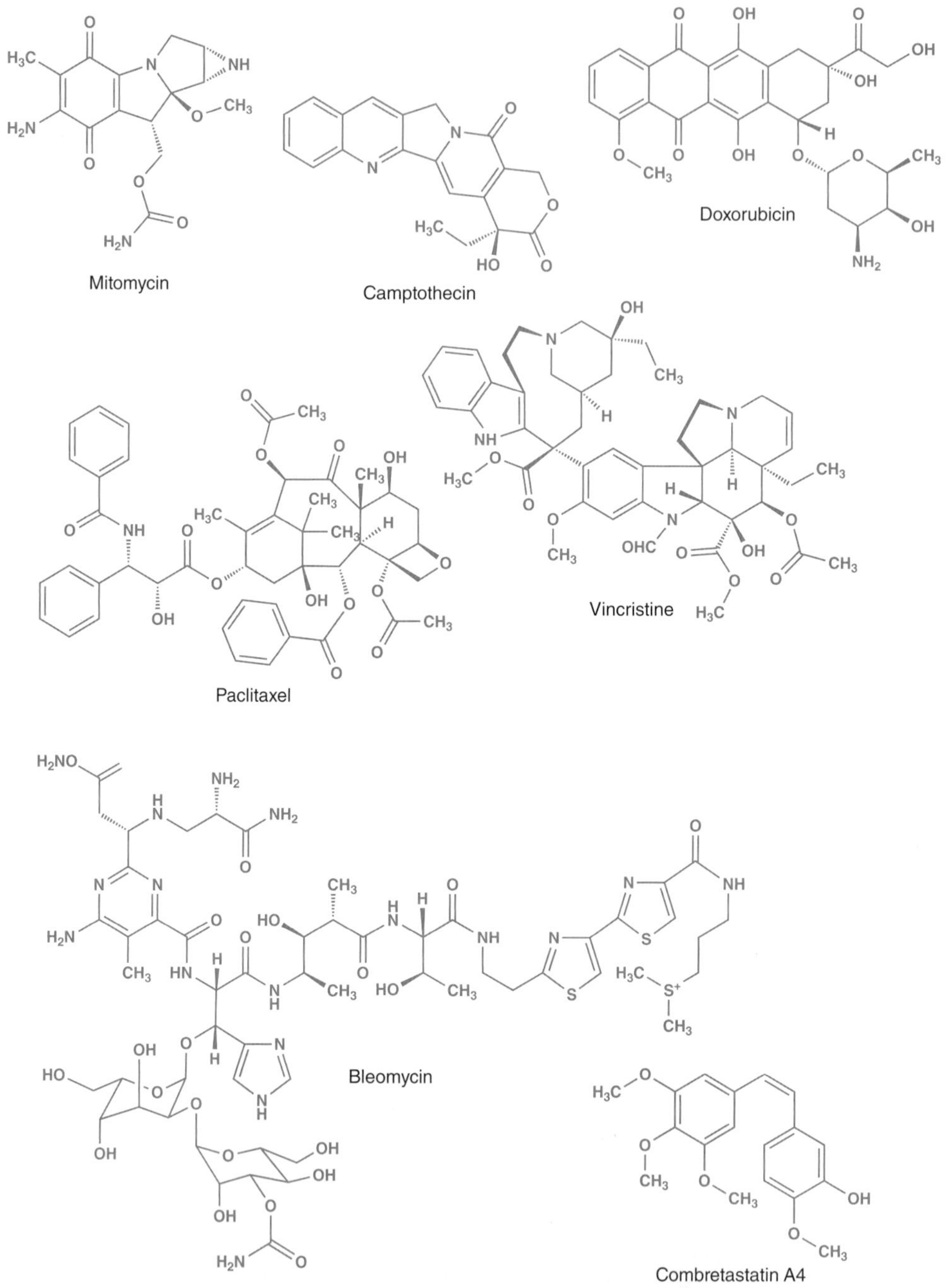

Mitomycin

Camptothecin

Doxorubicin

Paclitaxel

Vincristine

Bleomycin

Combretastatin A4

Self-check 13.10

Can you identify the number of chiral centres and types of functional groups in the anti-cancer compounds in Figure 13.6? Can you identify the different hybridization states of the atoms in those molecules and predict which parts of the molecules are planar?

Anti-cancer drugs which interact with DNA

The structures of bleomycin (which is dispensed as a mixture of bleomycin A_2 and B_2), doxorubicin and mitomycin, are all very different and complex; they are natural products after all! Despite their structural differences, they all act as anti-cancer agents by interacting with DNA.

Bleomycin is a very complex three-dimensional molecule isolated from the soil bacterium *Streptomyces verticillus*. It causes breaks in the strands of DNA, which ultimately leads to cell death—a good thing for a cancer cell! It is used intravenously or intramuscularly to treat, amongst other things, certain types of skin cancer.

Doxorubicin is also derived from a soil bacterium, *Streptomyces peucetius*, but, in contrast to bleomycin, doxorubicin has four fused rings in which fourteen of the eighteen carbon atoms are sp^2 hybridized, meaning they are planar (i.e. flat). The planar structure means that doxorubicin is able to slip in between the base pairs of DNA. This process is called intercalation, and it prevents DNA replication and ultimately leads to cell death. Doxorubicin is used to treat acute leukaemias, lymphomas and a variety of solid tumours.

Mitomycin, another *Streptomyces* product, has yet another way to interact with DNA and kill cancer cells. The mechanism by which mitomycin works is rather complex and beyond the scope of this book; its interesting structure enables it to alkylate DNA. It is used for the treatment of upper gastrointestinal cancer, as well as breast cancer. It is one of the most toxic anti-cancer drugs in clinical use, causing delayed bone-marrow toxicity, and it can result in permanent bone-marrow damage if used for long periods of time.

> For the structure of DNA, refer to Chapter 9, 'Nucleic acids'. Chapter 5 'Alcohols, phenols, ethers, organic halogen compounds, and amines' provides details of some simpler alkylating agents. Refer to Chapter 8, 'Inorganic chemistry in pharmacy', for an account of cisplatin—an inorganic anti-cancer agent that interacts with DNA.

Anti-cancer drugs which act on important proteins

There are huge numbers of important proteins in our bodies (see Box 13.2). Enzymes and receptors are (normally) proteins, and both are used as targets for a range of therapies in a number of therapeutic areas. Paclitaxel, combretastatin A4 and vincristine (Figure 13.6) are naturally occurring anti-cancer agents which induce cell death by interfering with a crucial structural protein called tubulin. Paclitaxel is a member of the taxane group of drugs and was originally derived from the Pacific yew tree, but is now produced from sustainable sources (see Section 13.3). It can be used to treat ovarian, breast, and non-small cell lung cancers and is administered by intravenous infusion. Combretastatin A4, from the South African bush willow, is in clinical trials for the treatment of thyroid cancer. Vincristine and related compounds from the Madagascan periwinkle plant also interfere with tubulin and are used to treat a variety of cancers including leukaemias, lymphomas and some solid tumours such as breast and lung cancer. Like paclitaxel, they are administered intravenously. Inadvertent intrathecal (injection into the spinal cord) administration of vincristine sometimes occurs because the drug is often given in combination with intrathecal medicines. This is usually fatal.

> Anti-cancer agents treat cancer using a number of different mechanisms, and hence they are structurally quite different.

Box 13.2   The Human Genome Project

The Human Genome Project has shown that humans have about 27,000 genes. It used to be thought that one gene was responsible for one protein, but we now know that proteins can be modified in so many ways that one human gene may give rise to perhaps ten different protein molecules. So we do not know how many different proteins there are in the body, but it is more than 27,000.

Hormones

Many naturally occurring hormones are used as medicines; Figure 13.7 shows some of these. In many cases the hormone (or a simple derivative of it) simply 'tops up' the patient's own reserves of the naturally occurring molecule and restores normal function to the body. A dose of the hormone in a level similar to that found in the body is called a physiological dose, whilst a dose that exceeds that found in the body is a pharmacological dose. The effects on the body of a physiological dose and a pharmacological dose may be quite different, and this difference has been exploited in the development of useful therapies.

The most commonly prescribed hormones are the oestrogen and progestagen steroids, which are prescribed for contraception and for menstrual disorders (see, for example, estradiol and progesterone in Figure 13.7A and B). Other steroids produced by our bodies are used for treating

Self-check 13.11

Can you identify the structural similarities between the three steroids in Figure 13.7? What shape do you think these molecules will have? Hint: Refer to Chapter 3.

Figure 13.7   Naturally occurring hormone drugs

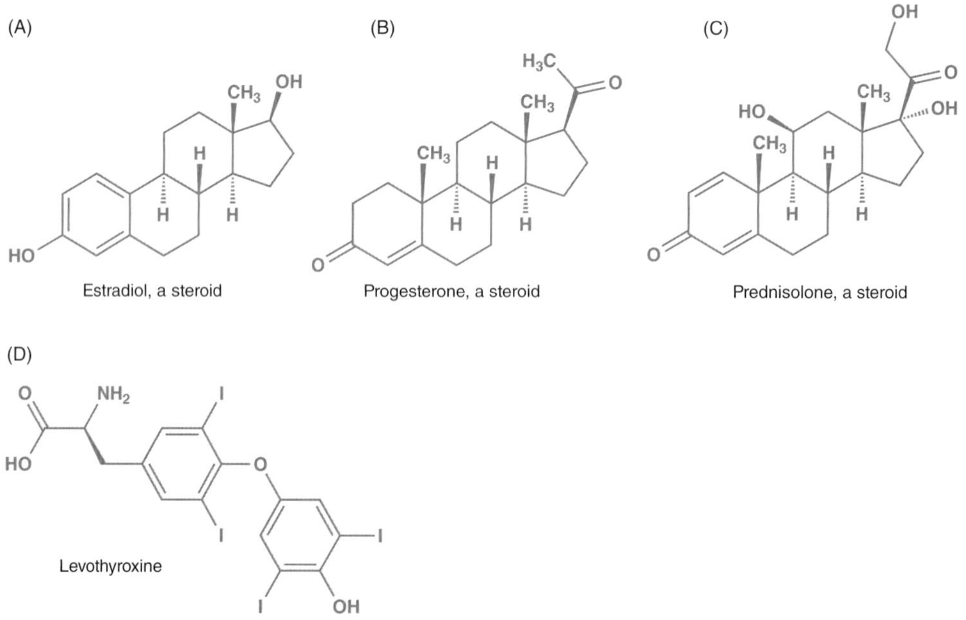

(A) Estradiol, a steroid

(B) Progesterone, a steroid

(C) Prednisolone, a steroid

(D) Levothyroxine

a range of inflammatory and allergic disorders such as autoimmune diseases, skin disorders and respiratory problems, including asthma. For example, prednisolone (see Figure 13.7C) may be taken orally as an immune suppressant, as a cream for the topical treatment of skin disorders, or by inhaler for the treatment of asthma.

The common hormone thyroxine (Figure 13.7D) is sold with the name levothyroxine. The prefix *levo* indicates that the drug is enantiomerically pure and rotates the plane of polarized light anticlockwise. Levothyroxine is used as a maintenance treatment for hypothyroidism (underactive thyroid). Hypothyroidism typically leads to tiredness, weight gain and a general slowing down of metabolism. Thyroxine is the major hormone produced by the thyroid gland, and patients taking levothyroxine do so in order to 'top up' the levels of thyroxine in their bodies to ensure that normal function is maintained.

Insulin (a peptide containing fifty-one amino acids; see Figure 13.8) plays an important role in the regulation of carbohydrate, fat and protein metabolism. Insulin is used as a therapy for the treatment of Type 1 diabetes—a disease by which a patient's own body destroys the insulin-producing cells of the pancreas. The subsequent lack of insulin then leads to an increase in blood and urine glucose, and if untreated the condition is usually fatal. Insulin is sensitive to both stomach acid and digestive enzymes in the intestine, so patients with Type 1 diabetes have to inject the hormone regularly.

〉 Enantiomers are discussed in more detail in Chapter 3, 'Stereochemistry and drug action'.

13.3 SEMI-SYNTHETIC DRUGS

As we have seen in Section 13.2, many drugs can be isolated from natural sources. These compounds, however, did not evolve in nature to benefit humans, but to provide the plants and micro-organisms that produce them with a competitive advantage. We would therefore expect there to be a limit to their efficiency as drugs, both in terms of activity and toxicity. Luckily, with the aid of chemistry we are able to take the natural product and alter its chemical structure appropriately to make similar compounds (**analogues**) to the natural structure with the aim of improving activity, reducing toxicity or introducing some other desired property.

Figure 13.8   The structure of the human insulin monomer. Insulin monomers tend to aggregate as hexamers, but the monomer is the active form

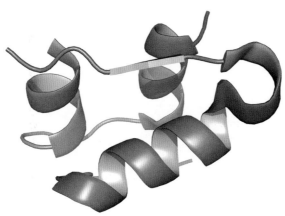

Self-check 13.12

Think back again to the sections on the analgesics and antibiotics. Why do similar structures have similar activities?

The process of manipulating the structure of a naturally occurring compound in the laboratory is called semi-synthesis. Semi-synthesis may produce the natural product itself. Usually, however, the process will produce new compounds in the hope that they are better drugs than the parent natural product. There is a lot of trial and error in this process. Lots of analogues are prepared and tested before the best analogue is progressed further. The 'best analogue' is judged on its overall activity, toxicity, aqueous solubility and many other factors. The examples in Figure 13.9 show some of these analogues alongside their naturally occurring 'parent' structure.

Figure 13.9 Semi-synthetic analogues of natural products

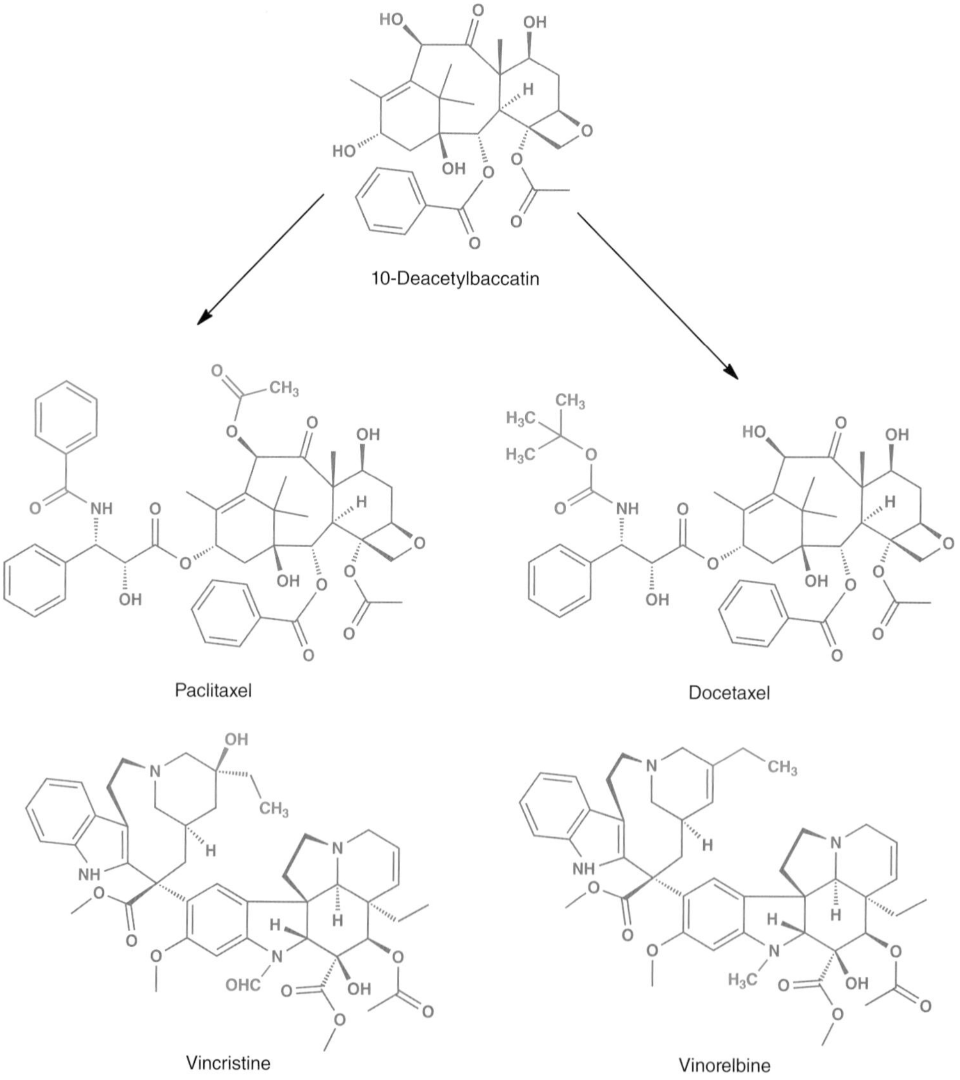
10-Deacetylbaccatin
Paclitaxel
Docetaxel
Vincristine
Vinorelbine

Semi-synthetic paclitaxel and its analogues

Paclitaxel, mentioned in Section 13.2, was originally isolated from the bark of the Pacific yew tree during a project aimed at finding new anti-cancer agents. Intense research ultimately led to paclitaxel in minute quantities, but unfortunately, the extraction of 300 mg (0.3 g) of the compound (about a single dose for a cancer patient) required an entire 100-year-old yew tree. Obviously, there are simply not enough trees to meet this demand, and it would be far too slow to plant and grow more trees. One potential solution to this problem came about when it was found that the needles and twigs of the European yew tree contained a molecule called 10-deacetylbaccatin (Figure 13.9), which could be converted into paclitaxel relatively easily in the laboratory using semi-synthesis. Needles and twigs can be harvested without killing the tree; they are a renewable source that allowed relatively large quantities of paclitaxel to be produced. Nevertheless, to meet the huge demand on this new drug, chemists set about trying to synthesize this huge molecule 'from scratch'. This required many synthetic steps, but was achieved by two independent research groups in 1994. As is often the case, the synthetic route was not economical on a large scale, and paclitaxel is still manufactured by semi-synthesis from deacetylbaccatin.

Now that a semi-synthetic paclitaxel had been developed, analogues could be made to see if its biological properties as an anti-cancer agent could be improved. Docetaxel is one such analogue, and its structure can be seen in Figure 13.9 alongside paclitaxel. Both compounds inhibit tubulin depolymerization, but docetaxel has greater water solubility than paclitaxel. The small difference between these two structures (shown in green) means that although both docetaxel and paclitaxel can be used for the treatment of metastatic breast cancer and non-small cell lung cancer, of the two, only paclitaxel can be used to treat ovarian cancer.

Semi-synthetic penicillins

The penicillin antibiotics are quite reactive. The four-membered ring (the square containing nitrogen, see Figure 13.10) in the middle of the structure is primed to pop open, and this reactivity enables it to act as an antibiotic. Unfortunately, such reactivity means that it is difficult to make in the laboratory. In 1957, John Sheehan's persistence paid off when he managed to make a small amount of penicillin V (Figure 13.10). His synthesis also enabled him to make 6-aminopenicillanic acid (see Figure 13.10), the precursor that would ultimately enable chemists to make a range of penicillin analogues.

Once again, however, a brilliant piece of organic synthesis did not prove to be an economical way of producing a compound with several chiral centres. In 1958, the Beecham company announced the isolation of 6-aminopenicillanic acid from *Penicillium* fungi. The free amine function is a good nucleophile and can be used to make numerous amides. This technology was developed and optimized to allow the synthesis of new penicillins at will, and the limitations of the only existing penicillin on the market in 1958—benzylpenicillin (penicillin G) (see Figure 13.4)—could be tackled. You only have to consider the enormous number of penicillin antibiotics on the market today to see what a huge discovery this was (see Figure 13.10).

Self-check 13.13

Vinorelbine is a semi-synthetic derivative of vincristine. What do you think are the clinical indications for vinorelbine?

Figure 13.10   Semi–synthetic penicillins

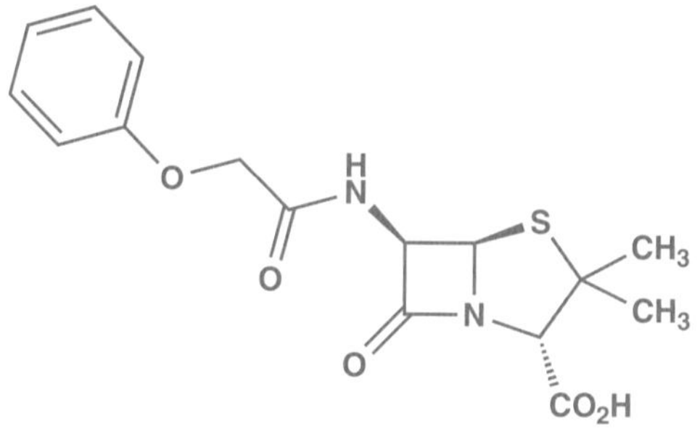

PenicillinV
(aka phenoxymethylpenicillin)

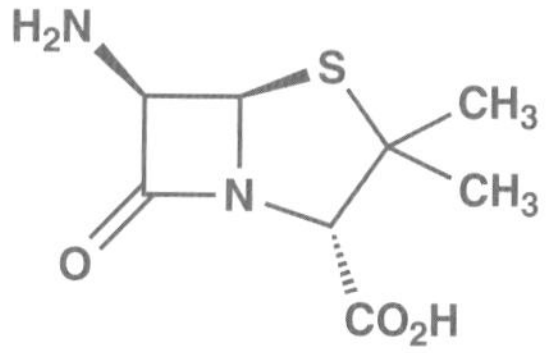

6-Aminopenicillanic acid
(6-APA)

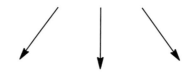

Meticillin, Phenoxymethylpenicillin,
Oxacillin, Cloxacillin, Flucloxacillin,
Ampicillin, Amoxicillin, Carbenicillin, Ticarcillin etc

Self-check 13.14

Look up the structures of the penicillins named in Figure 13.10. Can you identify their structural similarities?

Self-check 13.15

How would you synthesize benzylpenicillin (penicillin G) from 6-aminopenicillanic acid? Draw the reagents and mechanism for the amide formation. (Hint: if you are struggling, refer to Chapter 6.)

Semi-synthetic drugs are made by chemical modification of natural products. Semi-synthesis is often used to improve the properties of a drug, but it may also be used to produce a natural product in an economical or sustainable way.

13.4 SYNTHETIC DRUGS

As you have seen throughout this chapter, natural products can be very complex structures indeed; you should be able to spot one at a thousand paces by now! Some of these complicated structures possess amazing properties that can lead to diseases being cured.

Natural products do not, however, provide for all our medicinal needs. A huge number of drugs have been designed and made entirely in the chemical laboratory. Such drugs can be termed 'synthetic', and as you will see, their chemical structures are much simpler than those of natural products. Figure 13.11 shows some of today's synthetic drugs. These compounds are completely novel, so how did the chemists think them up? What inspired their thinking?

Figure 13.11   Some examples of the drugs made by total synthesis

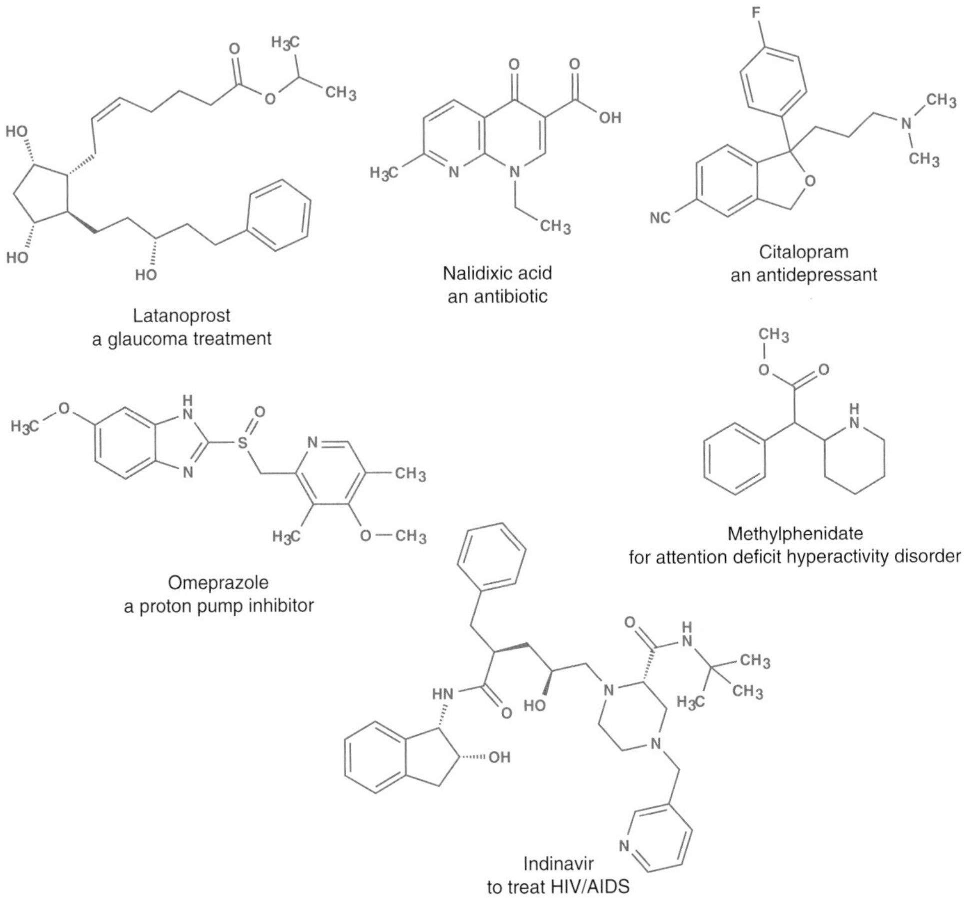

Latanoprost
a glaucoma treatment

Nalidixic acid
an antibiotic

Citalopram
an antidepressant

Omeprazole
a proton pump inhibitor

Methylphenidate
for attention deficit hyperactivity disorder

Indinavir
to treat HIV/AIDS

Self-check 13.16

Count the chiral centres in each of the molecules in Figure 13.11. Whenever you meet a drug for the first time, you should also look up its BNF entry.

The strategy of simplification

Natural products are very complex, and the biological activity of a natural product may reside in just a small part of that molecule. Drugs can be prepared by simplifying natural products; identifying the important part of the structure and synthesizing it, thus stripping away all of the molecular fragments that are not important for biological activity. This essential core can be optimized further as some complexity is added back to the core structure with the aim of making a new drug. These drugs are totally synthetic molecules. Figure 13.12 depicts a number of drugs which have been prepared by such a 'simplification' strategy.

Figure 13.12 Drugs designed by a simplification strategy. (A) Methadone, derived from morphine; (B) simplification of cocaine to give procaine (the insert shows how the two drugs can be overlaid—they have the same shape); (C) Lovastatin is found in oyster mushrooms
istock

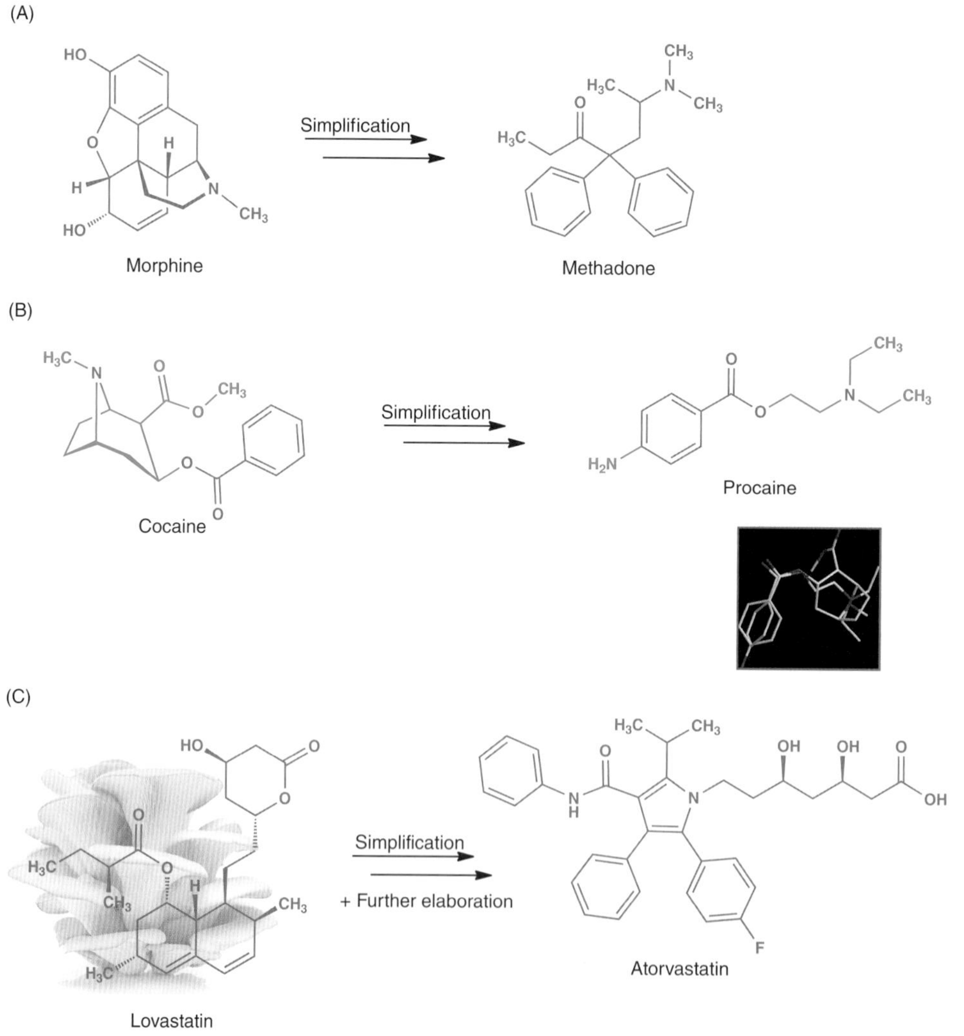

(A)

Morphine → Simplification → Methadone

(B)

Cocaine → Simplification → Procaine

(C)

Lovastatin → Simplification + Further elaboration → Atorvastatin

Methadone and procaine were developed from morphine and cocaine respectively. Figure 13.12 shows how procaine and cocaine overlay one another in three dimensions. The structural requirements which give cocaine its good anaesthetic properties (i.e. the benzene ring, ester and amine shown in blue) are also present in procaine *in the same orientation in space* thus giving it similar properties.

Atorvastatin is discussed in Chapters 1, 3 and 10. At first sight it does not look simpler than the natural product lovastatin, but actually it has many fewer chiral centres. Statins are used to lower cholesterol levels.

Synthetic drug structures inspired by nature

If a new drug cannot be developed from a natural product itself and if a simplification strategy cannot be used, nature can still help to *inspire* new drug structures.

Figure 13.13 shows a number of drugs (in blue) and the natural inhibitor that inspired their development (in purple). The drug and the natural product differ substantially because the drugs have undergone a huge amount of development before they made it on to the market. Such development includes:

- Simplification of the natural product, if possible.
- Optimization of the number, type and orientation of functional groups remaining once simplification has taken place.
- Optimization of aqueous or lipid solubility.
- Minimization of toxicity.

Why would these development steps be carried out? There may be a number of reasons:

- Simplification to remove unnecessary parts of the molecule.
- Optimization of the functional groups to give the best fit into the drug target.
- Modification of drugs that are either too hydrophobic or too hydrophilic to easily get through membranes and biological fluids to their sites of action.
- The minimization of toxicity to avoid harming the patient.

Here we will briefly consider some examples of drugs inspired by nature. Drugs such as captopril and enalapril were inspired by a very toxic xenobiotic, whereas both cimetidine and salbutamol were inspired by compounds found in the body.

Xenobiotic-inspired drugs

The venom from the Brazilian pit viper was found to inhibit angiotensin converting enzyme (ACE), reducing blood pressure. Uncontrolled lowering of blood pressure leads to death, and pit viper venom was historically used as an arrow poison. But the understanding of the mode of action to this poison led to the development of ACE inhibitors like captopril and enalapril, which can be used as drugs to combat hypertension.

> You can read more about the development of captopril in Chapter 6, 'The carbonyl group and its chemistry', and Chapter 8, 'Inorganic chemistry in pharmacy'.

Figure 13.13 Some drugs inspired by natural products: captopril and enalapril were inspired by teprotide, a constituent of Brazilian pit viper venom *Source*: https://commons.wikimedia. org/w/index.php?title=Special:Search&limit=500&offset=0&profile=default&search=timber+ rattlesnake&advancedSearch-current={}&ns0=1&ns6=1&ns12=1&ns14=1&ns100=1&ns106=1#/ media/File:Crotalus_horridus_(1).jpg

Camptothecin

Irinotecan

Topotecan

Podophyllotoxin

Etoposide

Teniposide

Glu-Trp-Pro-Arg-Pro-Gln-Ile-Pro

Teprotide

Enalapril

Captopril

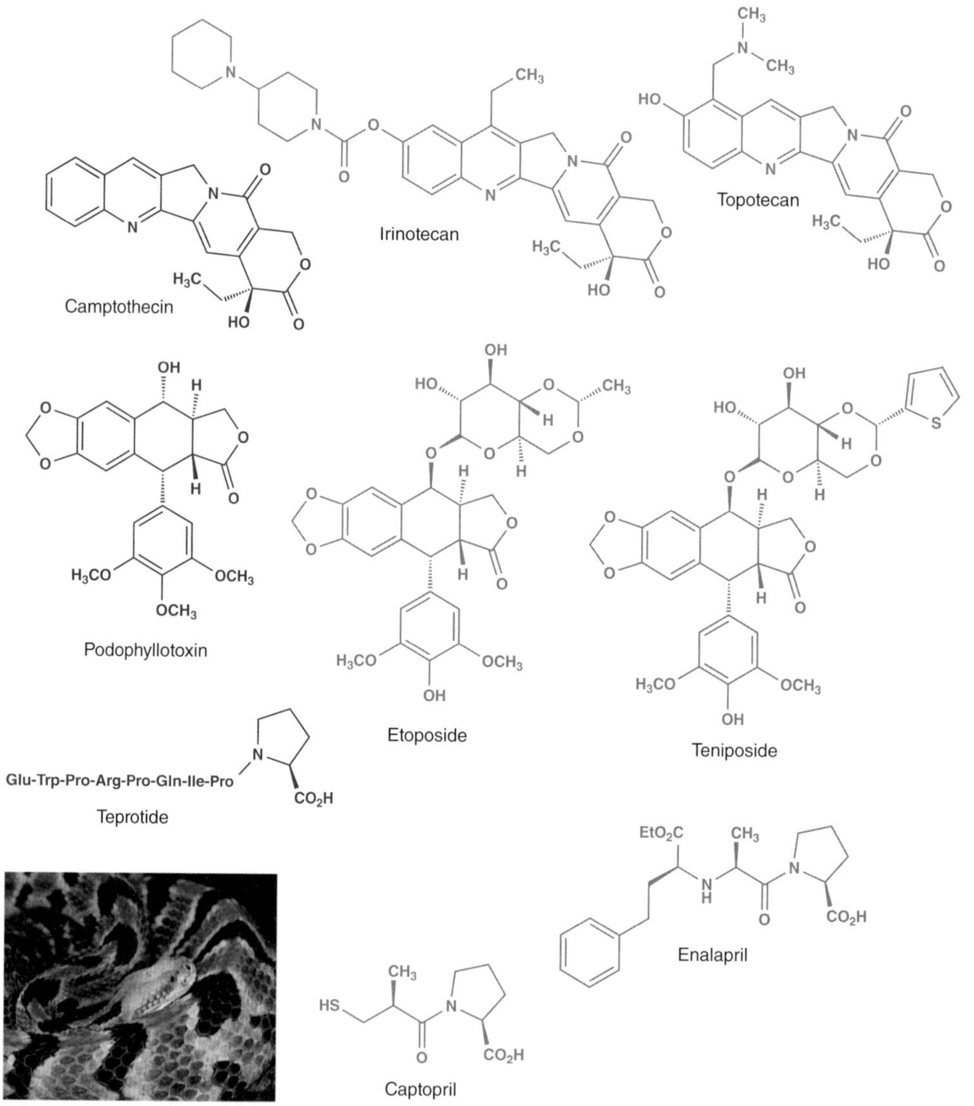

Drugs inspired by compounds found in the body (endogenous compounds)

Figure 13.14 shows the chemical structures of salbutamol, the asthma medication, and cimetidine, used for the treatment of peptic ulcers. Alongside their structures are the natural compounds from which they were developed.

Figure 13.14   Drugs inspired by natural ligands

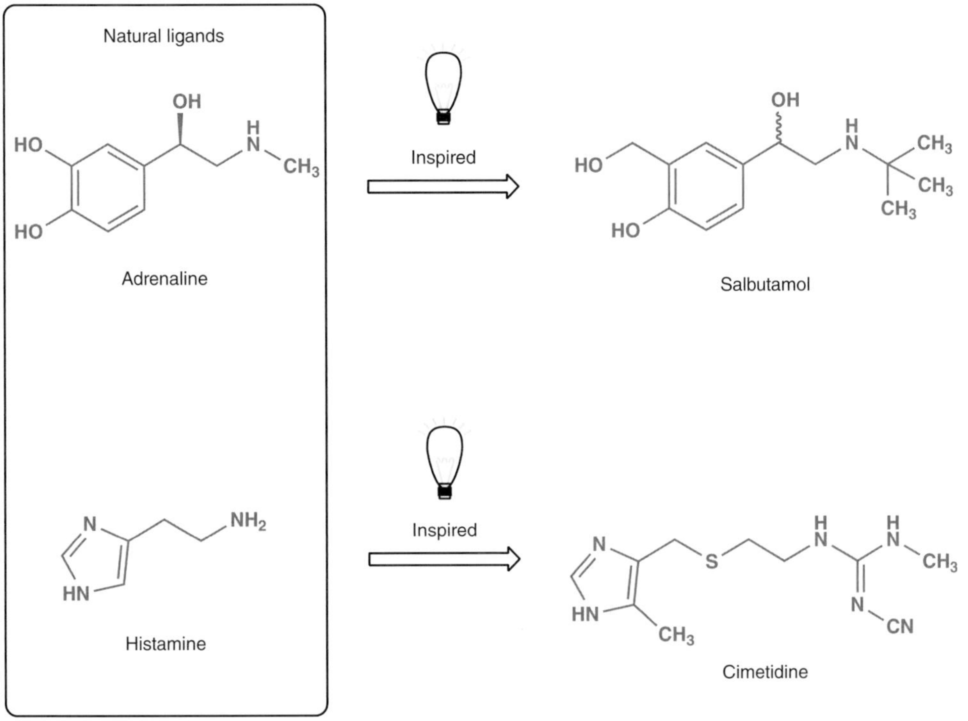

Cimetidine was inspired by a natural compound found in the stomach: histamine (see Figure 13.14). Histamine stimulates the production of gastric acid, which is a problem for patients with peptic ulcers, causing pain and inflammation. Nothing was known about the physiological site of action of histamine, so how could scientists design a drug to interact with it and stop the production of the problematic acid? The answer was ingenious. Histamine binds to the site, so chemists used the structure of histamine as a starting point. Their aim was to produce a new drug that would compete with histamine for the active site but would bind more strongly to it, and would suppress, rather than trigger, acid secretion. The structure of cimetidine was developed after much experimentation, both by computer (*in silico*) and in the laboratory. For several years, cimetidine was the number one selling prescription product in several countries, with worldwide annual sales of $1,000 million.

Self-check 13.17

Look at the structures in Figure 13.14. Can you imagine how the natural ligand led to the development of the popular drugs?

Totally synthetic drugs have often been inspired by the biological activity of a complex natural product.

Salbutamol synthesis

The asthma treatment salbutamol (see Figure 13.15) has an aromatic core; its structure is, in fact, a modified form of adrenaline. Adrenaline is a hormone that forms an important component of the '*fight or flight*' response, and has been used to treat asthma because it causes dilation of the bronchial airways.

   However, the effects of adrenaline on the body are dramatic and short-lived. It would be more desirable for an anti-asthma drug to exhibit greater selectivity for the β_2-adrenoreceptors to maximize dilation of the bronchial tree (while minimizing the detrimental cardiovascular interactions), and also to have an increased duration of action. Two modifications to adrenaline fulfil these objectives:

- Increasing the steric bulk on the amine by replacing a methyl group with a *tert*-butyl group enhances selectivity for the β_2-adrenoreceptor.

- The installation of a CH_2 between the aromatic ring and the hydroxyl group methylated by catechol-O-methyltransferase (COMT) reduces the activity of that enzyme on the drug and so increases its duration of action.

The synthetic route, illustrated in Figure 13.16, starts with aspirin. Treatment with $AlCl_3$ initiates a reaction known as the Fries rearrangement, which involves formation of an acylium ion (the active electrophile in the Friedel–Crafts acylation), and an electrophilic aromatic substitution reaction, equivalent to a Friedel–Crafts acylation, ensues. The *ortho-, para*-directing effect of the oxygen of the aluminium alkoxide is dominant, but the *meta*-directing carboxyl group also favours substitution at carbons 3 and 5. So where will the electrophile attach? Both substituents direct the incoming electrophile to positions 3 and 5, but a 1,2,3-trisubstituted benzene is sterically congested, so 5-substitution is favoured and the major product by far is the isomer shown in Figure 13.16.

   When the acid is treated with methanol in the presence of catalytic acid, the expected ester is formed. Bromination of the ketone with bromine in chloroform gives the mono bromide by reaction *via* the enol form (aided by traces of acid in the chloroform and bromine). (Refer to Chapter 6 if this is not clear.) The addition of *N*-benzyl-*N*-*tert*-butylamine by nucleophilic substitution of bromide installs the amine functionality.

   The benzyl group ($PhCH_2-$) may seem unnecessary as it does not feature in the final product, but it serves to prevent addition of the amine to more than one bromoketone molecule in

Figure 13.15   Structures of adrenaline and salbutamol

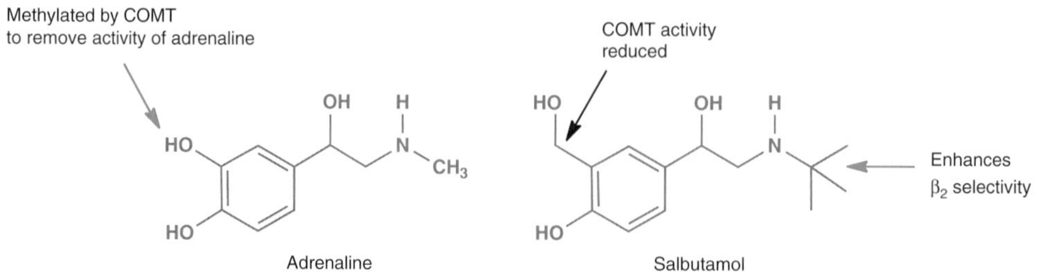

Figure 13.16 Synthesis of salbutamol and the structure of salmeterol

Racemic salbutamol (the (R)-isomer is nearly 70 times more active than the (S)-isomer)

Salmeterol

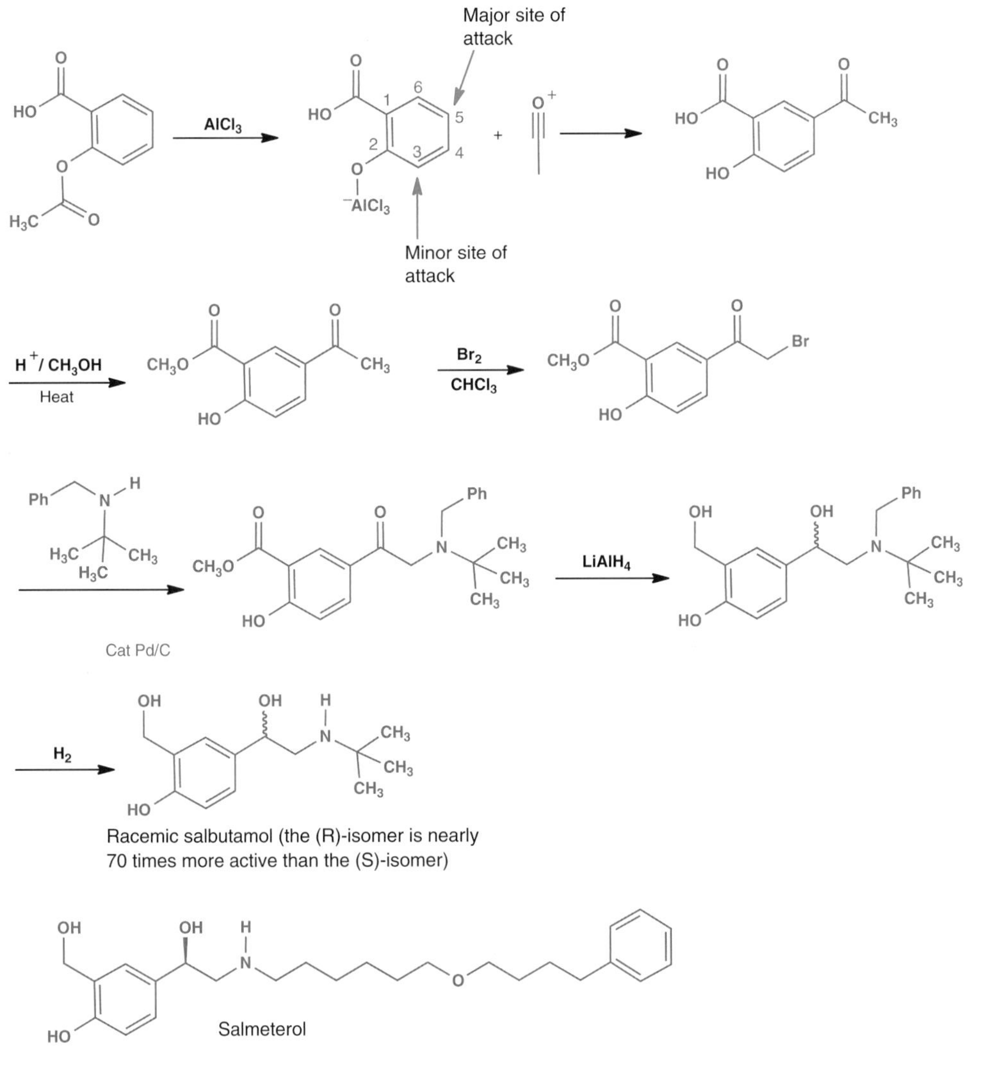

this step and can be cleanly removed later. Over-alkylation of nitrogen is a common problem in synthesis. Reduction of the ketone and ester with lithium aluminium hydride, followed by the removal of the benzyl group with hydrogen and palladium on charcoal catalyst, generates salbutamol in racemic form.

Although salbutamol is an extremely effective asthma treatment (most people will have seen the blue inhalers), its duration of action is shorter than ideal. Further work on the side-chain led to the production of salmeterol, which has an extended duration of action (around 16 hours) compared with 4 hours for salbutamol. Notice how the aromatic core has remained intact in the structure of salmeterol.

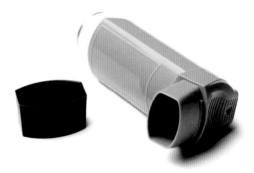

This coloured inhaler is used for salbutamol; other asthma drugs are provided in different co-loured inhalers.

> Amine alkylation is discussed in more detail in Chapter 5, 'Alcohols, phenols, ethers, organic halogen compounds, and amines'.

> More details on reactions of ketones can be found in Chapter 6, 'The carbonyl group and its chemistry'.

Computer-aided drug design

Some drugs are designed entirely on a computer, using what we call 'computational chemistry'. Provided they start with good quality information provided by competent scientists, comput-ers can make a huge contribution to the design of drugs, by designing or selecting compounds for testing against a desired biological target (see Box 13.3). We can use computers to predict molecular properties such as aqueous solubility and shape. Sophisticated programs now enable us to predict the ability of a molecule to bind to biomolecules, including proteins, lipids and nucleic acids. This can then help to speed up the drug discovery process.

Captopril—a clinically important antihypertensive drug inspired by Brazilian pit viper venom—was one of the first drugs to be designed logically with the aid of computers in the 1970s. During its development, scientists at the Squibb Research Institute in the USA made use of a hypothetical model of the active site of the angiotensin–converting enzyme (ACE) to guide the design and synthesis of specific inhibitors. Using the model, they were able to propose which amino acids in the active site of ACE were important in binding inhibitors, leading to the

---

Box 13.3   The Lifesaver Screensaver Project

The Lifesaver Screensaver project (2003–09) harnessed 3.5 million home computers in more than 200 countries to help with synthetic drug design. The project built a database of bil-lions of small drug-like synthetic molecules, and tried to fit them into important biological macromolecules. The main diseases under study were cancer, anthrax and smallpox. Up to 10% of the molecules that the computers predicted to have activity were verified by scien-tists under experimental conditions.

preparation and biological testing of a **lead compound**, which supported their hypothesis. Optimization of this lead compound ultimately led to the development of captopril (see Figure 13.13).

'Me-too' drugs

'Me-too' is a peculiar but useful name. One definition of a 'me-too' drug is: a drug which follows an initial therapy and works through essentially the same mechanism. Once a new drug has proved itself so that it passes all the biological tests, clinical trials and regulatory issues, it is relatively easy for other companies (or the same company even) to make similar molecules that do a similar thing. Ideally, these new molecules will have improved properties compared with the existing drug. Patent protection will be in place to stop unscrupulous copying of structures, but patent protection can only cover so many analogues and it is often possible to develop new compounds that have similar or better biological profiles without infringing the original patent. Figure 13.17 shows some examples of 'me-too' drugs. We have already met the proton pump inhibitor omeprazole, the antidepressant citalopram, and cimetidine, used to treat peptic ulcers. Esomeprazole, escitalopram and ranitidine are 'me-too' drugs resembling these.

Figure 13.17   'Me-too' drugs

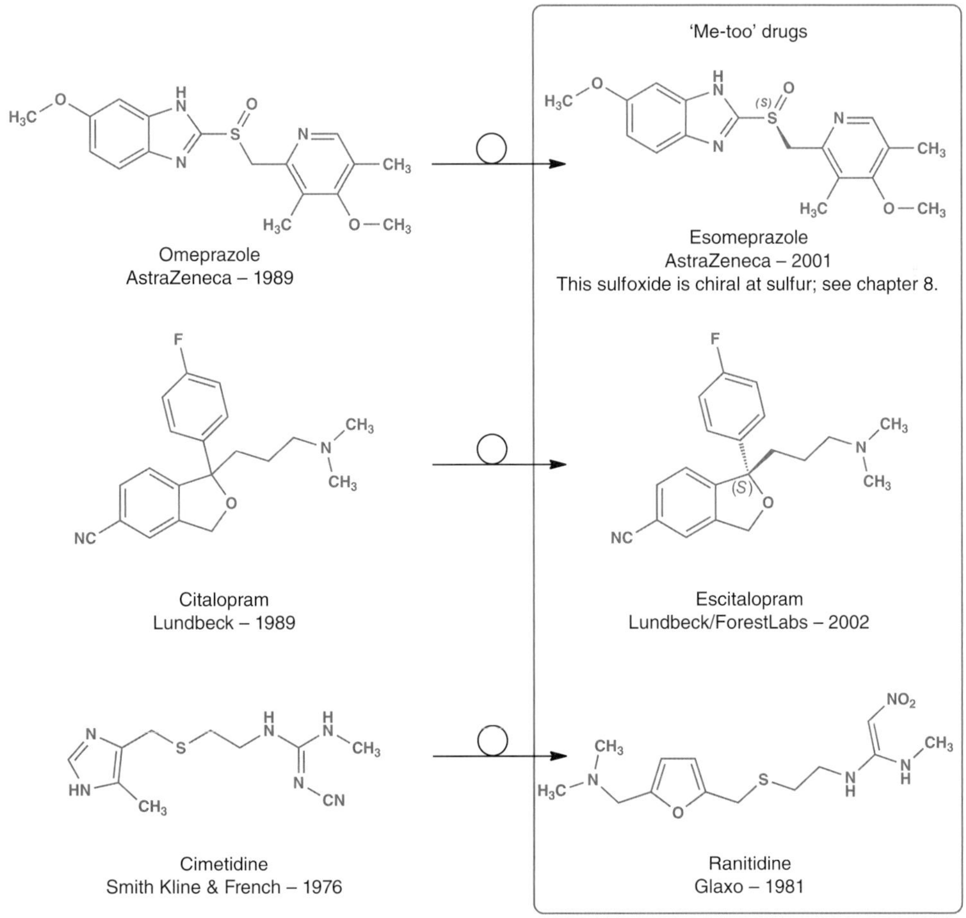

High-throughput screening is a method that enables a large number of compounds (typically thousands) to be **screened** in an automated fashion and on a small scale. Activity needs to be easily detected: for example, a colour change caused by enzyme action. While high-throughput screening itself may not result in a blockbuster drug, it can help find new lead compounds for further optimization by medicinal chemists.

Library screening

Some drug companies possess large banks of compounds (often up to several hundred thousand) which they can potentially screen against any disease (see Box 13.4). To develop a new drug they screen the entire library to see if any of the molecules in it has any activity, no matter how small, against their disease of choice. If a 'hit' is identified, the chemists then make hundreds of analogues of it to optimize its activity. Several rounds of analogue preparation and optimization then takes place to see if these new structures have the potential to become the next marketable drug.

13.5 GENETIC ENGINEERING AND FERMENTATION (BIOTECHNOLOGY) FOR THE PRODUCTION OF DRUGS

Biotechnology means using living systems and organisms to develop or make products. In the context of this chapter, 'products' refers to medically useful drugs and drug intermediates. An early example of a pharmaceutical process using biotechnology was the synthesis of hydrocortisone in the 1940s by whole-cell hydroxylation. In this particular instance, the cells are used to insert a single hydroxyl group into one of the cyclohexane rings (see Figure 13.18). Notice how selective the reaction is; the hydroxyl group is only inserted in that exact position, and with that precise stereochemistry. Such selectivity is the speciality of enzyme–catalysed reactions and biotechnology. To perform such a selective reaction using traditional organic synthesis alone would be almost impossible. Nowadays, a biocatalyst (enzyme) exists for the selective hydroxylation of every position on the steroid framework.

Unfortunately, finding a whole cell that can perform the precise reaction you want is not easy. The enzyme within the cell may not be expressed at a high enough level to be useful, or there

Figure 13.18 Selective steroid hydroxylation

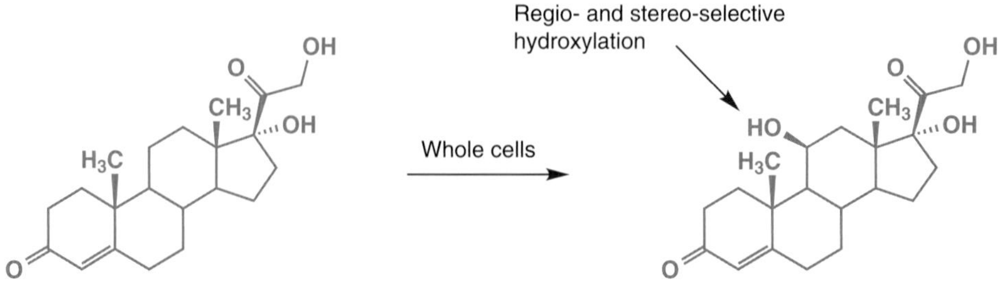

may be other enzymes in the cell that compete for your substrate, producing unwanted side products. Importantly, 30–40 years ago, advances in genetic engineering techniques meant that scientists can now transfer the DNA which codes for a protein into a microorganism which can grow in a fermenter and produce large quantities of the required enzyme. Such procedures are called recombinant DNA technologies, and the commercial value of the medicinal products generated is significant (several hundred million dollars per year).

Further advances in molecular biology over the past few years have now meant that scientists can use genetic engineering to help produce important molecules, particularly important proteins, regularly. By cloning specific genes and incorporating them into the DNA of fast-growing cells (such as bacteria or yeast), we can use the cells as a kind of 'factory' to produce large quantities of proteins and other molecules. Such genetic engineering processes are currently used for the mass production of numerous drugs, including insulin, human growth hormones, human albumin, monoclonal antibodies and vaccines.

Genetic engineering is such a flexible method of drug preparation because it is possible to manipulate the genetic information so that bacteria or yeast produce not just natural compounds but analogues of the natural compounds for us too. The first genetically engineered drug made in this way and approved was human insulin for the treatment of diabetes.

It is very easy to purify genetically engineered proteins, and this substantially reduces the risk of contamination by viruses, such as HIV, or by disease-causing proteins, such as those causing Creutzfeldt–Jakob disease.

Since the introduction of genetically engineered insulin, the insulin gene has been manipulated to produce analogues of insulin. Figure 13.19 shows normal human insulin together with two clinically useful analogues, which help diabetics maintain near-normal insulin activity. Insulin lispro is a fast-acting insulin, and insulin glargine is a long-acting insulin, useful for maintaining constant insulin levels.

In addition to insulin, other human proteins that have been made from genes cloned in bacteria and/or eukaryotic cells include somatostatin and somatotropin (used in the treatment of growth disorders), interferon-α, β, γ and interleukins (used in the treatment of cancer and

Figure 13.19 Genetically engineered insulins. Differences between insulin analogues and normal human insulin are shown in red

```
Human Insulin

GIVEQCCTSICSLTQLENYCN
      |             /
FVNQHLCGSHLVEALYLVCGERGFFYTPKT

Insulin lispro

GIVEQCCTSICSLTQLENYCN
      |             /
FVNQHLCGSHLVEALYLVCGERGFFYTKPT

Insulin glargin

GIVEQCCTSICSLTQLENYCG
      |             /
FVNQHLCGSHLVEALYLVCGERGFFYTPKTRR
```

immune disorders), erythropoietin (used in the treatment of anaemia), serum albumin (used as a plasma supplement) and monoclonal antibodies.

In addition to the recombinant synthesis of therapeutic proteins, biotechnology can also be used for the production of small-molecule drugs.

> Refer to the semi-synthetic penicillins section of this chapter for an example of biotechnology being used to produce small molecule drugs.

Other examples of biotechnology being used for the production of small-molecule drugs can be seen in research carried out in the United States. In 2011, Pfeifer and co-workers developed a process using an *E. coli* strain to ultimately deliver a process that was capable of the simultaneous production of precursors to both paclitaxel (see Figure 13.6) and erythromycin (see Figure 13.4), at synthetically useful concentrations, and with straightforward purification processes.

CHAPTER SUMMARY

- The structure of a drug is important. It must have the correct functional groups in the correct orientation to interact with its biological target and initiate a response.
- Drugs can originate from a range of sources, including nature, chemical laboratories or a combination of the two.
- Even drugs from nature are sometimes made in a chemical laboratory so that enough of the active ingredient is available.
- Nature can be used as an inspiration to chemists when developing new drugs.
- Many analogues of new drugs have to be made before the best candidate is found.
- Organic chemistry is used to make most small-molecule drugs.
- Genetic engineering and fermentation (biotechnology) can be used for the production of protein-based drugs.

FURTHER READING

Awan, A. R., Blount, B. A., Bell, D. J., Shaw, W. M., Ho, J. C. H., McKiernan, R. M. and Ellis, T., 'Biosynthesis of the antibiotic nonribosomal peptide penicillin in baker's yeast', *Nature Communications* 2017, 8:15202.
This article shows that baker's yeast (*S. cerevisiae*) can be used to synthesize nonribosomal peptide antibiotics.

Clayden, J., Greeves, N. and Warren, S. *Organic Chemistry*, 2nd edn. Oxford University Press, 2012.
An excellent reference work about all aspects of organic chemistry.

Elander, R. P., 'Industrial production of ß-lactam antibiotics', *Appl. Microbiol. Biotechnol.* 2003, 61:385–92.
An excellent review on the production of ß-lactam antibiotics.

Fu, Y., Li, S., Zu, Y., Yang, G., Yang, Z., Luo, M., Jiang, S., Wink, M. and Efferth, T., 'Medicinal chemistry of Paclitaxel and its analogues', *Current Medicinal Chemistry* 2009, 16:3966–85.

An in-depth account of the state-of-the-art medicinal chemistry of paclitaxel and its analogues.

Graham Richards, W., 'Virtual screening using grid computing: the screensaver project', *Nature Reviews Drug Discovery* 2002, 1:551–5.

A description of how massively distributed computing using screensavers has allowed databases of billions of compounds to be screened against protein targets in a matter of days.

Mann, J. *Murder, Magic and Medicine*, 2nd edn. Oxford University Press, 2000.

A very readable book outlining the evolution of modern medicines from their origins in nature and their uses as poisons, hallucinogenics and medicines.

Moroder, L. and Musiol, H. J., 'Insulin: from its discovery to the industrial synthesis of modern insulin analogues', *Angewandte Chemie-International Edition* 2017, 56(36):10656–69.

A review describing a number of both synthetic and biotechnology approaches to obtaining therapeutically useful insulin analogues.

Newman, D. J. 'Natural products as leads to potential drugs: an old process or the new hope for drug discovery?, *J. Med. Chem.* 2008, 51:2589–99.

Presents a concise account of the influence of natural products on drug discovery.

Nicolaou, K. C., Yang, Z., Liu, J. J., Ueno, H., Nantermet, P. G., Guy, R. K., Claiborne, C. F., Renaud, J., Couladouros, E. A., Paulvannan, K. and Sorensen, E. J., 'Total synthesis of Taxol', *Nature* 1994, 367:630–4.

One of the first total syntheses of taxol.

Patrick, G. L. *An Introduction to Medicinal Chemistry*, 6th edn. Oxford University Press, 2017.

Presents a very in-depth account of medicinal chemistry and includes an excellent section on drug discovery, design and development.

387

Self-check

For the answers to the Self-Check questions in Chapter 13, visit the online resources which accompany this textbook.

ABSORPTION, DISTRIBUTION, METABOLISM AND EXCRETION

Chris Rostron

In order for a drug to have an effect on the physiological processes within the body, it has to be able to enter the body, reach its intended target, and remain in the body for as long as is necessary for it to achieve its desired effect. However, most drugs are xenobiotics, i.e. molecules foreign to the body, and, as such, the body has complex mechanisms to prevent xenobiotics from entering the body and to remove them when they do get inside the body. A vital part of drug design and development is dedicated to overcoming or exploiting these mechanisms. This is the science of pharmacokinetics, which is commonly divided into absorption, distribution, metabolism and excretion, often represented by the acronym ADME. This chapter intends to provide only an overview of the science of pharmacokinetics in order to allow you to understand the basic concepts. For a more detailed treatment of this complex subject, refer to the Further Reading at the end of the chapter.

Learning objectives

Having read this chapter you are expected to be able to:

- appreciate the routes by which drugs enter the body
- understand the mechanisms of drug absorption from the gastrointestinal tract
- identify the factors affecting drug absorption
- understand the physicochemical properties which affect drug distribution to the tissues
- identify the reactions by which a drug can be metabolized
- appreciate the role of cytochrome P450 enzymes and other endogenous molecules in drug metabolism
- describe the routes of drug excretion from the body.

14.1 ABSORPTION

Absorption can be defined as the passage of a drug from its site of administration into the plasma. Therefore, it must be taken into account for all routes of administration except the intravenous route, where administration is directly into the systemic circulation. The main routes of administration are shown in Table 14.1, together with the organ to which they are administered. Most drugs are administered by the oral route, with other routes usually being employed for specific purposes referred to in Table 14.1. Because of this, this chapter will deal largely with drug absorption from the gastrointestinal tract.

The fraction of the dose of a drug that is present in the body and thus available to bring about the desired physiological response is referred to as the bioavailability of the drug. Bioavailability is often linked to the route of administration, that is, which epithelial tissues are involved in the absorption process. For example, for a drug that is administered by intravenous injection, the bioavailability is 100%. The vast majority of drugs administered via the gastrointestinal tract have bioavailability values lower than 100%. Although bioavailability is a useful concept, it has certain limitations, being dependent not only on the route of administration, but also on levels of metabolic enzyme activity, gastric pH or gastrointestinal motility, all of which can vary between individuals.

> The oral route of administration is the main route for most drugs, although other routes may be used in specific circumstances.

Table 14.1 Routes of administration.

Route	Organ	Examples of reason for use
Enteral—Oral	GI tract	Most convenient route
Sublingual	Tongue	Drug degraded in GI tract
Buccal	Oral mucosa	Drug degraded in GI tract
Rectal	GI tract	Patient cannot swallow
Parenteral—Intravenous	Bloodstream	Immediate entry to systemic circulation
Intramuscular	Muscle	Low oral availability
Subcutaneous		Low oral availability
Topical—Dermal	Skin	Treatment of skin conditions
Transdermal	Skin	Avoids first pass metabolism
Ocular	Eye	Treatment of eye disorders
Otic	Ear	Treatment of ear disorders
Nasal	Nose	Mainly local effect
Pulmonary	Lungs	Mainly local effect

Self-check 14.1

Name nine routes of administration where the site of administration of the dosage form is at a particular body location.

Absorption from the gastrointestinal tract

Drugs (and other molecules) can be absorbed from the gastrointestinal tract by passive diffusion, facilitated diffusion or active transport. Most drugs are, however, absorbed by passive diffusion whereas very few drugs are absorbed by facilitated diffusion. Active transport is often a mechanism of absorption for drugs which structurally resemble naturally occurring molecules, such as some amino acids, which are actively transported.

The first requirement for passive diffusion of a drug through a lipid membrane, such as the lining of the gastrointestinal tract, is that it is present in solution—a drug that is not soluble cannot diffuse. The process of passive diffusion involves the partitioning of the drug from the gastrointestinal fluid (aqueous in nature) into the lipid membrane, diffusion across the lipid membrane, and partitioning from the lipid membrane into the bloodstream (aqueous in nature). This process is based on concentration gradients, with diffusion taking place from regions of higher concentration to regions of lower concentration. Initially the drug concentration in the gastrointestinal fluid is high and the concentration in the lipid membrane is low, so the drug partitions into the membrane. Because, initially, there is no drug in the bloodstream, the drug diffuses from the membrane into the bloodstream. As the drug is carried away by the bloodstream (thus the concentration remains low), diffusion continues from the gastrointestinal fluid to the blood. This is the situation which occurs with non-polar and uncharged molecules. Thus the most important molecular property with respect to passive diffusion is the partition coefficient i.e. the balance between lipid and aqueous solubility. The size and shape of the molecule is of little relevance. Most drugs given orally have sufficient water solubility to undergo passive diffusion and so passive diffusion depends largely on lipid solubility (see Box 14.1 Aminoglycoside antibiotics).

The situation with molecules which can ionize is, however, quite different. As many drugs are either weak acids or bases, this situation is important. Here the extent of passive diffusion depends on both the lipid solubility of the unionized species and the degree of ionization at the appropriate physiological pH. On this basis you would expect weak acids like aspirin (pKa 3.5) to be unionized in the stomach (pH 2) and to be mainly absorbed from there, rather than from the small intestine (pH 6). However, the vastly greater available surface area for absorption in the small intestine compared with the stomach, means that weakly acidic drugs like aspirin are mainly absorbed from the small intestine rather than the stomach.

Facilitated diffusion and active transport both utilize a transport protein to carry molecules across a membrane. Facilitated diffusion operates from a region of high concentration to one of low concentration and so does not require energy. Active transport operates against a concentration gradient and so is an energy-requiring process. Normally the transport proteins carry very structurally specific molecules across the membranes, e.g. amino acids. Consequently, for a drug to be absorbed via a carrier protein it has to be structurally very similar to the normal substrate for the carrier protein, and so few drugs are absorbed by this process.

Factors affecting absorption

In addition to the abovementioned lipid solubility and degree of ionization, gastrointestinal motility and the nature of the formulation can also affect drug absorption. The timing of drug dosage with respect to food intake can also be important with respect to absorption. For example, a drug taken after a meal is often more slowly absorbed because of delayed gastric emptying.

Drugs can be absorbed from the gastrointestinal tract by passive diffusion, facilitated diffusion or active transport, with passive diffusion being the most common method.

Box 14.1   Aminoglycoside antibiotics

The aminoglycoside group of antibiotics (including streptomycin, gentamicin and neomycin) all have complex structures (see Figure) and, despite their large molecular weight, are all highly water-soluble, due mainly to the large number of polar groups in their structures. They are so highly water-soluble that their absorption from the gastrointestinal tract is very poor and they are mainly administered by injection. Streptomycin is used by intravenous injection to treat tuberculosis and intravenous gentamicin is used to treat a range of serious bacterial infections. Neomycin is used topically to treat bacterial skin infection and occasionally orally to treat bacterial infections of the gastrointestinal tract (because it is not absorbed from there). Because of the toxicity profile of the aminoglycosides (in particular **nephro- and oto-toxicity**) it is recommended that the blood levels of these drugs are closely monitored.

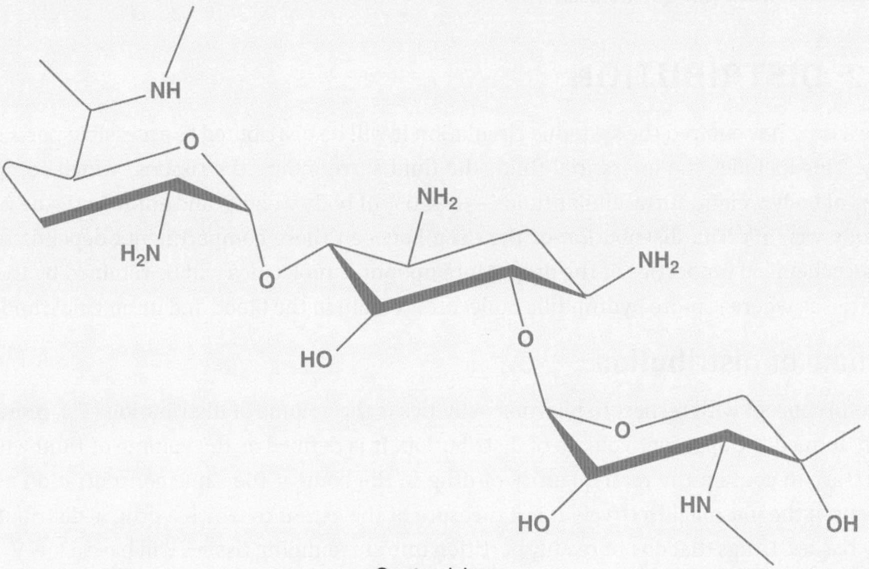

Gentamicin

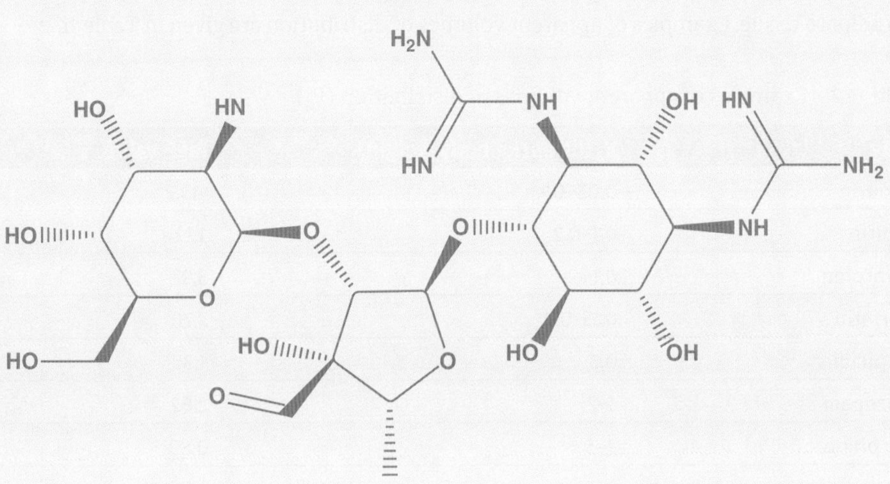

Streptomycin

⚷ Factors affecting drug absorption include lipid solubility, degree of ionization, gastrointestinal motility and the nature of the drug formulation.

Self-check 14.2

Which of the following drugs would you expect to have a high oral bioavailability: codeine, propranolol, morphine, sumatriptan, vancomycin, and why?

An enormous amount of effort goes into the development of formulations which will optimize drug absorption. Thus formulations can be utilized to delay absorption (capsules and tablets with resistant coatings), to speed up absorption (fast release tablets which have reduced particle size to enhance absorption), or to achieve a controlled absorption over a period of time (sustained release (SR) formulations).

14.2 DISTRIBUTION

Once a drug has entered the systemic circulation it will be distributed to accessible parts of the body. This includes the interstitial fluid (the fluid surrounding the tissues) which comprises ~16% of body weight, intracellular fluid (~30–40% of body weight) and adipose tissue (~20% of body weight). The distribution of the drug between these compartments depends on the physicochemical properties of the drug. More lipophilic molecules will be retained by the adipose tissue whereas more hydrophilic molecules remain in the blood and interstitial fluid.

Volume of distribution

A useful concept with respect to pharmacokinetics is the volume of distribution (V_d), more correctly termed the apparent volume of distribution. It is defined as the volume of fluid which is necessary to contain the total quantity of drug in the body at the same concentration as that present in the plasma. Effectively it is a measure of the extent to which a drug is distributed to body tissues. Drugs that do not readily partition into surrounding tissues will have a low V_d value whereas drugs that are highly lipophilic will have high V_d values because of their partitioning into adipose tissue. Examples of apparent volumes of distribution are given in Table 14.2.

Table 14.2 Examples of apparent volumes of distribution (V_d).

Drug	V_d (litres/kg body weight)	logP value
Heparin	0.05–0.1	-13.2
Aspirin	0.1–0.2	1.19
Ibuprofen	0.14	3.97
Warfarin	0.15–0.2	2.70
Ampicillin	0.3	1.35
Diazepam	1–2	2.82
Morphine	2–5	0.89
Digoxin	2–5	1.26
Chlorpromazine	2–5	5.41

Volume of distribution is a measure of the extent to which a drug is distributed to the body tissues.

Plasma protein binding

Drugs which enter the systemic circulation are in a position to bind to proteins circulating in the blood. The extent to which a drug is bound to plasma protein has an influence on its therapeutic activity because a bound drug cannot reach its intended site of action, nor can it be metabolized and eliminated from the body.

Albumin is the most important plasma protein with respect to drug binding, binding weakly acidic drugs such as aspirin. Weakly basic drugs, for example diazepam, bind mainly to α-acid glycoprotein. The nature of the binding to protein is reversible, with both free and bound forms forming an equilibrium situation in the blood (see Figure 14.1 and Box 14.2 Extent of plasma protein binding). The binding interactions may be electrostatic interactions, hydrogen bonding, dipole–dipole interactions and van der Waals interactions—in other words, similar to those involved in drug-receptor interactions.

Figure 14.1   Plasma protein binding

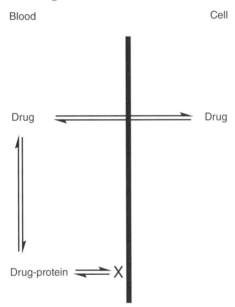

 The binding of drugs to plasma proteins affects their availability to their site of action, their metabolism and their excretion.

Self-check 14.3

Which of the following drugs are highly plasma-protein bound: warfarin, codeine, ibuprofen, isoniazid, midazolam, lithium?

> **Box 14.2   Extent of plasma protein binding**
>
> Many drugs bind to plasma proteins, but the % bound and the % of potential protein bind-
> ing sites occupied can vary enormously. Diazepam is 98% protein bound at therapeutic con-
> centrations, but less than 1% of the available protein binding sites are occupied, whereas
> aspirin is only 50% protein bound at therapeutic concentrations but occupies 50% of the
> available protein binding sites. The % of binding sites occupied does not relate to the ease
> of displacement by another drug. Diazepam, occupying less than 1% of available sites, can
> be displaced from those sites by another drug such as sodium valproate, more than dou-
> bling the amount of free diazepam in the plasma.

14.3 METABOLISM

Drug metabolism can be defined as the chemical alteration of a drug by a biological system, with
the principal objective of eliminating the drug from that system. Metabolism is a protective mechanism by which the body can remove potentially toxic foreign molecules from the body and is often
called xenobiotic metabolism. As most drugs are molecules which are foreign to the body, they are
subjected to these metabolic processes. A significant factor controlling the concentration of a drug
reaching its site of action will be how much of it will be metabolized before it reaches its site of
action. The design of a new drug, therefore, demands an understanding of the metabolic processes
for that drug and, equally importantly, the biological activity of any products of that metabolism.

   Excretion by the kidneys (renal excretion) is enhanced by increased water solubility. As most
drugs are quite lipid soluble, metabolism is designed to increase the water solubility of drugs
and so increase their rate of removal from the body by renal excretion. The majority of metabolic reactions are enzyme controlled and, as such, exhibit many of the features of enzyme
controlled reactions such as substrate specificity, control by substrate concentration and ste-
reoselectivity. Often metabolism of a drug will involve different reaction routes, giving rise to a
number of different products (metabolites). These metabolites may have no biological activity,
reduced activity, increased activity, or even a different biological activity, potentially leading to
unwanted side-effects or toxicity.

   As xenobiotic metabolism is a process designed to protect the body from ingested molecules
which might be toxic, it makes sense for it to take place as soon after absorption as possible.
Consequently, the majority of drug metabolism occurs in the liver, although drug metabolism
can take place in a number of other body tissues (see Table 14.3).

Table 14.3   Sites of drug metabolism.

Site of metabolism	Example of drugs metabolized at this site
Liver	Main site for most drugs
Gastrointestinal tract	Suxamethonium hydrolyzed by esterases
Lungs	Prodrugs of inhaled steroids metabolized to active drug by esterases
Blood	Procaine hydrolysed by plasma esterases
Skin	Prodrugs of topical steroids by esterases
Kidneys	Glucuronidation of prostaglandins

🔑 Metabolism is a process within the body which aims to increase the water solubility of a drug (or any xenobiotic) in order to facilitate its excretion via the kidney.

The majority of drugs are delivered orally, and drug absorption can take place immediately after ingestion in the gastrointestinal mucosa. However, not all drugs absorbed into the gastrointestinal mucosa reach the general blood circulation. **P-glycoprotein**, which is an ATP-dependent efflux pump for xenobiotics, can secrete drugs such as digoxin from the intestinal mucosa back into the lumen of the gastrointestinal tract, thus being responsible for decreased drug accumulation in the blood. Additionally, certain esterases present in the intestine can hydrolyse esters and amides. However, most drugs are absorbed relatively unchanged through the intestinal wall into the bloodstream. The gastrointestinal blood supply (portal blood supply) passes through the liver before distribution to the rest of the body. It is in the liver that the vast majority of drug metabolism occurs, and this is often referred to as 'first pass metabolism'. This process can greatly affect the **bioavailability** of a drug and, in extreme cases, may require an alternative route of administration to avoid the initial hepatic metabolism (see Box 14.3 Lidocaine and Figure).

Although the liver is the major site of drug metabolism, other sites in the body may be involved (see Table 14.3). The metabolic processes which occur in these alternative tissues tend to be rather more substrate-specific than those which take place in the liver. For example, ester and amide hydrolysis takes place via esterases and related enzymes in the plasma. The metabolic processes taking place in the liver can occur in various cell tissues, such as the mitochondria and the cytosol. However, the vast majority of metabolic reactions involve **cytochrome P450 enzymes** which are associated with the **endoplasmic reticulum** of the liver cells (see Box 14.4 Cytochrome P450 enzymes).

Phase I metabolism

Drug metabolic reactions are conveniently classified into Phase I and Phase II reactions. Phase I metabolism involves the conversion of a drug to a more water-soluble molecule. Improved water-solubility requires a functional group with a good hydrogen bonding capacity and involves the introduction of such a group or the unmasking of such a group (for example, the conversion of an ester to a carboxylic acid). If the metabolites are now sufficiently water-soluble, renal excretion can occur. Phase I metabolic reactions are classified as oxidation, reduction and hydrolysis. The Phase I metabolites may still not be sufficiently water-soluble to be readily excreted. In this situation, Phase II metabolism may take place.

Oxidative reactions are the most important reactions of Phase I metabolism. They generally involve the introduction of a hydroxyl (OH) group (hydroxylation), the oxidation of a sulfur or nitrogen atom (S- or N- oxidation), or the removal of an alkyl group from nitrogen or oxygen

🔑 Drug metabolism can take place in a number of body tissues, but the liver is the primary site of metabolism.

🔑 Drug metabolism takes place in two steps: Phases I and II. Phase I introduces or unmasks a group with increased water solubility. Phase II involves a reaction to further increase water solubility if necessary.

Box 14.3 Lidocaine

Lidocaine was originally designed as a local anaesthetic but is also a very useful **antiar-rhythmic** drug. It is the drug of choice for the emergency treatment of **ventricular arrhythmia**. It is very useful in this regard because of its rapid metabolism, because the therapy can be rapidly modified in response to changes in the patient's status. Lidocaine can only be used as an antiarrhythmic when administered parenterally. Activity is not seen after oral administration because of the rapid first pass metabolism. Knowledge of the metabolism of lidocaine has also led to the production of tocainide, which also has antiarrhythmic activity but is orally active. The plasma half-life of tocainide is about 12 hours, compared with about 15 minutes for lidocaine.

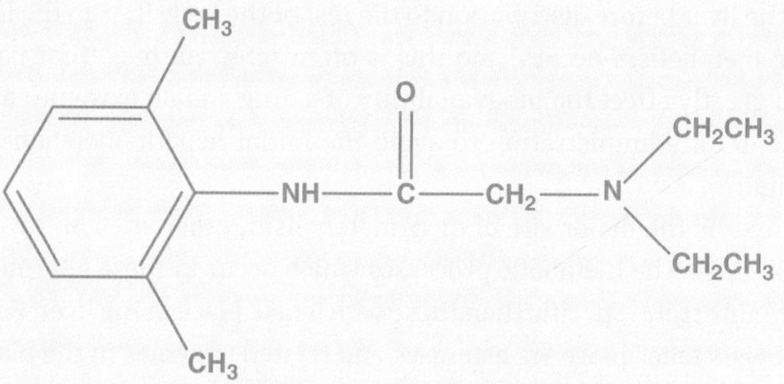

Lidocaine

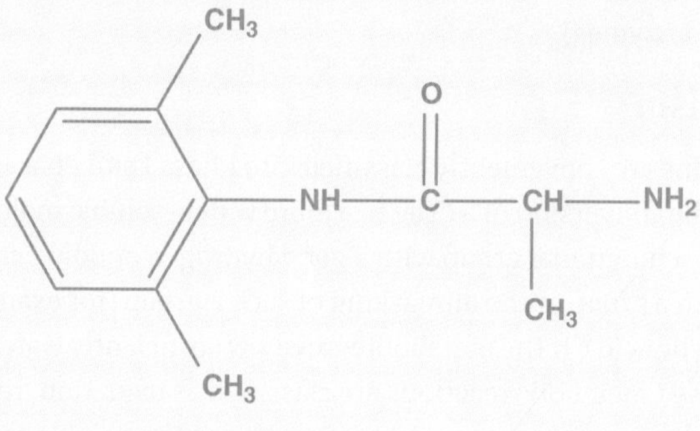

Tocainide

(N- or O-dealkylation) (see Figure 14.2). These oxidative reactions occur in a series of steps, and cytochrome P450s are involved in one or more of these steps. Whatever the oxidation metabolic product, CYP450 enzymes will be involved.

Reductive metabolic reactions usually involve specific reductase enzymes. Although reductive reactions are less common than oxidative ones, they involve some important drug metabolic reactions such as reduction of aldehydes and ketones to alcohols and, less commonly, the

Many oxidative metabolic reactions involve cytochrome P450 enzyme systems.

Box 14.4   Cytochrome P450 enzymes

Cytochrome P450s are a family of enzymes that have an important role in metabolism of xenobiotics. The title P450 arises from the fact that they complex with carbon monoxide and the complexes absorb light of about 450nm. They all have a similar structure, having an iron atom (Fe^{2+}) which forms coordinate bonds with four nitrogen atoms of haem and the thiol group of a cysteine residue in a globin protein (see Figure which appeared earlier in Chapter 8 and is reproduced below). The final coordination position is occupied by water or other ligands which are easily exchanged. The nomenclature of cytochromes can appear quite complex but is actually relatively straightforward. The letters CYP represents the cytochrome system. This is followed by the cytochrome family number (CYP1, CYP2 etc.). This is then followed by an upper-case letter representing the sub-family (CYP1A, CYP2B etc.). Specific enzymes which catalyse a specific reaction are indicated by a final number (CYP1A1).

Haem

Water molecule which can be replaced by oxygen

Cytochrome

Reductive metabolic reactions usually involve drugs with ketone or nitro groups.

reduction of nitro groups to amines. Aldehydes are relatively easily oxidized and so reduction is less often involved. Ketones, however, are resistant to oxidation and so are often reduced to secondary alcohols. Reduction of ketones often leads to the formation of a new asymmetric carbon atom and, therefore, two stereoisomers (see Figure 14.3). This situation can have significant consequences for biological activity and is often a consideration in drug design and development.

Hydrolytic metabolic reactions involve largely ester and amide groups (see Figure 14.4). Ester hydrolysis can take place by non-specific esterases in the liver, kidney and other tissues, and also by pseudocholinesterases in the plasma. Amide hydrolysis usually involves non-specific amidases, carboxypeptidases and aminopeptidases. Ester hydrolysis is usually more rapid than amide hydrolysis.

Hydrolytic metabolic processes mainly involve drugs containing an ester or amide group.

Phase II metabolism

In this process a functional group present in the drug, or its metabolites, reacts with an endogenous substance and forms a highly polar (water-soluble) conjugate. Phase II metabolism
is also known as conjugation. The endogenous substances include glucuronic acid, sulfate,
acetic acid and a number of amino acids. Phase II metabolism is often the final step in drug
metabolism, and the conjugates are excreted in the urine and/or the bile. Conjugates are usually biologically inactive, with few exceptions, whereas phase I metabolites can retain some
biological activity.

Reaction with glucuronic acid is the most important of the phase II reactions. The body
has plenty available glucuronic acid, and reaction (glucuronidation) can take place with alcohols, phenols, thiols, amines and carboxylic acids within drugs or their metabolites (see
Figure 14.5).

Figure 14.2 Examples of oxidative drug metabolism: (a) hydroxylation; (b) S-oxidation; (c)
N-oxidation; (d) N-dealkylation; (e) O-dealkylation

(A) Hydroxylation

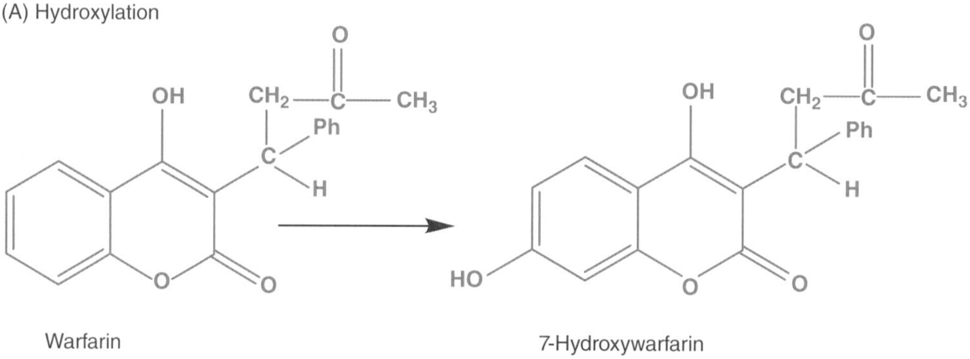

Warfarin

7-Hydroxywarfarin

(B) S-oxidation

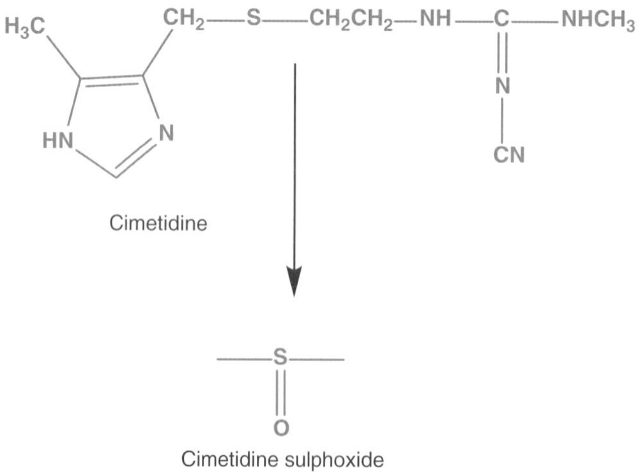

Cimetidine

Cimetidine sulphoxide

Figure 14.2 *continued*

(C) N-oxidation

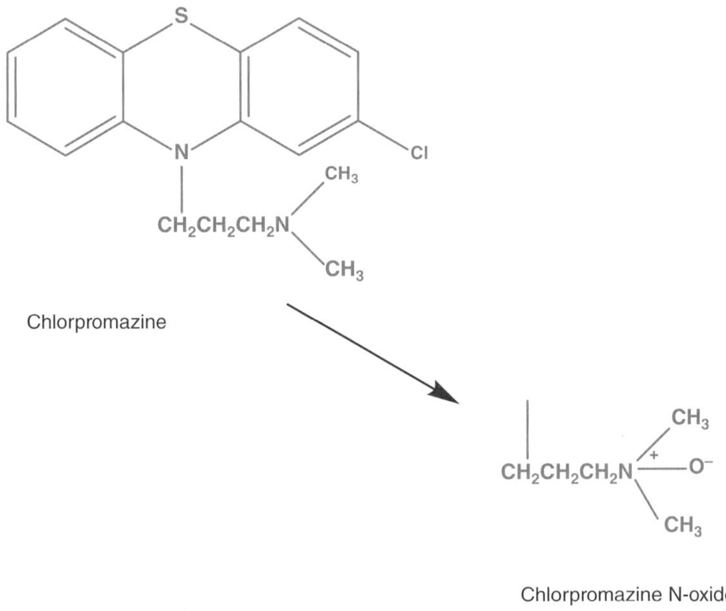

Chlorpromazine

Chlorpromazine N-oxide

(D) N-dealkylation

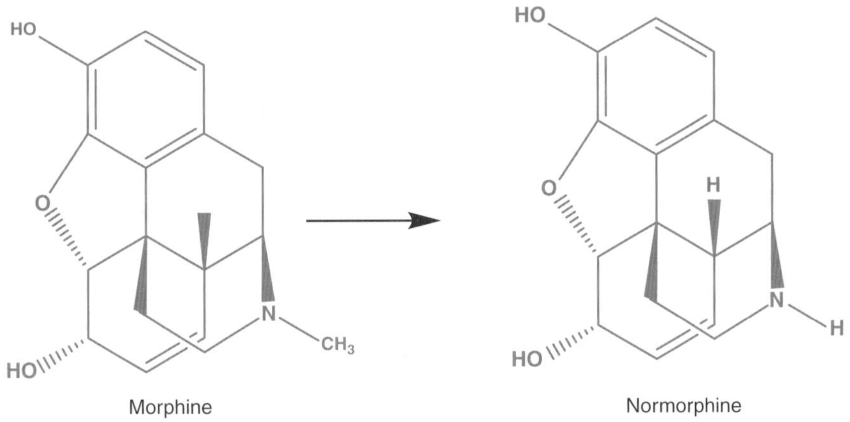

Morphine

Normorphine

(E) O-dealkylation

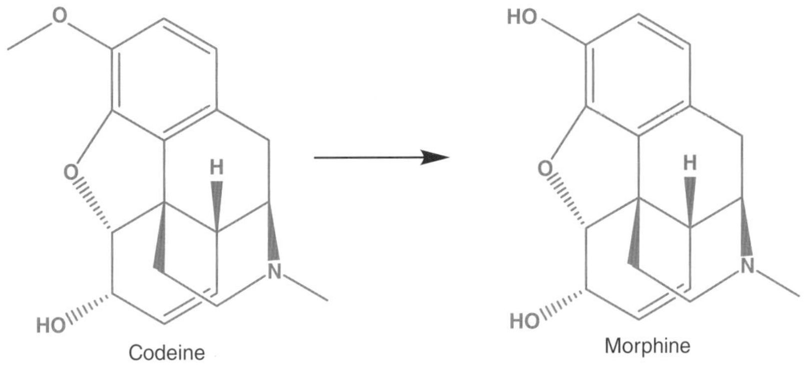

Codeine

Morphine

Figure 14.3 Example of metabolic reduction of ketone-producing stereoisomers

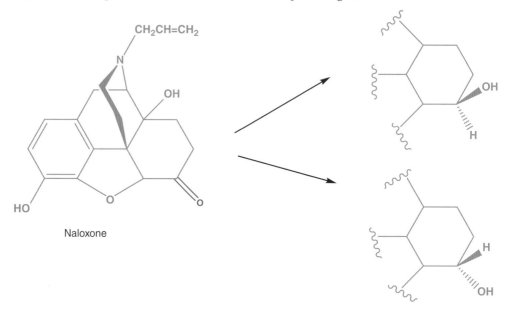

Naloxone

Sulfate formation is a metabolic route for phenols and, occasionally, alcohols and amines (see Figure 14.6).

Acetylation—or rather, reaction with activated acetate (acetylCoA)—usually involves amines or alcohols. Probably the best known example is the metabolism of the anti-tubercular drug isoniazid (see Figure 14.7).

Conjugation with an amino acid is an important metabolic route for carboxylic acids. The reaction takes place in a series of steps. The carboxylic acid reacts with ATP to form an AMP intermediate. This intermediate is converted to an active CoA intermediate, and this activated intermediate undergoes nucleophilic displacement with the amino acid. The most common amino acid used by humans is glycine, but glutamine conjugates are also formed although glycine conjugates are more common (see Figure 14.8). Species other than humans use different amino acids—birds use ornithine and rodents use alanine. Humans also use glutathione (GSH), which is a tripeptide consisting of the amino acids glycine, cysteine and glutamic acid. In this

> Phase II metabolism involves reaction with an endogenous substance to form a highly water-soluble conjugate. The endogenous compounds are mainly glucuronic acid, sulfate, acetylCoA, amino acids and glutathione.

Self-check 14.4

Suggest possible metabolic routes for the following drugs: pethidine, amphetamine, ibuprofen, lidocaine, trimethoprim. Compare your suggestions with the known metabolic routes for these drugs.

Figure 14.4 Examples of hydrolytic drug metabolism

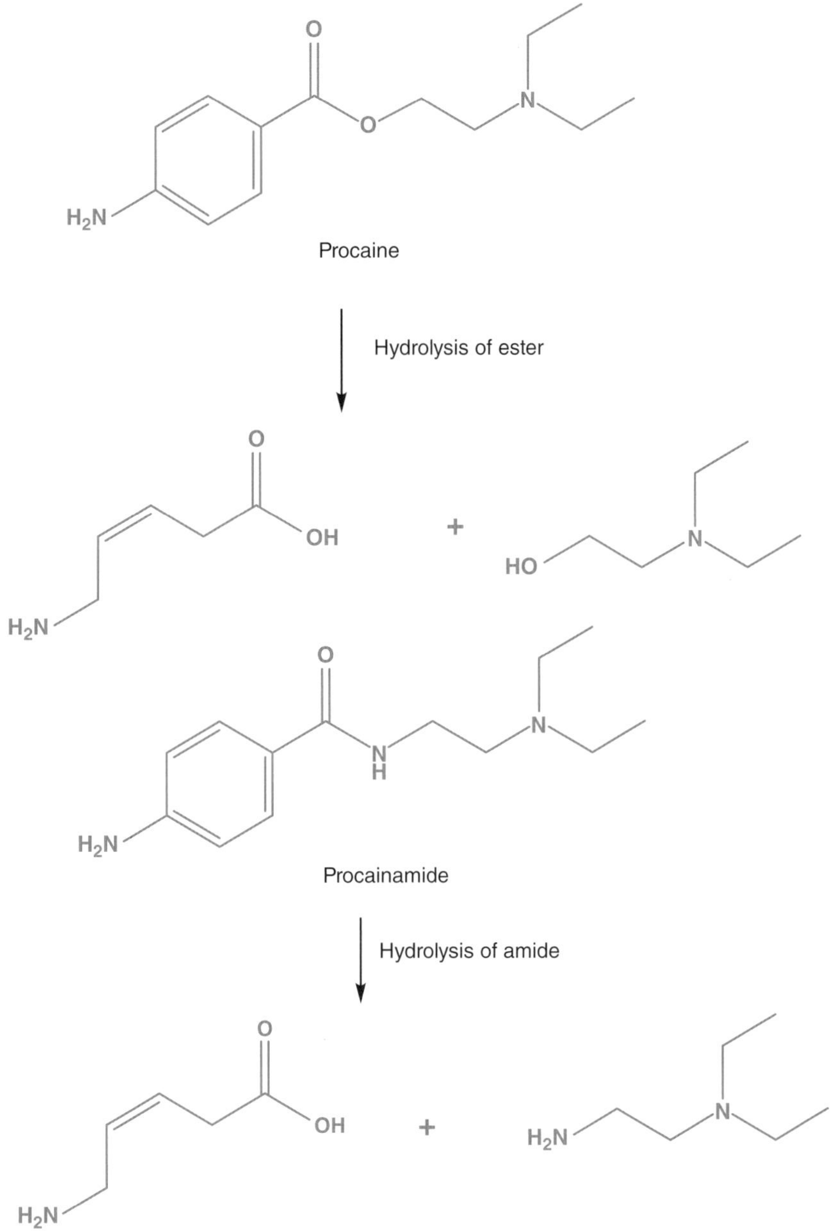

process, however, it is the thiol (SH) group of the cysteine which reacts. This thiol group is very nucleophilic and undergoes conjugation with molecules containing electrophilic centres such as epoxides or haloalkanes. Glutathione conjugates are formed and then converted to mercapturic acids which are excreted in the urine (see Figure 14.9).

Figure 14.5 Example of glucuronidation

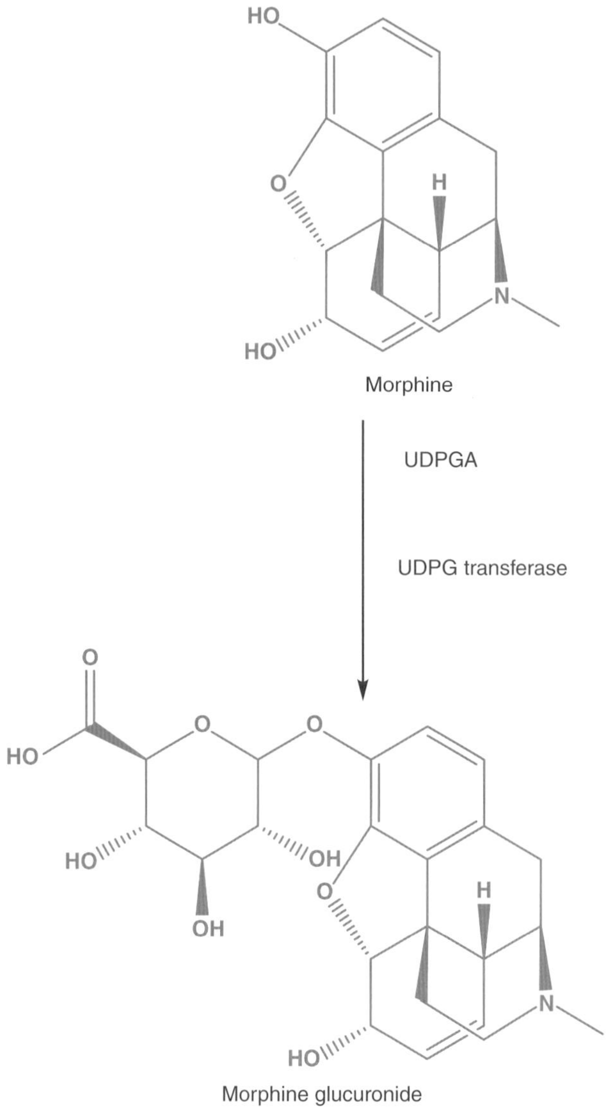
HO
O
H
N
HO
Morphine
UDPGA
UDPG transferase
O
HO
O
O
HO
OH
O
OH
H
N
HO
Morphine glucuronide

Figure 14.6 Example of sulfation

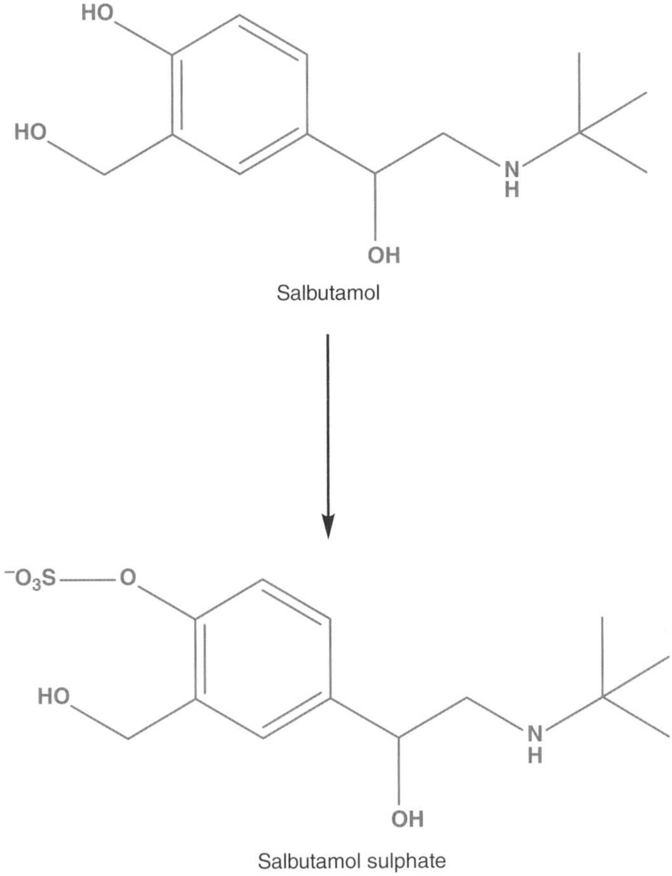
HO
HO
N
H
OH
Salbutamol
$^{-}O_3S$—O
HO
N
H
OH
Salbutamol sulphate

Figure 14.7 Example of acetylation

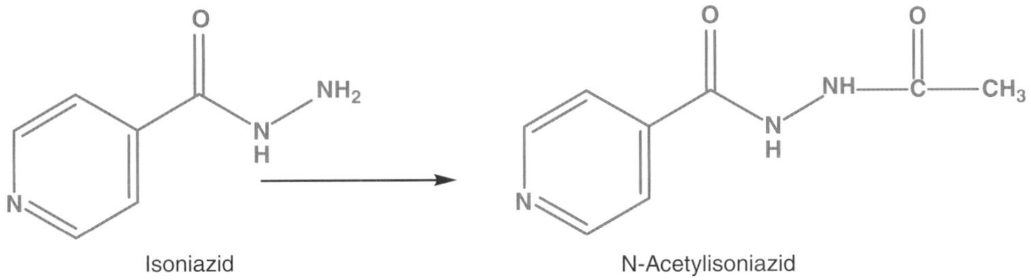
O
NH_2
N
H
N
Isoniazid
O
O
NH—C—CH_3
N
H
N
N-Acetylisoniazid

Figure 14.8 Example of amino acid conjugation

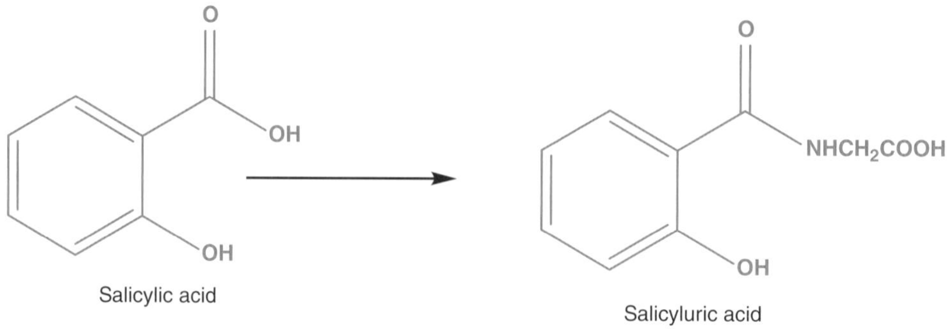

Salicylic acid

Salicyluric acid

Figure 14.9 Example of glutathione conjugation

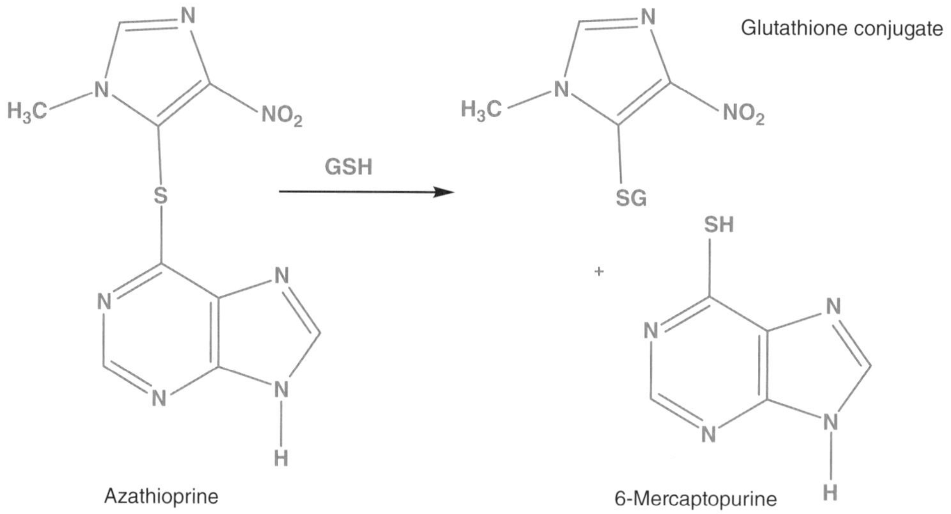

Glutathione conjugate

GSH

Azathioprine

6-Mercaptopurine

14.4 EXCRETION

Excretion is the removal of a drug and its metabolites from the body and is an irreversible process. The primary excretion route for most drugs and their metabolites is via the kidney and into the urine. There are other routes of excretion such as the faeces, lungs, sweat and the bile. Usually only the last of these has any general significance.

Renal excretion

Drugs are excreted via the kidney by two processes: glomerular filtration and tubular secretion. The capillaries of the glomeruli act as a filter and allow the passage of water, ions and small molecules (such as drugs and their metabolites). Large molecules like proteins are retained, including any drug-protein complexes. Glomerular filtration is essentially a passive diffusion process. On the other hand, secretion into the renal tubules (tubular secretion) is an active transport process and thus requires energy. The carrier systems are relatively non-selective, and there are two systems which transport drugs into the renal tubules—one which handles acidic drugs, and a separate system which handles basic drugs. However, some molecules are reabsorbed from the tubules. This is a process which is normally used to return compounds vital to the body such as glucose and amino acids. The process can, however, return drug molecules to the body. As this reabsorption is mainly by passive diffusion, it is mainly the more lipid-soluble drug molecules which will be reabsorbed.

Tubular reabsorption is dependent upon the pH of the urine, and the extent of reabsorption of a drug can be changed by changing the urinary pH. Making the urine more alkaline will lead to greater excretion of acidic drugs. Making the urine more acidic will increase the excretion of basic drugs. This control of urinary pH can be of value in drug overdose situations.

Most drugs are excreted via the kidney, either by glomerular filtration of tubular secretion.

Drugs which are converted to glucuronides in the liver are sometimes excreted in the bile.

Biliary excretion

Some molecules which have been metabolized by the liver during phase II metabolism, particularly those where the glucuronide has been formed, are transported to the bile. These conjugates are concentrated in the bile and passed into the intestine. If the glucuronide is hydrolysed in the intestine, the free drug is available to be reabsorbed via the enterohepatic cycle, and in some cases this can prolong the drug action. This process is known as 'enterohepatic recirculation', and examples of drugs where this can be significant are morphine and ethinyloestradiol.

Half-life and clearance

The half-life of a drug ($t_{1/2}$) is the time it takes for the plasma concentration of the drug to decrease by 50%. Knowledge of the half-life is important when determining the duration of action of a drug and its dosage regimen. The half-life will be affected by the volume of distribution (V_d), because if a large proportion of the drug is not in the plasma (a large V_d) the time taken to reduce its concentration will be longer. The half-life of a drug is inversely proportional to clearance (more correctly, total clearance) of the drug. Total clearance (C_T) is the volume of blood that is cleared of the drug per unit time by all available routes. The main contributors to total clearance are renal clearance and hepatic clearance (i.e. representing excretion and metabolism). Table 14.4 gives some examples of drug clearance and half-life values. Clearance is affected by numerous factors such as weight, age, renal and hepatic disorders, genetic predisposition and drug–drug interactions.

Table 14.4   Examples of drug clearance values.

Drug	Total clearance (C_T) ml/min/kg	Half-life (hours)
Heparin	0.43	1.5
Ranitidine	10	2.8–3.1
Vancomycin	1.0	4–11
Warfarin	0.02–0.065	21–89
Morphine	20–30	2–4
Chlorpromazine	11	30

The half-life and clearance of a drug are key pharmacokinetic parameters used in determining the dosage regimen of a drug.

Self-check 14.5

What is the difference between hepatic clearance and renal clearance?

Case study 14.1

Mr Ford had been prescribed simvastatin, a cholesterol-lowering drug, to help bring his blood cholesterol levels down to a more appropriate value. His GP had told him that he must avoid grapefruit and grapefruit juice whilst taking this drug. When he visited Tu's pharmacy to collect his prescription he asked Tu about not consuming grapefruit and whether it was really important. Tu told Mr Ford that it was important, as consuming grapefruit juice could increase the likelihood of any side-effects associated with this drug. Mr Ford said that that was a pity, because he really enjoyed a big glass of grapefruit juice with his breakfast every morning.

Reflection questions

1. Why would grapefruit juice consumption increase the likelihood of side-effects from taking the simvastatin?

2. Is there any way that Mr Ford can continue to enjoy his daily grapefruit juice and still benefit from the cholesterol-lowering activity of a statin drug?

For answers, visit the online resources which accompany this textbook.

CHAPTER SUMMARY

- The absorption of a drug into the body is important for all routes of administration except intravenous injection where the drug enters the bloodstream directly.

- Absorption from the gastrointestinal tract can be by passive diffusion, facilitated diffusion or active transport.

- Factors which can affect drug absorption are the lipid solubility and degree of ionization of the drug and the formulation of the drug.

- The distribution of a drug into the body tissues is largely dependent upon the physico-chemical properties of the drug, particularly the solubility characteristics.

- The apparent volume of distribution gives an indication of the extent to which a drug is distributed to the body tissues.

- Many drugs bind to plasma proteins, and this affects the amount of drug available to the site of action, their metabolism and excretion.

- The principal objective of drug metabolism is aiding the removal of the drug from the body by increasing its water solubility.

- The liver is the most important site of drug metabolism, although drug metabolism can take place in other tissues.

- Drug metabolism takes place in two phases: phase I and phase II. Both phases are designed to produce metabolites with increased water-solubility.

- Phase I metabolism involves the introduction or unmasking of a group with increased water-solubility.

- Phase II metabolism involves reaction of a drug and/or its phase I metabolite with an endogenous molecule to produce a highly water-soluble conjugate.

- The most important phase I reactions are oxidation reactions, mainly catalysed by cytochrome P450 enzymes. Other phase I reactions are reduction and hydrolysis.

- The endogenous molecules involved in phase II reactions are glucuronic acid, sulfate, acetylCoA, amino acids and glutathione.

- The main route of drug excretion is via the kidney into the urine.

- Renal excretion involves glomerular filtration and tubular secretion.

- Two useful pharmacokinetic parameters are the half-life of a drug and its clearance value. Knowledge of these values informs the dosage regimen of a drug.

FURTHER READING

Coleman, M. *Human Drug Metabolism: An Introduction*, 2nd edn. Wiley, 2010. ISBN 978-0-470-74217.

An accessible text dealing with all aspects of drug metabolism, including a number of case studies.

Rowe, P. H. *Pharmacokinetics*, 2012, Bookboon.com (a free e-book). ISBN 978–87-403-0090-1.

All the basic concepts of pharmacokinetics are covered in a user-friendly fashion, with lots of worked examples.

Thomas, G. *Medicinal Chemistry: An Introduction*, 2nd edn. Wiley, 2008. ISBN 978-0-470-02597-0.

A general medicinal chemistry text which contains a detailed chapter on drug metabolism

Self-check

For the answers to the Self-check questions in Chapter 14, visit the online resources which accompany this textbook.

GLOSSARY

Absorption (*verb*, **to absorb**) The taking up of electromagnetic radiation by matter.

ACE inhibitor Angiotensin-converting enzyme inhibitors inhibit the conversion of angiotensin I to angiotensin II; they may be used to treat heart failure and hypertension.

Acetylcholinesterease An enzyme that catalyses the hydrolysis of acetylcholine.

Achiral molecules An achiral molecule is a non-chiral molecule. It is a molecule without chiral centres. Glycine is the only achiral amino acid in nature.

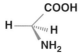

Acid dissociation constant An acid dissociation constant is the equilibrium constant for the dissociation of an acid in aqueous solution. It is a measure of acid strength.

Activating Effect of substituents that stabilize the cationic intermediate in electrophilic substitution and hence increase the rate of reaction.

Active transport Active transport of a metabolite involves transporting the molecule against a concentration gradient, using energy in the process. The term is used more loosely with drugs, to describe the movement across a membrane by hijack of an active transport system. Natural products can sometimes do this.

Acylation A reaction in which an acyl group is added to a molecule.

Addition reaction A reaction where a π bond is broken and two new σ bonds are formed.

Adenosine-5'-triphosphate (ATP) High-energy phosphate molecule that is a product of respiration and a source of energy for cellular processes. Its hydrolysis to ADP (adenosine-5'-diphosphate) and inorganic phosphate can yield up to about $50 \, \text{kJmol}^{-1}$.

Adipose tissue Connective tissue that acts as the main site of storage for fat.

Agonist An agonist is a molecule that activates a particular receptor to produce a specific response.

Aldose Sugar containing one aldehyde (CH=O) group per molecule.

Aliphatic An organic compound whose structure does not contain benzene or a similar structure.

Alkanes Saturated hydrocarbons, containing only single bonds.

Alkenes Hydrocarbons containing one or more carbon–carbon double bonds.

Alkylation A reaction in which an alkyl group is added to a molecule.

Alkynes Hydrocarbons containing one or more carbon–carbon triple bonds.

Allosteric A type of receptor binding that involves a change in the shape and activity of an enzyme when a drug binds at a site other than the binding site of the endogenous ligand.

Amino acid Molecule that has an amine group, a carboxylic acid group and a side-chain. Amino acids are essential for life as they are the building blocks of protein.

Amphiphilic or Amphipathic The property (attributed to a molecule) of both polar and non-polar characteristics (literally loving both hydrophobic and hydrophilic environments).

Anaerobes Organisms that do not require oxygen to live. Metronidazole is an effective drug for treating anaerobic bacteria.

Analgesic Reduces or even eliminates pain through a pharmacological action.

Analogue A compound that differs from another in a small, carefully considered way. Analogues of an active compound are often made in order to optimize activity.

Angstrom (abbreviation Å) An angstrom is a unit of length equivalent to 0.1 nm, or 10^{-10} m. This non-standard unit is very convenient because it is of the same order of magnitude as a bond length. A C–C bond is about 1.5 Å, a hydrogen bond about 2.7 Å, for example.

Animals Major group of eukaryotic multicellular organisms.

Antagonist An antagonist is a molecule that binds to a receptor but does not trigger the usual response, and can block the binding of, and activation by, an agonist at the same receptor.

Antiarrhymic agent A drug which is used to control cardiac arrhymias.

Antiperiplanar Term used to describe the A-B-C-D bond angle in a molecule where the dihedral angle is 180° (more strictly between +150° and −150°).

Antipyretic An antipyretic relieves a fever (which is sometimes called pyrexia) by reducing a higher-than-normal body temperature, through a pharmacological action.

Assay A method of quantitative analysis.

Autosomal Relating to a chromosome that is not a sex chromosome.

ATP Adenosine triphosphate is the universal currency of energy in biological systems. Its hydrolysis to ADP (adenosine diphosphate) and inorganic phosphate can yield up to about 50 kJ mol^{-1}.

API Active pharmaceutical ingredient.

Axial In a chair conformation of a six-membered ring the axial substituents stick up or down, as shown by the red and blue positions in the diagram.

Bacterial DNA gyrases Enzymes responsible for introducing supercoils into the DNA double helix so that it can replicate.

β-lactam antibiotic A class of antibiotic drugs which include the penicillins and cephalosporins that have a β-lactam ring at the heart of their structure. They work by inhibiting the enzymes responsible for the synthesis of bacterial cell walls.

β-lactamase An enzyme capable of deactivating a β-lactam antibiotic (such as a penicillin or cephalosporin) by hydrolysing it.

β-globin Polypeptide that forms part of the haemoglobin protein in the blood.

Bilayer A physical structure, typically of a cell membrane, that consists of two layers of molecules facing each other.

Bioavailability The proportion of an administered drug which reaches the systemic circulation unchanged.

Biochemistry The study of biology from a chemical/molecular perspective.

Biologics An emerging class of drugs consisting of high-molecular-weight biological molecules such as proteins or nucleic acids.

Biopolymer A polymeric molecule produced within a biological system.

Biosynthesis The synthesis of a compound by a biological system.

Biosynthetic precursor A substance that occurs early in the production pathway of a molecule prepared within a biological system.

Boat conformation The boat conformation of a six-membered ring has minimal torsional strain, but eclipsed substituents mean that it is less favoured than the chair form. Its shape is as shown.

Bonding interactions Weak bonds, especially hydrogen bonds and non-polar bonds, which frequently occur within biological macromolecules (intramolecular) or between a drug and its target (intermolecular).

Bronchial tree The airways within the lungs.

Bronchodilation A widening of the air passages in the windpipe (trachea) which allows increased airflow in and out of the lungs.

Brønsted acids Species that can act as proton donors.

Cancer A number of diseases characterized by abnormal growths and uncontrolled cell division and often with the ability to spread (metastasize) to other tissues of the body.

Carbocation A positively charged carbon atom, also known as a carbonium ion.

Carcinogenesis The process of initiating and promoting cancer.

Catalyst A compound that increases the rate of reaction without being consumed in the process.

Catalytic hydrogenation A reaction between molecular hydrogen and another molecule in the presence of a catalyst.

Chair conformation The chair conformation of a six-membered ring is the conformation in which torsional and steric strain are minimized. Its shape is as shown.

Chelating agent A ligand which has more than one functional group that can form a dative bond with a metal ion.

Chemical dipole moment The measure of polarity of a chemical bond.

Chiral A chiral carbon has four different groups bonded to it. These groups may be hydrogen, groups based on carbon or on another element, such as oxygen or nitrogen. If a molecule contains a chiral carbon it cannot be superimposed on its mirror image.

Cholinesterase A family of enzymes that catalyze the hydrolysis of acetylcholine into choline and acetate.

Chromatogram A visible record showing the separation of compounds by chromatography.

Chromophore The part of a molecule that is responsible for the absorbance of electromagnetic radiation (usually light or ultraviolet radiation). The term originated in the dyestuff industry, meaning the parts of the molecule responsible for colour.

Clinical trials Generally considered to be biomedical or health-related research studies in humans that follow a predefined method.

Coding strand The strand in a double-stranded DNA molecule that has the same sequence of bases as the transcribed mRNA (except that uracil (U) in RNA replaces thymine (T) in the DNA sequence). The other strand in the double-stranded DNA molecule is often referred to as the non-coding strand.

Co-enzyme A non-protein chemical compound that is bound to an enzyme and is required for the enzyme's biological activity.

Concerted In a concerted reaction, the movement of electrons involved in both bond-making and bond-breaking takes place at the same time. There is no formation of an intermediate carbocation (hence its being a one-step reaction).

Condensation reaction A bond-forming reaction that involves the loss of a molecule of water. It can also be described as a dehydration reaction.

Conformation The special arrangement or shape of a molecule.

Conjugates Compounds formed as a result of phase II metabolic transformation.

Conjugated Possessing a system of connected p orbitals with delocalized electrons with alternating double and single bonds.

Complex A metal ion or atom bound to one or more molecules, usually through covalent dative bonding.

Constitutional isomers Molecules that contain the same atoms but connected in different ways (i.e. their *connectivity* is different). They have different physical and chemical properties.

Covalent bond A strong form of chemical bonding that occurs when two different atoms share electrons.

Covalent dative bonding A covalent bond where both electrons come from the same atom.

3',5'-cyclic adenosine monophosphate (cyclic AMP) Derivative of ATP that acts as a second messenger in signal transduction within biological processes. Contains a ribose sugar with an adenine base attached to the 1' carbon atom of the sugar and a phosphate attached to both the 3' and 5' carbon atoms, giving a cyclic structure.

Cytochrome Membrane-bound proteins that contain haem and are involved in electron transport.

Cytochrome P450 enzymes A family of mono-oxygenase enzymes that have an iron-haem core and are responsible for many metabolic oxidations by association of molecular oxygen with the metal centre.

Cytotoxic Toxic to cells.

Daughter cells The two cells that result when one cell divides.

Deactivating Effect of substituents that destabilize the cationic intermediate formed during electrophilic substitution and hence decrease the rate of reaction.

Degenerate Atomic or hybrid orbitals that have the same energy; for example, the three 2p atomic orbitals, or the four sp^3 hybrid orbitals, are said to be degenerate.

Denaturation Irreversible damage to a protein structure, usually by heat.

Dependence A compulsive or chronic need to take a drug; an addiction.

Differentiate The process by which a cell such as a haematopoietic stem cell becomes a more specialized cell such as a red blood cell.

Dimerize To form a compound by combination of two identical molecules.

Dipole–dipole interactions The attraction between molecules as a result of the presence of a permanent dipole moment.

Directing effect A term used to describe how substituents on an aromatic ring can influence the regiochemistry of electrophilic aromatic substitution. The effect that a substituent has on the EAS reaction is determined by the effect it has on a positive charge on the carbon that carries it. There are three main classes:

- Electron-donating groups, which stabilize an adjacent positive charge and are *ortho/para*-directing and activating.

- Electron-withdrawing groups, which destabilize an adjacent positive charge and are *meta*-directing and deactivating.

- The halogens, which are *ortho/para*-directing.

Disaccharide A carbohydrate composed of two monosaccharides.

Divalent In the case of carbon, forming two covalent bonds to other atoms. (Note that the word is also used when referring to ions. A divalent cation, for example Ca^{2+}, has two fewer electrons than the atom in its elemental state, while a divalent anion, for example O^{2-}, has two more electrons than the atom in its elemental state.)

Double helix The spiral-like structure that results from two closely associated strands coiled about a central axis.

Downstream Toward the 3' end of a DNA molecule relative to a particular position in the molecule.

Eclipsed In an eclipsed conformation, two atoms bonded to adjacent carbon atoms are as close together as possible. This is best illustrated with a diagram.

Electron-donating group A group which donates electron density to a conjugated π system via a mesomeric or inductive effect.

Electronegativity The ability of an atom, or group of atoms, to attract electrons, or electron density, towards it.

Electron-withdrawing group A group which removes electron density from a conjugated π system via a mesomeric or inductive effect.

Electrostatic interaction The attraction between a charged group on one molecule and an oppositely charged group on another molecule.

Elute To remove a bound substance in a solvent, typically to remove a substance from a chromatography column.

Emulsifying agent A substance that prevents the coagulation of colloidal particles.

Enantiomers A pair of chiral molecules that are non-superimposable mirror images of each other. They have identical physical and chemical properties, but they rotate the plane of polarized light in opposite directions.

Endofacial Facing towards the interior of a cell.

Endogenous compound Compound found in the body.

Endoplasmic reticulum A series of folded membranes within the cytoplasm of the cell which are associated with protein synthesis and storage.

Enterohepatic cycle A process by which bile acids and other molecules are reabsorbed from the lower small intestine, returned to the liver and reused.

Enzyme Protein catalyst that increases the rate of biochemical reactions in the body.

Epithelial cells Group of cells that are often arranged in layers that cover our external and internal surfaces to form the epithelium. The cells that make up our skin are epithelial cells.

Equatorial In a chair conformation of a six-membered ring, the equatorial substituents stick out sideways, as shown in yellow on the diagram.

Excipients Excipients are combined with the API (defined elsewhere) to produce a medicine. They can help in the delivery of the API to the receptor and during the manufacturing of the dosage form.

Exofacial Facing away from the interior of a cell.

E,Z system The IUPAC preferred system for describing the stereochemistry of a double bond.

Formulate To develop a preparation of a drug.

Formulation The science of converting a drug into a form that is suitable for presentation to a patient.

Free radical scavenger A compound that reacts with free radicals in a biological system.

Functional group A group of atoms within a molecule that is responsible for certain properties of the molecule.

Fungi A subgroup of eukaryotic organisms, including moulds, yeasts and mushrooms, that have a cell wall containing a substance called chitin.

Geminal dihalides Compounds that have both halogen atoms on the same carbon.

Gene A sequence of DNA that codes for a functional substance such as a protein or for one of the different forms of RNA molecule.

Genetic code The code describing the translation of the sequence of nucleotides found in nucleic acids into a sequence of amino acids. It is written in a series of base-sequence triplets (codons) of the nucleotides. There are sixty-four possible codons in the genetic code, which can act as signals or codes for amino acids.

Genus A level of taxonomic classification of living and fossilized organisms (*plural*, genera).

Geometric isomers Compounds which differ from each other in the arrangement of groups with respect to a double bond, ring or other rigid structure.

Germ cells An egg or sperm cell. These cells have half the normal number of chromosomes, but the full complement of chromosomes is restored at the point of conception, when two germ cells unite.

Glucagon A peptide hormone released from the pancreas. It causes the liver to release stored glucose into the bloodstream.

Glycogen Complex branched carbohydrate molecule consisting of glucose units, used as storage of energy in the cell.

Glycosidic bond A covalent bond that joins a carbohydrate molecule to another functional group.

Gram-negative bacteria and Gram-positive bacteria Gram-positive and Gram-negative bacteria can both be stained with Gram stain (crystal violet). The stain can be easily removed from Gram-negative bacteria by washing with acetone, but the cell walls of Gram-positive bacteria retain the stain. Gram-negative cell walls are much thicker than Gram-positive cell walls and are resistant to many antibiotics. The quinolones are unusual in targeting Gram-negative bacteria, preferentially. Examples of Gram-negative bacteria are *Salmonella* and *Escherichia coli.* Examples of Gram-positive bacteria include *Staphylococcus aureus* and *Streptococcus pneumoniae.*

'Green' synthesis A chemical synthesis with little waste, especially of carbon.

Heterocyclic A carbon-containing (organic) ring system that contains one or more atoms other than carbon (commonly nitrogen and/or oxygen).

High-performance liquid chromatography An instrumental technique for the separation of mixtures of compounds. It may be used for purification, identification or quantification.

Homonuclear bond A bond connecting two atoms of the same element.

Hydrogen bond A non-covalent bond between an electron-deficient hydrogen and an electronegative atom such as oxygen or nitrogen.

Hydrolysis The addition of water to a substance, causing the breaking of a chemical bond.

Hydrophilic Water-attracting.

Hydrophobic Water-repelling.

Hygroscopicity The ability to absorb moisture, particularly from the atmosphere.

Imine A compound which contains a C=N–R group, where R is an alkyl group or just a hydrogen atom. They are typically formed by the reaction of a carbonyl group (C=O) in an aldehyde or ketone with ammonia or an amine, leading to loss of a water molecule and the formation of a C=N double bond.

Immune system The mechanism by which the body protects itself from pathogens such as bacteria, viruses, fungi and parasites.

Inductive effect Arises as a result of a difference in electronegativity between atoms and is transmitted through σ bonds.

Infrared spectroscopy Involves irradiation of a compound with light of the infrared region of the electromagnetic spectrum. Molecules absorb infrared radiation of different frequencies according to their structure. The presence of functional groups can be identified by their characteristic absorption wavelengths.

Intercalating drug A flat (planar) molecule capable of interacting with DNA by insertion between the base-pairs of the DNA ladder.

Isomer Two isomers have the same chemical formulae but different structural formulae. *Cis*-retinal and *trans*-retinal are isomers of one another, so *cis*-retinal can be isomerized to *trans*-retinal.

Isomerization The reaction in which a molecule is transformed into a different molecule with the same atoms but rearranged. The product is called an isomer.

Ketose A sugar containing one ketone group per molecule.

Lactone A cyclic ester.

Lead compound A compound that shows a desired pharmacological property, which is then developed further through the synthesis of analogues to optimize its activity.

Leaving group A fragment of the molecule that leaves. Good leaving groups are neutral or bear a stabilized negative charge.

Lewis acid A species that can accept a pair of electrons, e.g. a metal ion.

Lewis base An atom or group that can donate a pair of electrons, e.g. a nitrogen atom.

Ligand An ion or molecule that binds to a metal ion or atom to form a coordination complex.

Lipids Biomacromolecules, including fats which function within the body as energy storage, structural elements within the cellular membrane and signalling molecules.

Liposomes Microscopic artificial lipid bilayer spheres that enclose an aqueous core and are sometimes used to deliver drugs or other substances to cells.

Metabolism A range of biochemical reactions, vital for life, in which substances are produced or broken down.

Meta-**directing effect** The propensity of a functional group on an aromatic ring to direct an electrophile to the *meta*-position in an electrophilic aromatic substitution reaction.

Microtubules Hollow cylindrical proteins, found in the cytosol of eukaryotic cells, which give structural support to cells.

Miscible Capable of being mixed in all proportions.

Mitochondrial electron transport chain The pathway in which electron transfer is coupled to proton transfer across a membrane. This results in an electrochemical proton gradient, which is used in the mitochondria to generate energy in the form of ATP.

Molar Unit of concentration meaning the number of moles per unit volume; for example, mol/litre.

Mole Unit of measurement to describe the amount of a chemical. One mole of an element contains 6.02×10^{23} atoms of that element. One mole of a molecule contains 6.02×10^{23} formula units of that molecule. 6.02×10^{23} is Avogadro's constant.

Monograph An entry in a pharmacopoeia, which contains the specifications for a particular drug or drug preparation.

Monomer A small molecule that when bonded to other molecules of a similar type creates a polymer.

Monosaccharide A simple carbohydrate, often containing five or six carbon atoms. Used as building blocks for larger carbohydrates.

Nephrotoxicity Toxicity to the kidneys.

Nicotinamide adenine dinucleotide (NAD⁺) A coenzyme whose role is to accept hydride ions produced by enzyme-controlled oxidation reactions. The NAD⁺ is reduced to NADH.

Non-covalent bonds Weaker than covalent bonds and include electrostatic interactions, hydrogen bonds, hydrophobic interactions and van der Waals interactions.

Non-stereogenic A non-stereogenic (or achiral) carbon has four groups bonded to it, at least two of which are the same. These groups may be hydrogen, groups based on carbon or on another element, such as oxygen or nitrogen. If a molecule contains only non-stereogenic carbons, it can be superimposed on its mirror image.

Nuclear spin Some atomic nuclei behave as if they were spinning, and because they are charged they create a magnetic field.

Nucleosides A nucleobase (adenine, guanine, thymine, uracil, cytosine) bound to a sugar (ribose or deoxyribose).

Nucleus Organelle containing the genetic material of a cell.

Oil-water interface An interface forming the boundary between the two immiscible liquids oil and water.

Orbital A region of space near the nucleus of an atom in which there is a high probability (frequently taken as a 95% probability) of finding an electron. Note that we may refer to atomic orbitals (the pure, unaltered orbitals surrounding an isolated atom in its lowest energy state), hybrid orbitals (the combination of these atomic orbitals described in Section 2.4) and molecular orbitals (where the orbitals embrace more than one atom, or even a whole molecule, when they are involved in interatomic bonding).

Organelles Structures within the cytoplasm of a cell that carry out specialized functions.

Ortho/para-**directing effect** The propensity of an element or functional group on an aromatic ring to direct an electrophile to the ***ortho***- or ***para***-position in an electrophilic aromatic substitution reaction.

Osmotic pressure Pressure required to stop the tendency of a solvent (usually water) from passing from one area to another through a semipermeable membrane (via osmosis).

Ototoxicity Toxicity to the ears.

Oxidation A reaction in which the oxygen content of a compound or the number of bonds to oxygen is increased.

Oxidation number The number of electrons that an atom has lost or gained means that it has lost electrons and has gained electrons.

Oxidizing agent A substance that oxidizes another substance, itself being reduced in the process.

Patent Newly developed drugs need to be protected to prevent other companies benefiting from the invention, time and money spent in developing a new drug. This protection takes the form of a legally binding patent.

Peptide bond An amide bond specifically linking two amino acids to form a peptide backbone.

Peroxide A compound containing an oxygen–oxygen bond.

P-glycoprotein A protein which pumps many foreign substances out of cells.

Pharmacopoeia A reference book containing specifications for drugs and drug preparations.

Physicochemical properties The properties relating to a system's physical state that influence chemical behaviour.

Plant Multicellular eukaryotic organisms that can carry out photosynthesis

Polarized A polarizable atom or molecule is one which is neutral, though the electron cloud around it can be distorted so that there are now regions of positive and negative charge existing at the same time (a dipole); the atom or molecule is then said to be polarized. Generally this is easier with larger atoms, for example argon rather than neon, or the iodide ion rather than the chloride ion, where the electrons are further from the nucleus and so are more weakly held.

Polymers Compounds formed of many repeated simpler molecules (monomers).

Polypeptide A chain of amino acids (usually greater than ten) that are linked by peptide bonds.

Polysaccharide A large, complex carbohydrate that comprises many monosaccharide monomers.

Pro-drug A compound that is not itself a drug but is converted to a drug in the body.

Protecting group A protecting group reversibly modifies a functional group to prevent it taking part in a reaction.

Proteins Large biomolecules that contain one or more chains of amino acids. The folding of these chains gives proteins three-dimensional shapes and dictates their activity. The sequence of amino acids is defined by the nucleotide sequence within the relevant gene.

Protists Class of eukaryotic organisms that include protozoa, algae and some slime moulds.

Proximate carcinogens A chemical or physical agent that initiates a sequence of reactions leading to carcinogenesis.

Pseudocholinesterase (plasma cholinesterase) An enzyme present in the blood and other organs which hydrolyses acetylcholine more slowly than acetylcholinesterase.

Pyranose A six-membered ring consisting of five carbon atoms and one oxygen atom.

Racemate (racemic mixture) An equimolar mixture of enantiomers.

Racemization The process of forming a racemate from a single enantiomer.

Receptors A biochemical structure or site (often found on the surface of a cell or sometimes within a cell), such as a protein or nucleic acid, that can be activated by natural molecules and drugs to cause a specific effect.

Reduction potential (also known as redox potential) A measure of the tendency of chemical species to acquire electrons and thereby be reduced. Reduction potential is measured in volts (V) or millivolts (mV). Each species has its own intrinsic reduction potential; the more positive the potential, the greater the species' affinity for electrons and tendency to be reduced.

Regioselective The preference for one direction of making or breaking a chemical bond over other possibilities.

Resolution The separation of a racemic mixture into its component enantiomers.

Resonance hybrid See 'resonance structures'.

Resonate To exhibit resonance when two or more structures have an identical arrangement of atoms but a different arrangement of electrons.

Resonance structures and canonical forms Frequently, the structures of compounds, or reaction intermediates, are written showing a formal arrangement of double and single bonds and positive or negative charges, trying to complete the octet of eight electrons around a p block element. Often this can be done in more than one way, though no individual one of these structures represents the compound completely accurately. These are referred to as *resonance structures* or *canonical forms*. The actual structure of the compound or intermediate is an average of these and is referred to as a *resonance hybrid*. An illustration of this is given in Figure 2.26, where different representations of the ethanoate (acetate) ion are shown, as well as the 'average' or resonance hybrid.

Retrosynthesis The process of designing the chemical synthesis of a target molecule by starting at the target and working backwards to readily available compounds.

Ring flip The interconversion of cyclic conformations.

Screening The testing of a particular compound or sample for biological activity.

Selective toxicity The injury of one kind of living matter without harming another with which it is in intimate contact.

Serendipity A 'happy accident' or 'pleasant surprise'; specifically, the accident of finding something good or useful without looking for it.

Severe combined immunodeficiency disease (SCID) Disease in which children are born with a non-functioning immune system, making them extremely vulnerable to severe infections.

Sigma conjugation Also known as hyperconjugation, it is a stabilizing overlap between a pi orbital and a sigma orbital.

Sigmoid curve S-shaped curve.

Single helix A spiral-like structure created when a strand of material coils about a central axis.

Somatic cells Any cell of a living organism other than the reproductive cells.

Specific rotation [α] The observed angle of optical rotation when plane-polarized light is passed through a sample of standard concentration and path length at standard temperature in a defined solvent.

Spectroscopic techniques Experimental methods that measure the interaction between matter and radiation intensity as a function of wavelength.

Staggered In a staggered conformation, two atoms bonded to adjacent carbon atoms are as far apart as possible. This is best illustrated with a diagram.

Stereogenic A stereogenic centre is an alternative name for a chiral centre.

Steric Effects due to the size of substituents are called steric effects.

Structure Activity Relationship (SAR) study A tactic to assess the importance of particular areas of a biologically active molecule. Portions of the molecule in question are altered systematically with the aim of discovering the important structural features within a molecule and trying to improve them.

Substitution reaction A reaction where one atom of a group is replaced by another atom or group.

Suicide substrate A compound that interacts with the active site of an enzyme and undergoes a transformation to produce a compound that forms an irreversible complex with an enzyme itself, often by means of a covalent bond.

Target A target for a drug is a biological molecule, usually a protein or a nucleic acid, that interacts with that drug.

Tautomers A special case of structural isomerism; they are isomers which differ only in the position of a hydrogen atom and bonding electrons. Tautomers are in equilibrium with each other.

Tetravalent Forming four covalent bonds to other atoms.

Thioester An ester in which one of the oxygen atoms is replaced by a sulfur (−COSR). A thioester is more reactive than the corresponding oxygen ester.

Thiol and thioether Functional groups analogous to alcohol and ether in which the oxygen has been replaced with a sulfur, i.e. R−S−H and R−S−R. 'Thio' refers to sulfur, so an ether becomes a thioether and a thioalcohol is shortened to thiol.

Tolerance A term used to indicate that repeat doses of a drug give rise to a smaller biological effect. Larger doses are needed for the same pharmacological effect.

Topical A drug applied locally, to the skin or the eye or the ear, for example. It is not systemic (applied to the whole body by the oral route or by injection).

Torsional Effects due to bond twisting are called torsional effects.

Triacylglycerol Major energy reserve found in animals, which is an ester derived from glycerol with three fatty acids.

tRNA (transfer RNA) Ribonucleic acid (RNA) converts the genetic code (DNA) into proteins. Transfer RNA is one of three types of RNA involved in this process.

Upstream Toward the 5' end of a DNA molecule relative to a particular position in the DNA molecule.

Van der Waals interaction Weak interactions between two molecules as a result of temporary dipoles.

Ventricular arrhymia A disturbance of the normal conduction impulses within the ventricles of the heart.

Vicinal dihalides Compounds that have halogen atoms on adjacent carbons.

Viruses Simple infectious agents that are parasitic to living cells and can only multiply within them. Many viruses are harmless, but some are responsible for a range of diseases such as colds, influenza and some cancers.

Xenobiotic A substance in the blood stream that is not normally found there. Xenobiotics are often processed in the liver.

Xenobiotic-metabolizing enzymes Enzymes that control the metabolic pathways that modify xenobiotic molecules, foreign to an organism's normal biochemistry

INDEX

Index

nucleotides 285
nucleus 281
nystatin 11–13, 106
  structure 13

O

Oblivon 41
oestradiol 352, 370
oestrogens 236–237
oestrone 236, 237
ofloxacin 86
oleic acid 347
oligosaccharides 332–334
omeprazole 270, 272, 375, 383
opioid analgesics 362–363
opium 362
opsin 4
optical isomerism 68–70
organelles 282–284
organic chemistry 26–27
ortho substitution 223
orthophosphoric acid 260
oxacillin 179, 181
oxalic acid 27
oxidation 8, 246
  alcohols 8, 143–146
  alkenes 119–120
  alkynes 129–130
  amines 163
  linoleic acid 132–133
  medicine stability and 132–133
  oxidative drug metabolism 395–396,
    398–399
  phenols 150
  see also combustion
oxidation states 246
oxidative cleavage 120
oxidative stress 152
oxiranes *see* epoxides
oxygen 137
  see also oxidation
ozone 120

P

P-glycoprotein 395
paclitaxel 368, 369, 372, 373
  analogues 373
palmitic acid 348
palmitoleic acid 348
papaverine 70

para substitution 223
para-aminobenzoic acid 23
paracetamol 232, 238
  isomers 56, 57
    separation of 233
  structure 3–4, 41, 211
  synthesis 233–234
pargyline 41
penicillamine 30
penicillins 13–15, 166, 322, 364–365
  allergies 365
  biosynthesis 14
  semi-synthetic 373–374
  synthesis from acyl chlorides
    179, 181
pentane 96–97
pentobarbital 131, 276
pentoses 330
pepsin 203
peptide bonds 9–10, 202–204, 310
peptides 311
peptidoglycans 282
pericyclic reactions 46
periodic table 244–245
permanent dipole 43
peroxides 154, 155
pethidine 61
  conformation 62
petrol 108
pharmacokinetics 388
phase I metabolism 395–397
phase II metabolism 398–401
α-phellandrene 111
phenolate 148, 149
phenols 148–152
  acidity 148–150
  as antioxidants 151–152
  bromination 227
  reactions 150–151
phenyl ring 61–62
phenylalanine 309
phenyldiazonium chloride 232
pheromones 111
phosphate esters 166, 261–264
phosphatidylcholine 350
phosphodiesters 261, 285
phosphofructokinase 343
3-phosphoglycerate 146–147
phospholipids 264–265, 349–351
phosphomonoesters 261
phosphoric acid 260–261